Praise for

The System of Care Handbook

"We know that comprehensive, community-based, coordinated care is the gold standard for children, youth, and families. This handbook provides a practical guide for how to implement quality mental health services in communities across the nation."

—**Rosalynn Carter**
Former First Lady and Chair
The Carter Center Mental Health Task Force

"As Surgeon General of the United States, I identified the unmet need for children's mental health services as a public health crisis. This excellent handbook provides comprehensive information that begins to address this crisis and build systems of care for children's mental health."

—**David Satcher, M.D., Ph.D.**
16th Surgeon General of the United States

"As Secretary of the U.S. Department of Health and Human Services, our department, through the Substance Abuse and Mental Health Services Administration under the leadership of Charley Curie, invested significant resources in the development of systems of care in communities. This book will help ensure that quality mental health services are provided to children, youth, and families across America."

—**The Honorable Tommy G. Thompson**
Former Secretary, U.S. Department of Health and Human Services

"We face daunting and persistent challenges in designing effective service systems for children with mental health needs. This volume comprehensively summarizes our experiences with systems of care for children's mental health, providing a 'hands on' perspective on the most vexing and important challenges in designing services that work. We must capitalize on these insights to finish the job of transforming our service systems. Lost opportunities translate to lost lives. One more is too many."

—**David L. Shern, Ph.D.**
President and CEO, Mental Health America

"Our mission is to keep kids at home, in school and out of trouble. *The System of Care Handbook* gives the leaders and staff of behavioral health organizations tools to help accomplish our mission. The case studies inspire us, while the programs and services described in the handbook offer interventions for effectively treating and supporting children and their families. Well done and much needed!"

—**Linda Rosenberg, M.S.W.**
President and CEO
National Council for Community Behavioral Healthcare

**Systems of Care for
Children's Mental Health**

Series Editors:
Beth A. Stroul, M.Ed.
Robert M. Friedman, Ph.D.

The System
of Care Handbook

Other Volumes in This Series

The System of Care Handbook

Transforming Mental Health Services for Children, Youth, and Families

edited by

Beth A. Stroul, M.Ed.
President
Management & Training Innovations, Inc.
McLean, Virginia

and

Gary M. Blau, Ph.D.
Chief
Child, Adolescent and Family Branch
Center for Mental Health Services
Substance Abuse and Mental Health Services Administration
Rockville, Maryland

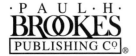

Baltimore • London • Sydney

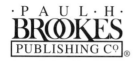

Paul H. Brookes Publishing Co.
Post Office Box 10624
Baltimore, Maryland 21285-0624
USA

www.brookespublishing.com

Typeset by Integrated Publishing Solutions, Grand Rapids, Michigan.
Manufactured in the United States of America by
Sheridan Books, Inc., Chelsea, Michigan.

The individuals described in this book are composites or real people whose situations are masked and are based on the authors' actual experiences. Real names and identifying details are used by permission.

The content of this publication does not necessarily reflect the views, opinions, or policies of the Center for Mental Health Services, the Substance Abuse and Mental Health Services Administration, the U.S. Department of Health and Human Services, the National Institute of Disability and Rehabilitation Research, or the U.S. Department of Education.

Library of Congress Cataloguing-in-Publication Data
The system of care handbook : transforming mental health services for children, youth, and families / edited by Beth A. Stroul and Gary M. Blau.
    p.   ; cm. — (Systems of care for children's mental health)
Includes bibliographical references and index.
ISBN-13: 978-1-55766-962-9 (hardcover)
ISBN-10: 1-55766-962-7 (hardcover)
    1. Child mental health services—United States.   2. Family—Mental health—United States.
I. Stroul, Beth A.   II. Blau, Gary M.   III. Title.   IV. Series.
[DNLM: 1. Mental Health Services—organization & administration—United States.
2. Mental Health Services—trends—United States.   3. Adolescent—United States.
4. Child—United States.   5. Family—United States.   6. Quality of Health Care—organization & administration—United States.   7. Quality of Health Care—trends—United States.   WM 30 S9977 2008]
RJ501.A2S97 2008
362.198'9289—dc22   2008008320

British Library cataloguing in Publication data are available from the British Library.

2012   2011   2010   2009   2008
10   9   8   7   6   5   4   3   2   1

Contents

Series Preface

In 1982, Knitzer's seminal study, *Unclaimed Children,* was published by the Children's Defense Fund. At that time, the field of children's mental health was characterized by a lack of federal or state leadership, few community-based services, little collaboration among child-serving systems, negligible parent involvement, and little or no advocacy on behalf of youth with emotional disorders. Since that time, substantial gains have been realized in both the conceptualization and the implementation of comprehensive, community-based systems of care for children and adolescents with serious emotional disorders and their families.

A vast amount of information has emanated from the system-building experiences of states and communities and from research and technical assistance efforts. Many of the trends and philosophies emergent in recent years have now become widely accepted as "state of the art" for conceptualizing and providing services to youth with emotional disorders and their families. There is now broad agreement surrounding the need to create community-based systems of care throughout the United States for children and their families, and the development of these systems has become a national goal. Such systems of care are based on the premises of providing services in the most normative environments, creating effective interagency relationships among the key child-serving systems, involving families and youth in all phases of the planning and delivery of services, and creating service systems that are designed to respond to the needs of culturally diverse populations.

A major need is to incorporate these concepts and trends into the published literature. This need stems from the critical shortage of staff who are appropriately trained to serve youth in community-based systems of care, with new philosophies and new service delivery approaches. Of utmost importance is the need to provide state-of-the-art information to institutions of higher education for use in the preservice education of professionals across disciplines, including the social work, counseling, psychology, and psychiatry fields. Similarly, there is an equally vital need for resources in the in-service training of staff in mental health, child welfare, education, health, early childhood, and juvenile justice agencies to assist staff in working more effectively with youth with emotional disorders and their families.

This book series, *Systems of Care for Children's Mental Health,* is designed to fulfill these needs by addressing current trends in children's mental health service delivery. The series has several broad goals:

- To increase awareness of the system of care concept and philosophy among current and future mental health professionals who will be providing services to children, adolescents, and their families

- To broaden the mental health field's understanding of treatment and services delivery beyond traditional approaches to include innovative, state-of-the-art approaches and evidence-based practices

- To provide practical information that will assist the mental health field to implement and apply the philosophy, services, and approaches embodied in the system of care concept

Each volume in the continuing series addresses a major issue or topic related to the development of systems of care. The books contain information useful to planners, program managers, policy makers, practitioners, families, youth, teachers, researchers, and others who are interested and involved in improving systems of care for children with emotional disorders and their families. As the series editors, it is our goal for the series to provide an ongoing vehicle and forum for exploring critical aspects of systems of care as they continue to evolve.

Beth A. Stroul   *Robert M. Friedman*

Editorial Advisory Board

About the Editors

Beth A. Stroul, M.Ed., President, Management & Training Innovations, Inc., 7417 Seneca Ridge Drive, Suite 100, McLean, Virginia 22102

Ms. Stroul is a consultant in the area of mental health policy and has completed numerous research, evaluation, policy analysis, and technical assistance projects related to service systems for children and adolescents with emotional disorders and their families. As one of the architects of the concept of community-based systems of care, she has published extensively in the children's mental health field and is co-editor of the *Systems of Care for Children's Mental Health* ongoing book series. She is a senior consultant to the National Technical Assistance Center for Children's Mental Health at Georgetown University and to the national evaluation of the Comprehensive Community Mental Health Services for Children and Their Families Program. She served on the mental health working group of the President's Task Force on Health Care Reform and more recently served as a consultant to the President's New Freedom Commission on Mental Health. She has been honored by the Federation of Families for Children's Mental Health with the Claiming Children Award and by the American Psychological Association with the Distinguished Contribution to Child Advocacy Award.

Gary M. Blau, Ph.D., Chief, Child, Adolescent and Family Branch, Division of Services and Systems Improvement, Center for Mental Health Services, Substance Abuse and Mental Health Services Administration, 1 Choke Cherry Road, Room 6-1045, Rockville, Maryland 20857

Dr. Blau is a clinical psychologist and chief of the Child, Adolescent and Family Branch of the Center for Mental Health Services. In this role, he provides national leadership for children's mental health and for creating systems of care across the country. Previously, Dr. Blau was the bureau chief of quality management and the director of mental health at the Connecticut Department of Children and Families. He has received several awards, including the Pro Humanitate Literary Award for literary works that best exemplify the intellectual integrity and moral courage required to transcend political and social barriers to promote best practice in the field of child welfare, the Governor's Service Award, the Phoebe Bennet Award for outstanding contribution to children's mental health in Connecticut, and the Making a Difference Award presented by Connecticut's Federation of Families for Children's Mental Health. He has numerous publications and has been the editor of several books, including the recently published *Handbook of Childhood Behavioral Issues: Evidence Based Approaches to Prevention and Treatment* (with co-editor Thomas P. Gullotta, Taylor & Francis, 2008). He received his doctorate from Auburn University in 1988 and currently holds a clinical faculty appointment at the Yale Child Study Center.

About the Contributors

Ignacio David Acevedo-Polakovich, Ph.D., M.S., Assistant Professor, Louis de la Parte Florida Mental Health Institute, University of South Florida, 13301 Bruce B. Downs Boulevard, Tampa, Florida 33612. Dr. Acevedo-Polakovich's research and professional activities focus on the promotion of development opportunities for youth and families from historically underprivileged backgrounds. He also pursues research and professional work in cultural training and in culturally competent approaches to psychosocial assessment.

Mary Armstrong, Ph.D., Assistant Professor and Director, Division of State and Local Support, Department of Child and Family Studies, Louis de la Parte Florida Mental Health Institute, University of South Florida, 13301 Bruce B. Downs Boulevard, Tampa, Florida 33612. Dr. Armstrong has more than 25 years of experience in children's behavioral health, public sector managed care, and child welfare services. She is responsible for the administration of the Division of State and Local Support, including the direction of evaluation and research activities, policy analysis, and specialized consultation, training, and technical assistance to public sector entities nationally and in Florida.

Karen A. Blase, Ph.D., Research Professor, Louis de la Parte Florida Mental Health Institute, University of South Florida, 13301 Bruce B. Downs Boulevard, Tampa, Florida 33612. Dr. Blase, together with her colleague, Dean Fixsen, is co-director of the National Implementation Research Network (http://nirn.fmhi.usf.edu). Her work in human services focuses on practice and program improvement in children's mental health, education, child welfare, and juvenile justice with a focus on system change, scale-up of evidence-based interventions, development of innovative practices, and the science and practice of implementation.

Freda Brashears, M.S.W., Senior Project Manager, Macro International Inc., 3 Corporate Square, Suite 370, Atlanta, Georgia 30329. Ms. Brashears has more than 30 years of social work experience in public social services, private practice, and education. She works primarily on national multisite evaluations in the area of children's mental health and plays a significant role in the national evaluation of the Comprehensive Community Mental Health Services for Children and Their Families Program.

Eric J. Bruns, Ph.D., Associate Professor, University of Washington School of Medicine, Division of Public Behavioral Health and Justice Policy, 2815 Eastlake Avenue East, Suite 200, Seattle, Washington 98102. Dr. Bruns's major research focus is on developing and evaluating community-based services and supports for families and children. He co-directs the National Wraparound Initiative and has several National Institute of Mental Health–funded research projects related to implementation of the wraparound process.

Joyce L. Burrell, M.S., Deputy Commissioner, New York State Office of Children and Family Services, 52 Washington Street, Suite 130 North, Rensselaer, New York 12144. Ms. Burrell has more than 20 years of experience in juvenile justice and currently is deputy commissioner of New York's Office of Children and Family Services, Division of Juvenile Justice and Opportunities for Youth. Previously, she led large urban juvenile justice systems in Washington, D.C., and Philadelphia; served as project director for the National Evaluation and Technical Assistance Center for the Education of Children Who are Neglected, Delinquent or At Risk; and provided juvenile justice–related technical assistance to system of care communities funded by the Comprehensive Community Mental Health Services to Children and Their Families Program.

Myrna Carpenter is a young adult who has worked first as an advocate in her own life and in recent years advocating for others. She currently is living in Minneapolis, Minnesota, and hoping to pursue a degree in child psychology.

Hewitt B. "Rusty" Clark, Ph.D., Professor, Department of Child and Family Studies, Louis de la Parte Florida Mental Health Institute, University of South Florida, 13301 Bruce B. Downs Boulevard, Tampa, Florida 33612. Dr. Clark is the director of the National Center on Youth Transition for Young People with Emotional/Behavioral Difficulties. Over the course of his career, he has developed and researched various innovative programs and has published extensively, with 3 books and more than 110 publications to his credit.

Joseph J. Cocozza, Ph.D., Vice President for Research, Policy Research Associates, 345 Delaware Avenue, Delmar, New York 12054. Dr. Cocozza is the director of the National Center for Mental Health and Juvenile Justice (NCMHJJ), located within Policy Research Associates. He has held a number of policy-oriented research, academic, and administrative positions and has authored a number of professional publications and reports.

Nicole Deschênes, M.Ed., Faculty, Department of Child and Family Studies, Louis de la Parte Florida Mental Health Institute, University of South Florida, 13301 Bruce B. Downs Boulevard, Tampa, Florida 33612. Ms. Deschênes is the co-director of the National Center on Youth Transition, which dedicates itself to improving practice, systems, and outcomes for youth and young adults with emotional and behavioral difficulties. She has more than 30 years of experience as a community mental health nurse, educator, consultant and researcher, and, throughout her career, has assisted local, national, and international organizations in developing improved supports and services for individuals with emotional and behavioral issues.

Joan M. Dodge, Ph.D., Senior Policy Associate, National Technical Assistance Center for Children's Mental Health, Georgetown University Center for Child and Human Development, 3300 Whitehaven Street NW, Suite 3300, Washington, DC 20007. Dr. Dodge is responsible at the National Technical Assistance Center for Children's Mental Health for implementing a series of Policy Academies for selected states and territories that are interested in creating policies to build and sustain systems of care for children, youth, and their families. Most recently, she has assisted in the implementation of a Tribal Policy Summit to address the issue of youth suicide within tribal communities, focusing specifically on prevention, intervention, and healing.

Timothy P. Dollard, M.S., L.P.C.-S., Director, Children's Services, Jefferson-Blount-St. Clair Mental Health/Mental Retardation Authority, 940 Montclair Road, Suite 200, Birmingham, Alabama 35213. As director of children's services for the Jefferson-Blount-St. Clair Mental Health/Mental Retardation Authority, Mr. Dollard coordinates mental health services for children with serious emotional disturbances and their families. He served as the project director for the federally funded system of care operated by the nonprofit organization Jefferson County Community Partnership, with responsibilities including the management of interagency collaboration, service agreements, contracts, and staff for direct service delivery to children and their families.

Christina M. Donkervoet, M.S., RN, Director, Care Coordination and Patient Flow, Queens Medical Center, 1301 Punchbowl Avenue, Honolulu, Hawaii 96813. Ms. Donkervoet was the chief of the Child and Adolescent Mental Health Division in Hawaii for 10 years. In her position, she provided leadership for the development of the statewide evidence-based system of care for Hawaii's children and youth with the most serious and challenging mental health concerns.

Albert J. Duchnowski, Ph.D., Professor and Deputy Director, Research and Training Center for Children's Mental Health, Louis de la Parte Florida Mental Health Institute, University of South Florida, 13301 Bruce B. Downs Boulevard, Tampa, Florida 33612. Dr. Duchnowski conducts research, consultation, and training activities aimed at improving outcomes for children who have emotional disturbances and their families. He is one of the founders of the Federation of Families for Children's Mental Health.

Holly Echo-Hawk, M.S., Principal, Echo-Hawk & Associates, 16715 Leaper Road, Vancouver, Washington 98686. Ms. Echo-Hawk is a former director of community mental health services with nearly 30 years of experience in the administration of child and family services. A member of the Pawnee Nation, she has specialized knowledge of the development of systems of care in American Indian and Alaska Native communities and provides extensive consultation across the country in culturally competent system implementation.

Caraleen M. Fawcett, Operations Coordinator, Counseling & Consulting Services, 2430 East 6th Street, Tucson, Arizona 85719. Ms. Fawcett resides in Tucson, Arizona, with her 8-year-old daughter. She is pursuing her degree in law with the hopes of becoming an attorney so that she can work for parents involved in the child welfare and juvenile justice systems.

Sylvia Kay Fisher, Ph.D., Director of Evaluation, Child, Adolescent and Family Branch, Division of Services and Systems Improvement, Center for Mental

Health Services, Substance Abuse and Mental Health Services Administration, 1 Choke Cherry Road, Room 6-1047, Rockville, Maryland 20857. Dr. Fisher is project officer for the national evaluation of the Comprehensive Community Mental Health Services for Children and Their Families Program. Formerly, she was a research psychologist at the U.S. Bureau of Labor Statistics, Office of Survey Research Methods; a senior study director at Westat, Inc.; and a counselor and psychological evaluator with diverse clinical populations.

Robert M. Friedman, Ph.D., Professor, Department of Child and Family Studies, Louis de la Parte Florida Mental Health Institute, University of South Florida, 13301 Bruce B. Downs Boulevard, Tampa, Florida 33612. Since 1984, Dr. Friedman has served as principal investigator and director of the Research and Training Center for Children's Mental Health at the University of South Florida. Dr. Friedman's areas of specialization are the development, implementation, and evaluation of systems of care and child mental health policy overall.

Stephen A. Gilbertson, M.S., Consulting and Clinical Psychologist/Clinical Coordinator, Wraparound Milwaukee, 9201 Watertown Plank Road, Milwaukee, Wisconsin 53226. Mr. Gilbertson is a psychologist with more than 20 years of experience working with youth and families and the systems with which they interact. A system of care devotee, his clinical and consulting practice, applied research, and training have contributed to the promotion of credible community-based alternatives for youth considered at high risk for institutional placement.

Sybil K. Goldman, M.S.W., Senior Advisor, National Technical Assistance for Children's Mental Health, Georgetown University Center for Children and Human Development, 3300 Whitehaven Street NW, Suite 3300, Washington, DC 20007. For over 15 years, Ms. Goldman directed the National Technical Assistance Center for Children's Mental Health at Georgetown and for 4 years served as the senior advisor on children to the administrator of the federal Substance Abuse and Mental Health Services Administration. She has extensive experience in child mental health at national, state, and local levels and has provided assistance to major policy forums including the President's New Freedom Commission on Mental Health, the Surgeon General's National Action Agenda for Children's Mental Health, and the President's Health Care Reform Task Force.

Melanie E. Green, Consumer Support Specialist, Clark County Department of Community Services, Post Office Box 5000, Vancouver, Washington 98666. Ms. Green was involved in the Options program in Clark County, Washington, from the very beginning—using her experience as a youth living with mental illness and her passion for improving the lives of others to help design, implement, and operate the program as its youth coordinator. Ms. Green uses her unique expertise to present at regional and national conferences and provide consultation across the country on various topics, including the need for and components of quality transition services and the role and value of youth voice.

Mario Hernandez, Ph.D., Professor and Chair of the Department of Child and Family Studies, Louis de la Parte Florida Mental Health Institute, University of South Florida, 13301 Bruce B. Downs Boulevard, Tampa, Florida 33612. Dr. Hernandez is a psychologist and professor at the University of South Florida, Tampa. He has published various articles and book chapters on developing theories of change for children's mental health and cultural competence.

Regenia Hicks, Ph.D., Project Director, Technical Assistance Partnership for Child and Family Mental Health, American Institutes for Research, 1000 Thomas Jefferson Street NW, Washington, DC 20007. Dr. Hicks has a 24-year history of providing services to children in outpatient and inpatient settings as well as experience in planning, program development, and administration at the state and federal level. She currently serves as the project director for the Technical Assistance Partnership for Child and Family Mental Health, which provides technical assistance and support to all of the federally funded system of care communities.

Sharon Hodges, Ph.D., M.B.A., Research Assistant Professor, Department of Child and Family Studies, Louis de la Parte Florida Mental Health Institute, University of South Florida, 13301 Bruce B. Downs Boulevard, Tampa, Florida 33612. Dr. Hodges is an applied organizational anthropologist and research assistant professor in the Department of Child and Family Studies at the University of South Florida. She is principal investigator for a study of Case Studies of System of Care Implementation, a 5-year investigation that is part of the Research and Training Center for Children's Mental Health.

Sarah Hoover, M.Ed., Faculty, University of Colorado at Denver and Health Sciences Center, 13121 East 17th Avenue, Post Office Box 6511, L28, 5111 JFK Partners C234, Aurora, Colorado 80045. For more than 15 years, Ms. Hoover has worked in the field of human services at the state and local level, with an emphasis on disabilities, social movements and advocacy, early care and education, family supports, early intervention, and interagency collaboration. She has developed and received multiple state and federal grants focusing on advocacy, public policy, early childhood, mental health, and family support.

Larke Nahme Huang, Ph.D., Senior Advisor on Children to the Administrator, Substance Abuse and Mental Health Services Administration (SAMHSA), 1 Choke Cherry Road, Rockville, Maryland, 20857. Dr. Huang, a licensed clinical-community psychologist, is senior advisor on children to the administrator at SAMHSA, where she provides leadership on national policy for mental health and substance use services for children, adolescents, and families and is also the agency lead on cultural competence and eliminating disparities. Over the past 25 years, she has worked as a practitioner, researcher, and policymaker at the local, state, and national level to improve mental health and substance abuse services for youth and their families. In 2003, Dr. Huang served as an appointed commissioner on the President's New Freedom Commission on Mental Health.

Barbara Huff, Family Involvement Coordinator, Federation of Families for Children's Mental Health, 9605 Medical Center Drive, Suite 280, Rockville, Maryland 20850. Ms. Huff is the former executive director of the Federation of Families for Children's Mental Health, a national family-run organization focused on the needs of children and youth with mental health needs and their families. She now represents the Federation as the family involvement coordinator for the Caring for Every Child's Mental Health Campaign. Ms. Huff is also a partner in Huff Osher Consulting Inc.

Charles Huffine, M.D., Medical Director, Child and Adolescent Programs, King County Mental Health, Chemical Abuse, and Dependency Services Division, Volunteer Youth Coordinator, Youth 'N Action, Private Practice, 3123 Fairview Avenue East, Seattle, Washington 98102. Dr. Huffine has devoted his 33 years of practice to the treatment of adolescents. He has been active within the system of care in his community and nationally in promoting youth voice.

Mareasa R. Isaacs, Ph.D., M.S.W., Executive Director, National Alliance of Multi-Ethnic Behavioral Health Associations (NAMBHA), 1220 Blair Mill Road, Suite 404, Silver Spring, Maryland, 20910. Dr. Isaacs has more than 25 years of experience in government and nonprofit organizations. She is currently the executive director of NAMBHA, a multicultural, multi-ethnic organization composed of multidisciplinary professionals, consumers, family members, and community providers.

Nathaniel Israel, Ph.D., Director, Evidence Based Training Academy, San Francisco Department of Public Health, 1380 Howard Street, Fifth Floor, San Francisco, California 94103. Dr. Israel is a systems researcher and implementer. He directs evidence-based performance improvement efforts within the San Francisco children's mental health care system and consults on system development and improvement efforts nationwide.

Vivian Hopkins Jackson, Ph.D., M.S.W., Senior Policy Associate, National Center for Cultural Competence, Georgetown University Center for Child and Human Development, 3300 Whitehaven Street NW, Suite 3300, Washington, DC 20007. Dr. Jackson provides training and technical assistance on cultural and linguistic competence to human services organizations and systems. She is co-editor of *Cultural Competency in Managed Behavioral Healthcare* (Manisses Communications, 1999) and recently led the development of the National Association of Social Workers' (2007) monograph, *Institutional Racism and the Social Work Profession: A Call to Action.*

Margaret Jefferson, Director, Families United of Milwaukee, Inc., 2501 West Vliet Street, Milwaukee, Wisconsin 53205. Ms. Jefferson is the director of Families United of Milwaukee, which has provided family advocacy and parent support services for Wraparound Milwaukee and Milwaukee County for 11 years. She has been an advocate for youth since the age of 14 and is dedicated to empowering the youth and families of Milwaukee County.

Bruce Kamradt, M.S.W., Director, Wraparound Milwaukee, 9201 Watertown Plank Road, Milwaukee, Wisconsin 53226. Mr. Kamradt has more than 22 years of mental health administrative experience and has focused on the development of comprehensive community-based systems of care for children with serious mental health needs. As director of Wraparound Milwaukee, he has fashioned a unique publicly operated managed care system with strength-based, family-focused, and pooled-funded components that have made it a national model in the care of children, adolescents, and their families.

Patrick J. Kanary, M.Ed., Director, Center for Innovative Practices, 800 Market Avenue North, Suite 1500-C, Canton, Ohio 44702. Since 2001, Mr. Kanary has been the director of the Center for Innovative Practices, a Coordinating Center of Excellence, supported in part by the Ohio Department of Mental Health. His previous positions include independent consultant, former chief of the Bureau of Children's Service for the Ohio Department of Health, associate director of a children's mental health agency, psychoeducation specialist, and special education teacher.

Roxane K. Kaufmann, M.A., Director, Early Childhood Policy, Georgetown University Center for Child and Human Development, 3300 Whitehaven Street NW, Suite 3300, Washington, DC 20016. Ms. Kaufmann has worked in the early childhood field for more than 30 years. As faculty at Georgetown University, she has been a strong advocate for the development of integrated services, supports, and systems for young children and their families.

Sandra Keenan, M.Ed., C.A.G.S., Senior Research Analyst, American Institutes for Research, 1000 Thomas Jefferson Street NW, Washington, DC 20007. Ms. Keenan is the education resource specialist to the Technical Assistance Partnership for Child and Family Mental Health. She also assists with leading the National Center for Mental Health Promotion and Youth Violence Prevention that provides technical assistance for Safe Schools/Healthy Students grantees.

Teresa King, B.A., Parent Lead, Cuyahoga Tapestry System of Care, 1400 West 25th Street, Fourth Floor, Cleveland, Ohio 44113. Ms. King is the parent lead for the Cuyahoga Tapestry System of Care and has a child of her own in the system of care. As the parent lead, she is committed to educating other parents about their rights, choices, and points of access to a range of developmental and supportive services.

Chris Koyanagi, Policy Director, Judge David L. Bazelon Center for Mental Health Law, 1101 15th Street NW, Suite 1212, Washington, DC 20005. Ms. Koyanagi is policy director for the Bazelon Center for Mental Health Law, a Washington-based legal advocacy organization. She has more than 30 years of experience in mental health public policy, with a particular focus on financing policy regarding community mental health services for children.

Anna Krivelyova, M.A., Research Associate, Macro International Inc., 3 Corporate Square, Suite 370, Atlanta, Georgia 30329. Ms. Krivelyova is an economist with a specialization in labor economics and applied econometrics. For Macro International Inc., she works as a research associate for the national evaluation team for the Comprehensive Community Mental Health Services for Children and Their Families Program.

Krista Kutash, Ph.D., Professor and Deputy Director, Research and Training Center for Children's Mental Health, Louis de la Parte Florida Mental Health Institute, University of South Florida, 13301 Bruce B. Downs Boulevard, Tampa, Florida 33612. Dr. Kutash is a mental health services researcher involved in improving outcomes for children with emotional and behavior disorders. She has been principal investigator on multiple federal grants and is currently co-editor of the *Journal of Emotional and Behavior Disorders.*

Stephanie Lane, M.S.W., Director, Office of Consumer Partnerships, Washington State Mental Health Division, 1221 Mottmon Road SW, Olympia, Washington 98512. Ms. Lane is a consumer survivor dedicated to youth/family/consumer and professional partnerships. She is the co-founder of Youth 'N Action! in Washington State; has won several awards for her work with youth, including the HERO award and the Governor's Excellence Award for Cultural Competence; and is on the Board of Directors for the System of Care Alumni Association.

Brigitte Manteuffel, Ph.D., Vice President, Applied Research Division, Macro International Inc., 3 Corporate Square, Suite 370, Atlanta, Georgia 30329. Dr. Manteuffel has been the principal investigator of the national evaluation of the Comprehensive Community Mental Health Services for Children and Their Families Program since 2001. She has more than 20 years of experience with health services research in mental health, public health, and nursing involving a range of study designs, with specialization in intervention research involving caregivers and children.

Ken Martinez, Psy.D., Principal Research Analyst, Mental Health Resource Specialist, American Institutes for Research, 1000 Thomas Jefferson Street NW, Washington, DC 20007. Dr. Martinez is the mental health resource specialist for the Technical Assistance Partnership for Child and Family Mental Health, where he provides support to federally funded system of care communities and is a clinical assistant professor of psychiatry at the University of New Mexico Health Sciences Center. Previously, he was the state children's behavioral health director in New Mexico and chair of the Children, Youth, and Families Division of the National Association of State Mental Health Program Directors. He is currently on the board of directors of the National Latino Behavioral Health Association in the National Alliance of Multi-Ethnic Behavioral Health Associates and a member of the National Network to Eliminate Disparities in Behavioral Health.

Marlene Matarese, M.S.W., Director, Training and Technical Assistance, Innovations Institute, University of Maryland School of Medicine, Department of Child

Psychiatry, 737 West Lombard Street, Baltimore, Maryland 21201. Ms. Matarese's previous experience as the youth resource specialist for the Technical Assistance Partnership for Child and Family Mental Health, combined with her experience working within systems of care both locally and nationally, lends to her dedication in supporting youth partnership in systems transformation.

John Mayo, M.A., LMHC, Deputy Executive Director, Success 4 Kids & Families, 1311 North Westshore Boulevard, Suite 302, Tampa, Florida 33607. Mr. Mayo has been the deputy executive director of Success 4 Kids & Families, a not-for-profit agency following system of care principles that provides community-based services to families of children with emotional disturbances, since April 2000. He has been a licensed mental health counselor since 1982 and has held a variety of positions including serving as a counseling supervisor at an adolescent day treatment program, a family builders therapist, a children's clinical case manager, a case review committee chairperson, and a member of the board of the Federation of Families for Children's Mental Health.

Jan McCarthy, M.S.W., Director of Child Welfare Policy, National Technical Assistance Center for Children's Mental Health, Georgetown University Center for Child and Human Development, 3300 Whitehaven Street NW, Suite 3300, Washington, DC 20007. Ms. McCarthy served as the director of child welfare policy at the National Technical Assistance Center for Children's Mental Health at Georgetown University from 1995 to 2008. She has also worked in state and local public and private child welfare, family service, and mental health agencies and in a university-based child welfare training center.

Janet S. McIntyre, M.P.A., Director, Choices TA Center, Choices, Inc., 4701 North Keystone Avenue, Suite 150, Indianapolis, Indiana 46205. Ms. McIntyre joined Choices in 1999 as systems and technical assistance coordinator for the Dawn Project, a federally funded system of care. In 2002, she was named co-director of Choices TA Center and, since 2006, has been director of the center.

Trina W. Osher, M.A., President, Huff Osher Consulting, Inc., is a recognized leader in the family movement who raised two children with special needs. Ms. Osher speaks with a family voice to policy makers, administrators, and practitioners in the mental health, education, child welfare, and juvenile justice communities. As president of Huff Osher Consulting, Inc., and the principle architect of the definition of family-driven care, she works to promote family-driven practice by building collaborative alliances between families and the programs, agencies, and systems that serve them.

Kayla Paulson is a high school student in King County, Washington. She has been involved in the mental health system for many years.

Marlene Penn, Family Technical Consultant, 8 Tudor Court, Medford, New Jersey 08055. Ms. Penn began to navigate the children's mental health system through efforts to care for her own son, and she subsequently became an advocate for other families. She was the founding executive director of the Family Support Organization of Burlington County and currently serves as a consultant on building family leadership within child serving systems to communities and universities throughout the country.

Deborah F. Perry, Ph.D., M.A., Director, Women's and Children's Health Policy Center, Johns Hopkins Bloomberg School of Public Health, Department of Population, Family and Reproductive Health, 615 North Wolfe Street, E4144, Baltimore, Maryland 21205. Dr. Perry's research focuses on reducing the risk for mental health problems in young children and their families. For more than a decade she served on the faculty of Georgetown University's Center for Child and Human Development, providing national technical assistance to states and communities seeking to build systems of care for infants, toddlers, preschoolers, and their caregivers.

Sheila A. Pires, M.P.A., Partner, Human Service Collaborative, 1728 Wisconsin Avenue NW, #224, Washington, DC 20007. Ms. Pires is a senior partner in the Human Service Collaborative, a policy and technical assistance group that works with states and communities to improve service delivery systems for children, youth, and families. She served in the Carter White House, advised President Clinton's Health Care Reform Task Force, and contributed to the children's subcommittee report for President Bush's New Freedom Commission on Mental Health. She was also deputy commissioner of social services for the District of Columbia.

Karabelle A. Pizzigati, Ph.D., Child and Family Policy Adviser, 3213 Fayette Road, Kensington, Maryland 20895. Dr. Pizzigati formerly led public policy for the Washington, D.C.–based Child Welfare League of America and earlier directed the staff of the Select Committee on Children, Youth, and Families of the U.S. House of Representatives. She has served on the Technical Work Group for the National Longitudinal Study of Child and Adolescent Well-Being and currently sits on several professional and policy boards.

Frank Rider, M.S., Regional Technical Assistance Coordinator, Federation of Families for Children's Mental Health, 9605 Medical Center Drive, Suite 280, Rockville, Maryland 20850. Mr. Rider supports numerous emerging systems of care in both rural and urban communities throughout the Midwest for the Technical Assistance Partnership for Child and Family Mental Health. As former director of the Children's Bureau for the Arizona Division of Behavioral Health Services, he co-founded the Arizona Institute for Family Involvement.

Vestena Robbins, Ph.D., Associate Director, Kentucky Department for Mental Health and Mental Retardation Services, Division of Mental Health and Substance Abuse, 100 Fair Oaks Lane, 4E-D, Frankfort, Kentucky 40621. Dr. Robbins is involved in research, evaluation, and practice improvement efforts for children and youth with mental health and co-occurring substance use challenges and their families. She is the evaluation director for Kentuckians Encouraging Youth to Succeed, the state's federally funded system of care community, and is principal investigator of Kentucky's National Institute of Mental Health–funded Evidence-Based Practices State Planning Grant.

Maria J. Rodriguez, B.B.A., President, Vanguard Communications, 2121 K Street NW, Suite 300, Washington, DC 20037. Ms. Rodriguez is the president and owner of Vanguard Communications, a full-service public relations firm committed exclusively to the marketing and promotion of social issues. With an extensive background in public relations, social marketing, and culturally competent communications, Ms. Rodriguez has managed many outreach and marketing programs for a broad spectrum of nonprofit organizations and government agencies.

Knute Rotto, ACSW, Chief Executive Officer, Choices, Inc., 4701 North Keystone Avenue, Suite 150, Indianapolis, Indiana 46205. Mr. Rotto is chief executive officer of Choices, Inc., a nonprofit organization that has developed cost-effective, comprehensive systems of care in Indiana, Ohio, and Maryland. He is a nationally recognized expert in creating high-fidelity wraparound programs; managing provider networks of strength-based, community-based services; and developing braided and flexible funding streams.

Lisa Rubenstein, M.H.A., Public Health Advisor, Center for Mental Health Services, Substance Abuse and Mental Health Services Administration, 1 Choke Cherry Road, Room 6-1046, Rockville, Maryland 20857. Ms. Rubenstein has almost 25 years of experience in social marketing and public health. She currently serves as the government project officer for the Caring for Every Child's Mental Health Campaign, a national social marketing campaign raising awareness about systems of care and addressing the issue of stigma related to children's mental health.

Jacquelyn P. Scales, M.A., J.B.S. Mental Health/Mental Retardation Authority, 940 Montclair Road, Suite 200, Birmingham, Alabama 35213. Ms. Scales is the parent of a child with severe emotional disturbance and a retired school teacher. She is also a parent advocate who has worked with parents of children at the Jefferson County Family Court in Birmingham for the past 9 years. Ms. Scales is the past president and present secretary/treasurer of Alabama Family Ties, the Alabama statewide family organization.

Jason Schiffman, Ph.D., Associate Professor, University of Hawaii, 2430 Campus Road, 110 Gartley Hall, Honolulu, Hawaii 96822. Dr. Schiffman is an associate professor of clinical psychology, co-director of the Center for Cognitive Behavior Therapy, and director of the Child and Adolescent Thought Disorders Program, all at the University of Hawaii. In addition, he serves as a mental health consultant for the Child and Adolescent Mental Health Division of the Hawaii Department of Health and as a member of the Mental Health Division's Evidence-Based Services Committee.

Celia Serkin, B.A., Executive Director, Montgomery County Federation for Children's Mental Health, 1299 Lamberton Drive, Suite 1B, Silver Spring, Maryland 20902. Ms. Serkin is the executive director of the Montgomery County Federation of Families for Children's Mental Health, a family organization that helps families who have children or youth with emotional, behavioral, and mental health challenges. Prior to joining the family organization, she directed the family component of Community Kids, a federally funded effort to create a family-driven, youth-guided, culturally competent, and community-based system of care in Montgomery County, Maryland.

Angela Sheehan, M.P.A., Assistant Deputy Commissioner, Office of Evaluation and Research, City of New York, Department of Social Services, 180 Water Street, New York, New York, 10017. Ms. Sheehan was a project manager for Macro International Inc. until June 2007 and developed the Continuous Quality Improvement (CQI) Progress Report as a tool to monitor progress toward meeting system of care goals and objectives. While at Macro International Inc., she served as the project director for the cross-site evaluation of the Garrett Lee Smith Suicide Prevention Program and worked with communities funded under the Comprehensive Community Mental Health for Children and Their Families Program in implementing the national evaluation.

DeDe Sieler, B.S., Youth Program Manager, Clark County Department of Community Services–Youth House, 1012 Esther Street, Vancouver, Washington 98666. Ms. Sieler has worked extensively in the system of care arena and served as the project manager for the Partnerships for Youth Transition grant in Clark County, Washington.

Kathleen R. Skowyra, B.A., Senior Consultant, National Center for Mental Health and Juvenile Justice (NCMHJJ), Policy Research Associates, 345 Delaware Avenue, Delmar, New York 12054. Ms Skowyra is the former associate director of the NCMHJJ, where she oversaw projects funded by the Office of Juvenile Justice and Delinquency Prevention, the Substance Abuse and Mental Health Services Administration, and the John D. and Catherine T. MacArthur Foundation. Prior to joining Policy Research Associates, she managed several juvenile justice initiatives for the New York State Department of Social Services and served as a policy analyst for the New York State Council on Children and Families.

Diane L. Sondheimer, M.S.N., M.P.H., CPNP, Deputy Chief, Child, Adolescent and Family Branch, Center for Mental Health Services, Substance Abuse and Mental Health Services Administration, 1 Choke Cherry Road, Room 6-1043, Rockville, Maryland 20857. Ms. Sondheimer is a nationally recognized leader with more than 2 decades of experience in developing, implementing, administering, and evaluating local, state, and national health and mental health programs designed to improve the quality of life for children, adolescents, and their families. She has contributed to the research literature in the areas of HIV/AIDS, adolescent head trauma, homeless youth, girls in the juvenile justice system, youth in transition to adulthood, and other issues pertaining to child and adolescent mental health.

Steve Sparks, M.S.W., Regional Program Manager, Family and Community Services, Idaho Department of Health and Welfare, 1720 Westgate Drive, Suite D,

Boise, Idaho 83704. Mr. Sparks has more than 20 years of experience directing and providing child welfare and behavioral health services on behalf of children and families in three state systems. He has developed innovative programs and systems of care at the state, multicounty, and community levels, and his experience includes program administration and management, social service planning, program development, public speaking, and consultation.

Sandra A. Spencer, B.A., Chief Executive Officer, National Federation of Families for Children's Mental Health, 9605 Medical Center Drive, Suite 280, Rockville, Maryland 20886. Ms. Spencer is the executive director of the National Federation of Families for Children's Mental Health. She has worked with national policy and program leaders, family members, youth, and children for more than a decade and has navigated a highly visible career path through local family organizing, state-level system of care development, advocacy, national meeting planning for both the Federation of Families for Children's Mental Health and the Technical Assistance Partnership for Child and Family Mental Health, and providing training and technical assistance to family-run organizations.

Robert L. Stephens, Ph.D., M.P.H., Technical Director, Macro International Inc., 3 Corporate Square, Suite 370, Atlanta, Georgia 30329. Dr. Stephens is a technical director at Macro International Inc., working primarily on national multisite evaluations in the area of children's mental health. He has more than 20 years of experience as a research psychologist in government, academic, and private-sector settings providing consultation on experimental design and statistical analysis of longitudinal data.

Chris Stormann, Ph.D., Project Director, Institute for the Study and Prevention of Violence, Kent State University, 230 Cartwright Hall, Post Office Box 5190, Kent, Ohio 44242. Dr. Stormann is evaluator for the Cuyahoga Tapestry (Cleveland) System of Care. Prior to this, he was the director of research and development at the Eureka! Ranch leading continuous quality improvement and new product development initiatives and co-invented a forecasting model named "Top 20 emerging technologies in America" by *Fortune Small Business.*

Keren S. Vergon, Ph.D., Assistant Professor, Department of Child and Family Studies, Louis de la Parte Florida Mental Health Institute, University of South Florida, 13301 Bruce B. Downs Boulevard, Tampa, Florida 33612. Dr. Vergon has 12 years of experience in the areas of older adults' and children's mental health. She has been a member of the evaluation team for two federal system of care grants and is currently the evaluator for a National Child Traumatic Stress Network grant in Florida.

Janet S. Walker, Ph.D., Director of Research and Dissemination, Research and Training Center on Family Support and Children's Mental Health, Senior Research Associate, Regional Research Institute, Portland State University, 1600 Southwest 4th Avenue, Suite 900, Portland, Oregon 97201. Dr. Walker's current research focuses on exploring how individuals and organizations acquire the capacity to implement and sustain high-quality practice in human service settings, describing key implementation factors that affect the ability of organizations and individuals to provide high-quality services, and developing and evaluating interventions to increase the extent to which youth with emotional and mental health difficulties are meaningfully involved in care and treatment planning. Together with Dr. Eric Bruns, she co-directs the National Wraparound Initiative.

Christine Walrath, Ph.D., M.H.S., Vice President, Applied Research Division, Macro International Inc., 116 John Street, Suite 800, New York, New York 10038. Dr. Walrath has more than 13 years of experience in children's mental health research and evaluation, which includes extensive experience in the design and implementation of multimethod approaches to mutisite process and impact evaluation. She is experienced in both local- and national-level research and evaluation, with a concentrated focus on the multilevel impact of children's mental health services initiatives.

Ed K.S. Wang, Psy.D., Director, Office of Multicultural Affairs, Massachusetts Department of Mental Health, 25 Staniford Street, Boston, Massachusetts 02114. Dr. Wang directs the Office of Multicultural Affairs for the Massachusetts Department of Mental Health and is a clinical instructor in the Department of Psychiatry at Harvard Medical School. He focuses on clinical competence in working with culturally diverse clients and on trauma and recovery. Dr. Wang is a member of the National Advisory Council for the Substance Abuse and Mental Health Services Administration and is vice president of the Governing Board of the National Asian American Pacific Islander Mental Health Association.

Gwendolyn White, M.S.W., Director, System of Care Initiative, County of Allegheny Department of Human Services, 304 Wood Street, Pittsburgh, Pennsylvania 15222. Ms White has worked with children and families for more than 25 years. She has developed programs in the pediatric, educational, child welfare, and mental health arenas and is dedicated to consumer-driven services and supports.

Ginny Wood, B.S., President and Founder, Family Support Systems, Inc., 20487 North 94th Avenue, Peoria, Arizona 85382. Ms. Wood has more than 25 years of experience in children's mental health advocating for her son and specializing in helping family members and system builders create family-driven organizations. She was the founding director of the statewide organization Families Together in New York State and co-founder of the Family Involvement Center located in Phoenix, Arizona.

Claudia Zundel, M.S.W., Early Childhood Mental Health Specialist, Colorado Department of Human Services, Division of Mental Health, 3824 West Princeton Circle, Denver, Colorado 80236. Ms. Zundel is principal investigator for Project BLOOM, a federally funded system of care for children from birth to 5 years. For more than 20 years, Ms. Zundel has worked on system change projects within state government. She serves on Colorado's Interagency Coordinating Council, a governor-appointed position.

Foreword

The Fantastic Voyage

When the conceptualization of a system of care for children and adolescents with serious emotional disturbance and their families began to emerge in the early 1980s, no one involved with that movement dared to think that it would still be alive after 25 years. History had demonstrated that there had been one child advocacy movement about every decade since the year 1900 and that each had failed to survive for longer than 5 years. The movement toward systems of care has been, in large part, an advocacy effort, and over two decades later in 2008, not only is the system of care movement still alive, but it is thriving!

The original federal program promoting systems of care was the Child and Adolescent Service System Program (CASSP), which brought the message to all 50 states that we needed to begin a process of changing how services and supports to the children with the most serious and complex needs and their families would be met. In the early 1980s, the prevailing manner in which these children and adolescents and their families received services was by obtaining care from one of several major public agencies: mental health, child welfare, juvenile justice, education, substance abuse, or health. The system of care concept grew out of the recognition that these individuals had more than one need and could not be adequately served by one agency in isolation. Rather, they had multiple needs that required integrated care from two, three, or even more of these agencies. CASSP set out to restructure the service system so that all of a child or adolescent's and family's needs could be met through one community-based process. In addition, system of care principles stated that children and adolescents needed to be served in their communities with their families—not in institutional facilities, which were not only typically out of their communities, but often many miles away out of state.

CASSP set out to change our way of approaching services for children and adolescents with the most serious and complex needs. First, a national cadre of professionals across disciplines, both in practice and government service, was energized to begin a process of systems change and to develop a broad array of home and community-based services within the framework of a coordinated system of care. Next, CASSP expanded to include families, creating a parent movement, which has taken on a life of its own and has led to the development of family advocacy and support organizations at the national, state, and community levels. All states and many communities now have active family groups providing advocacy and peer support for families of youth with mental health challenges supported by the national Federation of Families for Children's Mental Health. Third, CASSP generated the concept of cultural and linguistic competence for systems of care and the services provided within them. This has led to systems of care being more responsive to people of color and to the development of special grant programs supporting culturally competent service delivery approaches for Native American populations.

Following from the foundation created by these CASSP efforts, the Robert Wood Johnson and Annie E. Casey Foundations both funded community-based demonstrations to test approaches for translating system of care principles to the community, service delivery, and practice levels, where the individualized, "wraparound" approach has emerged as the child and family–level service delivery approach that best embodies the system of care philosophy.

The federal government then followed by initiating a multimillion dollar grant program to support communities in creating the infrastructure and services needed to develop systems of care nationwide, as well as a grant program to support the development of statewide family organizations. These programs have now had a demonstrable impact in every state as well as numerous counties, municipalities, and Native American communities. Throughout this process, first three, then four, and finally five centers of excellence have provided the research, policy analysis, and technical assistance needed to support all of this growth. They are the National Technical Assistance Center for Children's Mental Health at Georgetown University, the Research and Training Center on Children's Mental Health at the University of South Florida, the Research and Training Center on Family Support and Children's Mental Health at Portland State University, the Technical Assistance Partnership for Child and Family Mental Health, and the Statewide Family Networks Technical Assistance Center at United Advocates for Children and Families.

Most recently, there was a major shift in national mental health policy when the Surgeon General of the United States of America issued a report on the mental health of children, focusing heavily on the service delivery approaches inherent in the system of care framework, reifying the system of care approach as national policy. Similarly, the system of care philosophy and approach formed the basis for the child-, youth-, and family-focused recommendations of the President's New Freedom Commission on Mental Health.

This has all been a "Fantastic Voyage" to a destination that could not have been conceived of at the start. And, the journey is not over. The system of care concepts and philosophy have grown and matured. New technologies have advanced the application of these concepts to better organize communities in the delivery of care to children and families in need and to provide more appropriate, effective, and integrated services than ever before. Research has helped to understand, modify, and justify these technologies. This book leads you through the developmental history of system of care concepts, technologies, and research and provides practical and "how to" information that moves us from ideas to operational realities. The volume brings you up to date with where the system of care movement has come and provides more than a hint as to where the fantastic voyage may lead us next.

Ira S. Lourie, M.D.
Child Psychiatrist, Partner in the Human Services Collaborative
Medical Director of Pressley Ridge Maryland and AWARE Montana
Former Director of the Child and Adolescent Service System
Program of the National Institute of Mental Health

Foreword

Finding a Balance in Systems of Care

When I think about all of the effort it has taken to get the point where this book has emerged, I must also think about my own history and my role in the system of care movement. I grew up with systems of care, first as an early enrollee into the then federally funded grant program in my community, and later into the burgeoning youth movement, helping to lay the groundwork for youth-driven advocacy organizations within my state and at the national level. Along the way I have become a social worker, board member, youth coordinator, trainer, researcher, and social marketer, among other roles.

I believe in systems of care. This is not the belief born of debatable, static research that attempts to capture moments in the stream of people's lives (though we have plenty of that, too), but of a belief grounded in bearing witness to the lives that have been transformed in the process. My first example is always my own, as my local system of care helped me to accomplish things that the best professionals in my community once thought impossible: simple things like maintaining a job, finishing college, starting my own family, and living outside of an institutional setting. Next, I remember all the brilliant, powerful young people I have met across the country who are living better and feeling better, and, often, working to help other youth do the same. Finally, I am encouraged by the professionals who have made their own transformations, facing their doubts and fears about partnering with youth and families and growing in both skill and humanity in the process.

I am frequently asked how systems of care work. Of course, like many system-level issues, it is hard to pinpoint specific processes or practices that make the difference. But in my work around the country, I have come to see that this kind of change really is one in which the whole is greater than the sum of its parts. Surely, in places where the process is diluted, so are the results. However, one key principle (that is not found in the system of care *values and principles*) seems to be "balance." When communities find the balance between traditional approaches and emerging trends, the strengths of youth and adults, the expertise of families and professionals, and the wisdom learned from one's culture versus that of academia, real change starts to occur.

So where does this book come in? If systems of care are about changing entire communities, the knowledge must be accessible to those outside of the mental health system and to individuals beyond those who are already involved in system of care work. Systems of care truly are about "caring for every child's mental health," but to do that we must address the disengagement in one area in particular—academia and the education of mental health and social service professionals that occurs in academic settings.

As a college student, it was exceedingly frustrating to find that the work I was immersed in was not addressed in any of my undergraduate or graduate classes. If practice typically lags behind research by 10 years, and since academic research appears to be 10 years behind what is currently happening in the field, then it could take up to 2 decades for the benefits of our system of care work in communities to impact the preservice education of mental health and social service professionals, as well as greater society. As a mother, aunt, and professional, I find this lag unacceptable and hope that the use of this book in academia will shorten the delay.

Finally, this book is also about celebrating and honoring where we have come as a community of change makers. This road has its share of joy and tragedy, and we have come through it with tears, laughter, and, ultimately, hope for the future of our children, families, and communities. May the examples in this book inspire you to join us in this exciting journey.

Samantha Jo Broderick, M.S.W.
System Alumna and Board Member
Youth M.O.V.E. National
New Jersey

Foreword

Family-Driven Systems of Care

The voices of families raising children with serious behavioral, emotional, and mental health challenges were silent before the birth of systems of care. Historically, families were blamed for their child's mental health disabilities. The phrase *blamed and shamed* refers to the way families were treated. The system first blamed parents for all of the child's behaviors, and parents then felt ashamed for having caused such a bad thing to happen to their child. It was also a common practice for families of children with mental health issues to be labeled as "dysfunctional" families, again putting the blame on the family.

When the system of care concept emerged, a core value asserted that systems of care should be child and family focused, with the needs of the child and family dictating the types and mix of services provided. One of the 10 guiding principles for systems of care further stated that families and surrogate families of children with emotional disturbances should be full participants in all aspects of the planning and delivery of services. Systems of care began to use the language of partnership. The concept was that parents and other caregivers could be viewed as partners with providers in the care and treatment of their children.

The role of families in systems of care helped jumpstart what is known now as the family movement. This movement has evolved to ensure that children with serious emotional disturbances and their families have a voice. Critical to this movement is not just the voice of families, but also attention and responsiveness to the culture of each individual family. Systems of care recognize that one size does not fit all when it comes to treatment plans and service delivery systems. Systems of care provide individualized services and supports that allow for culturally and linguistically competent service approaches for youth and families.

In 1989, the National Federation of Families for Children's Mental Health was formed as a result of this movement. The federation became the national voice for children's mental health. This national family-run organization was formed by a group of family members who saw the need to provide a forum for the collective voices of families to have an impact on the children's mental health service delivery system. Through the leadership of the National Federation, family voice has become an integral component of systems of care.

The voices of families have also had an impact on the Guidance for Applicants (GFA) that supports federally funded systems of care through the Comprehensive Community Mental Health for Children and Their Families Program. The language of the GFA around family involvement has been strengthened over time. In 1999, *family involvement* was mandated in all grant applications. In 2000, *family–professional partnerships* were required, and families were invited to work hand in hand with professionals in developing their individualized service plans for their child and family, as well as in helping to shape the developing of systems of care. In 2003, a full-time position for a family member was mandated, requiring systems of care to hire a Key Family Contact. The role of the Key Family Contact was to ensure family involvement in planning, implementing, and evaluating the system of care. Each funded system of care community was also encouraged to support a family-run organization.

The concept of family-driven care was set forth in the 2003 President's New Freedom Commission Report on Mental Health: *Achieving the Promise: Transforming Mental Health Care in America,* with Goal 2 stating that mental health care must be consumer and family driven. In response, the National Federation of Families for Children's Mental Health was asked to develop a definition of the term *family-driven.* In 2005, *family-driven* was written in the GFA, and it was further suggested that financial support be provided to sustain family involvement throughout and beyond the federal funding period.

Systems of care have opened the door for emerging family leaders all across the country. Many family members have found gainful employment as consultants, family organization employees, and mental health service providers as a result of systems of care. In addition, an ever-increasing number of family-run organizations are being formed in communities to offer peer-to-peer support to families and to provide family voice to systems of care.

This book provides a historical context for systems of care and highlights promising strategies and practical approaches in many areas of system of care development, as well has offering readers a snapshot of where we are heading in the future. Systems of care improve the lives of children with serious emotional disturbances and their families. This book is a much-needed resource to keep this innovation alive and to further disseminate knowledge about the system of care philosophy and approach.

Sandra A. Spencer
Family Member
Executive Director of the National Federation of
Families for Children's Mental Health

Acknowledgments

We would like to acknowledge some important partners in the development of this book. First and foremost, we acknowledge youth who experience mental health challenges and their families. We hope and believe that this volume pays tribute to and honors their experiences, struggles, and successes. The book reflects our belief that, collectively, we need to redouble our efforts to ensure that youth and families receive all of the services and supports they need and deserve to lead healthy and productive lives.

We also acknowledge and congratulate the public and private providers, neighborhood and community partners, state and local policy makers and administrators, families and youth, technical assistance providers, researchers and evaluators, social marketers, youth coordinators, and other constituency groups who represent the backbone of systems of care. These individuals are working tirelessly to build and sustain systems of care across this nation and to overcome the difficult, real-world challenges inherent in achieving this vision. To assist them in accomplishing their goals, this book is full of practical examples for implementing the system of care approach in the real world.

We feel extremely fortunate to have amassed a collective of authors who not only represent diverse constituency groups, but who also are recognized leaders in the field. We are grateful to them for donating significant time and effort to share their extensive experience, wisdom, and "hands-on" strategies by contributing to this book. We are also lucky to have caring and understanding friends and family who support our efforts and allow us the freedom to turn ideas into realities.

For us, it has been a great privilege to work together to create this volume. There is so much dedication and passion in the field of children's mental health, and we are honored to produce a book that has, as its ultimate goal, to provide help and hope to children and youth who experience mental health challenges and their families. We all know someone who has, or has had, a mental health issue. The truth is that people with mental health challenges are our neighbors, our friends, and our families. Mental illnesses are real, and they are very treatable. We truly hope that this book will be used to educate, spread the word, and further the growth of systems of care—a proven strategy to improve lives.

Introduction

For the past two decades, systems of care have been transforming services across America, and we are happy to report that the "movement" to transform children's mental health services is alive and well. Historically, there have been calls for reform in children's mental health in the United States since the 1960s. In nearly all the reports and documents advocating system change, the major themes were the same. They were that:

- Most children in need simply weren't getting mental health services

- Those served were often in excessively restrictive settings

- Services were limited to outpatient, inpatient, and residential treatment—few, if any intermediate, community-based options were available

- The various child-serving systems sharing responsibility for children with mental health problems rarely worked together

- Families typically were blamed and weren't involved as partners in their child's care

- Agencies and systems rarely considered or addressed cultural differences in the population they served

The solution to these systemic problems has been to create comprehensive, coordinated, community-based systems of services and supports, that we call *systems of care*.

The system of care approach has evolved into a major organizing force shaping the development of children's mental health services across the United States. At its most fundamental level, this approach consists of the development of a comprehensive spectrum of mental health and other necessary services that is guided by a core set of values and guiding principles. Core values specify that systems of care are community based, child centered and family focused, and culturally and linguistically competent; principles call for services that are individualized, family driven and youth guided, provided in the least restrictive setting, and coordinated. Systems of care are undergirded by an infrastructure based on a clear locus of accountability for services to children with mental health challenges and their families and interagency collaboration in both system management and service delivery. The system of care concept and philosophy have influenced and guided the articulation of public policy that supports the improvement of mental health services for children and their families. Most notably, the system of care concept and philosophy formed the basis for the recommendations of the President's New Freedom Commission on Mental Health to "transform" mental health systems to enable children with emotional disorders to live, work, learn, and fully function in their homes and communities.

Though the system of care concept may sound self-evident, we now know from experience and from extensive research that has been conducted over the past two decades that implementing systems of care is a difficult and complex endeavor. Much of the knowledge base has emerged from the federal Comprehensive Community Mental Health Services for Children and Their Families Program, which has provided over one billion dollars in federal funding since 1993 for the development of local systems of care. The national focus on systems of care and the wide dissemination of information about them and their achievements set the stage for significant state and local investments in the development of systems of care, in many cases without federal financial support. Information learned through experience and evaluation of the federal program and related efforts offers a rich source of guidance for states and communities as they seek to further develop, improve, and sustain their systems of care and the component services and supports.

Although available information on the development and impact of systems of care is wide ranging, we identified the need for a single volume that captures the key lessons learned and provides a roadmap for those interested in developing and sustaining systems of care across the country. This book draws on information from federally funded systems of care and on available information on systems of care more generally as the approach has expanded. The result is a unique compendium of information that we hope will prove useful to a wide audience in all states and communities.

Thus, the purpose of this handbook is to provide a compendium of information on how to develop systems of care—a one-stop reference for those interested in understanding and applying effective strategies for system-building and service delivery. Throughout the book, "recommended practice" examples are incorporated, illustrating the implementation of critical elements of systems of care and offering a wealth of real-world experience. Evaluation results also are incorporated to illustrate the utilization of data to inform decision making at multiple levels, from providing services to individual children and families to system management. Key contextual issues and emerging trends affecting the development of systems of care are addressed, such as the current emphasis on implementing evidence-based practices. Core values and principles of systems of care such as individualized services, family and youth involvement, and cultural and linguistic competence serve as the foundation of the book and are incorporated into each chapter.

Our intention is that the audience for this handbook will include the multiple constituencies that are involved in building community-based systems of care for children and their families across the nation's states and communities. It is designed to meet the burgeoning demand for written resources, tool kits, books, and other practical materials on the structures and processes involved in creating effective systems and services. This demand comes from the front lines including families, youth, program developers, and service delivery personnel, as well as from policy makers from partner child-serving agencies at federal, state, and local levels. Importantly, this book is also intended to fulfill requests from higher education institutions for materials appropriate for preservice education across the mental health disciplines that provide cutting-edge information on the development and maintenance of systems of care and state-of-the-art service delivery approaches.

The creation of an effective and responsive system of care is always about teamwork, collaboration, and persistence. And, consistent with the system of care philosophy, this volume has quite literally taken a multitude of contributors. The book is dividend into five sections: Section I presents an overview of systems of care, including three chapters that outline the history, results, and components of this approach. The five chapters in Section II describe elements of systems of care, including critical structures and functions, along with strategies to incorporate individualized services, evidence-based practices, effective financing strategies, and approaches for sustaining systems of care over time. Section III provides practice examples at the system level, detailing practical approaches for implementing family-driven and youth-guided systems, enhancing cultural and linguistic competence, measuring fidelity, conducting social marketing, and incorporating evaluation and continuous quality improvement. Section IV provides practice examples at the service delivery level. Each chapter demonstrates how systems of care can improve outcomes for youth and families by providing strengths-based, individualized services; incorporating evidence-based practice elements; and by addressing the unique needs of young children; youth in transition to adulthood; youth in the child welfare, education, and juvenile justice systems; and youth from diverse communities. Finally, Section V discusses future directions for systems of care, focusing on the critical topics of workforce, policy, and research. Throughout these chapters, examples from the field are provided to illustrate the implementation of effective strategies and to outline challenges and strategies for overcoming these challenges.

Over the past 20 years, this country has seen tremendous progress. Yet we know that the journey is just beginning, and that there is much to be done. We hope that the unique focus on practical, *how to* information in this handbook will provide concrete guidance to shift the focus from the theoretical to the applied and to continue our work to develop systems of care in all of our nation's communities.

I

Overview

1

Systems of Care

A Strategy to Transform Children's Mental Health Care

BETH A. STROUL, GARY M. BLAU, AND DIANE L. SONDHEIMER

The need to reform children's mental health systems in the United States has been extensively documented. As early as 1969, the Joint Commission on Mental Health of Children concluded that only a fraction of the children in need were actually receiving mental health services and that the services being provided were largely ineffective. Subsequent policy studies documented similar conclusions: children were not receiving needed mental health services; services were often provided in excessively restrictive settings; services were limited to outpatient, inpatient, and residential treatment, with few intermediate, community-based options available; and coordination between child-serving systems was weak (Knitzer, 1982; President's Commission on Mental Health, 1978; U.S. Congress, Office of Technology Assessment, 1986). Furthermore, families were typically blamed for their children's problems and were not involved in decision making about their children's care, and little attention was paid to cultural and linguistic differences in service delivery (Friesen & Huff, 1996; Isaacs-Shockley, Cross, Bazron, Dennis, & Benjamin, 1996; U.S. Department of Health and Human Services, 2001). The proposed solution to these systemic problems was comprehensive community-based systems of services and supports that eventually became known as *systems of care*.

These initial reports served as a catalyst for bringing the federal government's attention to the issue of children's mental health. The first federal program, the Child and Adolescent Service System Program (CASSP), was launched by the National Institute of Mental Health in 1984 to assist states and communities in building the capacity to develop services targeted for children with serious emotional disturbances (SEDs) and their families. The goals of this program were to promote systems change; assist states and communities in the development of comprehensive community-based systems of care; and encourage collaboration among service providers, parents, advocates, and policy makers. CASSP's efforts resulted in the identification of dedicated staff assigned to children's mental health in all states and the District of Columbia; a substantial increase in the proportion of states with separate child mental health budgets (from 18% in 1982 to 70% in 1993); legislatively mandated interagency planning councils and interagency care review processes in approximately 50% of states; and increased family involvement in policy making, program planning, and service planning, which is now mandated in at least 22 states (Center for Mental Health Services, 1997). A major accomplishment of the CASSP initiative that has had a far-reaching effect nationwide was the development and definition of the concept of a system of care to serve as a framework for reform (Stroul, 2002; Stroul & Friedman, 1986, 1996). Such systems of care emphasize a wide array of services, individualized care, the least restrictive environments possible for service provision, the full participation of families and youth, coordination among child-serving agencies and programs, and cultural and linguistic competence.

This chapter defines and clarifies the system of care concept and philosophy, which has been used as the foundation for system reform for more than two decades. System of care development is explained as a complex, multilevel process with goals and outcomes at various levels of intervention. Systems of care are discussed as a strategy for transforming the approach to mental health care for children and their families. The chapter also provides an overview of federal programs supporting the development of systems of care for children with or at risk for emotional disorders and their families, highlighting the current Comprehensive Community Mental Health Services for Children and Their Families Program (i.e., the Children's Mental Health Initiative). Information is presented about the types of supports that have been provided by federal and state governments to assist in developing and sustaining systems of care (e.g., training and technical assistance, evaluation, social marketing). Finally, the chapter discusses the future directions of systems of care.

DEFINING THE SYSTEM OF CARE CONCEPT

System of Care Concept and Philosophy

First published in 1986, the definition of a system of care was stated as being a "comprehensive spectrum of mental health and other necessary services which are organized into a coordinated network to meet the multiple and changing needs of children and their families" (Stroul & Friedman, 1986, p. 3). In 2005, an updated definition was developed by a consortium of professionals, family members, and youth:

> A system of care is a coordinated network of community-based services and supports that are organized to meet the challenges of children and youth with serious mental health needs and their families. Families and youth work in partnership with public and private organizations to design mental health services and supports that are effective, that build on the strengths of individuals, and that address each person's cultural and linguistic needs. A system of care helps children, youth, and families function better at home, in school, in the community, and throughout life. (http://www.systemsofcare.samhsa.gov)

Although the system of care concept was originally crafted for children and youth with SEDs (diagnosable mental health disorders with extreme functional impairment that limit or interfere with one's ability to function in the family, school, and/or community), the applicability of the concept and philosophy to other populations, with appropriate modifications, has become apparent. The core values of the system of care philosophy specify that services should be community based, child centered, family focused, and culturally and linguistically competent. The guiding principles specify that services should be comprehensive and include a broad array of services, individualized to each child and family, provided in the least restrictive appropriate setting, coordinated at both the system and the service delivery levels, organized to involve families and youth as full partners, and designed to emphasize early identification and intervention (Stroul & Friedman, 1986, 1996) (Table 1.1).

The concept of family and youth involvement has been strengthened over time, and the new concept of family-driven, youth-guided care is gaining broad acceptance. *Family-driven* care means that families have a primary decision-making role in the care of their own children, as well as the policies and procedures governing care for all children in their community, state, tribe, and nation. Similarly, *youth-guided* care means that young people have the right to be empowered, educated, and given a decision-making role in their own care and in the establishment of policies and procedures governing care for all youth in their community, state, tribe, and nation (http://www.systemsofcare.samhsa.gov).

Rather than addressing mental health treatment needs in isolation, the system of care concept recognizes that children and families have needs in many domains. It thus promotes a holistic approach in which *all* life domains and needs are considered in serving children and their families. Accordingly, the system of care framework is organized around eight overlapping dimensions, each representing an area of need for the child and family (Holden & Blau, 2006; Stroul & Friedman, 1986, 1996) (Figure 1.1).

The mental health dimension is emphasized due to its obvious importance for children with emotional and behavioral disorders and includes a range of both nonresidential and residential services and supports. Experience has demonstrated the need to expand the definition of mental health services and has shown that additional services, such as respite care, therapeutic recreation, school-based mental health services, mental health consultation, behavioral aides, targeted financial assistance to meet basic needs, primary health care, after-school programs, transportation, and care management, are also essential (Blau & Brumer, 1996, 1999) (Table 1.2).

Several points emphasized about the mental health dimension in 1986 remain equally relevant today. First, all of the components are interrelated, making the effectiveness of any one component related to the availability and effectiveness of all other components. Because of this interdependence, it is important to consider the entire system, not just one or two of the services, when investing in service capacity. Second, an appropriate balance between the components of a ser-

Table 1.1. System of care values and principles

Core values

1. The system of care should be child centered and family focused, with the needs of the child and family dictating the types and mix of services provided.

2. The system of care should be community based, with the locus of services as well as management and decision-making responsibility resting at the community level.

3. The system of care should be culturally and linguistically competent, with agencies, programs, and services that are responsive to the cultural, racial, and ethnic differences of the populations they serve.

Guiding principles

1. Children with emotional disturbances should have access to a comprehensive array of services that address their physical, emotional, social, and educational needs.

2. Children with emotional disturbances should receive individualized services in accordance with the unique needs and potentials of each child and guided by an individualized service plan.

3. Children with emotional disturbances should receive services within the least restrictive, most normative environment that is clinically appropriate.

4. The families and surrogate families of children with emotional disturbances should be full participants in all aspects of the planning and delivery of services.

5. Children with emotional disturbances should receive services that are integrated, with linkages between child-serving agencies and programs and mechanisms for planning, developing, and coordinating services.

6. Children with emotional disturbances should be provided with case management or similar mechanisms to ensure that multiple services are delivered in a coordinated and therapeutic manner and that they can move through the system of services in accordance with their changing needs.

7. Early identification and intervention for children with emotional disturbances should be promoted by the system of care in order to enhance the likelihood of positive outcomes.

8. Children with emotional disturbances should be ensured smooth transitions to the adult service system as they reach maturity.

9. The rights of children with emotional disturbances should be protected, and effective advocacy efforts for children and adolescents with emotional disturbances should be promoted.

10. Children with emotional disturbances should receive services without regard to race, religion, national origin, sex, physical disability, or other characteristics, and services should be sensitive and responsive to cultural differences and special needs.

Reprinted from Stroul, B., & Friedman, R. (1986). *A system of care for children and youth with severe emotional disturbances* (Rev. ed., p. 17). Washington, DC: Georgetown University Child Development Center, National Technical Assistance Center for Children's Mental Health.

vice system is important, which is particularly significant in determining the balance between the more restrictive and the less restrictive services. It is imperative that the concepts of treatment intensity, treatment restrictiveness, and treatment setting not be confused, as intensive treatment interventions—even the *same* treatment interventions—can be offered in a variety of settings and through numerous service programs.

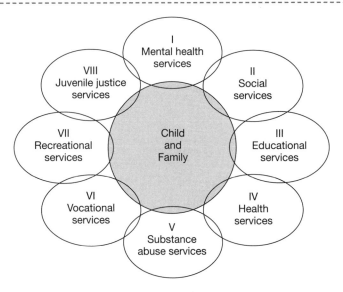

Figure 1.1. System of care framework. (Reprinted from Stroul, B. & Friedman, R. [1986]. *A system of care for children and youth with severe emotional disturbances* [Rev. ed., p. 30]. Washington, DC: Georgetown University Child Development Center, National Technical Assistance Center for Children's Mental Health.)

Systems of Care as Complex, Multilevel Processes

Over time, there have been a lot of interpretations of the term *system of care*. It has been referred to as a *model*, a *program*, and a *value*. People have tried to replicate it, operationalize it, measure it, evaluate it, and compare it with so-called traditional services. Essentially, a system of care can be best understood as a range of

Table 1.2. Mental health dimension

Nonresidential services	Crisis residential services
Prevention	Inpatient hospitalization
Early intervention	**Other essential services**
Assessment	Care management
Outpatient treatment	Respite services
Home-based services	School-based mental health
Day treatment	services
Crisis services	Behavioral aides
Residential services	Mental health consultation
Therapeutic foster care	Therapeutic recreation
Therapeutic group care	After school services
Therapeutic camp services	Flexible funds
Independent living services	Transportation
Residential treatment	

Source: Stroul & Friedman (1986).

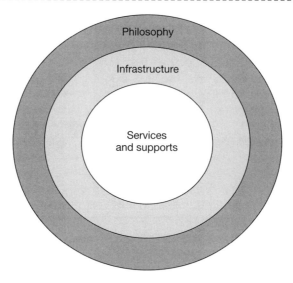

Figure 1.2. System of care concept.

treatment services and supports guided by a philosophy and supported by an infrastructure. It is an organizing framework based on a set of principles that seeks to develop and implement services to improve the lives of children and adolescents with serious mental health challenges, as well as their families (Figure 1.2).

It is essential to recognize that developing a system of care is a multifaceted, multilevel process that involves making changes:

1. In state policies, financing mechanisms, workforce development, and other structures and processes to support systems of care

2. At the local system level to plan, implement, manage, and evaluate the system

3. At the service delivery level to provide a broad array of effective, state-of-the-art treatment services and supports to children and families in an individualized and coordinated manner

Thus, developing a system of care is a difficult and complex process that presents many challenges at each of these levels.

In an effort to clarify the meaning of the system of care concept, Friedman (2001) emphasized that developing a system of care is neither a specific nor a simple intervention. It can be seen as a general statement of policy indicating a desire to establish a complex system targeted at a specific population of children and families based on a widely agreed-on set of principles and values. Hernandez and Hodges (2002) suggested that a system of care may be better thought of as a cluster of organizational change strategies based on a set of values and principles that are intended to shape policies, regulations, funding mechanisms, services, and supports. These interpretations also emphasize the complexity of the system of care concept and the fact that intervention occurs on multiple levels.

Further complication in defining the system of care concept is created by several of its basic characteristics that have become more apparent over time. First, the system of care concept is a framework and a guide, not a prescription. The concept of a system of care was never intended to be a discrete model to be replicated; rather, it was intended to serve as an organizing framework and value base. Flexibility to implement the system of care concept and philosophy in a way that fits the particular state and community is inherent in the approach. Therefore, different communities have implemented systems of care in very different ways— no two are alike. It is the philosophy (the value base) that remains constant. Hernandez and Hodges (2002) captured this by stating that a system of care is "not a clean package," adding that what is commonly called a system of care can vary considerably from community to community, both within and across states, and that these systems are not "single, bounded, well-defined units." Each community must employ its own strategy to plan, implement, and evaluate its system of care based on its particular needs, goals, priorities, and environment.

Another complication is that systems of care are not static but continue to change and evolve over time. The policies, organizational arrangements, service delivery approaches, and treatments modify and adapt to changing needs, opportunities, and environmental circumstances in states and communities, both positive and negative. Furthermore, because a system of care is not a clean package, it is very difficult to definitively conclude that one community has one and another does not. It is more appropriate to define the level of development of a system of care. Many communities in the nation have some elements of the system of care philosophy and services in place, even if they are in the earliest stages along the developmental pathway.

Researchers continue to assess the effectiveness of systems of care, but in some cases, they have failed to consider the basic characteristics:

- Systems of care are multifaceted, multilevel interventions, making them difficult to measure. They are probably more complex, challenging, and time consuming to implement than most researchers would anticipate.

- The services in systems of care are difficult to measure because children are likely to be receiving multiple services as part of a package of flexible, individualized services and supports, as opposed to a single treatment that can be isolated.

- Systems of care do not involve a unitary approach but rather are substantially different in every community. Thus, it is difficult to group them together and measure them in the same way.

- They are not static interventions. Every system of care is in a constant state of development and evolution.

- Most communities have some elements of the philosophy and services in place, making it difficult to compare those that have a system of care with those that do not.

Given these complexities and variations, evaluating systems of care is a significant challenge. The central issue in evaluating the effectiveness of systems of care is to recognize that there are goals and desired outcomes at each level of the intervention, all of which are important and all of which should be considered and measured appropriately. System-level changes cannot be examined and measured simply by looking at clinical and functional outcomes. Such outcomes must be linked to what occurs at the service delivery or practice level, and improved clinical and functional outcomes cannot be reasonably expected if the intervention only involves system-level changes, such as building an infrastructure or system coordination. Care must be taken to ensure that the outcomes being measured are reasonably linked to the level and the aspect of the intervention that is being assessed.

Rosenblatt (1998) emphasized this point by stating that it is important to match the measurement of a system of care to its proximal organizational intentions in order to avoid inappropriate assessment of the results of systems of care. Hernandez and Hodges (2002) raised a similar point when they stated that the system of care concept has been framed by some researchers as a clinical intervention, leading to the erroneous expectation that a system can be implemented and evaluated as a discrete unit intended to directly improve the emotional and behavioral status of children. They further suggested that child-specific clinical outcomes are best understood as resulting from the specific treatments or treatment clusters made available through systems of care (Figure 1.3).

An important challenge for the field of children's mental health as a community is to address the ways it can improve the systems of care that serve children with emotional disorders and their families, as well as the services and treatment interventions embedded within them, to achieve better outcomes. Are systems of care serving their intended populations? Are they providing the intended services and supports in the intended manner? Did children and families experience the

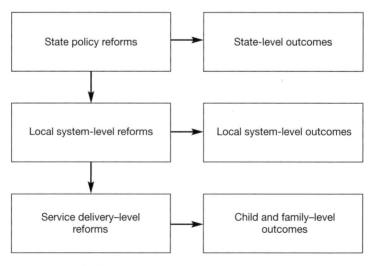

Figure 1.3. Levels of system of care development.

services and supports in the anticipated way? Which elements and characteristics of systems and treatment interventions are associated with positive outcomes at each level? These are the questions that will continue to move the field forward.

SYSTEMS OF CARE AS A FRAMEWORK FOR TRANSFORMATION

Since the 1980s, there has been a growing movement to change the way providers, administrators, and families think about the delivery of human services to children and adolescents with serious mental health needs and their families (Osher, Osher, & Blau, in press). To put these changes into context, it is important to understand that change in human services is not a new concept. During the past century, mental health providers have experienced a number of philosophical shifts that have led to many advances in methods for working with individuals and families. From the popularity of the introspective approaches by Freud and Jung, to the focus on maximizing potential brought forth by Carl Rogers, to the behavioral focus of B.F. Skinner, change in the approaches used by mental health practitioners has evolved over time (de Voursney, Mannix, Brounstein, & Blau, 2007; Gullotta, in press). On a broad policy and system level, federal efforts have led the way in transforming mental health care in America.

Comprehensive Community Mental Health Services for Children and Their Families Program

Following the implementation of CASSP, the Comprehensive Community Mental Health Services for Children and Their Families Program was established in 1992 by the Substance Abuse and Mental Health Services Administration (SAMHSA) with administrative oversight placed within the Child, Adolescent, and Family Branch (CAFB). Considered the next evolution of CASSP, this program was funded at an initial level of $4.9 million, offering grants to communities to develop, implement, and sustain systems of care for children and youth with SEDs and their families. Nearly 15 years later, as of federal fiscal year 2007, 126 communities across all 50 states and the territories of Guam and Puerto Rico have received at least one of these transformative grants. With the support of the President and the help of Congress, this program has grown to an annual budget of more than $104 million.

These are now 6-year grants with a federal investment of up to $9 million during the 6-year funding period. There are also local match requirements. Specifically, in Years 1–3 of the grant, the funded community must provide, through either cash or in-kind support, 1 local dollar for every 3 federal dollars. In Year 4, this increases to 1 local dollar for every federal dollar, and in Years 5 and 6, the local contribution must be 2 dollars to 1 federal dollar. This match requirement is legislatively mandated with the rationale of promoting local and state commitment and investment to ensure that the developing service delivery system is sustained beyond the federal funding (Figure 1.4).

System of Care Communities of the Comprehensive Community Mental Health Services for Children and Their Families Program

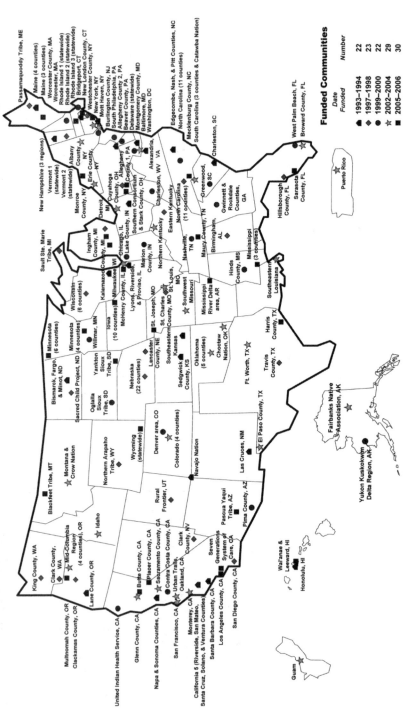

Figure 1.4. System of care communities of the Comprehensive Community Mental Health Services for Children and Their Families Program. (Reprinted from Center for Mental Health Services. *Mental Health Directory, 2000,* compiled by Manderscheid, R.W.; Atay, J.E.; Brown, D.; and Henderson, M.J. DHHS Pub. No. [SMA]01-3503. Washington, DC: Superintendent of Documents, U.S. Government Printing Office, 20402.)

Child, Adolescent, and Family Branch

Transforming mental health services for children, youth, and families requires first and foremost a commitment to operate from an organizational vision and mission that is consistent with the values and principles espoused by systems of care. The vision and mission at the CAFB reflects a shared commitment to developing community-based systems of care that assist children and their families to live, learn, work, and participate fully in their communities where they experience joy, health, love, and hope. The CAFB mission statement epitomizes this vision:

> Through investment and partnerships in home and community-based systems of care, the Child, Adolescent and Family Branch promotes the potential and well-being of children and youth who have, or are at-risk for having, a serious emotional or behavioral disturbance, and their families. (http://www.systemsofcare.samhsa.gov)

Strategically, the guiding framework for transformation efforts can be evidenced through the Transformation Equation:

$$T = (V + B + A) \times (CQI)^2$$

This equation is composed of the following elements: *Transformation* = (*Vision* plus *Beliefs* plus *Action*) multiplied by (*Continuous Quality Improvement*) squared.

Vision provides the direction for the work (e.g., all children and their families can live, learn, work, and participate fully in communities where they experience joy, health, love, and hope). Beliefs guide the work (system of care values and principles). Actions must be taken to turn beliefs into reality. Continuous quality improvement ensures that the actions reflect the wishes and needs of the individuals and communities being served, and it is squared to illustrate the importance of this feedback and input. The system of care model remains a transformation strategy because it is constantly evolving, new ideas and concepts continue to be developed, and new actions are continually taken to push the envelope toward the provision of better services and the achievement of better outcomes.

Other Federal Efforts Guided by the System of Care Philosophy

In addition to the Comprehensive Community Mental Health Services for Children and Their Families Program, the federal government has developed and implemented other children's mental health initiatives that incorporate the system of care values and principles.

Partnerships for Youth Transition   In 2002, the Center for Mental Health Services (CMHS) of SAMHSA, in partnership with the Office on Special Education Programs of the Department of Education, awarded approximately $2.5 million per year for 4 years for the Partnerships for Youth Transition (PYT) initiative. The PYT program was established to address the specific developmentally based service needs of youth ages 16–25 in a coordinated, individualized manner. The initiative funded five sites across the nation to develop and implement transition systems for youth with mental and emotional difficulties as they enter adulthood. These five sites were the Utah Department of Human Services; the Clark County Department of Community Services and Corrections in Vancouver, Washington; the PACT-4 Families Collaborative in Willmar, Minnesota; the Department of Behavioral and Development Services of the Spring Harbor/ Maine Medical Center Mental Health Network and the Department of Vocational Services at Maine Medical Center, under contract with the State of Maine Department Health and Human Services in Augusta, Maine; and the Allegheny County Department of Human Services Department in Pittsburgh, Pennsylvania.

The PYT sites worked with youth and community services to reach out to young people with serious mental health needs; align services to fit their needs; maintain continuity of care; and offer opportunities to engage young people with caring, responsible adults in planning and preparing for adulthood and their future. The services offered by these sites were youth-guided, supportive of appropriate family involvement, individualized, developmentally appropriate, appealing to the target population, and designed to reach the hardest-to-reach young people. PYT has allowed for the unique development of service delivery approaches that contribute to an enhanced understanding of how to best address the needs of youth in transition to adulthood in the context of systems of care.

Statewide Family Networks   Forty-two statewide family organizations receive federal grants to provide information, referrals, and support to families of children and youth with or at risk of experiencing SEDs. These grantees also participate in the development of policies, programs, and quality assurance activities related to the mental health of children and adolescents with SEDs and their families in the states in which they live. This grant program is designed to increase the capacity of statewide family organizations and to strengthen coalitions among family members, policy makers, and service providers. The essence of knowledge application is achieving change with the recognition that family members are the best and most effective change agents. Technical assistance is provided to the grantees through the United Advocates for Children and Families.

Child and Adolescent Mental Health and Substance Abuse State Infrastructure Grants   Child and Adolescent Mental Health and Substance Abuse State Infrastructure Grants (CA-SIG) strengthen the capacity of states, territories, and Native American tribal governments to develop and sustain substance abuse and mental health services at the local level, including early intervention, treatment, and continuing services and supports, for children, adolescents, and youth in transition to adulthood (i.e., birth to 24 years old) with SEDs, substance abuse disorders, or co-occurring disorders, while also providing supports to their families. Grantees are expected to use the funds to build the infrastructure necessary to promote, support, and sustain local service and treatment intervention capabilities for the target population across service delivery systems. The program is intended to provide sufficient flexibility and scope to enable states or tribal governments to determine whether they will focus on the entire target population or specific demographic or geographic subsets of the population. Grants are provided over 5 years to strengthen the capacity of states, territories, and American Indian tribal governments. They are jointly administered by the SAMHSA Centers for Substance Abuse Treatment and Mental Health Services.

Circles of Care The Circles of Care initiative represents the collective vision of American Indian and Alaska Native (AI/AN) tribal members, service providers, advocates, and federal agency representatives who developed the concept of Circles of Care planning grants for federally recognized tribes and urban Indian programs as defined by the Indian Self-Determination and Education Assistance Act of 1975 (PL 93-638) and the Indian Health Care Improvement Act of 1976 (PL 94-437). The Circles of Care grants provide funds and technical assistance for AI/AN communities to support the development of culturally appropriate system of care models to achieve their selected emotional, behavioral, educational, vocational, and spiritual outcomes for their children. The grants seek to increase the capacity for tribal programs to reduce the disparity between the disproportionate levels of suicide, substance abuse, and behavioral disorders and the availability and appropriateness of prevention and treatment resources. A third set of grants was awarded in 2005. Through partnerships with the Indian Health Service and National Institutes for Health, technical assistance for program development, process evaluation, needs assessment, and publication is provided by the National Indian Child Welfare Association, based in Portland, Oregon, and the National Center for American Indian and Alaska Native Mental Health Research at the University of Colorado.

Federal Supports for Developing and Sustaining Systems of Care

In addition to grant programs, the federal government has also created a variety of technical assistance and evaluation supports designed to provide education and information about recommended practices and lessons learned.

Technical Assistance Partnership for Child and Family Mental Health Partnership The Technical Assistance Partnership operates under a contract with the federal CMHS to provide community-driven technical assistance to system of care communities funded by the Comprehensive Community Mental Health Services for Children and Their Families Program. The goal of the Technical Assistance Partnership is to support states and local communities in their efforts to successfully develop and implement systems of care. The Technical Assistance Partnership is a collaboration between two organizations—the American Institutes for Research, which is committed to improving the lives of families and communities through the translation of research into the recommended practice and policy, and the Federation of Families for Children's Mental Health, which is dedicated to effective family leadership and advocacy to improve the quality of life of children with mental health needs and their families.

This partnership models the family–professional relationship, an essential value in systems of care. Families share leadership roles in planning, implementing, and evaluating systems of care in their communities. The Technical Assistance Partnership provides a staff of family members in key roles and professionals with extensive practice experience grounded in an organization with vast research experience.

National Technical Assistance Center for Children's Mental Health

The National Technical Assistance Center for Children's Mental Health at the Georgetown University Center for Child and Human Development is dedicated to helping states, tribes, territories, and communities discover, apply, and sustain innovative and collaborative solutions that improve the social, emotional, and behavioral well-being of children and families. System of care values and principles have guided the center's work with states and communities since its inception in 1984.

The National Technical Assistance Center focuses on priority areas for developing and implementing comprehensive service delivery systems; that is, policy development, leadership development, strategic planning, interagency collaboration, family involvement, cultural and linguistic competence, early intervention, early childhood mental health systems of care, evaluation, interagency management information systems, evidence-based and promising practices, financing and managed care, workforce development, and mediation and negotiation training. The center's activities reach diverse stakeholders, including state and local policy makers, administrators of all child-serving systems, service providers, families, youth, advocates, researchers and evaluators, and educators. One of the center's most important activities involves organizing biennial training institutes that provide practical, hands-on training on various aspects of system of care development to more than 2,000 attendees.

Research and Training Center for Children's Mental Health

The Research and Training Center for Children's Mental Health works to strengthen the empirical foundation for effective systems of care through an integrated set of research, training, consultation, and dissemination activities. The center is part of the Department of Child and Family Studies of the Louis de la Parte Florida Mental Health Institute at the University of South Florida in Tampa.

First funded in 1984, the Research and Training Center is jointly supported by the Center for Mental Health Services of the U.S. Department of Health and Human Services and the National Institute on Disability and Rehabilitation Research of the U.S. Department of Education. The center also receives financial support from the Department of Child and Family Studies.

Both the center and the Department of Child and Family Studies employ a diverse team of researchers, evaluators, policy makers, administrators, parents, and practitioners. The center and department are committed to interdisciplinary approaches in their work and specialize in the use of multiple methods to conduct in-depth studies of important issues in system of care development and implementation. The center's research is based in complex, real-world environments, and findings are disseminated in formats suitable for a variety of audiences. Although the center's primary mission is to develop and disseminate new knowledge on implementation of effective systems of care through its research, its team is available to communities and states around the country for consultation and technical assistance. It has implemented a multidisciplinary degree program in systems of care, as well as web-based training programs for practitioners and students.

Research and Training Center on Family Support and Children's Mental Health   Established in 1984, the Research and Training Center on Family Support and Children's Mental Health at Portland State University is dedicated to promoting the well-being and full community participation of children, youth, and families affected by mental health difficulties. The center pursues its mission through collaborative research, technical assistance, and knowledge-sharing partnerships with family members, youth, service providers, policy makers, and other concerned individuals and organizations. The center's research is designed to promote the transformation of mental health care by increasing knowledge of supports, services, and policies that build on family strengths. These services are community based, family driven, and youth guided. They also promote cultural competence and are based on evidence of effectiveness.

The center produces a variety of publications, training materials, and other products that are designed to be relevant and accessible to diverse audiences. These products are related to current projects and ongoing research themes, including:

- Effective wraparound processes and the organizational and system attributes that support the wraparound approach

- Roles and supports for family members and youth in evaluation and policy making

- Culturally competent policies and practices, along with strategies for effective family support

Caring for Every Child's Mental Health Campaign   The Caring for Every Child's Mental Health Campaign supports system of care communities through the strategic use of social marketing and communications strategies. Funded by a contract with the CAFB, the campaign operates through a partnership among the National Association of State Mental Health Program Directors (NASMHPD), Vanguard Communications (Vanguard), and the Federation of Families for Children's Mental Health (the Federation). The team works to address the needs of diverse system of care communities using social marketing and communications techniques that are youth and family driven, culturally competent, and responsive to individual community needs.

Founded in 1959, NASMHPD is a nonprofit organization that represents the $23 billion public mental health service delivery system serving 6.1 million people annually in all 50 states, four territories, and the District of Columbia. Vanguard, a Hispanic female–owned firm specializing in public education, social marketing, and culturally competent communications on behalf of social issues, has supported the campaign since its inception. The Federation is a national family-run organization dedicated exclusively to helping children and youth with mental health needs and their families achieve a better quality of life.

Increasing awareness of children's mental health has been one of the core goals of the Caring for Every Child's Mental Health Campaign since its inception in 1994. The initially developed core messages and themes, materials, and products still play a significant role in national public education initiatives. Now in its third phase, the expanded campaign is working with system of care communities across the country to reach new audiences and forge partnerships in the public and private sectors to further refine the national agenda on children's mental health.

The overarching purpose of the campaign is to stimulate support for a comprehensive system of care approach to children's mental health services. To accomplish this, the campaign has set the following primary goals:

- Reduce the stigma associated with mental illness and promote mental health.

- Use social marketing strategies to help increase the likelihood that children and youth with SEDs and their families are appropriately treated and served.

- Increase awareness of mental health needs and services for children and youth among mental health care providers, system of care communities, intermediary groups and organizations, and the public.

- Demonstrate to communities that the mental health needs of children and youth with SEDs are best met through the utilization of systems of care.

- Use social marketing strategies to help build capacity within system of care communities to sustain services and support to children and youth with SEDs and their families.

National Evaluation of the Comprehensive Community Mental Health Services for Children and Their Families Program   The National Evaluation Team is a partnership comprising Macro International Inc. and Walter R. McDonald & Associates, Inc. This partnership is supported by evaluation partners from the Federation of Families for Children's Mental Health and the Research and Training Center for Children's Mental Health.

Macro International Inc. (Macro) is a research, management consulting, and information technology firm that supports businesses and governments worldwide. It provides survey and market research, policy analysis and evaluation, performance improvement, training, and technology support. Walter R. McDonald & Associates, Inc. (WRMA) is a leading provider of consulting services to human services agencies and organizations, providing managerial and technical consulting in the education, juvenile justice, health, and human services fields to improve the lives of children and families.

CMHS has contracted with Macro and WRMA to conduct a national multisite evaluation of the implementation of systems of care in federally funded communities. The evaluation has several goals:

- Describe the children and families served by the CMHS-funded systems of care.

- Determine the nature and extent of clinical and functional outcomes for children and families served in systems of care.

- Examine how children and families experience services within systems of care and how they use services and supports (i.e., utilization patterns).

- Estimate the cost of serving children in systems of care.

- Examine the development of systems of care as each community moves toward offering integrated and comprehensive services.

- Assess the extent to which funded systems of care are sustainable and continue to be sustained postfunding.

- Assess the effectiveness of the system of care approach compared with usual service delivery approaches.

- Assess the effectiveness of evidence-based treatments within systems of care.

- Provide technical assistance to grantee communities to enhance community-level evaluation capacity and support data collection for the national evaluation.

- Provide feedback to CMHS about program progress at the grantee level to support targeted technical assistance and continuous quality improvement of the program.

FUTURE DIRECTIONS FOR SYSTEMS OF CARE

The changes taking place within the children's mental health field, especially in the first few years of the 21st century, are far beyond any singular innovation in working with individuals and families decades ago. The values and principles inherent in systems of care are nothing short of a monumental transformation in how we think about the design, delivery, and evaluation of services provided to youth with serious mental health needs and their families. Never before has the meaningful involvement of families and communities on the front end of designing and delivering services been more prominent. Never before has the meaningful involvement of youth been more critical. Never before have practitioners and policy makers had such an extensive array of choices available to them when considering which services to offer. Never before has there been as much empirical support for evidence-based practices or promising information on practice-based evidence. There are, however, five main areas of transformation that must continue to develop within the system of care framework as practitioners look toward the future—family-driven care, youth-guided care, cultural and linguistic competence, evidence-based practice and practice-based evidence, and workforce development and leadership. These future directions were emphasized by the Surgeon General's report on mental health and the ensuing national action agenda for children's mental health, as well as in the recommendations of the President's New Freedom Commission on Mental Health (President's New Freedom Commission on Mental Health, 2003; U.S. Department of Health and Human Services, 1999; U.S. Public Health Service, 2000).

Family-Driven Care

In 2003, the President's New Freedom Commission on Mental Health issued its report, *Achieving the Promise: Transforming Mental Health Care in America.* Goal 2 of that report called for consumer- and family-driven care. The report cited research showing that hope and self-determination play a key role in recovery. The commissioners insisted that families "must stand at the center of the system of care" (p. 35). They also said that the needs of children, youth, and families must "drive the care and services that are provided" (p. 35). In a family-driven system, families take the lead in choosing supports, services, and providers; set goals; design and implement programs; and monitor outcomes. If done well, the power of decision making will shift from the sole right of providers to a shared power between providers and families. Two excellent sources of information on this area of focus can be found at the web sites of the Portland State University Research and Training Center (http://www.rtc.pdx.edu) and the Federation of Families for Children's Mental Health (http://www.ffcmh.org). There is a continued need for families to take leadership roles and have decision-making authority at all levels of systems of care.

Youth-Guided Care

A national youth movement in mental health has been growing since 2005. There are three levels of youth-guided care based on the developmental readiness of individual youth. The first level, called *youth-guided* care, allows young people to participate in the development of their own service and support plan and gives them a voice when it comes to deciding on activities. The second level, called *youth-directed* care, is reached when young people have more knowledge about services and systems. They can then actively assist in service delivery decisions or take on voting roles on community boards or committees. The third level, called *youth-driven* care, is reached when young people can set their own goals, identify their own outcomes for service delivery, or develop policy and implement programs for systems of care. Youth are more actively participating in the transformation of services, a fact that is clearly evidenced in the emerging national organization Youth Motivating Others through Voices of Experience (Youth M.O.V.E.). This is also evidenced by the emergence of youth coordinators across the country who are involved in organizing youth and ensuring that they participate in system of care development. Youth empowerment will become even more critical in the years to come.

Cultural and Linguistic Competence

Transforming mental health services means eliminating disparities and enhancing cultural and linguistic competence among policy makers, administrators, and service providers. Each system of care community represents a rich mosaic of cultures and ethnicities, and it is vital that service providers increase awareness and knowledge of factors that contribute to disparities. This activity will require strong efforts to enhance organizational capacities for cultural and linguistic competence. Thus, organizations will have to address their own needs for self-assessment and ensure that the workforce is sensitive and responsive to the cultural and linguistic needs of the populations served.

Evidence-Based Practice and Practice-Based Evidence

The literature describing which services are effective in supporting child, youth, and family mental health has grown tremendously in recent years and will continue to do so in the future. However, in addition to focusing on specific service strategies, it will become increasingly important that individuals, agencies, and systems create a culture of evidence. Such a culture will value data and regularly engage in the review of outcomes and performance (i.e., continuous quality improvement). Clinical practices within the systems of care that work and are supported by quality research must continue to be promoted and advanced. This means providing the necessary training and education about the most effective treatment practices. Equally important is the need to educate administrators of mental health programs about practice-based evidence (i.e., practices that may be nontraditional, culturally based, or clinically supported but still lack a strong evidence base). Families should also be knowledgeable about which services have proven to be the most effective with their children. The combination of a trained clinical staff, families, administrators, and knowledgeable policy makers will go a long way toward building a solid foundation for effective systems of care.

Workforce and Leadership

The fact that there is an inadequate supply of well-trained providers of child, youth, and family mental health services has been extensively documented. In fact, less than 20% of the estimated 14 million children and adolescents with mental health challenges actually receive the treatment they need (President's New Freedom Commission, 2003). Some refer to this as a public health crisis, and much has been written on how to address this shortage (see http://www .annapoliscoalition.org). Clearly, it will become increasingly important to recruit and retain a qualified workforce, but this alone will not be enough. In the future, it will be necessary to build services and supports around the concept of consumer-directed care. This type of care includes family-to-family support and peer support models. New ways of training and reimbursement will also have to be developed. Telehealth approaches will have to expand as services need to become more available in rural, remote, and frontier regions of the country. The future of systems of care and all other issues regarding children's mental health must include a concerted effort to address the workforce shortfall and create future leaders. Recruitment will likely need to start in high schools with guidance counselors to promote careers in children's mental health service delivery. Finally, compensation levels will need to provide a living wage so that the best and the brightest practitioners can be attracted and remain in the field.

CONCLUSION

The ultimate goal for the future of systems of care is not to create or sustain a program per se, but rather a philosophy of care for children, youth, and families that improves lives and endures. It is clear that systems of care are most effective when there is fidelity to the values and principles, but much more work is needed to achieve successful transformation and to bring these efforts to scale. The purpose of this book is to provide an updated foundation from which systems of care can continue to evolve, address the multidimensional aspects of developing a comprehensive system, and identify the pockets of excellence and the recommended practices that can be models to improve service delivery. It is hoped that this information will promote the implementation of systems of care across America and beyond.

REFERENCES

Blau, G.M., & Brumer, D. (1996). Comments on adolescent behavior problems: Developing coordinated systems of care. In G.M. Blau & T.P. Gullotta (Eds.), *Adolescent dysfunctional behavior: Causes, intervention, and prevention* (pp. 284–292). Thousand Oaks, CA: Sage Publications.

Blau, G.M., & Brumer, D. (1999). Developing integrating service delivery systems for children and families: Opportunities and barriers. In T.P. Gullotta (Ed.), *Children's health care: Issues for the year 2000 and beyond* (pp. 283–308). Thousand Oaks, CA: Sage Publications.

Brannan, A., Baughman, L., Reed, E., & Katz-Leavy, J. (2002). System of care assessment: Cross-site comparison of findings. *Children's Services: Social Policy, Research, and Practice, 5,* 37–56.

Burns, B., & Hoagwood, K. (2002). *Community treatment for youth: Evidence-based interventions for severe emotional and behavioral disorders.* New York: Oxford University Press.

Burns, B., Hoagwood, K., & Mrazek, P. (1999). Effective treatment for mental disorders in children and adolescents. *Clinical Child and Family Psychology Review, 2,* 199–254.

Center for Mental Health Services. (1997). *Final report: Local level infrastructure development grant program evaluation* (Contract #282-92-0042). Rockville, MD: Author.

de Voursney, D., Mannix, D., Brounstein, P., & Blau, G.M. (2007). Childhood growth and development. In T.P. Gullotta & G.M. Blau (Eds.), *Handbook of childhood behavioral issues: Evidence based approaches to prevention and treatment* (pp. 19–39). New York: Routledge Press.

Friedman, R. (2001). The practice of psychology with children, adolescents, and their families: A look to the future. In J.N. Hughes, A.M. LaGreca, & U.C. Conoley (Eds.), *Handbook of psychological services for children and adolescents* (pp. 3–22). New York: Oxford University Press.

Friesen, B., & Huff, B. (1996). Family perspectives on systems of care. In B.A. Stroul & R.M. Friedman (Series Eds.) & B.A. Stroul (Vol. Ed.), *Systems of care for children's men-*

tal health series: Children's mental health: Creating systems of care in a changing society (pp. 41–68). Baltimore: Paul H. Brookes Publishing Co.

Gullotta, T.P. (in press). From theory to practice: Treatment and prevention possibilities. In T.P. Gullotta & G.M. Blau (Eds.), *Family influences on childhood behavior and development: Evidence based prevention and treatment approaches.* New York: Routledge Press.

Hernandez, M., & Hodges, S. (2002). *Building upon the theory of change for systems of care.* Manuscript submitted for publication.

Holden, E.W., & Blau, G.M. (2006). An expanded perspective on children's mental health. *American Psychologist, 61,* 642–643.

Indian Health Care Improvement Act of 1976, PL 94-437, 90 Stat. 1400.

Indian Self-Determination and Education Assistance Act of 1975, PL 93-638, 88 Stat. 2203.

Isaacs-Shockley, M., Cross, T., Bazron, B., Dennis, K., & Benjamin, M. (1996). Framework for a culturally competent system of care. In B.A. Stroul & R.M. Friedman (Series Eds.) & B.A. Stroul (Vol. Ed.), *Systems of care for children's mental health series: Children's mental health: Creating systems of care in a changing society* (pp. 23–40). Baltimore: Paul H. Brookes Publishing Co.

Joint Commission on the Mental Health of Children. (1969). *Crisis in child mental health.* New York: Harper & Row.

Knitzer, J. (1982). *Unclaimed children: The failure of public responsibility to children and adolescents in need of mental health services.* Washington, DC: Children's Defense Fund.

Osher, T.W., Osher, D., & Blau, G.M. (in press). Families matter. In T.P. Gullotta & G.M. Blau (Eds.), *Family influences on childhood behavior and development: Evidence based prevention and treatment approaches.* New York: Routledge Press.

President's Commission on Mental Health. (1978). *Report of the sub-task panel on infants, children, and adolescents.* Washington, DC: Author.

President's New Freedom Commission on Mental Health. (2003). *Achieving the promise: Transforming mental health care in America. Final report* (DHHS Publication No. SMA-03-3832). Rockville, MD: Author.

Rosenblatt, A. (1998). Assessing the child and family outcomes of systems of care for youth with serious emotional disturbance. In M. Epstein, K. Kutash, & A. Duchnowski (Eds.), *Outcomes for children and youth with behavioral and emotional disorders and their families* (pp. 329–362). Austin, TX: PRO-ED.

Stroul, B. (2002). *Issue brief—System of care: A framework for reform in children's mental health.* Washington, DC: Georgetown University Child Development Center, National Technical Assistance Center for Children's Mental Health.

Stroul, B., & Friedman, R. (1986). *A system of care for children and youth with severe emotional disturbances* (Rev. ed.). Washington, DC: Georgetown University Child Development Center, National Technical Assistance Center for Children's Mental Health.

Stroul, B., & Friedman, R. (1996). The system of care concept and philosophy. In B.A. Stroul & R.M. Friedman (Series Eds.) & B.A. Stroul (Vol. Ed.), *Systems of care for children's mental health series: Children's mental health: Creating systems of care in a changing society* (pp. 1–22). Baltimore: Paul H. Brookes Publishing Co.

U.S. Congress, Office of Technology Assessment. (1986). *Children's mental health: Problems and services: A background paper.* Washington, DC: Author.

U.S. Department of Health and Human Services. (1999). *Mental health: A report of the Surgeon General.* Rockville, MD: U.S. Department of Health and Human Services, Substance Abuse and Mental Health Services Administration, Center for Mental Health Services, and National Institutes of Health, National Institute of Mental Health.

U.S. Department of Health and Human Services. (2001). *Mental health: Culture, race, and ethnicity—A supplement to mental health: A report of the Surgeon General.* Rockville, MD: Author.

U.S. Public Health Service. (2000). *Report of the Surgeon General's Conference on Children's Mental Health: A national action agenda.* Washington, DC: Author.

2

Evaluation Results and Systems of Care

A Review

Brigitte Manteuffel, Robert L. Stephens,
Freda Brashears, Anna Krivelyova, and Sylvia Kay Fisher

Providing mental health services and supports for children and youth with serious emotional disturbance and their families in a coordinated manner across multiple service providers in systems of care requires change at multiple levels. Service system change affects agency relationships and structures, service provider practices, and the experiences and well-being of the children, youth, and families who receive services in systems of care. Evaluation of the complex characteristics, development, and outcomes of systems of care needs to address the multiple levels of system of care development and relationships among systems, service delivery, and child or youth and family outcomes.

This chapter provides a review of the results of research and evaluation regarding systems of care. Beginning with a review of previous research, the chapter focuses on the results of the national evaluation implemented in communities funded by the federal Comprehensive Community Mental Health Services for Children and Their Families Program to implement systems of care. Conducted since 1993 with more than 81,000 children and youth from 126 communities funded since the inception of this program, the national evaluation represents the largest effort to date to understand the characteristics and outcomes of efforts to

This study was funded by contracts 280-97-8014, 280-00-8040, 280-99-8023, 280-03-1603, and 280-03-1604 from the Center for Mental Health Services at the Substance Abuse and Mental Health Services Administration, U.S. Department of Health and Human Services.

Since the inception of the national evaluation in 1993, a broad range of national evaluation team members at Macro International Inc., consultants, and collaborators at various institutions have contributed to designing and conducting the national evaluation, as well as interpreting and reporting evaluation findings. We cannot name all of these individuals here, but we would like to acknowledge the contributions made to unpublished summary reports by Susan Zaro, E. Wayne Holden, Robin Soler, Kara Riehman, and Jennifer Dewey.

Disclaimer. The views expressed in this chapter do not necessarily reflect the official policies of the U.S. Department of Health and Human Services, nor does any mention of trade names, commercial practices, or organizations imply endorsement by the U.S. Government.

serve children and youth with serious mental health needs and their families through a system of care approach. The characteristics of children, adolescents, and families receiving services in systems of care are briefly reviewed. Results are highlighted at the various levels of system of care development—the system level, the service delivery level, the practice level, and the child and family level. Factors related to improved outcomes are discussed.

PAST RESEARCH ON CHILDREN'S MENTAL HEALTH SERVICES AND SYSTEMS OF CARE

Since the 1984 funding by the National Institute of Mental Health (NIMH) of 10 states through the Child and Adolescent Services System Program (CASSP) to help build their capacity to serve children, several research efforts have sought to understand the mental health needs of children and adolescents, the extent to which they receive needed services, service delivery characteristics, system change, costs associated with change, and child and family outcomes. Epidemiological studies provided information about prevalence rates, the need for services, and those who receive mental health services (Costello, 1997; Greenbaum et al., 1996; Greenbaum, Prange, Friedman, & Silver, 1991; Silver et al., 1992). Comparison studies have been conducted using various designs including pre- and postcomparisons (Salazar, Sherwood, & Toche, 1997), matched communities with and without systems of care (Bickman et al., 1995; Bickman, Summerfelt, & Noser, 1997; Glisson, 1994), comparison of data from system of care demonstration communities to other counties within a state (Rosenblatt & Attkisson, 1993), and randomized trials such as the one conducted in Stark County, Ohio, that compared groups served under the system of care or treatment as usual (Bickman, Summerfelt, Firth, & Douglas, 1997; Bickman, Noser, & Summerfelt, 1999) and examined clinical outcomes in the context of system change. Other studies examined specific treatments relevant to systems of care such as case management[1] (Burns, Farmer, Angold, Costello, & Behar, 1996), mentoring (Owley & Sternweis, 1997), and wraparound (Bruns, Leverentz-Brady, & Walker, 2007), or focused on caregivers (Brannan, Baughman, Reed, & Katz-Leavy, 2002), service experience (Heflinger, Sonnichsen, & Brannan, 1996), service use (Lambert, Brannan, Heflinger, Breda, & Bickman, 1998), and cost savings (Eggers, Delp, Lazear, Wells, & Alonso-Martinez, 1997; Rosenblatt, Attkisson, & Fernandez, 1992).

Studies examining system implementation and system change generally found that systems do change as efforts are made to implement systems of care. Positive change in systems and system-level outcomes were found in the Robert Wood Johnson demonstration program (Cole & Poe, 1993; Friedman, 1993) and

---

[1]The term *case management* is used throughout this chapter. The following description of *case management* is used in the national evaluation: "Case management or service coordination involves finding and organizing multiple treatment and support services, and may also include preparing, monitoring, and revising service plans; and advocating on behalf or the child and family. Case managers may also provide supportive counseling" (from Multi-Sector Service Contacts form developed for the national evaluation.)

in the Fort Bragg system of care demonstration (Heflinger et al., 1996); however, variation in system change was found across multiple sites of a single demonstration program (Johnson, Morrisey, & Colloway, 1996). In addition, systems change very slowly (Harra & Ooms, 1995; Wilhite, 1996), and implementing system change based on system of care principles takes time and often meets with resistance (Tannen, 1997). Consequently, it became clear that an adequate study time frame is needed to assess change and determine overall impact (Friedman & Burns, 1996).

Applying system of care values and principles has affected service delivery and use. The effects found in research have included improved timeliness of service delivery, increased use of services, shifts in the types of services used, and increased lengths of stay in the service system. For example, system of care implementation in Fort Bragg, a very early attempt to implement some of the features of a system of care, yielded more timely receipt of services (Summerfelt, Foster, & Saunders, 1996), and studies of supportive services found that children receiving case management (Burns et al., 1996) stayed in systems longer, used more community-based services, and used fewer inpatient days. Children who received mentoring services were also less likely to be placed in residential settings (Owley & Sternweis, 1997). When families were linked with a paraprofessional mentor, they experienced improved access to services and increased family empowerment (Koroloff, Elliot, Koren, & Friesen, 1996). Services that met family needs were most utilized when they were offered in a warm, hospitable environment (Tannen, 1997).

Studies that assessed differences in outcomes of children served in systems of care compared with those served in other systems yielded mixed results. Pre- and postexamination of juvenile recidivism found significant declines in felony and misdemeanor offenses among wards in systems of care when compared with the prior reporting period (Salazar et al., 1997). A 6-month comparison study of outcomes in Tennessee found that children had greater improvements in psychosocial functioning in the system of care (Glisson, 1994), whereas little difference was found in short-term clinical outcomes in the Fort Bragg study, which was limited to military families and compared children in the Fort Bragg system of care with other military communities offering traditional CHAMPUS mental health services (Bickman et al., 1995). The Fort Bragg study involved a sample of 984 children living at Fort Bragg and two other military installations in Kentucky and Georgia. The findings of this investigation yielded equivocal results and have been debated extensively in the literature (Bickman et al., 1999; Friedman & Burns, 1996). Perhaps the greatest limitation of this study was that the demonstration lacked key features of the system of care, involved large between-site differences at baseline, and lacked cost offset data from other child-serving systems. Few differences in clinical and functional outcomes were found in a study comparing youth in a system of care in Stark County with a matched comparison county (Bickman et al., 1997; Bickman et al., 1999), although the majority of children in this study had minimal functional impairment, and the small numbers limited analyses.

The complexity of service systems and the difficulty of obtaining unequivocal answers about the best approaches to children's mental health service delivery have challenged researchers examining service delivery and outcomes. These challenges include limitations of study designs to account for the range of factors potentially affecting child outcomes (Rugs & Kutash, 1994), and barriers to obtaining access to comprehensive service and cost data due to the disparate location of these data in multiple management information system (MIS) databases for children served across systems (Foster & Connor, 2005a). In particular, difficulties encountered with comparison studies have included a lack of control over changing system characteristics, unsuccessful matching of children in each condition, and the inability to make random assignments. Children and youth enter system of care services with a range of diagnoses, risk factors, past service experience, and severity of problems, as well as a range of family risk factors, school and community-based experiences, and other circumstances. Children come from diverse cultures, linguistic groups, geographic regions, socioeconomic circumstances, living situations, and family compositions. The ability to control for variability through random assignment or data analysis after a study is completed is difficult, and the number of children needed to control for all potential factors in one study can be enormous and costly. Debate on the best methods for examining outcomes in the varied contexts in which system change occurs—and among the children and families served—produced calls for a research agenda specifically focused on children's mental health at the national level (Burns, 1999). The need for improved methods for examining system change and outcomes was also recognized (Kuperminc & Cohen, 1995; Kutash, Duchnowski, Johnson, & Rugs, 1993).

EVALUATION OF THE COMPREHENSIVE COMMUNITY MENTAL HEALTH SERVICES FOR CHILDREN AND THEIR FAMILIES PROGRAM

Building on past efforts for mental health service system reform, the legislative authorization of the Comprehensive Community Mental Health Services for Children and Their Families Program (Children's Mental Health Initiative or CMHI) in 1992 (the ADAMHA Reorganization Act, PL 102-321) provided the means to develop systems of care for children with serious emotional disturbance and their families according to the values and principles articulated by Stroul and Friedman (1986). The program's legislation mandates program evaluation and that annual reports of evaluation findings be delivered to Congress. The national evaluation that addresses this mandate provides information about program performance; system and service characteristics; and the children, youth, and families served (see Table 2.1). Evaluation findings inform Congress about the program, and they contribute to annual program performance reporting to the Office of Management and Budget for the Government Performance and Results Act of 1993 (PL 103-62), as well as the literature and public dialogue about service provision and children's mental health outcomes. These documented findings contributed to the growth of the program from an annual budget of $4.9 million in 1993 to a budget of nearly $105 million in 2007. Funding has supported 126 grants for 5

Table 2.1. National evaluation response to evaluation requirement of PL 102-321

Describe the children and families served by the system of care initiative.

Assess how systems of care develop and what factors impede or enhance their development.

Measure whether children served through the program experience improvement in clinical and functional outcomes, whether those improvements endure over time, and why.

Determine whether the consumers are satisfied with the services they receive.

Measure the costs associated with the implementation of a system of care and determine its cost effectiveness.

years or cooperative agreements for 6 years beginning in 2002 in all 50 states, Guam, Puerto Rico, and 15 American Indian and Alaska Native communities (see Figure 2.1).

Design of the CMHI National Evaluation: A Response to Early Research Findings

Building on the framework for system change provided by the system of care principles outlined by Stroul and Friedman (1986), the program's authorizing legislation and logic model (Center for Mental Health Services [CMHS], 1999, 2001, 2003b; Hernandez & Hodges, 2005), and the approaches and recommendations of earlier studies, the national evaluation was developed to assess change in systems of care at multiple levels. The initial evaluation design, informed by an expert advisory panel composed of researchers and program developers specializing in children's mental health, was implemented with communities funded in 1993 and 1994 (CMHS 1997, 1998, 1999; Holden, Friedman, & Santiago, 2001; Manteuffel, Stephens, & Santiago, 2002). Subsequently, research questions, methodology, approaches to data collection, and instrumentation were revised based on experience with the evaluation, the limitations encountered, the need for new or additional information for the program, and input from federal and community level program staff, family members, and researchers.

National Evaluation Design and Components

The evaluation design has included five core components from its inception: 1) assessment of system development, 2) study of characteristics of children and families receiving services, 3) longitudinal assessment of child and family outcomes, 4) assessment of service experience and satisfaction, and 5) assessment of services received and costs. Assessment of sustainability was added in 2000 to address program reporting requirements. Figure 2.2 provides a timeline of the years of program funding and the phases of the national evaluation that correspond to funded cohorts of communities.

Initially, a comparison study design, comparing funded systems of care to traditional service systems in similar communities was a core component of the

Phase I (grants awarded in 1993 and 1994)

Arizona, New Mexico, and Utah: *K'é Project*, Navajo Nation
California: *Children's Systems of Care/California 5*, Riverside, San Mateo, Santa Cruz, Solano, and Ventura counties
California: *Multiagency Integrated System of Care (MISC)*, Santa Barbara County
California: *Sonoma-Napa Comprehensive System of Care*, Sonoma and Napa counties
Hawai'i: *Hawai'i 'Ohana Project*, Wai'anae Coast and Leeward Oahu
Illinois: *Community Wraparound Initiative*, Lyons, Riverside, and Proviso townships
Kansas: *COMCARE*, Sedgwick County
Kansas: *KanFocus*, 13 southeastern counties
Maine: *Wings for Children and Families*, Piscataquis, Hancock, Penobscot, and Washington counties
Maryland: *East Baltimore Mental Health Partnership*, East Baltimore, Maryland
New Mexico: *Olympia (formerly Doña Ana County Child and Adolescent Collaborative)*, Doña Ana County
New York: *Families Reaching in Ever New Directions (FRIENDS)*, Mott Haven
North Carolina: *Pitt-Edgecombe-Nash Public-Academic-Liaison Project (PEN-PAL)*, Pitt, Edgecombe, and Nash counties
North Dakota: *Partnerships Project*, Minot, Bismarck, and Fargo regions
Ohio: *Stark County Family Council and Southern Consortium*, Stark County and 10 southeastern counties
Oregon: *New Opportunities*, Lane County
Pennsylvania: *South Philadelphia Family Partnership Project*, South Philadelphia
Rhode Island: *Project REACH Rhode Island*, Statewide
South Carolina: *The Village Project*, Charleston and Dorchester counties
Virginia: *City of Alexandria System of Care*, City of Alexandria
Vermont: *ACCESS*, Statewide
Wisconsin: *Wraparound Milwaukee*, Milwaukee County

Phase II (grants awarded in 1997 and 1998)

Alabama: *The Jefferson County Community Partnership*, Jefferson County
California: *Children's Mental Health Services Initiative*, San Diego County
Florida: *Tampa-Hillsborough Integrated Network for Kids (THINK) System*, Hillsborough County
Kentucky: *Kentucky Bridges Project*, 3 Appalachian regions
Maine: *Kmihqitahasultipon ("We Remember") Project*, Passamaquoddy Tribe Indian Township
Michigan: *Mno Bmaadzid Endaad ("Be in good health at his house")*, Sault Sainte Marie Tribe of Chippewa Indians and Bay Mills Ojibwa Indian Community; Chippewa, Mackinac, and Schoolcraft counties
Michigan: *Southwest Community Partnership*, Detroit
Missouri: *Partnership With Families*, St. Charles County
Nebraska: *Families First and Foremost*, Lancaster County
Nebraska: *Nebraska Family Central*, 22 central counties
Nevada: *Neighborhood Care Centers*, Clark County
North Carolina: *North Carolina Families and Communities Equal Success (FACES)*, Blue Ridge, Cleveland, Guilford, and Sandhills
North Dakota: *Sacred Child Project*, Fort Berthold, Standing Rock, Spirit Lake, and Turtle Mountain Indian reservations
Oregon: *Clackamas Partnership*, Clackamas County
Pennsylvania: *Community Connections for Families*, Allegheny County
Rhode Island: *Project Hope*, Statewide
Texas: *The Children's Partnership*, Travis County
Utah: *Utah Frontiers Project*, Beaver, Carbon, Emery, Garfield, Grand, and Kane counties
Vermont: *Children's UPstream Services*, Statewide
Washington: *Children and Families in Common*, King County
Washington: *Clark County Children's Mental Health Initiative*, Clark County

Figure 2.1. System of care communities funded through the Comprehensive Community Mental Health Services for Children and Their Families Program 1993–2006. (Reprinted from Macro International Inc. [2007]. *Final report: Phase III of the Comprehensive Community Mental Health Services for Children and Their Families Program, grant communities funded in 1999–2000.* Manuscript in preparation.)

Wisconsin: *Northwoods Alliance for Children and Families,* Forest, Langlade, Lincoln, Marathon, Oneida, and Vilas counties

Wyoming: *With Eagle's Wings,* Wind River Indian Reservation

Phase III (grants awarded in 1999 and 2000)

Alaska: *Yuut Calilriit Ikaiyuquulluteng ("People Working Together") Project,* Delta region of southwest Alaska

Arizona: *Project MATCH (Multi-Agency Team for CHildren),* Pima County

California: *A-KO-NES Wraparound System of Care,* Humboldt and Del Norte counties

California: *Spirit of Caring Project,* Contra Costa County

Colorado: *Colorado Cornerstone System of Care Initiative,* Denver, Jefferson, Clear Creek, and Gilpin counties

Delaware: *Families and Communities Together (FACT) Project,* Statewide

Florida: *Family HOPE (Helping Organize Partnerships for Empowerment),* West Palm Beach

Georgia: *Kidsnet Rockdale,* Rockdale and Gwinnett counties

Indiana: *Circle Around Families,* East Chicago, Gary, and Hammond

Indiana: *Dawn Project,* Marion County

Maryland: Community Kids, Montgomery County

Massachusetts: *Worcester Communities of Care,* Worcester

Minnesota: *PACT (Putting All Communities Together) 4 Families Collaborative,* Kandiyohi, Meeker, Renville, and Yellow Medicine counties

Mississippi: *COMPASS (Children of Mississippi and Their Parents Accessing Strength-Based Services),* Hinds County

New Hampshire: *CARE NH: Community Alliance Reform Effort,* Manchester, Littleton, and Berlin

New Jersey: *Burlington Partnership,* Burlington County

New York: *Westchester Community Network,* Westchester County

North Carolina: *North Carolina System of Care Network,* 11 counties

South Carolina: *Gateways to Success,* Greenwood County

South Dakota: *Nagi Kicopi–Calling the Spirit Back Project,* Oglala Sioux Tribe, Pine Ridge Indian Reservation, Pine Ridge

Tennessee: *Nashville Connection,* Nashville

West Virginia: *Mountain State Family Alliance,* 12 counties

Phase IV (grants awarded in 2002, 2003, and 2004)

Alaska: *Ch'eghutsen' A System of Care,* Fairbanks Native Association

California: *Glenn County Children's System of Care,* Glenn County

California: *La Familia Sana,* Monterey County

California: *OASIS (Obtaining and Sustaining Independent Success),* Sacramento County

California: *San Francisco Children's System of Care,* San Francisco

California: *Urban Trails,* Oakland

Colorado: *Project BLOOM,* El Paso, Fremont, and Mesa counties, and the City of Aurora

Connecticut: *Partnership for Kids (PARK) Project,* Statewide

Florida: *One Community Partnership,* Broward County

Guam: *I'Famagu'onta (Our Children),* Territorywide

Idaho: *Building on Each Other's Strengths,* Statewide

Illinois: *System of Care Chicago,* Chicago

Kentucky: *Kentuckians Encouraging Youth to Succeed (KEYS),* Boone, Campbell, Carroll, Gallatin, Grant, Kenton, Owen, and Pendleton counties

Louisiana: *Louisiana Youth Enhanced Services for Children's Mental Health (LA–YES),* Jefferson, Orleans, Plaquemines, St. Bernard, and St. Tammany parishes

Missouri: *Show Me Kids,* Barry, Christian, Green, Lawrence, Stone, and Taney counties

Missouri: *Transitions,* St. Louis County and City

Montana: *Missoula Kids Integrated Delivery System Management Authority (KMA),* Statewide and Crow Indian Nation

New York: *Families Together in Albany County,* Albany County

(continued)

Figure 2.1. *(continued)*

New York: *Family Voices Network,* Erie County
New York: *Coordinated Children's Services Initiative (CCSI) / The Family Network,* New York City
Ohio: *Tapestry,* Cuyahoga County
Oklahoma: *Choctaw Nation CARES,* Choctaw Nation of Oklahoma
Oklahoma: *Great Plains Systems of Care,* Beckham, Canadian, Kay, Oklahoma, and Tulsa, counties
Oregon: *Columbia River Wraparound,* Gilliam, Hood River, Sherman, and Wasco counties
Puerto Rico: *Puerto Rico Mental Health Initiative for Children,* Llorens Torres Housing Project in San Juan, Municipality of Gurabo
South Carolina: *YouthNet,* Chester, Lancaster, and York counties and Catawba Indian Nation
Texas: *Border Children's Mental Health Collaborative,* El Paso County
Texas: *Community Solutions,* Fort Worth
Washington, District of Columbia: *D.C. Children Inspired Now Gain Strength (D.C. CINGS),* Districtwide

---

Phase V (grants awarded in 2005 and 2006)

Arizona: *Sewa Uusim (Flower Children): Our Hope, Our Light, Our Future,* Pascua Yaqui Tribe of Arizona
Arkansas: *ACTION for Kids (Arkansas Collaborating to Improve Our Network),* Craighead, Lee, Mississippi, and Phillips counties
California: *Connecting Circles of Care,* Butte County
California: *Seven Generations System of Care,* Los Angeles County
California: *Project ABC (About Building Connections for Young Children and Families),* Los Angeles County
California: *Placer County SMART System of Care (Systems Management, Advocacy, and Resource Team),* Placer County
Connecticut: *Building Blocks,* New London County
Florida: *Sarasota Partnership for Children's Mental Health,* Sarasota County
Hawai'i: *Project Ho'omohala (Transition to Adulthood),* Honolulu
Illinois: *McHenry County Family CARE (Child/Adolescent Recovery Experience),* McHenry County
Iowa: *Community Circle of Care,* 10 northeastern counties
Maine: *Thrive,* Androscoggin, Franklin, and Oxford counties
Massachusetts: *Central Massachusetts Communities of Care,* Worcester County (excluding the City of Worcester)
Michigan: *Impact,* Ingham County
Michigan: *Kalamazoo Wraps,* Kalamazoo County
Minnesota: *Children Succeed Initiative: A Six-County Children's Health System of Care,* Kittson, Mahnomen, Marshall, Norman, Polk, and Red Lake counties
Minnesota: *STARS for Children's Mental Health (System Transformation of Area Resources and Services),* Benton, Sherburne, Stearns, and Wright counties
Mississippi: *CommUNITY Cares,* Forrest, Lamar, and Marion counties
Mississippi: *Circle of H.O.P.E. (Home, Opportunities, Parents & Providers, Empowerment),* Andrew and Buchanan counties
Montana: *Blackfeet Po'Ka Project, System of Care,* Blackfeet Reservation
New York: *Monroe County Achieving Culturally Competent and Effective Services and Supports (Monroe County ACCESS),* Monroe County
North Carolina: *MeckCARES,* Mecklenburg County
Oregon: *Wraparound Oregon: Early Childhood,* Multnomah County
Pennsylvania: *Starting Early Together (SET),* Allegheny County
Pennsylvania: *Beaver County's System of Care: Optimizing Resources, Education and Supports (BCBSCORES),* Beaver County
Rhode Island: *Rhode Island Positive Education Partnership,* Statewide
South Dakota: *Tiwahe Wakan (Families as Sacred),* Yankton Sioux Reservation
Tennessee: *Mule Town Family Network: A System of Care for Maury County,* Maury County
Texas: *Systems of Hope,* Harris County
Wyoming: *The SAGE Initiative,* Statewide

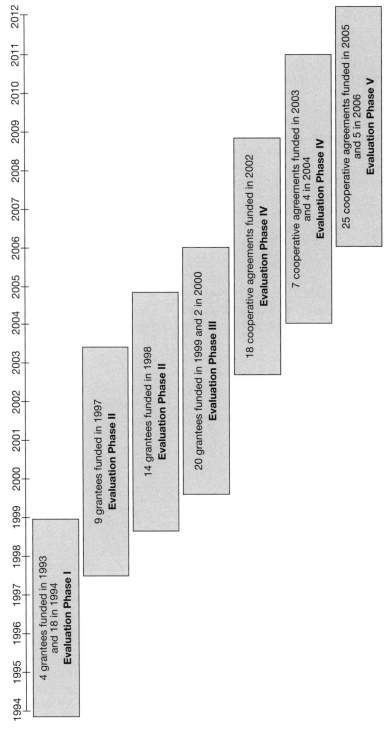

Figure 2.2. Timeline of system of care funding and phases of the national evaluation. (*Sources:* Center for Mental Health Services, 2000, 2001.)

33

national evaluation. Comparison studies that used quasi-experimental designs were conducted in three funded and three matched nonfunded communities in Phase I (Foster, Qaseem, & Connor, 2004; Stephens, Connor, et al., 2005), and in two funded and two matched communities in Phase II (CMHS, 2001, 2002, 2003b). Additional studies addressed specific aspects of service delivery systems such as cultural competence (Brashears, Santiago, Sgro, & Gilford, 2005), evidence-based practice (Aarons, MacDonald, Sheehan, & Walrath-Greene, 2007; Sheehan, Walrath-Greene, Fisher, Crossbear, & Walker, 2007; Sheehan, Walrath, & Holden, 2006; Walrath, Sheehan, Holden, Hernandez, & Blau, 2006), effectiveness of evidence-based treatments (Johnson, Manteuffel, Sukumar, & McBride, 2007), provider attitudes and practices (Manteuffel, Grossman, & Stephens, 2005), tribal financing (CMHS, 2007), managed care (Stroul, Pires, & Armstrong, 1998), primary care provider involvement with mental health (Manteuffel, Krivelyova, Laygo, Brashears, & Grossman, 2006), and conflict management (Evans, Blanch, Boothroyd, Boustead, & Chen, 2007). A brief description of each evaluation component is shown on Box 2.1.

FINDINGS FROM THE NATIONAL EVALUATION OF SYSTEMS OF CARE

Each phase of the national evaluation has contributed to broader understanding of system implementation; service delivery; children and families served; clinical, behavioral, and functional outcomes; and program sustainability. Findings from core components and special studies of the national evaluation have been shared through reports to Congress, a range of publications, and presentations at conferences. Putting all of the pieces together to understand how systems, services, and child and family outcomes interact effectively to meet the needs of children, youth, and families is complex. This chapter summarizes what has been learned from communities funded from 1993 to 2000 about the children, youth, and families served in systems of care; system of care infrastructure and service delivery; services provided and the providers and agencies providing them; family and youth service experience; and the sustainability of systems of care. Information from subsequently funded communities is incomplete as evaluation efforts are ongoing during funding years. Some comparative trends are noted as appropriate.

Implementation of Systems of Care at the System Level

The system-level assessment examined whether each grant community had established formal structures and organizational arrangements that supported service delivery practices guided by system of care principles. A system-level assessment has been part of the national evaluation since its inception. The original protocol used with grant communities funded in 1993 and 1994 assessed attributes expected to be found in the infrastructure and in the service delivery of systems of care. Data were collected through periodic site visits that involved interviews with multiple key informants and document reviews to determine the status of system development over time.

Box 2.1. National Evaluation Components and Measures

SYSTEM OF CARE ASSESSMENT

Using a combination of semi-structured interviews with multiple stakeholders, review of randomly selected case records, document review, and follow-up telephone interviews as needed, this study assesses the extent to which systems are implemented according to system of care principles and documents system development. Respondents include project directors, representatives from core child-serving agencies, representatives from family organizations, local program evaluators, care coordinators, direct service providers, youth coordinators, caregivers, and youth served by the system of care. A *systemness* index to score communities on system development used in Phase I of the study was completely revised in Phase II with the development of a stable measure that assesses the extent to which infrastructure and service delivery are family driven, individualized, culturally competent, and coordinated, with services available in the community and in the least restrictive service environments. Two interviews to assess youth involvement were added in Phase IV.

CROSS-SECTIONAL DESCRIPTIVE STUDY

This study collects demographic, descriptive, and diagnostic information on all children served from caregiver report and chart review at service intake. A shorter web-based form was added in Phase IV that could be completed at the clinic level from the child's chart in an effort to improve data quantity and quality on all children served. Additional descriptive information is collected from caregivers and youth in the Longitudinal Child and Family Outcome Study.

Measures

Domain	Instrument	Phases Used
Descriptive characteristics	Descriptive Information Questionnaire (DIQ)*	II–III
	Record abstraction	I–V
	Enrollment and Demographic Information Form (EDIF)*	IV–V

LONGITUDINAL CHILD AND FAMILY OUTCOME STUDY

To examine outcomes for children, youth, and their families, caregivers and youth age 11 and older are interviewed using clinical and functional measures. Assessment periods and instruments have changed over multiple funding phases. Baseline assessments occur within 30 days of service intake. In Phase I, follow-up occurred at 6, 12, and 18 months after intake as long as the child was in services. Subsequently, follow-up has occurred every 6 months after intake for each child in and out of services for up to 36 months.

Measures

Domain	Instrument	Phases used
Descriptive measures		
Descriptive characteristics	Caregiver Information Questionnaire (CIQ)*	IV–V
	Youth Information Questionnaire (YIQ)*	IV–V

(continued)

Box 2.1. *(continued)*

Domain	Instrument	Phases used
Child-related measures		
Child functioning	Child and Adolescent Functional Assessment Scale (CAFAS; Hodges, 1990)	I–III
	Columbia Impairment Scale (CIS; Bird et al., 1993)	IV–V
Child behavioral and emotional problems	Child Behavior Checklist (CBCL; Achenbach, 1991; Achenbach & Reschorla, 2000, 2001)	I–V
	Youth Self Report (YSR; Achenbach & Edelbrook, 1987)	II–III
Childhood anxiety	Reynolds Childhood Manifest Anxiety Scale (RCMAS; Reynolds & Richmond, 1978)	IV–V
Adolescent depression	Reynolds Adolescent Depression Scale 2 (RADS-2; Reynolds, 1986)	IV–V
Child behavioral and emotional strengths	Behavioral and Emotional Rating Scale (BERS; Epstein & Sharma, 1998)	II–III
	Behavioral and Emotional Rating Scale-2 (BERS-2; Epstein, 2004) Caregiver and youth versions.	IV–V
Child development	Vineland Screener (VS; Sparrow, Carter, & Cicchetti, 1993)	IV–V
Child living situations	Restrictiveness of Living Environments Scale (ROLES; Hawkins, Almeida, Fabry, Reitz, 1992)	I
	Restrictiveness of Living Environments Scale–Revised (ROLES-R)	II–III
	Living Situations Questionnaire*	IV–V
Education	Education Questionnaire*	II–V
Delinquency	Delinquency Survey*	II–V
Youth substance use	Substance Use Survey*	II–III
Substance dependency	GAIN Quick-R (Titus & Dennis, 2005)	IV–V
Family Measures		
Family empowerment	Family Empowerment Scale (FES; Koren, DeChillo, & Friesen, 1992)	I
Family functioning	Family Assessment Device (FAD; Epstein, Baldwin, & Bishop, 1983),	II–III
Family life	Family Life Questionnaire (FLQ)*	IV–V
Caregiver strain	Caregiver Strain Questionnaire (CGSQ; Brannan et al., 1998)	II–V
Family resources	Family Resource Scale (FRS; Dunst & Leet, 1985)	II–IIII

SERVICE EXPERIENCE STUDY

Information is collected at follow-up outcome assessments from caregivers and youth on characteristics of services received, the extent which services met family needs, cultural and linguistic competence of service providers, and satisfaction with services. A caregiver report measure of service use was developed in Phase II and revised in Phase IV. The FSQ was revised from Phase I to Phase II, and youth were assessed with a corresponding YSQ in Phases II and III. The YSS was adopted in Phase IV, and a caregiver's assessment of provider cultural competence was developed.

Measures

Domain	Instrument	Phases used
Services received	Multi-sector Service Contacts Form*	II–V
Service experience and satisfaction	Family Satisfaction Questionnaire (FSQ) and Youth Satisfaction Questionnaire (YSQ) (Brunk, Santiago, Ewell, & Watts, 1997)	I–III
	Youth Services Survey (YSS) and Youth Services Survey–Family (YSS–F) (Brunk, Koch, & McCall, 2000)	IV–V
Cultural competence	Culturally Competent Service Provision (CCSP)*	IV–V

SERVICES AND COSTS STUDY

Using existing cost data in agency management information systems and budgets, this study describes the types of services used by children and families, their utilization patterns, and the associated costs. Changes were made to this study after 2005 to provide communities with standard templates for data about flexible fund expenditures and to further standardize the delivery of cross-agency service and cost data. Because access to service and cost data varies among communities, this study has used a tiered approach that accommodates availability of information from a single child-serving system and from multiple child-serving systems.

SUSTAINABILITY STUDY

Added in 2000 to assess communities 5 years postfunding, this study obtains information about 1) availability of specific services in the system of care, 2) implementation of system of care principles, 3) achievement of objectives related to system of care implementation, 4) roles and impact of various factors on the development or maintenance of the system of care, and 5) effectiveness of various general and financing strategies for sustaining systems of care. Phase I communities were assessed 5 years postfunding, and communities funded in 1997 were assessed in their final year of funding, both with a web-survey and telephone interviews with key individuals in the communities and at the state level. Communities funded in 1998–2000 were assessed with the web survey in their final year of funding; communities funded from 2002 to 2006 were assessed during the fiscal years in which the federal-local funding match requirements change (Years 3 and 4), and in their final year.

(continued)

Box 2.1. *(continued)*

COMPARISON STUDIES

Comparison studies using quasi-experimental designs were conducted in three funded communities in Phase I (Stephens, Connor, et al., 2005) and two in Phase II (CMHS, 2001, 2003b) and matched communities. Nonfunded communities were chosen by similar geographic and population characteristics, as well as their willingness to participate in the project. The design called for enrollment of the same number of children in the funded community and in the corresponding community, who were matched by age, gender, severity of behavioral and emotional problems, and functional impairment. Measures used in the descriptive and outcome studies were used in the comparison studies with some additions. The Phase II comparison study included substudies of service experiences and provider characteristics.

TREATMENT EFFECTIVENESS STUDIES

Treatment effectiveness studies to examine evidence-based treatment implementation and outcomes in systems of care were implemented with three different treatments in six communities. Children received diagnostic assessments to screen for diagnoses treated by the evidence-based treatment; children accepted into the study were randomly assigned to treatment and service as usual groups. A study of family education and support to build evidence for a practice utilized in systems of care is under way.

---

*Instrument developed for the National Evaluation of the Comprehensive Community Mental Health Services for Children and Their Families Program.

Results of this study found that systems developed incrementally over time and that the use of case management showed the most growth of all measured system of care attributes. This growth was accomplished through training, outstationing case management staff in partner agencies, and using a multidisciplinary cross-agency team approach to service planning. By the final grant year, all sites offered case management, and respondents across sites indicated that case management was considered one of the strongest and most important components of their systems of care (Vinson, Brannan, Baughman, Wilce, & Gawron, 2001).

Building on what was learned in the first study, a revised assessment tool was developed for the national evaluation of subsequently funded grant communities. This assessment tool was developed according to a conceptual framework that included two domains—the system infrastructure and the service delivery process. The system infrastructure domain referred to the organizational arrangements and procedural framework that supported and facilitated service delivery. The service delivery domain involved the activities and processes undertaken to provide services to children and families that addressed the emotional and behavioral challenges experienced by children. The tool assessed the extent to which system of care principles were manifest in each of the four subunits within the two domains. Indicators of achievement were developed for each cell in the framework (Figure 2.3).

Periodic on-site assessments were conducted over the 6-year funding period for each grant community to determine system development and adherence to system of care principles over time. Information was collected through face-to-face interviews with multiple key informants coupled with document review. In-

	Infrastructure domain				Service delivery domain			
	Governance	Management and operations	Service array	Quality monitoring	Entry into system	Service planning	Service provision	Case review
Family focused								
Individualized								
Culturally competent								
Interagency								
Collaborative/coordinated								
Accessible								
Community based								
Least restrictive								

Figure 2.3. System-level assessment framework matrix. (*Source:* Brannan, Baughman, Reed, & Katz-Leavy, 2002.)

terviewers used responses from individual informants to rate system achievement on the indicators on a 5-point scale (1 being the lowest and 5 the highest) using established criteria for items that mapped to framework indicators. Therefore, the qualitative data collected in the semi-structured interviews were used to produce ratings for each of the 118 indicators. Responses from the various informants were rated separately. This approach, which based numerical ratings on qualitative data, used comparisons within and between grant communities and then generated quantitative ratings, along with rich descriptive information.

Community Characteristics   Across all funding years (i.e., 1993–2000), grants were awarded to systems of care in a variety of geographic locales, including urban, small city or county, rural, and American Indian settings. Some were located in large urban areas, whereas others were located in rural or frontier communities. Some systems of care were responsible for residents living in catchment areas that covered thousands of square miles, and others were responsible for a single city neighborhood.

Most grant communities had a strong base of existing services and resources from which to draw at the time of their grant funding. In fact, in some of the grant communities, systems were built on structures and service arrays that existed well before the infusion of grant funds. For example, several communities had received CASSP grants from NIMH that formed the basis for system of care development within their state systems, and others were located in states that had passed legislation mandating interagency collaboration, intensive case management, and mental health services aimed at maintaining children in their home communities. Some grant communities operated within systems that had instituted statewide reform of public agencies from the state level to the local level to increase interagency collaboration and to enhance the provision of individualized and family-focused services.

Management structures of grant programs varied among grantees. In some communities, state-level mental health agencies were the official grantees. They either directly managed the programs or contracted them to the local region or county mental health agencies. In other communities, county-level mental health agencies were the grantees and managed the systems of care. Among American Indian grant communities, tribal governments or councils had the ultimate authority over grant funds.

All grant communities served children with serious emotional disturbance and their families, but program specifics differed regarding the ages of children served, the focus of the service delivery programs, and the point at which intervention began. Some systems of care provided early intervention services to children from birth to 6 years of age, whereas others served children from 5 to 8 years of age. Some were school based, whereas others focused on children involved in the juvenile justice system or on "stepping-down" children and youth from residential treatment or institutional placements. Programs serving American Indian children sought to provide services that used tribal culture and traditions to create and maintain tribal identity and self-sufficiency, often for all community members, as well as for identified children who entered the system of care.

Implementing System of Care Principles at the Infrastructure Level There was a general upward trend in ratings across grant communities for most system of care principles assessed. Figures 2.4, 2.5, 2.6, and 2.7 illustrate ratings of grant communities funded in 1998. The trends depicted in these figures were similar to those found in communities funded in 1997, 1999, and 2000.

Grant communities were usually rated in the 3–4 range, with incremental improvements at each assessment point. In general, communities obtained their highest ratings in infrastructure development in their final year of funding, although no grant community attained an overall rating of 5 in any principle at any assessment point. Across all assessment points, communities typically performed better in implementing the principle of family-focused care than any other principle (i.e., high 4s). Communities generally had more difficulty implementing and adhering to the principles of cultural competence and interagency collaboration than other principles across their grant funding cycle in that their ratings were consistently lower in these principles than in others. Communities, however, made the most dramatic improvement in their ratings over time in implementing the principles of cultural competence, collaboration/coordination, and accessibility than in other principles, increasing their ratings an entire point or more (from 2s to 3s).

Implementing System of Care Principles at the Service Delivery Level As with the infrastructure domain, ratings in the service delivery domain showed a general upward trend across most system of care principles. On the whole, grant communities performed somewhat better in the service delivery domain than they did in the infrastructure domain, although none achieved an over-

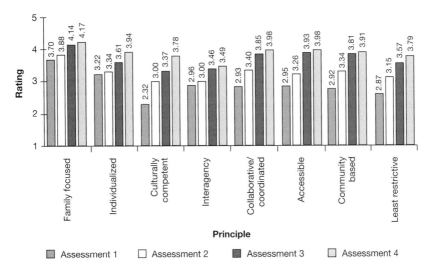

Figure 2.4. Average infrastructure ratings for communities funded in 1998 across assessment points. (Reprinted from Macro International Inc. [2007]. *Final report: Phase II of the Comprehensive Community Mental Health Services for Children and Their Families Program, grant communities funded in 1997–98.* Manuscript in preparation.)

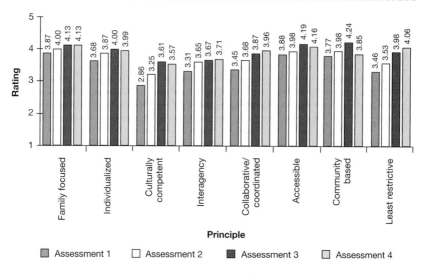

Figure 2.5. Average service delivery ratings for communities funded in 1998 across assessment points. (Reprinted from Macro International Inc. [2007]. *Final report: Phase II of the Comprehensive Community Mental Health Services for Children and Their Families Program, grant communities funded in 1997–98.* Manuscript in preparation.)

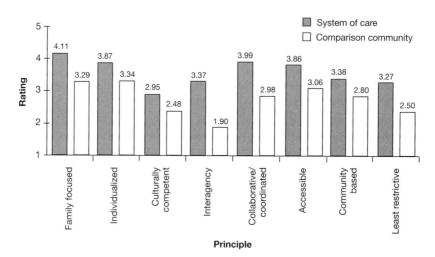

Figure 2.6. Overall system-level assessment ratings for Region III and Region IV, Nebraska. (Reprinted from Macro International Inc. [2007]. *Final report: Phase II of the Comprehensive Community Mental Health Services for Children and Their Families Program, grant communities funded in 1997–98.* Manuscript in preparation.)

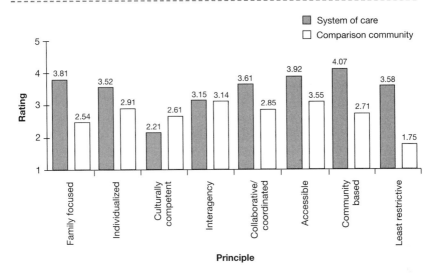

Figure 2.7. Overall system-level assessment ratings for Birmingham and Montgomery, Alabama. (Reprinted from Macro International Inc. [2007]. *Final report: Phase II of the Comprehensive Community Mental Health Services for Children and Their Families Program, grant communities funded in 1997–98.* Manuscript in preparation.)

all rating of 5 in any principle at any assessment point. Communities typically were more successful at providing family-focused, individualized, and accessible care (i.e., high 3s to low 4s), and least successful at providing culturally competent care (i.e., 2–3). The most dramatic improvements across the grant-funding cycle were in the principles of culturally competent care (i.e., a near 1-point increase from a mid-2 to a mid-3 rating), as well as in collaborative/coordinated care and least restrictive care (i.e., from mid-3 to 4).

Funded Systems of Care and Comparison Communities　The Phase I comparison study was conducted in three systems of care funded in 1993 and 1994 (East Baltimore, Maryland; Stark County, Ohio; and Santa Cruz, California) and three comparison communities (West Baltimore, Maryland; Mahoning County, Ohio; and Austin, Texas). Findings from this study were that funded systems generally demonstrated greater adherence to system of care principles than did their matched comparison sites (Brannan, Baughman, Reed, & Katz-Leavy, 2002).

The Phase II comparison study was conducted with two systems of care funded in 1997 (Birmingham, Alabama, and the Mental Health Service Region III in Nebraska) and two comparison communities (Montgomery, Alabama, and the Mental Health Service Region IV in Nebraska). Overall, the funded system of care communities performed better than the comparison communities in implementing system of care principles. The system of care communities were rated higher on their efforts to provide family-focused care, develop individualized care plans, support collaborative activities, provide adequate access to care, and offer services in the community and in the least restrictive setting possible. In Nebraska and Alabama, both the system of care and comparison communities received consistently low ratings for their efforts to provide culturally competent care. The system of care and comparison communities in Nebraska differed most on ratings of efforts to develop interagency partnerships and to provide coordinated/collaborative care. In Alabama, system of care and comparison communities differed most on ratings of efforts to provide community-based services in the least restrictive setting possible.

Summary   System of care assessment findings generally indicated that system of care principles were implemented and adhered to across the board. No grant community consistently scored below the midpoint of 3 on the 5-point assessment scale across time or across principles. Even in the early grant-funded years, performance was at or above the midpoint in all principles except cultural competence, which was generally rated 2. The relatively high level of performance by the second year of funding when the first assessments took place, the relative stability over time for some principles, and the dramatic improvements shown in others suggest that, as a set of guiding principles, the system of care philosophy has become status quo within funded communities.

The upward trend in ratings appears to support the underlying philosophy of the program and study hypothesis that implementing and adhering to system of care principles are developmental activities that will demonstrate continuing improvement over time. The general upward trend in the ratings suggests that in the effort to effect system change, progress is incremental and uneven. The ratings also indicated that across all principles in all communities, efforts were made to develop and manage systems of care according to the principles in each year of funding with at least some measure of effective results.

Overall, funded systems of care were successful in developing and implementing infrastructure and service delivery systems according to system of care principles, and they made incremental but progressive improvement across the funding cycle. Funded systems of care were more successful in providing family-focused, individualized, and culturally competent services in accessible, community-based, and least restrictive environments through interagency coordination and collaboration than were nonfunded comparison communities in almost all areas.

Children and Families Served in Systems of Care

From 1993 to 2007, more than 81,000 children and youth and their families have received services in systems of care. Although the extent and nature of descriptive information collected has varied, consistent patterns and variations have been observed among funded groups of communities, as well as individual communities.

Gender and Age   Funded systems of care have served more boys than girls, a finding that is consistent with earlier studies (Silver, Unger, & Friedman, 1993), with averages ranging from about 60% in the 1993 and 1994 funded sites to about 66% in sites funded from 1997 to 2000. These proportions represent the youth the programs serve, and thus they cannot be interpreted to represent relative levels of need among boys and girls. The average age of children and youth served ranges from 11.1 years among communities funded from 1997 to 1998 to 12.4 years and 12.1 years in those funded from 1993 to 1994 and 1999 to 2000, respectively. Most children are school age, ranging from 7 to 18 years. Ages vary across communities, largely because program funding in many instances is targeted for specific age ranges (e.g., children younger than age 6 years, children between the ages of 12 and 18 years), although across programs, all age groups from birth to 22 years are represented.

Race and Ethnicity   Across phases from 1993 to 2000, the percentage of children identified as White ranged from 51% to 64%. African American children served ranged from 16% to 33%, children of Hispanic origin ranged from 11% to 25%, and American Indian or Alaska Native children ranged from 2% to 10%. Variations in these percentages across funded groups of communities are generally indicative of the locations of funded systems of care and the variation in regional distributions among these groups. Thus, communities in states with larger Hispanic populations served more Hispanic children and youth, whereas urban locations served more African American families. Tribal grantees served the American Indian or Alaska Native children and families in their communities.

Poverty and Resource Needs   There is a high level of poverty among families served in federally funded systems of care. According to the U.S. Department of Health and Human Services guidelines appropriate to the period of data collection, poverty levels range from 54% to 60%. Because funding for systems of care goes to public mental health agencies that largely see families who do not have access to private services or whose children are eligible for Medicaid, it is not unexpected that high proportions of families served are living in poverty. Approximately half of all children are living in mother-maintained households, and between 35% and 42% lived in multiple settings before entering systems of care. Families frequently have multiple needs, including limited financial resources, and caregivers also have needs for additional support and resources in caring for their children and alleviating some of their worries and anxieties. Reimbursement for services largely occurs through public sector resources. More than 75% of children served received support from Medicaid in communities funded from 1999 to 2000; the State Children's Health Insurance Program, Temporary Assistance to Needy Families, and Supplemental Security Income were each sources of support for services for about one fifth of children (CMHS, 2006).

Mental Health Risk Factors   Many children participating in systems of care have been traumatized—often more than once in various ways—as indicated by their history of risk factors and the risk factors associated with their family lives. Results indicate that among children served in Phase II grant communities, more than 33% of youth had run away, 24% had a previous psychiatric hospitalization, 27% had been physically abused, 21% had been sexually abused, and 24% had a history of substance abuse. Although these proportions vary somewhat for children enrolled in Phase I and Phase III grant communities, the trend is similar regarding the prevalence of risk factors in the history of many participating children. Among family risk factors, the percentage of children who had experienced three or more risk factors ranged from 20% to more than 60%. Family characteristics such as a history of mental health disorders, family violence, and felony convictions also are believed to be associated with child and adolescent emotional disturbance (Friedman, Kutash, & Duchnowski, 1996). Child experiences of risk were related to low school performance at intake (Table 2.2).

Diagnoses and Challenges Mood disorders, oppositional defiant disorders, and attention-deficit/hyperactivity disorders have been the most common field diagnoses assigned to children served in systems of care. Adjustment disorders, post-traumatic stress disorders, and conduct-related disorders are in the next tier of frequently assigned diagnoses. Youth self-report of delinquency and substance use indicated than many of these children had trouble with the law and had various substance abuse problems prior to entering systems of care. Diagnoses of substance abuse were less frequently made, and these did not account for all youth who either self-reported substance use or showed impaired functioning due to substance use when rated on the Child and Adolescent Functional Assessment Scale (CAFAS; Hodges, 1990) (Stephens, Brannan, Holden, & Soler, 2005). Although most children attended school regularly at entry into services, their performance levels were below average. The addition of the Behavioral and Emotional Rating Scale (BERS; Epstein & Sharma, 1998), a strengths-based instrument, in Phase II showed that children generally had below-average strengths when they entered systems of care.

Referrals Because collaboration among child-serving agencies is a critical component of systems of care, the extent to which referrals are made to mental health services from other sectors is important to understanding where mental health needs are identified and how children enter services. Because some systems of care outstation mental health staff to other settings such as schools and courts,

Table 2.2. Examples of child and family risk factors

Child risk factors	Family risk factors
Physical abuse	Family history of mental illness
Sexual abuse	Family member psychiatric hospitalization
Suicide attempt	Family violence
Running away	Family member substance abuse
Substance use	Family member convicted of a crime
Psychiatric hospitalization	Sibling in institution
Sexually abusive	Sibling in foster care

defining a referral source can become less clear for communities as collaboration among agencies develops. Referrals from mental health agencies have varied from 22% in Phase I to 43% in Phase III communities funded in 1999–2000. Referrals from schools, about 20% among communities funded from 1993 to 1998, were lower among Phase III communities. Interestingly, in Phase IV (sites funded in 2002–2004), schools are the largest referral source. Child welfare referrals have ranged from 12% to 14%, with Phase IV referral rates averaging above 16%. Referrals from the juvenile justice sector have ranged from 11% to 19%. Referrals are made in smaller numbers from health care agencies, caregivers, self-referrals, substance abuse treatment programs, residential programs, and other site-specific programs. An ongoing concern among grantees is the low level of collaboration with health care providers, which is also reflected by low numbers of referrals from health agencies.

Children and youth served in systems of care have generally received prior services, with more than 60% receiving mental health services, more than 50% receiving school-based services, and more than one fourth of the services provided in residential settings as assessed in communities funded from 1997 to 2000.

Summary In general, youth served in systems of care are most often school-age boys, and the average age of youth has been gradually increasing across the federal funding cycles. Youth served are disproportionately members of minority races and ethnicities and from impoverished families. These youth, who are referred into services from multiple sources—primarily mental health agencies and schools—experience high rates of risk factors and present with a variety of diagnoses, severe clinical symptoms, and functional impairment. This information about child and family characteristics contributes to the understanding of the similarities and differences among the children served, as well as the extent to which these factors may be related to services received, family service experiences, changes in children's emotional and behavioral problems, changes in their social functioning, and changes in caregiver strain and family functioning over time.

Child and Youth Clinical and Functional Outcomes

With respect to clinical outcomes, the national evaluation has found that youth participating in systems of care generally showed improvement in clinical and functional outcomes, which are important indicators of recovery and quality of life. They exhibited significant improvement in behavioral and emotional strengths, and reductions in behavioral and emotional problems and functional impairment following intake into services. They also improved with regard to other important functional indicators (e.g., better school performance and attendance, fewer contacts with law enforcement, more stable living arrangements) following entry into systems of care.

Clinical Outcomes In communities initially funded between 1993 and 2000, functional impairment and behavioral and emotional symptoms were assessed by the CAFAS, the Child Behavior Checklist (CBCL; Achenbach, 1991), and the Youth Self-Report (YSR, for children 11 years of age and older; Achenbach & Edelbrock, 1987). The evaluation of grant communities initially funded in 1997–2000 added the BERS, a standardized, norm-referenced scale, to assess children's behavioral and emotional strengths (Epstein & Sharma, 1998).

In a report of preliminary results based on children served in communities initially funded in 1993–1994, children who left the evaluation 6 months after intake—and presumably left system of care services—had lower levels of functional impairment and behavioral problems at intake than those who remained in services 6 months (CMHS, 1997). Thus, remaining in the evaluation and continuing to participate in system of care services were indicative of greater levels of impairment and symptoms at intake. Roughly half of children remaining in services for 2 years in these communities exhibited clinically significant improvements in behavioral and emotional problems and functional impairment (Manteuffel et al., 2002).

For children enrolled in the evaluation of the 1997–1998 funded communities, functional impairment and behavioral and emotional symptoms improved significantly over time following entry into systems of care, with the greatest improvement typically occurring during the first 6 months of services, a trend that has continued across funding cohorts for children served in 1999–2000 funded communities (CMHS, 1997, 1998, 1999, 2000, 2001). On average, children's CBCL Total Problems scores improved at a rate of more than 13 points per year (i.e., > 1 standard deviation per year), but suicidal ideation at intake and a longer duration in services were associated with slower rates of improvement, and higher functional impairment at intake was associated with faster rates of improvement (Gilford & Stephens, 2002).

When changes in symptoms and strengths are conceptualized in terms of improvement or deterioration, children's CBCL Total Problems scores and BERS strength quotients were more likely to deteriorate from intake to 6 months if the children were members of a minority race or ethnic group, had a history of substance use, or had previously been in an out-of-home placement. A lower probability of deterioration in symptoms and strengths was related to higher levels of functional impairment, higher levels of caregiver strain, and poorer academic functioning at intake (Walrath, Ybarra, & Holden, 2006). One explanation for this finding may be that the children and youth who enter services with the greatest problems are able to make the greatest levels of improvement. The evaluation of 1993–1994 funded communities similarly found that children and youth with the most severe functional impairment received the largest number and the greatest variety of services, and made the greatest improvements during the first 6 months in systems of care (CMHS, 1998). Nearly half of all children served in systems of care show clinically significant improvement in their functioning (CAFAS) and behavioral and emotional problems (CBCL) in the first 12 months of services, but these improvements vary significantly across communities (Holden, 2000).

Over years of program development within funded communities, nearly half of the children enrolled each year showed clinically significant improvements in their strengths 12 months after enrolling in system of care services. About half of all children enrolled in each year also showed clinically significant decreases in their behavioral and emotional problems and their functional impairment during the 12 months following entry into services (CMHS, 2005).

The previously described comparison studies provided useful information regarding the relative effectiveness of systems of care. Findings from these studies indicated that clinical and functional outcomes improved over time for children served in both systems of care and comparison service delivery systems (Foster, Stephens, Krivelyova, & Gyamfi, 2007; Stephens et al., 2005; Stephens, Holden, & Hernandez, 2004). Youth served in systems of care showed greater reductions in functional impairment than youth served in the traditional, unfunded, comparison service delivery systems, but this finding was inconsistent across the pairs of comparison study communities (Foster et al., 2007; Stephens et al., 2005). When children served in the comparison communities experienced higher levels of services that were more consistent with system of care principles, they exhibited lower clinical symptom severity 1 year after intake than those who experienced lower levels of services; this suggests that a relationship exists between the experience of system of care principles at the practice level and reduced symptoms (Stephens et al., 2004). Differences in the relative effectiveness of systems of care across sites may reflect differences in system implementation, especially with regard to service provision (Foster et al., 2007).

Education Outcomes School attendance and grade performance are two important indicators of adjustment to the demands placed on children by caregivers and others in the community, with positive school adjustment and high performance indicative of subsequent life success. Children served in systems of care have consistently shown improvements in school performance and attendance (CMHS, 1997, 1998, 1999, 2000, 2001). Furthermore, regular school attendance was associated with a four-times greater likelihood of passing school performance at 6 months (Doucette-Gates, Hodges, & Liao, 1999). Below-average school performance and poor attendance were associated with greater functional impairment, emphasizing the importance of affecting clinical outcomes as they relate to functional indicators such as educational outcomes (Hodges, Doucette-Gates, & Liao, 1999).

Justice-Related Outcomes Although most youth served in systems of care do not have any contacts with law enforcement, those who do consistently experienced decreased law enforcement contacts (CMHS, 1997, 1998, 1999, 2000, 2001; Manteuffel et al., 2002). Based on findings from MIS data in the comparison studies, receiving mental health services in systems of care was more effective in reducing the risk of subsequent juvenile justice involvement than the receipt of services in comparison service delivery systems (Foster et al., 2004).

Living Situations Systems of care seek to provide services in less restrictive environments in part to establish residential stability for children and youth, and fewer residential changes are indicative of overall residential stability. Consistently, at intake into services, about one third of youth have experienced multiple living situations in the prior 6 months. Among those with multiple living arrangements at intake, about half reported having a single living arrangement after 6 months of services (CMHS, 1997, 1998, 1999, 2000, 2001).

Substance Use Youth who were 11 years or older at intake were asked to report on their substance use beginning with grant communities initially funded in 1997. Self-reported use of cigarettes, alcohol, and marijuana all showed reductions during the first 6 months of services (CMHS, 2001). Among youth with secondary diagnoses of substance use disorders, functional impairment at intake was significantly worse than for youth without substance use disorders. Youth with secondary diagnoses of substance use disorders showed significantly greater rates of improvement over the first year of services (CMHS, 1999).

System Characteristics and Child Outcomes Because the system of care principles emphasize the process of care (Burns, 1996), successful implementation of system of care principles is expected to produce improved clinical outcomes. Previous studies have shown that positive clinical outcomes are related to successful implementation of system of care principles (Burns et al., 1996; Clark, Lee, Prange, & McDonald, 1996). National evaluation data provide the opportunity to examine the relationship of individual- and system-level factors as predictors of improved outcomes for children and families. Results of these analyses indicate that more successful implementation at the system level of the principle that services should be individualized to meet the needs of each child and family—as measured by the previously described system of care assessment scores—resulted in greater improvement in functional impairment over the 18 months following intake. Children served in grant communities with high scores for the individualized principle improved at significantly faster rates than those children served in grant communities that were less successful at providing individualized care. In addition, more successful implementation of the principle that services should be easily accessible resulted in greater improvement in terms of CBCL Total Problems scores. Children served in grant communities with high scores for the accessible principle improved at a significantly faster rate than those children served in grant communities that were less successful at providing accessible services (CMHS, 2003a).

Summary Participation in systems of care resulted in meaningful outcomes related to recovery and quality of life for the children and youth served. Children and youth generally experienced meaningful improvement in important clinical and functional indicators. Their strengths, behavioral and emotional symptoms, and functioning were significantly improved following intake into services. Improvements in functional indicators were also observed. Children exhibited better school performance and attendance and fewer contacts with law enforcement following entry into systems of care.

Family Outcomes

In general, caregivers also benefited from the experience of system of care services. Caregivers of children served in systems of care experienced reduced strain associated with caring for children with a serious emotional disturbance, improved adequacy of resources for their families, and improvement in overall family functioning.

A number of standardized measures have been included in the national evaluation longitudinal outcome study to assess family outcomes such as family resources, caregiver strain, and family functioning. The Family Resources Scale (FRS; Dunst & Leet, 1985) measures the adequacy of a variety of resources needed by households with young children. The Family Assessment Device (FAD; Epstein, Baldwin, & Bishop, 1983) is a self-report measure of family functioning designed to measure how families interact, communicate, and work together. The Caregiver Strain Questionnaire (CGSQ; Brannan, Heflinger, & Bickman, 1998) assesses the extent to which caregivers experience additional difficulties, strains, and other negative effects as the result of their caregiving responsibilities in the 6 months prior to assessment.

Outcomes from Intake to 6 Months Based on initial analyses of data from families served in 1997–1998 funded communities, caregivers at entry into services considered their family resources to be adequate (CMHS, 2000), but they generally felt that the adequacy of resources improved significantly over the first 6 months of services (CMHS, 2001). Family functioning also improved (CMHS, 2001), and caregiver strain was significantly reduced during that period. Objective strain (e.g., interruption of personal time, missing work, financial strain) and subjective externalizing strain (e.g., anger, resentment, embarrassment) showed the largest reductions, but findings indicated significant improvement in the reduction of all dimensions of strain (CMHS, 2000, 2001).

Employment outcomes for caregivers have been explored (Brennen & Brannan, 2005; Krivelyova & Stephens, 2005). Findings indicate that caregivers of children with emotional and behavioral disorders are less likely to work if they do not have access to adequate child care (Brennen & Brannan, 2005); however, the services provided by systems of care can benefit various employment-related aspects of caregivers' lives. Caregivers reported that the mental health services that their child and family received helped them develop job-related, educational, and vocational skills, and, in turn, earn more money. Services also helped them miss fewer hours and days of work (Krivelyova & Stephens, 2005).

Family Resources, Family Functioning, and Caregiver Strain The data collected by the national evaluation on various characteristics of the caregivers and families of children with mental health challenges are providing insight into how factors such as family resources, caregiver strain, child problems, child strengths, and family functioning may interact. When family resources other than income are greater (e.g., time to be alone, time to be with children, child care), caregiver strain has been found to be lower, independent of the severity of children's problems and the family's income (Pullmann, Savage, & Koroloff, 2003). Differences have been found in the strain experienced by single mothers, grandmothers, and caregivers as compared with that of caregivers when there are two parents in the household. Although single mothers experienced the greatest amount of caregiver strain, family functioning and family resources were important considerations in the level of strain experienced by each type of caregiver (Sukumar, Manteuffel, Soler, & Sgro, 2003). Child strengths were greater among families with higher levels of resources; however, when families were functioning well, child strengths were less likely to be low even when family resources were low (Price, Gyamfi, Pope, & Lockaby, 2003). These findings are relevant to the ways in which services are used to support families and the effectiveness of the family support approach utilized in systems of care.

Summary   Participation in systems of care has resulted in significant positive outcomes for families and other caregivers. Caregivers experienced reduced strain associated with caring for a child with a serious emotional disturbance, improved adequacy of resources for their families, and improved family functioning.

Service Delivery and Service Experience

Federally funded systems of care are expected to have in place a mental health service array required by the program's authorizing legislation. Care managers coordinate services, keep families informed about their children's progress, facilitate procedures related to financial supports for services, and ensure receipt of appropriate services. Providers across agencies are expected to meet and communicate with each other and with the child and family about the child and family's needs. With increased emphasis on the availability and delivery of evidence-based treatments in systems of care, knowledge about evidence-based treatments and practices is also expected to be present. Use of services may vary according to the needs of individual children or youth and their families, the focus on a particular population by the system of care, geography, and other factors that may affect the availability or selection of services.

Services Used   On average, children and families used approximately six different kinds of services in their first 6 months in systems of care as reported by caregivers (CMHS, 2000). The services most often used were case management, individual therapy, and assessment. Case management and individual therapy were used by about 75% of children and families in the first 6 months. Although all families are expected to receive case management, not all families may need or want it. The percentage of children receiving medication management services in the first 6 months has varied from a high of 69% in communities funded from 1999 to 2000 to 45% in communities funded from 2002 to 2004. Among children receiving services for 24 months, nearly the same percentage consistently received medication management services as their use of other services decreased.

There were variations in the use of different types of support services. Family support services were received by just under one third of families, and recreation services were reported for slightly more than one third of the children among communities funded from 1997 to 2000. Transportation, flexible funds, and behavioral or therapeutic aides were used by at least one fifth of children and families. Respite was reported to be used by 11%–17% of families. Independent living and transition services intended for older adolescents were used by the smallest percentage of service recipients. In general, the use of each type of service decreased as children and youth progressed in systems of care. This finding should be anticipated when improvements in outcomes are obtained. These decreases are not seen for services associated with transition to adulthood (e.g., vocational training). These services become increasingly necessary as youth reach adulthood, and increases in age may be related to the increased utilization of these services (Macro International Inc., 2007a, 2007b; Manteuffel, Stephens, Sondheimer, & Fisher, in review).

Residential and inpatient services were used at lower levels than other types of services. Use of inpatient hospitalization and residential treatment ranged from approximately 7% to 13% across groups of communities funded from 1997 to 2004. Among children and youth receiving services to 24 months, use of inpatient hospitalization decreased somewhat, but use of residential treatment did not decline. Children and youth who remain in services for longer periods are also more likely to have more severe behavioral and emotional problems and may have a greater need for residential services. Therapeutic group homes, residential camps, and therapeutic foster care were used at lower levels than other services, including residential treatment and inpatient services. (Macro International Inc., 2007a, 2007b).

Service Experience   Youth and caregivers generally reported high levels of satisfaction with the services they received (CMHS, 1998, 1999, 2000, 2001). A consistent finding among systems of care is that youth reported higher levels of satisfaction with their own progress than that reported by their caregivers; however, youth have been generally less satisfied with their involvement in planning services and with the times when they were asked to participate in meetings. Considerable improvement is seen, however, in youth reports of satisfaction with involvement in service planning from their first 6 months in services to 36 months after service entry for those youth who continue to receive services. Increased youth satisfaction with involvement in treatment is consistent with changes in systems of care with regard to emphasizing youth-guided care.

After being enrolled in systems of care for 36 months, nearly 80% of caregivers reported that they were satisfied with services, and their reports of satisfaction with services were largely consistent over time. Youth satisfaction with services at 36 months was slightly lower at just under 75%, but their satisfaction varied over time and was higher at 36 months than at 6 months. Caregivers and youth were generally highly satisfied with their providers' understanding of their families' traditions, their involvement in service planning, and the times when they were asked to participate in meetings. Caregivers were less satisfied with their providers' ability to find services and were least satisfied with their children's progress. The relatively high rates of satisfaction among caregivers are consistent with those that have been typically found in the children's mental health literature (e.g., Heflinger et al., 1996).

Findings from the family-driven study, which involved focus groups with and surveys of family members, indicated that families were engaged through participation in treatment, family organization activities, team meetings, involvement with providers, and social activities (Macro International Inc., 2007b). Family members found that engagement in treatment led to greater levels of family support and empowerment, as well as improved care and services. The two greatest barriers to engagement reported were lack of access to services and funding and inadequate or inaccurate information.

Differences in services used and experiences with services in the systems of care and comparison communities in the Phase II comparison study showed that more children served in the systems of care received outpatient and support services and that they were more likely to receive case management and medication monitoring services (Macro International Inc., 2007a) without adjustments for differences in the samples in the matched communities. In Nebraska, families in the system of care were more likely to use family support services and receive services in a variety of locations, whereas children in the comparison community were more likely to receive restrictive services, spend more days in restrictive placements, and receive more episodes of nonrestrictive services. Caregivers in systems of care rated their experiences of case management as more consistent with system of care principles than caregivers in comparison communities.

Service Providers   Surveys were conducted with providers about their use of evidence-based practices, and providers in the Phase II comparison communities were assessed on their adherence to system of care principles in their service delivery. The mental health providers, child welfare case workers, special education teachers, and probation officers surveyed did not differ across systems of care and comparison communities in their responses about application of system of care principles in their work. Providers did, however, differ in their responses between states and by provider type. Special education teachers and probation officers were less likely to deliver services that were family focused, accessible, and culturally competent (Manteuffel et al., 2005).

Service providers reported variations in their knowledge of evidence-based practices, and they reported a range of barriers related to use of evidence-based treatments. The implementation of evidence-based treatments in systems of care encountered a range of obstacles generally consistent with issues found to be associated with the transfer of treatments to community settings. Buy-in by providers and agencies, the ability of family members to receive services at recommended levels, the availability of services for Spanish-speaking families, and issues with reimbursement for services were a few of the concerns encountered.

Summary   Children and youth with serious emotional disturbance in systems of care consistently receive basic clinical services and management and monitoring services and have a significant need for support services that are central to the goals of systems of care to keep children and youth at home and in their communities. When compared with other service systems, funded systems of care are demonstrating that they are providing more services to address clinical, monitoring, and family support needs. The types of services used must be considered within the context of the severity of behavior and emotional problems, age of the child or youth, family circumstances, availability of services to address the level of need, and potential for third-party reimbursement. The ability of providers to deliver evidence-based treatments and to practice according to system of care principles must be considered within the context of agency-, system-, local-, and state-level factors that may influence their ability to change their practice.

Service Costs

A critical issue in assessing changes produced by implementing systems of care is their impact on service costs. Children with serious emotional disturbance and their families receive services in multiple settings, and costs are incurred across multiple child-serving agencies. Access to management information systems and cost data housed in these systems has varied in funded systems of care from no access, or access only to services paid directly by grant funds, to extensive cross-system data, although these data still may not comprehensively capture the costs of serving an individual child. Informal services not captured in any system, services paid for privately, and costs connected to residential treatment centers in another state are some types of information that may contribute to gaps in a fully comprehensive picture of service use and costs.

Despite these obstacles, most communities have attempted to integrate service and cost data with other child-serving agencies (CMHS, 2004, 2006). Among systems of care funded from 1998 to 2004, most advocated for information sharing by demonstrating the benefits of integrated data to relevant stakeholders; building overall cross-agency partnerships; and setting clear rules and procedures regarding informed consents, privacy, and data transfers. Among systems of care funded in 2005, the top strategy to ensure cross-agency information sharing was building data integration into their infrastructure, including working with a dedicated software development partner, colocating staff in other agencies to ensure data access, and purchasing data systems capable of integrating data (CMHS, 2006).

Average Per Child Costs   Variations in the costs of services reflect a range of factors, including differences among community-level referral patterns, severity of the mental health needs of the children and youth served, and state health care financing policies. Examination of Medicaid claims in four communities in North Carolina indicated that some of the variation in costs across systems

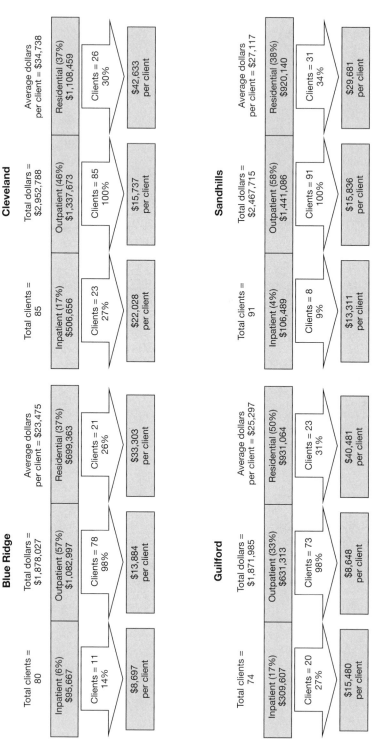

Blue Ridge

Total clients = 80

Average dollars per client = $23,475

| Inpatient (6%) $95,667 | Outpatient (57%) $1,082,997 | Residential (37%) $699,363 |

Total dollars = $1,878,027

Clients = 11 14%

Clients = 78 98%

Clients = 21 26%

$8,697 per client

$13,884 per client

$33,303 per client

Cleveland

Total clients = 85

Average dollars per client = $34,738

Total dollars = $2,952,788

| Inpatient (17%) $506,656 | Outpatient (46%) $1,337,673 | Residential (37%) $1,108,459 |

Clients = 23 27%

Clients = 85 100%

Clients = 26 30%

$22,028 per client

$15,737 per client

$42,633 per client

Guilford

Total clients = 74

Average dollars per client = $25,297

Total dollars = $1,871,985

| Inpatient (17%) $309,607 | Outpatient (33%) $631,313 | Residential (50%) $931,064 |

Clients = 20 27%

Clients = 73 98%

Clients = 23 31%

$15,480 per client

$8,648 per client

$40,481 per client

Sandhills

Total clients = 91

Average dollars per client = $27,117

Total dollars = $2,467,715

| Inpatient (4%) $106,489 | Outpatient (58%) $1,441,086 | Residential (38%) $920,140 |

Clients = 8 9%

Clients = 91 100%

Clients = 31 34%

$13,311 per client

$15,836 per client

$29,681 per client

Figure 2.8. Total Medicaid claims (January 2000–October 2002) in four North Carolina communities. (Reprinted from Macro International Inc. [2007]. *Final report: Phase III of the Comprehensive Community Mental Health Services for Children and Their Families Program, grant communities funded in 1999–2000.* Manuscript in preparation.)

56

of care can be explained by the differences in unit costs of services and the variation in utilization of restrictive services such as residential and inpatient care. In three of the four communities, average Medicaid expenditure costs per child decreased over time. Among significant predictors of Medicaid expenditures costs were the child's age and severity of the impairment (CMHS, 2003a; Macro International Inc., 2007a). Average per child costs ranged from $23,475 to $34,738. Differences in the rural and urban locations of these communities, and, therefore, access to services may be factors contributing to differences in the types of services used. Figure 2.8 provides details about the average cost per child in each of the four communities, as well as per client costs of inpatient, outpatient, and residential services.

As in other areas of health care, the analysis of cost data shows that a subset of children account for the lion's share of expenditures. When looking only at flexible funds, which are generally used to pay for basic needs such as housing, transportation, food, child care, camps and summer programs, and services not billable to Medicaid or other third-party payers in a sample of four grantee communities (i.e., located in Delaware, Massachusetts, New Hampshire, North Carolina), a small number of children accounted for the largest proportion of total costs (CMHS, 2006). The amount of flexible funds used, as well as the ways in which these resources were implemented, varied considerably by community, with some communities using flexible funds to fund certain types of services in larger amounts than others. In Delaware, the highest proportion of overall flexible funds was allocated to housing support (17.7%), and in North Carolina and New Hampshire the highest proportion was allocated to therapeutic camp (30.8% and 22.3%, respectively). Therapeutic camp also accounted for a large proportion of expenditures in Delaware (17.5%). In Massachusetts, after-school and summer programs accounted for the largest percentage of the total expended flexible funds (25.8%).

Cost Offsets Across Agencies   Systems of care are obligated to supply services in the community and in the least restrictive settings appropriate for each child's needs. Shifting treatment from residential and inpatient settings, where children are removed from their families, to community-based and outpatient services is a common goal for systems of care that is expected to have a considerable impact on cost reduction per child served. When inpatient costs and costs associated with arrests are examined across systems, significant reductions in costs are seen at the per child level (CMHS, 2005, 2006). These reductions in costs, however, are associated with individual services and may not be relevant to all systems. For example, those communities serving very young children would be less likely to find cost reductions for these services. A complete understanding of the costs and financing in systems of care involves understanding expenditures by other child-serving sectors or agencies (e.g., child welfare, juvenile justice, special education), as well as expenditures on mental health services funded by other payers. Examining cost data from individual systems of care has shown that the shift in resources from a collaborating agency to a mental health agency can appear to show increases in mental health expenditures if the overall increase in mental health resources resulting from transfer of resources from other systems is not understood. This was the case in the system of care in Milwaukee (i.e., Wraparound Milwaukee), where blended funding mechanisms developed with other child-serving agencies (e.g., juvenile justice, child welfare) were instrumental in increasing available funds and ensuring fiscal sustainability of the program (CMHS, 1999). With resources provided by these agencies, the system of care assumed responsibility for serving children at risk for out-of-home placement and youth referred by court order to residential treatment facilities, with a view toward shifting their care to home and community-based approaches. Wraparound Milwaukee has demonstrated that increased numbers of youth can generally be served with the same resources, resulting in significantly reduced costs to the child welfare and juvenile justice systems and a reduction in the cost per youth served.

Comparing Costs Between Systems   Analysis of comprehensive cost data was possible with one pair of communities participating in the Phase I comparison study. Per child expenditures were found to be higher in the Stark County, Ohio, system of care than in the Mahoning County, Ohio, comparison community (Foster & Connor, 2005b; Foster & Xuan, 2005); however, these higher costs reflected longer service episodes experienced by children served in the system of care community. When costs per day of treatment were considered, costs were found to be lower in the system of care because less costly forms of care were substituted for inpatient services. When expenditures in juvenile justice, special education, and child welfare systems were included in the analyses, it was found that although mental health costs were higher in the system of care, other agency costs were actually lower. These findings are supported by the reduced likelihood of juvenile justice involvement and a lower recidivism rate in the system of care than in the comparison community, with the greatest differences seen for youth who were the most serious offenders (Foster et al., 2004). Similar analysis using juvenile justice agency data from a more recent comparison study in Alabama revealed a significantly larger decrease in juvenile justice involvement for youth receiving services in the system of care compared with youth in the comparison community (Krivelyova, Matthews, & Stephens, 2006).

Summary   The costs of serving children with serious emotional disturbance and their families are affected by a range of factors at the individual child and family, community, system, and state levels. Costs of services and reductions in costs per child vary; however, these costs need to be considered across child-serving sectors to fully understand shifts in resources and changes in per child costs. Blending resources among child-serving providers has significantly increased total dollars available for mental health services in some communities. Access to service and cost information from agency MIS date is critical to fully understanding costs and developing strategies for sustainability.

Sustaining Systems of Care

Both qualitative information from the system of care assessment and the sustainability survey provide insight about program elements that are easier and more difficult to sustain and factors related to sustainability. Almost all of 1993–1994 programs were found to be sustained when assessed 5 years postfunding. Support services such as flexible funds, transportation, respite, and family support were more difficult to sustain. These services were generally paid for by grant dollars and were more difficult to replace with Medicaid or other resources. Increased availability of services was supported by partnerships among agencies, the ability to bill Medicaid for services, the availability of new or increased state funds, and the redirection of savings from reduced use of inpatient and residential treatment. Systems of care were able to continue to minimize the need for children to leave communities for treatment, reduce the number of children placed in residential settings, and achieve acceptance of the system of care philosophy among providers and system leaders.

Maintaining viable family organizations presented the greatest challenge at the system level. Other features, including an ongoing focal point for the system of care, capacity of services in the service array, and the use of evaluation data, represented additional challenges. Some communities have been successful in establishing family organizations as service providers so that family support services may be billed to third-party payers, but differences between states affect the ability to employ this approach. Institutionalizing the system of care philosophy at various levels (including legislation, policy, and service systems), continuity of leadership, and family advocacy were considered some of the elements critical to maintaining this philosophy (Stroul & Manteuffel, 2007).

Systems of care assessed in their last year of funding reported slightly different trends than those postfunding. Communities funded from 1998 to 2000 that were assessed at a later point in time chronologically differed in their responses about factors related to sustainability from assessment of the earlier cohorts (Stroul, Keens-Douglas, & Manteuffel, 2006). Some of these differences may have been due to changes in conditions external to funded programs but relevant to those programs. For example, the crisis in Medicaid funding was in the forefront at the time of the earlier assessment; however, adjustment to this issue had occurred by the later assessment. When asked in the middle of their funding period about general strategies relevant to sustaining their programs, systems of care funded in 2002–2003 reported training on the system of care approach, involving stakeholders, and cultivating strong interagency relationships as critical factors. In-kind space donations, pooling or blending funds from multiple agencies, obtaining grants, and acquiring new or increased local funds were reported as the most effective financing strategies used for sustainability (CMHS, 2007).

CONCLUSION

The data collected by the national evaluation provide a wealth of information about systems, services, and children and families served and their outcomes. Although a number of strategies have been used to examine system-level, service-level, and child-level characteristics in combination, these issues are complex, and more analyses are needed to understand the relationships among these levels. Systems of care serve children with a range of diagnoses who enter services in systems that differ considerably from one another, and they receive services tailored to their individual needs. To understand the extent to which system change, use of home and community-based services and supports in lieu of restrictive services, case management, or other features of systems of care account for differences in outcomes for children, youth, and their families presents significant challenges in data analyses.

Ongoing Evaluation Challenges

Conducting a large-scale multisite evaluation presents a range of challenges. The range of characteristics of children and families served, the unique circumstances and cultures within communities implementing systems of care, and differences in the specific objectives of systems of care across communities challenge the interpretation of findings at the aggregate level. Furthermore, assessing system of care effectiveness through quasi-experimental designs has had limited success. The use of comparison studies to assess system change is impeded by the practical realities that limit the ability of research to control the treatment environment of children and their families over an extended period through random assignment. Additional approaches to evaluation are being contemplated to address these challenges and to provide information about system development and outcomes needed to better understand what works best under which circumstances and for which children.

What Have We Learned?

Children experience reductions in their behavioral and emotional problems, increase their strengths, do better in school, and are less likely to be involved with the juvenile justice system after receiving services in systems of care. Caregivers make significant reductions in the strain they experience in caring for a child with a serious emotional disturbance and they continue to reduce their strain over multiple assessments. Caregivers improve their economic circumstances as their likelihood of employment increases.

Improvements for children, youth, and caregivers are greatest in the first 6 months in services, and they continue to improve over time, albeit more slowly. Children served for longer periods are also those children who have more severe problems. Because children continuing in services are also more likely to continue in the evaluation, longer-term outcomes generally reflect those of children with greater problems. Service use differs by level of severity of child functioning (CMHS, 1998), and rates of change in functioning differ by levels of functional impairment, as well as the amount and types of services received. Service experiences are largely consistent with system of care principles. Caregivers tend to be more satisfied with their involvement in services and less satisfied with their outcomes than youth, who express greater satisfaction with their own outcomes.

Future Evaluation Needs

There is a continuing need to test the effectiveness of systems of care and the relationship between their effectiveness and their various features. Given the extensive available data, additional effort is needed to use these data to model the relationships between features of systems, providers, services, and outcomes. Specific analyses can be used to examine a range of hypothesized relationships so a model of system change can be built empirically. The extensive analyses already conducted and reported in this chapter and elsewhere would benefit from meta-analyses to review what is already known and identify where gaps in understanding system change and outcomes exist. Implementation studies can provide more information about the efforts required to implement system change.

Continuous Quality Improvement

The use of evaluation data to inform program improvement—a key characteristic of the CMHI—continues to develop through efforts to foster technical assistance based on continuous quality improvement reports that summarize outcomes in key program areas. The use of evaluation data to inform and improve systems of care at the local and national levels has resulted in revisions to program requirements. Areas in which programs showed weaknesses in their implementation of system of care principles at the infrastructure and service delivery levels (e.g., cultural competence, family involvement) have resulted in increased requirements and increased attention in grant applications. Developing knowledge about sustainability postfunding is another area where evaluation findings have led to training efforts to enhance community understanding of obstacles that may be encountered when trying to achieve sustainability and actions that may improve it. Agency and provider-level barriers to implementing evidence-based treatments is also an area where new learning has led to new thinking about how to address these barriers. Systems of care continue to develop based on information obtained from both national and local evaluations (Substance Abuse and Mental Health Services Administration [SAMHSA], 2005).

Building the Future

The CMHI's experience with system change is an invaluable resource to the transformation agenda recommended by the President's New Freedom Commission (2003) and outlined in the *Federal Action Agenda* (SAMHSA, 2005). As a model for community-level care, the CMHI provides a successful and effective approach to coordinated service delivery for children and youth with serious emotional disturbances and their families. The community-level system transformation that began with federal funding continues to evolve in subsequent years. Facilitating collaboration among funded and previously funded communities, as well as building on the experience of both the individuals involved in these systems and the structures established among agencies within systems, are opportunities for furthering larger mental health system transformation. Communities that received federal funding to build systems of care have found that the 5- or 6-year period of federal grant funding is just a start and that long-range planning for 15 years or longer is needed to fully establish systems change. Evaluation data from these communities offers an important resource for understanding the evolution that occurs over the longer term, resulting in sustained transformation of mental health services for children, youth, and their families (CMHS, 2007).

REFERENCES

Aarons, G.A., MacDonald, E.J., Sheehan, A.K., & Walrath-Greene, C.M. (2007). Confirmatory factor analysis of the Evidence-Based Practice Attitude Scale (EBPAS) in a geographically diverse sample of community mental health providers. *Psychiatric Services, 34*(5), 465–469.

Achenbach, T.M. (1991). *Manual for the Child Behavior Checklist/4–18 and 1991 profile.* Burlington: University of Vermont, Department of Psychiatry.

Achenbach, T.M., & Edelbrook, C. (1987). *Manual for the Youth Self-Report and Profile.* Burlington: University of Vermont, Department of Psychiatry.

Achenbach, T.M., & Rescorla, L.A. (2000). *Manual for ASEBA Preschool Forms & Profiles.* Burlington: University of Vermont, Research Center for Children, Youth, and Families.

Achenbach, T.M., & Rescorla, L.A. (2001). *Manual for ASEBA School-Age Forms and Profiles.* Burlington: University of Vermont, Research Center for Children, Youth, and Families.

ADAMHA Reorganization Act, PL 102-321, 42 U.S.C. §§ 201 *et seq.*

Bickman, L., Guthrie, P.R., Foster, E.M., Lambert, W., Summerfelt, W.T., Breda, et al. (1995). *Evaluating managed mental health services: The Fort Bragg experiment.* New York: Plenum Press.

Bickman, L., Noser, K., & Summerfelt, W.M. (1999). Long-term effects of a system of care on children and adolescents. *Journal of Behavioral Health Services and Research, 26*(2), 185–202.

Bickman, L., Summerfelt, W., Firth, J., & Douglas, S. (1997). The Stark County evaluation project: Baseline results of a randomized experiment. In C. Nixon & D. Northrup (Eds.), *Evaluating mental health services* (pp. 231–258). Thousand Oaks, CA: Sage Publications.

Bickman, L., Summerfelt, W., & Noser, K. (1997). Comparative outcomes of emotionally disturbed children and adolescents in a system of services and usual care. *Psychiatric Services, 48,* 1543–1548.

Bird, H.R., Shaffer, D., Fisher, P., Gould, M.S., Staghezza, B., Chen, J.Y., et al. (1993). The Columbia Impairment Scale (CIS): Pilot findings on a measure of global impairment for children and adolescents. *International Journal of Methods in Psychiatric Research, 3,* 167–176.

Brannan, A.M., Baughman, L.N., Reed, E.D., & Katz-Leavy, J. (2002). System-of-care assessment: Cross-site comparison of findings. *Children's Services: Social Policy, Research, and Practice, 5*(1), 37–56.

Brannan, A.M., Heflinger, C.A., & Bickman, L. (1998). The Caregiver Strain Questionnaire: Measuring the impact on the family of living with a child with serious emotional disturbance. *Journal of Emotional and Behavioral Disorders, 5,* 212–222.

Brashears, F., Santiago, R.L., Sgro, G.M., & Gilford, J.W. (2005). Constancy and change in cultural competence in systems of care. In C. Newman, C.J. Liberton, K. Kutash, & R. M. Friedman (Eds.), *The 17th Annual Research Conference Proceedings, A system of care for children's mental health: Expanding the research base* (pp. 327–330). Tampa: University of South Florida, Louis de la Parte Florida Mental Health Institute, Research and Training Center for Children's Mental Health.

Brennan, E.M., & Brannan, A.M. (2005). Participation in the paid labor force by care-givers of children with emotional and behavioral disorders. *Journal of Emotional and Behavioral Disorders, 13*, 237–246.

Brunk, M., Koch, J.R., & McCall, B. (2000). *Report on parent satisfaction with services at community services boards.* Richmond: Virginia Department of Mental Health, Mental Retardation, and Substance Abuse Services.

Brunk, M., Santiago, R., Ewell, K., & Watts, A. (1997). Family satisfaction with level of cultural competence in systems of care: Development of a cultural competence scale. In C.J. Liberton, K. Kutash, & R. Friedman (Eds.), *The 10th Annual Research Conference Proceedings, A system of care for children's mental health: Expanding the research base* (pp. 113–118). Tampa: University of South Florida, Louis de la Parte Florida Mental Health Institute, Research and Training Center for Children's Mental Health.

Bruns, E.J., Leverentz-Brandy, K.M., & Walker, S. (2007, March). *Wraparound fidelity in systems of care and association with outcomes: Results of the national wraparound comparison study.* Presentation at the 20th Annual Research Conference, A System of Care for Children's Mental Health: Expanding the Research Base, Tampa, FL.

Burns, B.J. (1996). What drives outcomes for emotional and behavioral disorders in children and adolescents? In D.M. Steinwachs, L.M. Flynn, et al. (Eds.), *Using client outcomes information to improve mental health and substance abuse treatment: New directions for mental health services (No. 71*, pp. 89–102). San Francisco: Jossey-Bass.

Burns, B.J. (1999). A call for mental health services research agenda for youth with serious emotional disturbance. *Mental Health Services Research, 1*(1), 5-20.

Burns, B.J., Farmer, M., Angold, A., Costello, J., & Behar, L. (1996). A randomized trial of case management for youths with serious emotional disturbance. *U.S. Journal of Clinical Child Psychology, 25*(4), 476–486.

Center for Mental Health Services. (1997). *Annual report to Congress on the evaluation of the Comprehensive Community Mental Health Services for Children and Their Families Program, 1997.* Atlanta, GA: Macro International Inc.

Center for Mental Health Services. (1998). *Annual report to Congress on the evaluation of the Comprehensive Community Mental Health Services for Children and Their Families Program, 1998.* Atlanta, GA: Macro International Inc.

Center for Mental Health Services. (1999). *Annual report to Congress on the evaluation of the Comprehensive Community Mental Health Services for Children and Their Families Program, 1999.* Atlanta, GA: ORC Macro.

Center for Mental Health Services. (2000). *Annual report to Congress on the evaluation of the Comprehensive Community Mental Health Services for Children and Their Families Program, 2000.* Atlanta, GA: ORC Macro.

Center for Mental Health Services. (2001). *Annual report to Congress on the evaluation of the Comprehensive Community Mental Health Services for Children and Their Families Program, 2001.* Atlanta, GA: ORC Macro.

Center for Mental Health Services. (2002). *Annual report to Congress on the evaluation of the Comprehensive Community Mental Health Services for Children and Their Families Program, 2001.* Atlanta, GA: ORC Macro. Unpublished report.

Center for Mental Health Services. (2003a). *Annual report to Congress on the evaluation of the Comprehensive Community Mental Health Services for Children and Their Families Program.* Unpublished report, ORC Macro, Atlanta, GA.

Center for Mental Health Services. (2003b). *The Comprehensive Community Mental Health Services for Children and Their Families Program: Evaluation findings—Annual reports to Congress, 2002–2003.* Atlanta, GA: ORC Macro.

Center for Mental Health Services. (2004). *The Comprehensive Community Mental Health Services for Children and Their Families Program: Evaluation findings—Annual report to Congress, 2004.* Unpublished report, ORC Macro, Atlanta, GA.

Center for Mental Health Services. (2005). *The Comprehensive Community Mental Health Services for Children and Their Families Program: Evaluation findings—Annual report to Congress, 2005.* Unpublished report, ORC Macro, Atlanta, GA.

Center for Mental Health Services. (2006). *The Comprehensive Community Mental Health Services for Children and Their Families Program: Evaluation findings—Annual report to Congress, 2006.* Unpublished report, Macro International Inc., Atlanta, GA.

Center for Mental Health Services. (2007). *The Comprehensive Community Mental Health Services for Children and Their Families Program: Evaluation findings—Annual report to Congress, 2007.* Unpublished report, Macro International Inc., Atlanta, GA.

Clark, H.B., Lee, B., Prange, M.E., & McDonald, B.A. (1996). Children lost within the foster care system: Can wraparound service strategies improve placement outcomes? *Journal of Child and Family Studies, 5,* 39–54.

Cole, R.F., & Poe, S.L. (1993). *Partnerships for care: Systems of care for children with serious emotional disturbances and their families.* Washington, DC: Washington Business Group on Health.

Costello, E.J. (1997). Service needs and use for serious emotional disturbance: A community study. In C. Liberton, K. Kutash, & R. Freidman (Eds.), *The 9th Annual Research Conference Proceedings, A system of care for children's mental health: Expanding the research base, February 26–February 28, 1996* (pp. 406–407). Tampa: University of South Florida, Louis de la Parte Florida Mental Health Institute, Research and Training Center for Children's Mental Health.

Doucette-Gates, A., Hodges, K., & Liao, Q. (1999). Using the Child and Adolescent Functional Assessment Scale (CAFAS): Examining child outcomes and service use patterns. In J. Willis, C. Liberton, K. Kutash, & R. Friedman (Eds.), *The 11th Annual Research Conference Proceedings, A system of care for children's mental heath: Expanding the research base* (pp. 333–340). Tampa: University of South Florida, Louis de la Parte Florida Mental Health Institute, Research and Training Center for Children's Mental Health.

Dunst, C.J., & Leet, H.E. (1985). *Family Resource Scale: Reliability and validity.* Asheville, NC: Winterberry Press.

Eggers, T., Delp, W., Lazear, K., Wells, C., & Alonso-Martinez, M. (1997). Developing an effective statewide network: Outcomes of Florida's system of care for students with severe emotional disturbance. In C.J. Liberton, K. Kutash, & R.M. Friedman (Eds.), *The 9th Annual Research Conference Proceedings, A system of care for children's mental health: Expanding the research base, February 26–February 28, 1996* (pp. 195–198). Tampa: University of South Florida, Louis de la Parte Florida Mental Health Institute, Research and Training Center for Children's Mental Health.

Epstein, M.H. (2004). *Behavioral and Emotional Rating Scale: A strength-based approach to assessment. Examiner's manual* (2nd ed.). Austin, TX: PRO-ED.

Epstein, M.H., & Sharma, J. (1998). *Behavioral and Emotional Rating Scale: A strengths-based approach to assessment.* Austin, TX: PRO-ED.

Epstein, N.B., Baldwin, L.M., & Bishop, D.S. (1983). The McMaster Family Assessment Device. *Journal of Marital and Family Therapy, 9*(2), 171–180.

Evans, M.E., Blanch, A.K., Boothroyd, R.A., Boustead, R., & Chen, H.J. (2007, March). *Sources of conflict and conflict resolution in systems of care.* Paper presented at the 20th Annual Research Conference, A System of Care for Children's Mental Health: Expanding the Research Base, Tampa, FL.

Foster, E.M., & Connor, T. (2005a). A road map for costs analyses of systems of care. In M.H. Epstein, K. Kutash, & A. Duchnowski (Eds.), *Outcomes for children and youth with behavioral and emotional disorders and their families: Programs and evaluation best practices* (2nd ed., pp. 225–245). Austin, TX: PRO-ED..

Foster, E.M., & Connor, T. (2005b). The public costs of better mental health services for children and adolescents. *Psychiatric Services, 56,* 50–55.

Foster, E.M., Qaseem, A., & Connor, T. (2004). Can better mental health services reduce the risk of juvenile justice involvement? *American Journal of Public Health*, *94*, 859–865.

Foster, E.M., Stephens, R., Krivelyova, A., & Gyamfi, P. (2007). Can system integration improve mental health outcomes for children and youth? *Children and Youth Services Review*, *29*, 1301–1319.

Foster, E.M., & Xuan, F. (2005). An episode-based framework for analyzing health care expenditures: An application of reward renewal models. *Health Services Research*, *40*(6 Pt. 1), 1953–1971.

Friedman, R.M. (1993). *Clinical training and research for children's services in serving the seriously mental ill: Public academic linkages in services, research and training.* Washington, DC: American Psychological Association.

Friedman, R.M., & Burns, B.J. (1996). The evaluation of the Fort Bragg demonstration project: An alternative interpretation of the findings. *Journal of Mental Health Administration, 23*(1), 128–136.

Friedman, R.M., Kutash, K., & Duchnowski, A.J. (1996). The population of concern: Defining the issues. In B.A. Stroul & R.M. Friedman (Series Ed.) & B.A. Stroul (Vol. Ed.), *Children's mental health: Creating systems of care in a changing society* (pp. 69–96). Baltimore: Paul H. Brookes Publishing Co.

Gilford, J.W., & Stephens, R.L. (2002). Modeling change in caregiver reports of behavioral and emotional symptoms. In C. Newman, C.J. Liberton, K. Kutash, & R. Friedman (Eds.), *The 14th Annual Research Conference Proceedings, A system of care for children's mental heath: Expanding the research base* (pp. 13–16). Tampa: University of South Florida, Louis de la Parte Florida Mental Health Institute, Research and Training Center for Children's Mental Health.

Glisson, C. (1994). The effect of service coordination teams on outcomes for children in state custody. *Administrative Social Work, 18*, 1–23.

Government Performance and Results Act of 1993, PL 103-62, 31 U.S.C. §§ 1115 *et seq.*

Greenbaum, P.E., Dedrick, R.F., Friedman, R., Kutash, K., Brown, E., Lardieri, S., & Pugh, A. (1996). National adolescent and child treatment study (NACTS): Outcomes for individuals with serious emotional and behavioral disturbance. *Journal of Emotional and Behavioral Disorders, 4*, 130–146.

Greenbaum, P.E., Prange, M.E., Friedman, R.M., & Silver, S.E. (1991). Substance abuse prevalence and comorbidity with other psychiatric disorders among adolescents with severe emotional disturbances. *Journal of the American Academy of Child and Adolescent Psychiatry, 30*(4), 575–583.

Harra, S., & Ooms, T. (1995). *Children's mental health services: Policy implications of the new paradigm. Family Impact Seminar.* Washington, DC: Center for Mental Health Services.

Hawkins, R.P., Almeida, M.C., Fabry, B., & Reitz, A.L. (1992). A scale to measure restrictiveness of living environments for troubled children and youths. *Hospital and Community Psychiatry, 43*(1), 54–58.

Heflinger, C.A., Sonnichsen, S.E., & Brannan, A.M. (1996). Parent satisfaction with children's mental health services in a children's mental health managed care demonstration. *U.S. Journal of Mental Health Administration, 23*(1), 69–79.

Hernandez, M., & Hodges, S., (2005). *Crafting logic models for systems of care: Ideas into action. Making children's mental health services successful series* (Rev. ed., Vol. 1). Tampa: University of South Florida, Louis de la Parte Florida Mental Health Institute.

Hodges, K. (1990). *Child and Adolescent Functional Assessment Scale (CAFAS).* Ypsilanti, MI: Department of Psychology, Eastern Michigan University.

Hodges, K., Doucette-Gates, A., & Liao, Q. (1999). The relationship between the Child and Adolescent Functional Assessment Scale (CAFAS) and indicators of functioning. *Journal of Child and Family Studies, 8*, 109–122.

Holden, E.W. (2000). Outcomes of the national evaluation. In C. Liberton, C. Newman, K. Kutash, & R.M. Friedman (Eds.), *The 12th Annual Research Conference Proceedings, A system of care for children's mental health: Expanding the research base* (pp. 3–4). Tampa: University of South Florida, Louis de la Parte Florida Mental Health Institute, Research and Training Center for Children's Mental Health.

Holden, E.W., Friedman, R.M., & Santiago, R. (2001). Overview of the national evaluation of the Comprehensive Community Mental Health Services for Children and Their Families Program. *Journal of Emotional and Behavioral Disorders, 9*, 4–13.

Johnson, M.C., Morrissey, J.P., & Colloway, M.O. (1996). Structure and change in child mental health service delivery networks. *U.S. Journal of Community Psychology, 24*(3), 275–289.

Johnson, S.F., Manteuffel, B., Sukumar, B., & McBride, M. (2007, May). *Implementing Parent–Child Interaction Therapy (PCIT) in systems of care: Treatment outcomes and lessons learned from real world settings.* Paper presented at the Building on Family Strengths Conference: Research and Services in Support of Children and Their Families, Portland, OR.

Koren, P.E., DeChillo, N., & Friesen, B.J.(1992). Measuring empowerment in families whose children have emotional disabilities: A brief questionnaire. *Rehabilitation Psychology, 37*(4), 305–321.

Koroloff, N.M., Elliot, D.J., Koren, P.E., & Friesen, B.J. (1996). Linking low-income families to children's mental health services: The role of the family associate. *Journal of Emotional and Behavioral Disorders, 2*, 240–246.

Krivelyova, A., Matthews, S.K., & Stephens, R. (2006). Juvenile justice outcomes of youth in systems of care: Comparison study results. In C. Newman, C. Liberton, K. Kutash, & R.M. Friedman (Eds.), *The 18th Annual Research Conference Proceedings: A system of care for children's mental health: Expanding the research base* (pp. 433–436). Tampa: University of South Florida, Louis de la Parte Florida Mental Health Institute, Research and Training Center for Children's Mental Health.

Krivelyova, A., & Stephens, R. (2005). Caregivers of children in systems of care: Economic outcomes. In C. Newman, C.J. Liberton, K. Kutash, & R.M. Friedman (Eds.). *The 17th Annual Research Conference Proceedings, A system of care for children's mental health: Expanding the research base* (pp. 271–276). Tampa: University of South Florida, Louis de la Parte Florida Mental Health Institute, Research and Training Center for Children's Mental Health.

Kuperminc, G.P., & Cohen, R. (1995). Community mental health services for children and youth: What we know and what we need to learn. *Journal of Child and Family Studies, 4*, 147–175.

Kutash, K., Duchnowski, A., Johnson, M., & Rugs, D. (1993). Multistage evaluation for a community mental health system for children. *Administration and Policy in Mental Health, 20*(4), 311–322.

Lambert, E.W., Brannan, A.M., Heflinger, C.A., Breda, C., & Bickman, L. (1998). Common patterns of service use in children's mental health. *Evaluation and Program Planning, 2*, 47–57.

Macro International Inc. (2007a). *Final report: Phase II of the Comprehensive Community Mental Health Services for Children and Their Families Program, grant communities funded in 1997–1998.* Manuscript in preparation.

Macro International Inc. (2007b). *Final report: Phase III of the Comprehensive Community Mental Health Services for Children and Their Families Program, grant communities funded in 1999–2000.* Manuscript in preparation.

Manteuffel, B., Grossman, L.S., & Stephens, B. (2005). Provider attitudes and practices in system-of-care and non-system-of-care communities. In C. Newman, C.J. Liberton, K. Kutash, & R.M. Friedman (Eds.), *The 17th Annual Research Conference Proceedings, A system of care for children's mental health: Expanding the research base* (pp. 53–56). Tampa: University of South Florida, Louis de la Parte Florida Mental Health Institute, Research and Training Center for Children's Mental Health.

Manteuffel, B., Krivelyova, A., Laygo, R.M., Brashears, F., & Grossman, E. (2006). Characteristics of children with chronic physical illnesses, their service use and clinical outcomes in systems of care. In C. Newman, C. Liberton, K. Kutash, & R.M. Friedman (Eds.), *The 18th Annual Research Conference Proceedings: A system of care for children's mental health: Expanding the research base* (pp. 335–340). Tampa: University of South Florida, Louis de la Parte Florida Mental Health Institute, Research and Training Center for Children's Mental Health.

Manteuffel, B., Stephens, R.L., & Santiago, R. (2002). Overview of the national evaluation of the comprehensive community mental health services for children and their families program and summary of current findings. *Children's Services: Social Policy, Research, and Practice, 5*(1), 3–20.

Manteuffel, B., Stephens, R., Sondheimer, D., & Fisher, S. (in review). Characteristics, service experiences, and outcomes of transition-age youth: Policy implications. *Journal of Behavioral Health Services and Research.*

Owley, G.T., & Sternweis, J. (1997). Effectiveness of contracted services in individualizing and tailoring mentor programs for children with serious emotional disturbance in a public system. In C. Liberton, K. Kutash, & R. Freidman (Eds.), *The 9th Annual Research Conference Proceedings: A system of care for children's mental health, Expanding the research base, February 26–28, 1996* (pp. 29–32). Tampa: University of South Florida, Louis de la Parte Florida Mental Health Institute, Research and Training Center for Children's Mental Health.

President's New Freedom Commission on Mental Health. (2003). *Achieving the promise: Transforming mental health care in America. Final report.* (DHHS Pub. No. SMA-03-3832). Rockville, MD: Author.

Price, A.W., Gyamfi, P., Pope, A., & Lockaby, T. (2003). Family resources and children's strengths: Do families matter? In C. Newman, C. Liberton, K. Kutash, & R.M. Friedman (Eds.), *The 15th Annual Research Conference Proceedings, A system of care for children's mental health: Expanding the research base* (pp. 105–111). Tampa: University of South Florida, Louis de la Parte Florida Mental Health Institute, Research and Training Center for Children's Mental Health.

Pullmann, M., Savage, P., & Koroloff, N. (2003). More than money: Do family resources predict caregiver strain? In C. Newman, C. Liberton, K. Kutash, & R.M. Friedman (Eds.), *The 15th Annual Research Conference Proceedings, A system of care for children's mental health: Expanding the research base* (pp. 127–130). Tampa: University of South Florida, Louis de la Parte Florida Mental Health Institute, Research and Training Center for Children's Mental Health.

Reynolds, C.R., & Richmond, B.O. (1978). What I think and feel: A revised measure of children's manifest anxiety. *Journal of Abnormal Psychology, 6*(2), 271–280

Reynolds, W.M. (1986). *Reynolds Adolescent Depression Scale* (2nd ed.). Lutz, FL: Psychological Assessment Resources.

Rosenblatt, A., & Attkisson, C.C. (1992). Integrating systems of care in California for youth with severe emotional disturbance I: A descriptive overview of the California AB377 Evaluation Project. *Journal of Child and Family Studies, 1*(1), 93–113.

Rosenblatt, A., & Attkisson, C.C. (1993). Integrating systems of care in California for youth with severe emotional disturbance III: Answers that lead to questions about out-of-home placements and the AB377 Evaluation Project. *Journal of Child & Family Studies 2*(2), 1–33.

Rosenblatt, A., Attkisson, C.C., & Fernandez, A.J. (1992). Integrating systems of care in California with severe emotional disturbance II: Initial group home expenditure and utilization findings from the California AB377 Evaluation Project. *Journal of Child and Family Studies, 1*(3), 263–286.

Rugs, D., & Kutash, K. (1994). Evaluating children's mental health service systems: An analysis of critical behaviors and events. *Journal of Child and Family Studies, 3*(3), 249–262.

Salazar, J.J., Sherwood, D., & Toche, L.L. (1997). California's system of care model for reducing juvenile crime: Riverside County's successful interagency program. In C.J. Liberton, K. Kutash, & R.M. Friedman (Eds.), *The 9th Annual Research Conference Proceedings, A system of care for children's mental health: Expanding the research base, February 26–28, 1996* (pp. 211–215). Tampa: University of South Florida, Louis de la Parte Florida Mental Health Institute, Research and Training Center for Children's Mental Health.

Sheehan, A.K., Walrath-Greene, C., Fisher, S., Crossbear, S., & Walker, J. (2007). Evidence-based practice knowledge, use, and factors that influence decisions: Results from an evidence-based practice survey of providers in American Indian/Alaska Native communities. *American Indian and Alaska Native Mental Health Research, 14*(2), 29–48.

Sheehan, A.K., Walrath, C.M., & Holden, E.W. (2006). Evidence-based practice use, training, and implementation in the community-based service setting: A survey of children's mental health service providers. *Journal of Child and Family Studies, 16*(2), 169–182.

Silver, S.E., Duchnowski, A.J., Kutash, K., Friedman, R.M., et al., (1992). A comparison of children with serious emotional disturbance served in residential and school settings. *Journal of Child and Family Studies, 1*(1), 43–59.

Silver, S.E., Unger, K., & Friedman, R.M. (1993). *Transition to young adulthood among youth with emotional disturbance* (Report #839). Tampa: University of South Florida, Louis de la Parte Florida Mental Health Institute, Research and Training Center for Children's Mental Health.

Sparrow, S., Carter, A., & Cicchetti, D. (1993) *Vineland Screener: Overview, reliability, validity, administration, and scoring.* New Haven, CT: Yale University Child Study Center.

Stephens, R.L., Brannan, A.M., Holden, E.W., & Soler, R.E. (2005). Youth with emotional, behavioral and substance abuse disorders served in systems of care. In C. Newman, C.J. Liberton, K. Kutash, & R.M. Friedman (Eds.), *The 17th Annual Research Conference Proceedings, A system of care for children's mental health: Expanding the research base* (pp. 447–452). Tampa: University of South Florida, Louis de la Parte Florida Mental Health Institute, Research and Training Center for Children's Mental Health.

Stephens, R.L., Connor, T., Nguyen, H., Holden, E.W., Greenbaum, P., & Foster, E.M. (2005). The longitudinal comparison study of the national evaluation of the Comprehensive Community Mental Health Services for Children and Their Families Program. In M.H. Epstein, K. Kutash, & A.J. Duchnowski (Eds.), *Outcomes for children and youth with behavioral and emotional disorders and their families: Programs and evaluation best practices* (2nd ed., pp. 525–550). Austin, TX: PRO-ED.

Stephens, R.L., Holden, E.W., & Hernandez, M. (2004). System-of-care practice review scores as predictors of behavioral symptomatology and functional impairment. *Journal of Child and Family Studies, 13,* 179–191.

Stroul, B.A., & Friedman, R.M. (1986). *A system of care for children and youth with severe emotional disturbances* (Rev. ed.). Washington, DC: Georgetown University Child Development Center, CASSP Technical Assistance Center.

Stroul, B., Keens-Douglas, A., & Manteuffel, B. (2006, July). *The sustainability of systems of care: Lessons learned.* Poster presented at the Training Institutes: Developing Local Systems of Care for Children and Adolescents with Emotional Disturbances and Their Families: Family-Driven, Youth-Guided Services to Improve Outcomes, Orlando, FL.

Stroul, B.A., & Manteuffel, B.A. (2007). The sustainability of systems of care for children's mental health: Lessons learned. *Journal of Behavioral Health Services and Research, 34,* 237–259.

Stroul, B., Pires, S., & Armstrong, M. (1998). *Special study on managed care: Evaluation of the Comprehensive Community Mental Health Services for Children and Their Families Program.* Atlanta, GA: Macro International Inc.

Substance Abuse and Mental Health Services Administration, U.S. Department of Health and Human Services. (2005). *Transforming mental health care in America. Federal action agenda: First steps* (DHHS Pub. No. SMA-05-4069). Rockville, MD: Author.

Sukumar, B., Manteuffel, B., Soler, R., & Sgro, G. (2003). Caregiver strain among single mother, grandparent, and two-parent caregivers. In C. Newman, C. Liberton, K. Kutash, & R.M. Friedman (Eds.), *The 15th Annual Research Conference Proceedings, A system of care for children's mental health: Expanding the research base* (pp. 111–116). Tampa: University of South Florida, Louis de la Parte Florida Mental Health Institute, Research and Training Center for Children's Mental Health.

Summerfelt, W.T., Foster, E.M., & C. Saunders, R.C. (1996). Mental health services utilization in a children's mental heath managed care demonstration. *Journal of Mental Health Administration, 23*(1), 80–91.

Tannen, N. (1997). Families First in Essex County: A family designed and implemented system of care. In C. Liberton, K. Kutash, & R. Freidman (Eds.), *The 9th Annual Research Conference Proceedings: A system of care for children's mental health, Expanding the research base, February 26–28, 1996* (pp. 145–148). Tampa: University of South Florida, Louis de la Parte Florida Mental Health Institute, Research and Training Center for Children's Mental Health.

Titus, J.C., & Dennis, M.L. (2005). *Global Appraisal of Individual Needs–Quick (GAIN–Q): Administration and scoring guide for the GAIN–Q (version 2).* Retrieved August 30, 2006, from http://www.chestnut.org/LI/gain/GAIN_Q/GAIN-Q_v2_Instructions_09-07-2005.pdf

U.S. Department of Health and Human Services. (1999). *Mental health: A report of the Surgeon General.* Rockville, MD: Author.

Vinson, N., Brannan, A.M., Baughman, L., Wilce, M., & Gawron, T. (2001). The system-of-care model: Implementation in twenty-seven communities. *Journal of Emotional and Behavioral Disorders, 9,* 30–42.

Walrath, C.M., Sheehan, A.K., Holden, E.W., Hernandez, M., & Blau, G.M. (2006). Evidence-based treatments in the field: A brief report on provider knowledge, implementation, and practice. *Journal of Behavioral Health Services and Research, 33*(2), 244–253.

Walrath, C.M., Ybarra, M., & Holden, E.W. (2006). Understanding the prereferral factors associated with differential 6-month outcomes among children receiving system-of-care services. *Psychological Services, 3*(1) 35–50.

Wilhite, K.L. (1996). *Positive agents of change in the transformation of social systems: A role for education.* Indianapolis: Indiana University Press.

3

Integrating the Components into an Effective System of Care

A Framework for Putting the Pieces Together

Sharon Hodges, Robert M. Friedman, and Mario Hernandez

This chapter addresses critical factors in the implementation of systems of care. The main thesis is that the development of a local system of care must be anchored in a clear and widely held local vision that is achievable and that aims to provide an integrated, comprehensive, flexible system that attends as much to the connection between the separate components as it does to the presence and quality of each of its parts. This chapter assumes that the implementation of individual system components, such as wraparound services, evidence-based practices, interagency collaboration, blended funding, and cultural and linguistic competence, do not by themselves produce an effective local system of care. As reassuring as it may be to make progress in establishing a particular component, such efforts can be counterproductive to overall system implementation if they are not part of a strategy aimed at achieving a cohesive, integrated whole that is responsive to the strengths and needs of children, families, and the local community. By nature, the development of such a comprehensive local system is an iterative, constantly evolving, and challenging process, with a foundation and purpose based on a clear understanding and focus on the local population of concern.

EVOLUTION OF THE SYSTEM OF CARE CONCEPT

The publication of *Unclaimed Children* (Knitzer, 1982) decried the woeful condition of services and service sectors, as well as the resulting personal consequences for children with serious emotional disturbances and their families. In response to this book, the federal government, through the National Institute of Mental

71

Health (1983), launched an initiative designed to better serve these children and their families. This effort was based on the recognition that existing services were inadequate and that many children received no mental health services at all. When services were provided, they were typically inappropriately restrictive and uncoordinated among the multiple service sectors involved in the lives of these children and families. The population of concern for the federal initiative was loosely defined as children and adolescents with *Diagnostic and Statistical Manual* (American Psychiatric Association, 2000) diagnoses whose problems were of at least 6 months in duration and who required services from multiple service sectors. Of note in this definition was the mention of the multiple service sectors, including mental health, that provide services for this population of concern. This single mention of multiple service sectors has anchored the direction of service and system improvement efforts in the United States within a holistic process involving collaboration among community, state, and federal partners. Although little was known about this group of children and their families, Knitzer and the federal initiative that followed readily determined that their needs were enormous, their problems complex, and that solutions would require the development of a broad and coordinated range of cross-sector services and supports provided within homes, schools, and communities.

Based on the identification of unmet need and the tremendous social and personal consequences for children with serious emotional disorders, a national vision for change was articulated. This vision, known as *systems of care*, called for a community-based approach to tackling this unmet need. A *system of care* was defined as "a comprehensive spectrum of mental health and other necessary services which are organized into a coordinated network in order to meet the multiple and changing needs of severely emotionally disturbed children and adolescents" (Stroul & Friedman, 1986, p. iv). The system of care concept was first described in a monograph prepared by Stroul and Friedman (1986) on behalf of a number of child mental health leaders across the country. The monograph presented a set of values and principles to serve as the foundation for building systems of care, reviewed the research literature to offer guidance on what services had been shown to be effective, and offered a broad conceptual framework for organizing the work of creating change within multiple sectors for the purpose of keeping children within their communities. The concept of a *system*, as expressed in this monograph, assumed that it is not sufficient to have more and better services available within communities but that it is necessary that services be organized into a cohesive, interdependent, cross-sector whole in which system functioning is dependent on the success of each part.

Early efforts to conceptualize and implement systems of care shared a focus on the need to create systemic improvements in the infrastructure of child-serving organizations, in their interorganizational relationships, and in expanding and improving each sector's service delivery for the purpose of keeping children within their families and communities (Hernandez & Hodges, 2003; Lourie, Katz-Leavy, DeCarolis, & Quinlan, 1996). Knitzer, along with Stroul and Friedman, placed an emphasis on issues related to the changes in organizational relationships and system functioning needed to provide care in less restrictive settings. Systems of care focus on organizational change and the reduction of "bureaucratic turf and other organizational barriers" as a central concept intended to shape local strategies (Lourie et al., 1996, p. 105).

The conceptualization of systems of care has shifted and broadened over time. Stroul and Friedman (1994) captured some of these changes by including person- and family-first language in their definition of systems of care, as well as adding cultural competence to the core values that describe the operational philosophies of a system of care. More recently, the Center for Mental Health Services articulated a definition for systems of care that emphasizes family direction and youth involvement as well as cultural and linguistic competence (Child Adolescent and Family Branch, 2006). In another recent development, the Subcommittee on Children and Families of the President's New Freedom Commission on Mental Health also crafted a vision for children's mental health that is based on a system of care approach and calls for, "a broad array of services and supports to be provided in the child's home, school, and community, in partnership with the family and consistent with the culture, values, and preferences of the child, the youth, and the family" (Huang et al., 2005). This vision also calls for the application of a public health, population-based approach to the planning and delivery of services and supports to prevent child and adolescent mental health problems.

The system of care primer developed by Pires (2002) has been very useful in making the broad concepts more accessible to individuals wishing to implement local systems of care. A significant challenge of implementation, however, is often one of translating broad concepts into local action. The local conceptualization of a system of care and the operationalization of local system concepts affect how implementation is carried out by local stakeholders (Hernandez & Hodges, 2003; Hodges, Ferreira, Israel, & Mazza, 2007a). Because system of care solutions are anchored in a multisector context, the challenge to implementation is magnified by the conflicting mandates and funding restrictions within mental health, education, child welfare, and juvenile justice systems, as well as by policy and leadership changes that regularly occur throughout these service sectors. Moreover, when a local vision is not clearly articulated and widely held by stakeholders, policy and leadership changes wreak havoc on local system of care stability and sustainability. Such implementation challenges are not surprising because a review of the research literature on implementation suggests that good programs and policies often fail to fulfill their potential because of implementation challenges and deficiencies (Fixsen, Naoom, Blase, Friedman, & Wallace, 2005).

In addition, an approach that builds on knowledge of the population of concern is vital to the successful local implementation of a system of care. When local implementers have a clear understanding of those they intend to serve, their planning is more likely to select service and system strategies that are responsive to the needs and strengths of the identified local population of children and their families.

At its inception, the system of care movement identified a population of children with serious emotional disturbance who were involved with multiple service sectors (Stroul & Friedman, 1986). The federal population definition describes a group of children and youth younger than 22 years of age who have a diagnosable mental health disorder that results in reduced functioning in home, school, or community settings or that requires multiagency intervention. Also, this disability must have been present or is expected to be present for at least 1 year (Center for Mental Health Services, 2005). It should be noted, however, that communities adopt their own population definitions, sometimes choosing to focus on specific subgroups of particular concern within their communities. It has been suggested that the goal for the children's mental health field should be to provide access to effective care that is consistent with system of care values and principles for *all* children with or at risk for mental health challenges and their families (Friedman, 2005, 2007).

Although there is widespread support for system of care values and principles, system of care implementation is challenging and unpredictable work. Efforts to develop effective systems of care across the country have met with mixed success (Friedman, 2004b; National Institute on Disability and Rehabilitation Research, 2004). Part of this uneven success is due to the fact that system of care values and principles lack consistent definitions and operationalization at local, state, and federal levels. In addition, system of care implementation requires local knowledge of the population each system intends to serve, goals for system improvement, multisector strategies to reach these goals, and information required to determine if system improvement strategies are accomplishing change in the service of the identified children and their families (Hernandez & Hodges, 2005).

EVOLVING UNDERSTANDING OF SYSTEM IMPLEMENTATION

As the conceptualization of systems of care has evolved since the 1980s, there has been rich discussion of the benefits, accomplishments, and challenges related to systems of care. Since 1984, the Research and Training Center for Children's Mental Health (RTC) in the Department of Child and Family Studies at the University of South Florida has been funded to conduct research in children's mental health, much of it relating directly to systems of care, and has hosted 20 annual research conferences. At the same time, efforts to develop systems of care to effectively serve children with serious mental health challenges and their families across the country have grown, spurred in large measure by the federal Comprehensive Community Mental Health Services for Children and Their Families Program, referred to as the Children's Mental Health Initiative (CMHI) launched by the Center for Mental Health Services in 1993 (Center for Mental Health Services, 2002). The experience of researchers in the RTC, as well as their work with the national evaluation of the CMHI from 1999 to the present and the evaluation of the Annie E. Casey Mental Health Initiative for Urban Children from 1993 to 1999, has contributed to an evolving understanding of system implementation and has yielded six important lessons related to the understanding of system of care implementation. These lessons are related to: 1) thinking holistically, 2) informed decision making, 3) the importance of context, 4) the role of theories of change, 5) system implementation factors, and 6) leveraging system change. Together, they contribute to the implementation of a system that successfully integrates the individual components into a cohesive whole.

Thinking Holistically

In order to develop systems of care, strategies are needed to help local stakeholders organize service sectors into holistic service delivery systems. *Holism* refers to linkages across people, organizations, and service sectors that provide an integrated service response composed of multiple interconnected elements. Service integration across local agency partners is at the heart of the development of systems of care (Hernandez & Hodges, 2006). Proponents of service integration claim that to successfully resolve human services problems, a broad segment of the community must be involved in local problem solving and planning activities (Wandersman, 1984). Placer County, California's, system of care exemplifies service integration through the colocation and cross training of staff, the cross-sector supervision of staff, regular meetings at the executive and manager levels to create an effective collaborative service system, and the use of blended funding to allow system partners creativity in meeting families' needs. This investment in collaboration has built trust among system partners to the point where partners are able to, according to one senior administrator, "put their money on the table and their hands behind their backs." The ultimate benefit of this accomplishment is to orient the system away from self-preservation and perpetuation and toward the efficient service of families in ways that families can understand and appreciate (Hodges, Ferreira, Israel, & Mazza, 2006b).

Holistic thinking supports system linkage. It is also believed to support the capacity of the system to provide an individualized and nonlinear response to the needs of children and families, as well as service integration in system of care implementation efforts (Hodges, Ferreira, Israel, & Mazza, 2007c). A holistic approach to system implementation can be contrasted with the fragmentation and disconnectedness across people, agencies, and service sectors that exist in the absence of a system of care. Holistic thinking can also be contrasted with community efforts to implement a single component of a system of care (e.g., the development of a wraparound program, the creation of a vehicle for blended funding as a proxy for system change). Although such efforts can be important aspects of a system of care, these single actions cannot accomplish the goals of comprehensive system change.

The ability of system planners and implementers to think holistically is affected by whether they consider systems of care to be primarily a child-level intervention or an organizational change strategy. When systems of care are conceptualized primarily as clinical intervention entities, their success is determined by their ability to produce behavioral change at the individual child level. In contrast, when systems of care are conceptualized primarily as organizational change strategies, they can be expected to produce changes in access to an array of community-based services and supports that are individualized, family driven and youth guided, culturally and linguistically competent, and coordinated. Success in producing change at the level of individual children and families requires that the services and supports provided are effective. Although change at the system level may be necessary to make this happen, such changes alone are not sufficient. It is clearly the goal and hope of system planners that changes at both the system level and the child and family level will be achieved. The alignment of policy and system efforts with efforts to deliver effective services will ultimately benefit individual children by creating the systemic framework needed to support the provision of effective interventions at the child and family level.

Successful system implementation is, therefore, best measured by the ability to achieve systemwide goals, such as improved access and availability of services and supports and reductions in the use of restrictive services, than by clinical and behavioral outcomes at the individual child level (Hernandez & Hodges, 2003).

System implementers in Santa Cruz County, California, join representatives from the mental health, child welfare, juvenile probation, and education service sectors in their system-level planning. They focus attention on jointly pursuing and administering grants to fund innovative services, creating cross-disciplinary service teams, colocating staff across sectors, and creating opportunities for joint problem solving when differences in values or responses to families differ across the child-serving systems. The attitude of viewing the whole system as jointly accountable for child outcomes and jointly responsible to each component of the system for survival has allowed the system to survive and thrive, even during shifts in state and federal service and funding priorities (Hodges, Ferreira, Israel, & Mazza, 2006c).

In addition, holistic thinking better prepares system planners and implementers to bridge any conflict among stakeholders as to whether their efforts should be focused on child-level or organizational-level change strategies. Effective services and supports at the level of the individual child and family, as well as system changes that provide access to and availability of services and supports, are necessary for system implementation (Hodges, Ferreira, Israel, & Mazza, 2006a, 2006b, 2006c). As indicated, both must exist to achieve positive change for individual children and families.

Informed Decision Making

Early conceptualizations of system implementation recognized that there is an important need for access to information to mark the progress of system implementation efforts and guide their greater success. Hodges, Woodbridge, and Huang (2001) noted that a variety of initiatives undertaken by federal, state, and local officials since the 1980s have required public managers to provide evidence that their programs actually work. Similarly, funders in the nonprofit arena have become insistent in their requests for documentation of results. Beyond the demonstration of outcomes, however, improving system implementation through the examination of evaluation information involves taking action on what has been learned. Instead of measuring success to meet external accountability standards (e.g., contacts with clients, services provided, number of cases closed, average length of stay), system evaluation in support of system implementation should be driven by the needs of planners, implementers, and community stakeholders.

Informed decision making in service of system implementation suggests that system planners and implementers must look beyond the accountability functions and move forward with processes of internal evaluation that build opportunities for learning, self-correction, and quality control. For Region 3 Behavioral Health Services (BHS) in Central Nebraska, evaluation is an extremely high priority. There is a dual focus on clinical and administrative use of data. Region 3 BHS is unique in its ability to create reports that describe functioning at the system, program, and individual client levels. This capacity encourages people at all levels (e.g., frontline staff, families) to ask relevant questions, and evaluation staff are positioned to respond to these data-based requests. In addition, evaluation staff educate system stakeholders, including family members and other community partners, about evaluation results in order to support data-driven decisions in both short- and long-term time frames. This effort is made to ensure the best possible services for children with or at risk of serious emotional disturbance and their families. Data are also used to ensure that the system maintains its focus on the role of families and youth in the functioning of the system, the strengths of families served, and the diversity of families within this rural and frontier geographic area (Hodges, Ferreira, Israel, & Mazza, 2007a).

The focus on informed decision-making shifts system evaluation away from a summative approach to one that engages evaluators with community partners throughout implementation to identify and gather timely information of practical value. In this context, information can be viewed as an important tool for incremental change. Understanding how systems function in real time while trying to meet a community's needs requires an understanding of the local context. The Ecology of Outcomes model (Hernandez, Hodges, & Cascardi, 1998) was developed as part of a national study of outcome-based system accountability (Research and Training Center for Children's Mental Health, 1994b) that coincided with a growing national emphasis on outcome-based accountability within human services. The Ecology of Outcomes model offers a framework for outcome-based accountability efforts grounded in a local context. Based on this framework, agencies that serve children and families are encouraged to build and use outcome-oriented information systems to respond to their clients in a more flexible manner. The goal of this framework is to improve system implementation efforts by involving stakeholders in the identification of outcomes and in the utilization of results. The Ecology of Outcomes model emphasizes the integration of outcome information into a service system's decision-making process and the inclusion of client, stakeholder, and provider satisfaction information in evaluations.

Issues addressed by the Ecology of Outcomes model include the emphasis human service agencies place on rules compliance, the lack of feedback to program staff to allow for midcourse corrections, and the lack of input by key stakeholders in the identification of outcomes to be measured. The approach emphasizes the value of a planning process in which community stakeholders come together to clarify such basic and important questions as who is their population of concern, what are their goals for that population, and what do they believe it would take to achieve these goals. In this way, the Ecology of Outcomes model has also contributed to an early understanding of system implementation as an iterative and emergent process.

This context-informed decision making stands in contrast to decontextualized approaches to outcome accountability in which outcome measures are selected more because of their psychometric properties and acceptance in the field than because of their relevance to the population of concern or the goals of the system. The Hawaii system of care has developed a data collection and utilization process that is persistently focused on informing real-time, real-world problem solving at all levels of the system. An important marker of system accountability is the idea that any child at any point in time can be considered representative of system performance (Daleiden, Chorpita, Donkervoet, Arensdorf, & Brogan, 2006; Donkervoet, 2005). The focus on data-driven decision making has seeded the collection of data at time intervals and at levels of detail appropriate to issues encountered by system administrators, as well as decision makers involved in frontline care.

In addition, the use of quarterly and annual reports from Family Guidance Centers (lead agencies for children's mental health services) provided to governing bodies such as the state legislature reflect the ability to make data-based decisions about the allocation of resources at different levels within the system. The ability to track monthly service utilization and cost data is critical to the ability of the Hawaii system of care to act strategically during and across fiscal years. These reports also track system performance across a variety of management functions ranging from daily client-level service delivery decisions to broader interagency assessment of system outcomes. The performance reports help system implementers prioritize and assign resources where they are most needed. They also allow community members, funding authorities, and administrators to monitor system performance, take data-based corrective actions, and connect data to policy decisions.

For frontline care coordinators, the creation of a real-time dashboard of clinical services and clinical functioning reflects efforts to measure the effectiveness of practice for individual children and to support the ability to make on-the-spot, data-informed treatment decisions. These evaluation efforts are facilitated by the development of an attitude toward data as a way of asking meaningful questions about system performance. Stakeholders use data as a trigger for discussion of aspects of system functioning and dialogue about system improvement. This mindset enables the constructive application of data in fostering ongoing system improvement (Hodges et al., 2006a).

Importance of Context

Understanding the context in which outcomes occur is only one example of the importance of context during system implementation. To be successful, system implementation efforts must be simultaneously responsive to the needs and strengths of a local population of children and families in the context of the federal, state, and local policies of the multiple child-serving agencies responsible for this population. Variations in context within and across these levels mean that system implementation is rarely attempted in the same environment twice and that the implementation environment for systems of care changes over time.

Defining the local population of concern remains a critical aspect of local context. As noted, the system of care movement initially identified the population of focus as children with serious emotional disturbance (Knitzer, 1982; Stroul & Friedman, 1986), and the 2005 federal definition describes this population as children and youth younger than 22 years of age who have a diagnosable mental health disorder that results in reduced functioning in home, school, or community settings or requires multiagency intervention and whose disability must have been present or is expected to be present for at least 1 year (Center for Mental Health Services, 2005). These definitions are actually broad groupings of children that only provide basic parameters to guide local planning. Communities are expected to identify their own populations of children and families within these parameters. Initially, a community may choose to define the population of focus as a smaller subgroup of children within the juvenile justice, child welfare, or education systems who are of particular local concern. In addition, communities must make strategic decisions about where to begin their efforts and with which part of their local population of concern. This focus can help communities become better able to demonstrate local success to federal and state partners, as well as to think strategically about how to engage local service sectors in system planning efforts.

Placer County, California, provides a good example of a system in which partners have worked collaboratively to expand their population of concern over time. As one administrator noted, the target population had changed from "being system of care kids with serious emotional disturbance now to all kids in the county." This transition was not without challenges; one senior administrator noted, "There was a tension over expanding populations and shifting the financial power base to other agencies." Over time, the system has had to adjust service priorities in keeping with system capacity, but it has retained its focus on building the capacity to serve all children and youth with mental health needs and to serve them before their needs become chronic or severe. A growing amount of attention has been paid to the importance of building capacity to serve ethnically diverse families and very young children. These efforts indicate Placer County's ongoing awareness of the need to continually update the definition of the population of concern and to move toward generating the service capacity to effectively serve this evolving target population (Hodges et al., 2006b).

Responsiveness to context was a concept well-understood by colleagues in anthropology. For anthropologists, ethnographic field methods have always been adaptive and context specific by design, but they are less understood by those trained in more traditional psychological and mental health fields, as was seen in the earliest years of the system of care movement. The importance of cultural competence and family-driven, youth-guided care has brought the lessons of context home to many in the field of children's mental health (Cross, Bazron, Dennis, & Issacs, 1989; Stroul & Friedman, 1994). For successful implementation, system planners and implementers must understand that *mental health treatment* holds different meanings across communities; that children, youth, and families interpret behavior differently; and that family preferences for services and supports and the aspirations families hold for their children and themselves vary as well.

Drawing from their RTC study of community-based theories of change, Hernandez and Hodges (2003) concluded that what is commonly called a system of care can vary considerably from one community to the next and within and across states. Although system of care implementation across the country is based on a similar philosophy and is grounded in clearly articulated values and principles, the operationalization and implementation of these values and principles should reflect the unique needs and opportunities of the communities in which they develop. In this manner, local planning can be consistent with the value of anchoring the planning process around a population, rather than identifying a set of strategies and partners and then imposing them on the local population of concern.

When community planning is based on the knowledge of its own children and families, planners are more likely to select appropriate services and to affect the associated system structures and processes that influence the provision of services. This means that a local system of care must be built on a foundation of local population information. This foundation is what should drive system building and sustainability. Without this core knowledge of context, system planners are likely doomed to work in a manner that is disconnected from the needs and strengths of their local children and families and to proceed in a "business as usual" manner as they espouse system of care values and principles.

In Westchester County, New York, the system of care was developed from a grass roots effort in which community stakeholders came together to form local community networks that assist families whose needs span multiple systems (Hodges, Ferreira, Israel, & Mazza, 2007b). Westchester is a highly diverse county in which community needs vary considerably from one city or town to the next. The community network structure allows for true local problem solving and for individual communities as diverse as Mount Vernon and Peekskill to have a sense of genuine engagement in the system of care. System partners are involved in community-based problem solving around issues specific to their needs. This approach comports with the strong belief within Westchester that local networks drive the system of care and allow local community members to work together to solve problems in a responsive and timely manner. Particularly striking about the community-based networks within Westchester County is the fact that stakeholder participation is voluntary (Hodges et al., 2007b).

Role of Theories of Change

The impact of holistic thinking, informed decision making, and the consideration of context in system implementation is strengthened when system planners and implementers can clearly articulate goals for their community and the strategies they believe will best achieve those goals. Just as successful system implementation should be informed by evaluation data, meaningful implementation efforts must also be grounded in the underlying beliefs and assumptions (i.e., *theory of change*) of the system stakeholders (Chen, 1990; Patton, 1997; Weiss, 1995). The role of theory of change in system of care implementation was initially explored through the national evaluation of the Annie E. Casey Mental Health Initiative for Urban Children (Contreras et al., 2000) and further developed through the RTC (Hodges, Hernandez, Nesman, & Lipien, 2002; Research and Training Center for Children's Mental Health, 1994a, 1994b), as well as through the national evaluation of the Comprehensive Community Mental Health Services for Children and Their Families Program (Hernandez & Hodges, 2005). The expectation is that systems of care can meet the unique population needs of communities by adapting the application of the values and principles to the complex and constantly changing conditions that characterize local service delivery environments; however, the challenges of developing such a system can dissuade even the most inspired and willing advocates of community planning. One strategy for addressing this challenge is to develop a logic model for system of care implementation using a theory of change approach to planning. This process can bring consensus among interagency partners and other stakeholders for a shared overall strategy for system development. Theory of change logic models establish a context for articulating shared beliefs and strategies by having planning participants work together to establish logical connections among those who are expected to be served in their community, the strategies that are expected to be implemented, and the results that can be expected for the effort. The logic model graphically and succinctly depicts these connections, providing a roadmap for system implementation.

The experience of the system partners in Contra Costa County, California, illustrates how a theory of change approach to planning can build consensus across system sectors. System partners representing mental health, juvenile probation, education, and family members used this approach to organize service planning for a population of youth with mental health needs who had been arrested. The partners began their planning process with the assumption that they shared little in terms of values and beliefs. Using the theory of change approach to find common ground, they developed a communitywide and collaborative strategy for serving this population of youth. In doing so, they worked to integrate their independent agency missions into a collaborative vision that would serve their joint purposes while not detracting from their ability to carry out their established agency responsibilities (Hernandez & Hodges, 2006).

The goal of the theory of change approach is to provide a process for expressing and monitoring the link between the ideas or plans for system implementation to the corresponding actions taken by planners and implementers regarding how services and supports are actually deployed. The theory of change approach challenges key stakeholders to be clear about what they want to achieve and how they believe they can accomplish their goals. Through the process of developing theory of change logic models, stakeholders can explore the connection and relationship among the different components of system change. The theory of change process links community outcomes with planned activities and the assumptions or principles that underlie the community planning efforts. When complete, a theory of change logic model can serve as a guide for implementation, ensuring that community plans for service delivery remain true to their intent (Hernandez & Hodges, 2005).

The role of the evaluator in theory of change work departs from the traditional objective and detached evaluator role to one that supports community stakeholder implementation efforts. In Erie County, New York, a core group of planners that included the evaluator, project director, family director, youth coordinator, clinical director, and social marketer met weekly over the course of 4 months to create a theory of change logic model. They used their proposal for funding from the Comprehensive Community Mental Health Services for Children and Their Families Program to develop the logic model components including target population, challenges, assets, goals, and outcomes. In this process, they provided regular feedback on their progress to the management team, which included the governance body for the system of care. As described by their evaluator, the logic model became a tool for strategic planning, evaluation, and continuous quality improvement, with short- and long-term outcomes reviewed on a quarterly basis by the management team. Progress is noted; issues are discussed; and where appropriate, the infrastructure, service delivery, or child- and family-level changes are recommended and approved by consensus of the team (Hernandez & Hodges, 2007). Erie County's logic model is shown on Figure 3.1.

Theory of change development involves the visualization, description, and operationalization of system implementation efforts. Evaluators are encouraged to support the theory of change process by tracking data related to the identified population, system implementation strategies, and multiple levels of outcomes defined in the theory of change logic model. In this way, evaluators and system implementers become facilitators of a community process in which key stakeholders come together to plan their own approach to system change (Hernandez & Hodges, 2006). Theory of change logic models have provided a mechanism for helping stakeholders to clarify their target populations, the goals they intend to achieve, and the connections among the individual components of shared community strategies. They have also provided a mechanism for determining which ongoing data collection directly tied to local goals and strategies can best inform the system implementation efforts so that system planners and implementers can maximize intended gains.

System Implementation Factors

System of care values and principles have been widely accepted and recommended as the foundation for organizing services and supports in children's mental health care across the United States (Friedman, 2002; Huang et al., 2005; President's New Freedom Commission on Mental Health, 2003). Although systems of care have been found to positively affect the structure, organization, and availability of services (Hoagwood, Burns, Kiser, Ringeisen, & Schoenwald, 2001; Rosenblatt, 1998; Stroul, 1993), the implementation of these systems is significantly challenged by a lack of understanding regarding the factors that facilitate system development and how these factors interact to establish well-functioning systems of care (Hernandez & Hodges, 2003). The previously described lessons related to holistic thinking, informed decision making, and theory of change development led RTC researchers to the conclusion that system of care implementation is more challenging than originally anticipated, and traditional research methods have not yielded adequate practical information in support of system implementation.

In an effort to develop a better understanding of the process of system of care implementation, as well as to inform the efforts of communities to effectively accomplish this endeavor, the RTC proposed an implementation framework that emphasizes the importance of the connections among system components, along with a series of studies related to system of care implementation (Friedman, 2004a). The framework was based on a review of the research and theory on systems of care for children with serious emotional disturbance and their families, a review of research and theory in related fields, the experiences of the RTC over many years of conducting research within systems of care and in providing consultation and technical assistance to develop effective systems, and feedback on a preliminary draft of the framework from stakeholder groups (Friedman, 2006).

The framework emphasizes the importance of considering implementation from a systemic perspective rather than seeking to implement individual system components as if they were separate and isolated factors. The premise is that there are certain system implementation factors (e.g., collaboration, family voice and choice, an established provider network) that, when put into practice within communities, contribute to establishing well-functioning systems of care for children with serious emotional disturbances and their families. The 14 system implementation factors are as follows (Friedman, 2004a):

1. Values and principles

2. Population description

3. Theory of change

4. Implementation plan

5. Pathways to care

6. Range of effective services and supports

7. Financing structures and strategies

8. Provider network

9. Provider accountability

10. Family choice

11. Collaboration and family voice

12. Governance

13. Transformational leadership

14. Performance measurement system

Family Voices Network

Mission: Family Voices Network will provide individualized, integrated, comprehensive, culturally competent and cost-effective community-based services that support and promote self-sufficiency of children and families experiencing serious emotional and/or behavioral challenges.

Vision: Erie County will have a family-driven, strength-based integrated system of care that responds with appropriate coordinated services and effective partnering to support self-sufficiency. Services will be timely, flexible, individualized, reducing the need for out-of-home placement as well as shortening the length of stay when there is the need for placement.

Context	Goals	Strategies	Outcomes

Family, youth, and child involvement at each level of SOC

Population of concern

√ Children 5–17 and youth 18–21 in transition with serious emotional or behavioral challenges:

- At imminent risk for out-of-home, school, or community placement

√ And with severe functional impairments, with one or more of the following:

√ Achieve cross-system cultural change

√ Achieve fiscal stability

System strategies

Infrastructure

√ Work with Families CAN to develop youth and family involvement

√ Provide training in SOC principles to become culturally relevant

Service delivery

√ Embrace wraparound philosophy, principles, and values into daily practice

√ Develop integrated point of access

√ Identify gaps, barriers, and capacity service issues

System level

Infrastructure

√ Systemwide sustainability

√ System fiscal reform at local, state, and federal levels

√ Fully developed local SOC infrastructure

√ Increased community SOC knowledge, decreased stigma

84

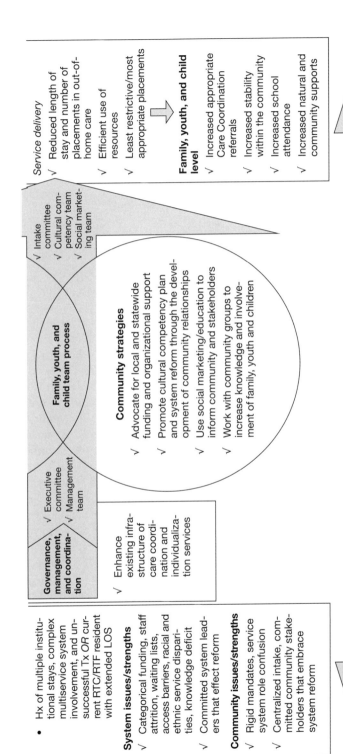

Figure 3.1. Context, goals, and strategies of the Family Voices Network of Erie County. (Reprinted by permission from Erie County Department of Mental Health.) (*Key:* CAN, Child Advocacy Network; Hx, history; LOS, length of stay; RTC/RTF, residential treatment center/facility; SOC, system of care; Tx, treatment.)

Of the 14 factors, four are considered to be the foundation for a system of care: 1) the description and understanding of the population of concern; 2) the development of a set of values and principles through a participatory process involving many stakeholders; 3) the development of a theory of change, also through a participatory process; and 4) the development of a performance measurement system to be used for purposes of ongoing assessment of system performance and continuous improvement.

One of the studies conducted through the RTC was designed, in part, to test the RTC premise that there are 14 system implementation factors that contribute to establishing well-functioning community-based systems of care for children with serious emotional disturbance and their families (Research and Training Center for Children's Mental Health, 2004). Case Studies of System Implementation is a holistic investigation of the iterative and relational aspects of system implementation in long-established systems of care. The investigation uses a multisite embedded case study design to examine the implementation experience of six established systems of care. This study represents a significant departure from previous research efforts that conceptualize system of care implementation as a predictable and step-wise system change. This study gathers data from multiple sources and through various methods in each community in an effort to capture the adaptive processes of system implementation. Established systems participating in Case Studies of System Implementation were identified through a national nomination process and were selected on the basis of having: 1) an identified local population(s) of youth with serious emotional disturbance, 2) clearly identified goals for this population that are consistent with system of care values and principles, 3) active implementation of strategies to achieve these goals, 4) outcome information demonstrating progress toward these goals, and 5) system sustainability that has been demonstrated over time.

The identification and definition of critical factors in local system of care implementation was an important aspect of data collection and analysis at each participating site. Local implementation factors were identified, defined, and validated by key stakeholders in each community through multiple methods, independent of the factors hypothesized by the RTC.

The core components of system implementation that were identified as critical by local stakeholders in Case Studies of System Implementation are remarkably similar across sites (Ferreira, 2007; Mazza, Ferreira, Hodges, Pinto, & Israel, 2006). Cross-site findings of locally identified implementation factors provide insight into the implementation experience of local system stakeholders and the methods by which they leveraged system change. These findings (Hodges, Ferreira, Israel, & Mazza, 2006d) are organized into four categories of implementation factors: 1) values and beliefs, 2) goals, 3) structures, and 4) information.

Values and Beliefs Factors   Values and beliefs shift the mindset of the system. Cross-site analyses indicate that factors related to the values and beliefs of system stakeholders incorporate three important characteristics:

1. Stakeholders share the values and beliefs that aligning service planning and delivery strategies with system of care principles will result in benefit to children and families.

2. Stakeholders share the values and beliefs that trust, commitment, and shared responsibility across system stakeholders is critical to system functioning.

3. Stakeholders share the belief that change is possible and that responsiveness and commitment to change make it possible to transcend the initial fragmented conditions of service delivery.

Goals Factors   System goals solidify stakeholder values and beliefs and orient system activity toward specific actions. Cross-site analyses indicate that as system of care values and beliefs begin to permeate the system, stakeholders set in motion the use of goal-related actions to establish shared expectations and intended outcomes for system change.

Structures Factors   Collaborative structures support system implementation. Data indicate that participating systems created structural changes related to specified roles, responsibilities, and authorities that enabled their systems to perform their functions. Structural changes were made in service of the articulated values and beliefs. These included the following:

1. Changes in the physical arrangement of services such as the colocation of cross-agency staff

2. Changes in the structures and budgetary authorities that facilitate interagency decision making regarding service eligibility and placement

3. Creation of an infrastructure that facilitates transition across service environments, such as home and school, as well as transitions to varying levels of services

Information Factors   Cross-site data indicate that information shapes the direction of system development. The structure and availability of information were strategically designed to support system development and reach specific agreed-on goals. Across systems, stakeholders were clear on the intent of their system activities, and they used information about system performance to shape the direction of system development. For each system, the structure and availability of system information created an informed responsiveness to local conditions. This allowed stakeholders to take action in response to local need and to make system modifications as local conditions or concerns changed.

Analyses of cross-site data suggest that the 14 theoretically-derived RTC implementation factors may well be characteristic of ideal and well-functioning systems of care. These characteristics consist of system structures, processes, and methods that support well-functioning systems of care. For example, factors such as a range of effective services and supports and an established provider network represent *structures* that are characteristic of ideal or well-functioning systems of care. Similarly, factors such as collaboration and family voice can be characterized as *processes* representative of a well-functioning system and having a widely-held theory of change or a shared foundation of values and principles are *methods* for supporting a well-functioning system of care.

Leveraging System Change

There is still much to learn about what factors are critical in bringing about system change and how these factors interact to establish well-functioning systems. The concept of leverage points is useful in understanding how local system developers have accomplished change and met the challenges inherent in planning and implementing their systems of care. *Leverage points* are defined as "places within a complex system where a small shift in one thing can produce big changes in everything" (Meadows 1999, p. 1). For systems of care, leverage points can be defined as places of influence where system planners and implementers strategically intervene in their existing system context to affect the development of their systems of care. The concept of leverage points is significant to system of care development for several reasons (Hodges et al., 2006d):

- The identification of leverage points specific to systems of care can illuminate key strategies for system development.

- The complex adaptive nature of systems of care makes it difficult for system planners and implementers to know which system interventions will produce desired change. Identification of leverage points will allow planners and implementers to better relate action to change.

- The identification of leverage points critical to system of care development can provide important strategies for expanding the capacity of systems to meet the needs of underserved and inappropriately served children and youth.

- The well-being of individual children with serious emotional disturbance and their families depends on the system of care's ability to provide access and availability of services and supports, so it is critical to maximize the advantage created by any system development efforts.

The identification of key leverage points can help system planners and implementers maximize that advantage.

Systems of care emerge from the choices and actions of stakeholders throughout the system, including family members, frontline staff, and community partners. Some of these choices and actions are the result of careful planning, whereas others emerge from the individuals in the system in an unplanned and unanticipated yet often very helpful way. The experiences of system of care implementers suggest the broad guidelines for leveraging system change (Hodges et al., 2007c):

1. Create an early and consistent focus on values and beliefs. The emphasis on values and beliefs provides a significant anchor for system development regardless of the challenges faced.

2. Translate shared beliefs into shared responsibility and shared action. Most importantly, share a commitment to the principle that things really can be done differently and that local stakeholders can be empowered to make change.

3. Recognize that opportunities to leverage change are not linear. Take advantage of opportunities to leverage system change whenever and wherever they occur.

4. Clearly articulate intended change and know that being concrete does not mean being static. Being concrete about values and strategic about action allows stakeholders to be flexible in system response and proactive in system development.

5. Undertake structural change only if the reason for doing so is solidly anchored in system values and beliefs; it is otherwise challenging to sustain the positive impact sought by system of care implementers.

NEW UNDERSTANDING OF SYSTEM IMPLEMENTATION

As Baum (1999) suggested, the real-world experience of system implementation includes contexts that reflect political change, government regulation, and linkages across community institutions. During the past 20 years, many in the field of children's mental health have come to understand that system of care implementation is a process of evolution and emergence that requires adaptation to changing conditions and opportunities. Increasingly, experience demonstrates that it is useful to ground system of care implementation in literature related to complexity theory (Capra, 2002; Holland, 1995) and systems theory (Checkland, 1993; Meadows, 1999). This grounding is helpful because it informs system implementation efforts by making conscious use of the concept of *wholeness* in an effort to conceptualize the complexity of the world around us.

Applying systems and complexity theory to system of care implementation provides a useful new direction because these theoretical perspectives serve as a reminder that a set of elements can come together in human organizations to form a whole that has different properties than those of the individual component parts (Checkland, 1993, 1999; Gharajedaghi, 1999). This theoretical grounding reminds us that system of care implementation need not be viewed as a linear process of achieving goals. Instead, the implementation of systems of care can be viewed as a process of continuous construction and reconstruction by individual stakeholders and community groups in an ongoing process that reflects the complexity of their experiences.

Assumptions, often implicit, about the nature of causal relationships can interfere with our understanding of system implementation. Experience reveals that system of care implementation has few well-defined linear relationships, making less viable the notion that a set of specific actions can produce a system of care in a predictable and measurable way. This understanding has significant implications because it suggests different ways of thinking about system development in the field of children's mental health (Friedman, 2007; Hodges, 2007). The process of relating real-world experience to action is a complex activity that requires holistic study to capture multifaceted and layered organizational processes. Understanding of system of care implementation will be enriched by the exploration and advancement of research methods that integrate scientific rigor with real-world experience because these are better suited for understanding the dynamic and complex environments of systems of care. The application of systems and complexity theory can teach stakeholders to anticipate that there will always be new patterns emerging within the realm system of care implementation.

CONCLUSION

This chapter emphasized the complexity and challenge involved in implementing effective systems of care, placing a particular focus on the need to develop systems of care in which all of the important components are integrated into a cohesive whole to make for a genuinely comprehensive system. Senge (1990) indicated that in a learning organization, it is essential to adopt a systemic framework in which individuals constantly consider the importance of the interrelationships among each of the components. Plsek (2001), placing similar emphasis on the importance of a systemic framework, indicated that rather than the power being in individual parts of a system, "the real power lies in the way the parts come together and are interconnected to fulfill some purpose" (p. 309). Senge (1990) also emphasized the importance within a learning organization of constantly examining the mental models or conceptual frameworks that are used to help make sense of complex information. As part of that process of examining the mental models, this chapter has offered adaptations to the system of care framework based on research, theory, and field experience for purposes of enhancing the effective implementation of systems of care.

REFERENCES

American Psychiatric Association. (2000). *Diagnostic and Statistical Manual of Mental Disorders, Fourth Edition, Text Revision* (DSM-IV-TR). Washington, DC: Author.

Baum, J. (1999). Organizational ecology. In S. Clegg & C. Hardy (Eds.), *Studying organization: Theory and method* (pp. 71–108). Thousand Oaks, CA: Sage Publications.

Capra, F. (2002). *The hidden connections: Integrating the biological, cognitive, and social dimensions of life into a science of sustainability.* New York: Doubleday.

Center for Mental Health Services. (2002). *Cooperative agreements for the Comprehensive Community Mental Health Services for Children and Their Families Program, Guidance for Applicants (GFA), No. SM-02-002 Part I: Programmatic Guidance.* Rockville, MD: Substance Abuse and Mental Health Services Administration.

Center for Mental Health Services. (2005). *Cooperative agreements for the Comprehensive Community Mental Health Services for Children and Their Families Program, request for applicants (RFA), No. SM-05-010.* Rockville, MD: Substance Abuse and Mental Health Services Administration. Retrieved November 3, 2006, from http://www.samhsa.gov/grants/2005/nofa/sm05010rfa_cmhi.pdf

Checkland, P. (1993). *Systems thinking, systems practice.* New York: Wiley.

Checkland, P. (1999). *Soft systems methodology: A 30-year retrospective.* New York: Wiley.

Chen, H.T. (1990). *Theory-driven evaluations.* Thousand Oaks, CA: Sage Publications.

Child Adolescent and Family Branch. (2006). *Helping children and youth with serious mental health needs: Systems of care.* Retrieved October 6, 2006, from http://systemsofcare.samhsa.gov/newinformation/docs/SOCfactsheet.pdf

Contreras, R., Friedman, R. M., Gutiérrez-Mayka, M., Hernandez, M., Joseph, R., Sengova, J., et al. (2000). *Systems reform in the Annie E. Casey Foundation Mental Health Initiative for Urban Children: Final evaluation report.* Tampa: University of South Florida, Louis de la Part Florida Mental Health Institute, Child and Family Studies.

Cross, T., Bazron, B., Dennis, K., & Issacs, M.R. (1989). *Towards a culturally competent system of care.* Washington, DC: Georgetown University Child Development Center, Child and Adolescent Service System Program (CASSP) Technical Assistance Center.

Daleiden, E.L., Chorpita, B.F., Donkervoet, C., Arensdorf, A.M., & Brogan, M. (2006). Getting better at getting them better: Health outcomes and evidence-based practice within a system of care. *Journal of the American Academy of Child and Adolescent Psychiatry, 45*(6), 749–756.

Donkervoet, C. (2005, March). *Hawaii's system of care: Lessons from the field*: Presentation at the 18th Annual Research Conference—A system of care for children's mental health: Expanding the research base, Tampa, FL.

Ferreira, K. (2007). Leveraging implementation in complex systems. In C. Newman, C. Liberton, K. Kutash, & R.M. Friedman (Eds.), *The 19th Annual Research Conference Proceedings—A system of care for children's mental health: Expanding the research base* (pp. 13–16). Tampa: University of South Florida, Louis de la Part Florida Mental Health Institute, Research and Training Center for Children's Mental Health.

Fixsen, D.L., Naoom, S.F., Blase, K.A., Friedman, R.M., & Wallace, F. (2005). *Implementation research: A synthesis of the literature* (FMHI Publication #231). Tampa: University of South Florida, Louis de la Parte Florida Mental Health Institute, The National Implementation Research Network.

Friedman, R.M. (2002, July). *Children's mental health: A status report and call to action.* Paper presented at the President's New Freedom Commission on Mental Health, Washington, DC.

Friedman, R.M. (2004a). *Application for a rehabilitation research and training center for developing and implementing integrated systems of care for children and adolescent mental health.* Tampa: University of South Florida, Louis de la Part Florida Mental Health Institute, Research and Training Center for Children's Mental Health.

Friedman, R.M. (2004b, March). *Systems of care: Present status and tomorrow's framework.* Presentation at the 17th Annual Research Conference—A system of care for children's mental health: Expanding the research base, Tampa, FL.

Friedman, R.M. (2005). *Transformation work group report.* Tampa: University of South Florida, Louis de la Parte Florida Mental Health Institute, Department of Child and Family Studies.

Friedman, R.M. (2006). A model for implementing effective systems of care. In C. Newman, C. Liberton, K. Kutash, & R.M. Friedman (Eds.), *The 18th Annual Research Conference Proceedings—A system of care for children's mental health: Expanding the research base* (pp. 3–9). Tampa: University of South Florida, Louis de la Parte Florida Mental Health Institute, Research and Training Center for Children's Mental Health.

Friedman, R.M. (2007, March). *Conceptualization and measurement of systems of care: Implications for maximizing the effectiveness of systems of care*: Presentation at the 20th Annual Research Conference—A system of care for children's mental health: Expanding the research base, Tampa, FL.

Gharajedaghi, J. (1999). *Systems thinking: Managing chaos and complexity.* Boston: Butterworth-Heinemann.

Hernandez, M., & Hodges, S. (2003). Building upon the theory of change for systems of care. *Journal of Emotional and Behavioral Disorders, 11*(1), 19–26.

Hernandez, M., & Hodges, S. (2005). *Crafting logic models for systems of care: Ideas into action* (Rev. ed.). Tampa: University of South Florida, Louis de la Parte Florida Mental Health Institute.

Hernandez, M., & Hodges, S. (2006). Applying a theory of change approach to interagency planning in child mental health. *American Journal of Community Psychology, 38*(3), 165.

Hernandez, M., & Hodges, S. (2007, May). The advantage of utilizing logic models. *Evaluation Update,* 1.

Hernandez, M., Hodges, S., & Cascardi, M. (1998). The ecology of outcomes: System accountability in children's mental health. *Journal of Behavioral Services and Research, 25*(2), 136–150.

Hoagwood, K., Burns, B., Kiser, L., Ringeisen, H., & Schoenwald, S. (2001). Evidence-based practice in child and adolescent mental health services. *Psychiatric Services, 52*(9), 1179–1184.

Hodges, S. (2007). *Conceptualization and measurement of systems of care: Case studies of system implementation.* Presentation at the 20th Annual Research Conference—A system of care for children's mental health: Expanding the research base, Tampa, FL.

Hodges, S., Ferreira, K., Israel, N., & Mazza, J. (2006a). *Leveraging change in the Hawaii system of care: Site report for case studies of system implementation.* Tampa: University of South Florida, Louis de la Parte Florida Mental Health Institute, Research and Training Center for Children's Mental Health.

Hodges, S., Ferreira, K., Israel, N., & Mazza, J. (2006b). *Leveraging change in the Placer County, California system of care: Site report for case studies of system implementation.* Tampa: University of South Florida, Louis de la Parte Florida Mental Health Institute, Research and Training Center for Children's Mental Health.

Hodges, S., Ferreira, K., Israel, N., & Mazza, J. (2006c). *Leveraging change in the Santa Cruz County, California system of care: Site report for case studies of system implementation.* Tampa: University of South Florida, Louis de la Parte Florida Mental Health Institute, Research and Training Center for Children's Mental Health.

Hodges, S., Ferreira, K., Israel, N., & Mazza, J. (2006d). *Strategies of system of care implementation: Making change in complex systems.* Tampa: University of South Florida, Louis de la Parte Florida Mental Health Institute, Department of Child and Family Studies, Research and Training Center for Children's Mental Health.

Hodges, S., Ferreira, K., Israel, N., & Mazza, J. (2007a). *Leveraging change in the Region III Behavioral Health system of care: Site report for case studies of system implementation.* Tampa: University of South Florida, Louis de la Parte Florida Mental Health Institute, Research and Training Center for Children's Mental Health.

Hodges, S., Ferreira, K., Israel, N., & Mazza, J. (2007b). *Leveraging change in the Westchester County, New York system of care: Site report for case studies of system implementation.* Tampa: University of South Florida, Louis de la Parte Florida Mental Health Institute, Research and Training Center for Children's Mental Health.

Hodges, S., Ferreira, K., Israel, N., & Mazza, J. (2007c). *System implementation issue brief #1—Lessons from successful systems: System of care definition.* Tampa: University of South Florida, Louis de la Parte Florida Mental Health Institute, Research and Training Center for Children's Mental Health.

Hodges, S., Hernandez, M., Nesman, T., & Lipien, L. (2002). *Creating change and keeping it real: How excellent child-serving organizations carry out their goals.* Tampa: University of South Florida, Louis de la Parte Florida Mental Health Institute, Research and Training Center for Children's Mental Health.

Hodges, S., Woodbridge, M., & Huang, L.N. (2001). Creating useful information in data-rich environments. In B.A. Stroul & R.M. Friedman (Series Eds.) & M. Hernandez & S. Hodges (Vol. Eds.), *Systems of care for children's mental health series: Developing outcome strategies in children's mental health* (pp. 239–256). Baltimore: Paul H. Brookes Publishing Co.

Holland, J.H. (1995). *Hidden order: How adaptation builds complexity.* Reading, MA: Helix Books.

Huang, L., Stroul, B., Friedman, R.M., Mrazek, P., Friesen, B., Pires, S., et al. (2005). Transforming mental health care for children and their families. *American Psychologist, 60*(6), 615.

Knitzer, J. (1982). *Unclaimed children: The failure of public responsibility to children and adolescents in need of mental health services.* Washington, DC: Children's Defense Fund.

Lourie, I.S., Katz-Leavy, J., DeCarolis, G., & Quinlan, W.A., Jr. (1996). The role of the federal government. In B.A. Stroul & R.M. Friedman (Series Eds.) & B.A. Stroul (Vol. Ed.), *Children's mental health: Creating systems of care in a changing society* (pp. 99–114). Baltimore: Paul H. Brookes Publishing Co.

Mazza, J., Ferreira, K., Hodges, S., Pinto, A., & Israel, N. (2006, February). *A piece of the puzzle: Identifying local system implementation factors.* Poster presentation at the 19th Annual Research Conference: A system of care for children's mental health: Expanding the research base, Tampa, FL.

Meadows, D. (1999). *Leverage points: Places to intervene in a system.* Hartland, VT: The Sustainability Institute.

National Institute of Mental Health. (1983). *Program announcement: Child and Adolescent Service System Program.* Rockville, MD: Author.

National Institute on Disability and Rehabilitation Research. (2004, March 25). Announcement of priorities. *Federal Register, 69*(58), 15308–15311.

Patton, M. (1997). *Utilization-focused evaluation: The new century text.* Thousand Oaks, CA: Sage Publications.

Pires, S.A. (2002). *Building systems of care: A primer.* Washington DC: National Technical Assistance Center for Children's Mental Health.

Plsek, P. (2001). Redesigning health care with insights from the science of complex adaptive systems. In Committee on Quality of Health Care in America and Institute of Medicine (Ed.), *Crossing the quality chasm: A new health system for the 21st century* (pp. 309–322). Washington, DC: National Academies Press.

President's New Freedom Commission on Mental Health. (2003). *Achieving the promise: Transforming mental healthcare in America. Final report* (DHHS Publication SMA-03-3831). Rockville, MD: Author.

Research and Training Center for Children's Mental Health. (1994a). *Community-based theories of change.* Tampa: University of South Florida, Louis de la Parte Florida Mental Health Institute, Research and Training Center for Children's Mental Health.

Research and Training Center for Children's Mental Health. (1994b). *System accountability study.* Tampa: University of South Florida, Louis de la Parte Florida Mental Health Institute, Research and Training Center for Children's Mental Health.

Research and Training Center for Children's Mental Health. (2004). *Accessibility of mental health services: Identifying and measuring organizational factors associated with reducing mental health disparities.* Tampa: University of South Florida, Louis de la Parte Florida Mental Health Institute, Research and Training Center for Children's Mental Health.

Rosenblatt, A. (1998). Assessing the child and family outcomes of systems of care for youth with serious emotional disturbance. In M. Epstein, K. Kutash, & A. Duchnowski (Eds.), *Outcomes for children and youth with behavioral and emotional disorders and their families* (pp. 329–362). Austin, TX: PRO-ED.

Senge, P.M. (1990). *The fifth discipline: The art and practice of the learning organization.* New York: Doubleday/Currency.

Stroul, B. (1993). *Systems of care for children and adolescents with severe emotional distur-bances: What are the results?* Washington, DC: Georgetown University Child Develop-ment Center, National Technical Assistance Center for Children's Mental Health.

Stroul, B., & Friedman, R.M. (1986). *A system of care for severely emotionally disturbed chil-dren and youth.* Washington, DC: Georgetown University Child Development Center, CASSP Technical Assistance Center.

Stroul, B., & Friedman, R.M. (1994). *A system of care for children and youth with severe emotional disturbances* (Rev. ed.). Washington, DC: Georgetown University Child De-velopment Center, CASSP Technical Assistance Center.

Wandersman, A. (1984). Citizen participation. In K. Heller, R. Price, S. Reinharz, S. Riger, & A. Wandersman (Eds.), *Psychology and community change: Challenges of the fu-ture.* (pp. 337–379). Homewood, IL: Dorsey Press.

Weiss, C.H. (1995). Nothing as practical as good theory: Exploring theory-based evalua-tion for comprehensive community initiatives. In J. Connel, A. Kubisch, L. Schorr, & C. Weiss (Eds.), *New approaches to evaluating community initiatives* (pp. 65–92). Wash-ington, DC: The Aspen Institute.

II

Building Systems of Care

4

Building Systems of Care
Critical Processes and Structures

SHEILA A. PIRES

Building anything, including systems of care, involves process and structures (Pires, 2002a). *Process* fundamentally entails the people involved in a system-building effort; the roles, rights, and responsibilities each stakeholder is accorded or assumes; and how these various players communicate, negotiate, and collaborate with one another. Process also has to do with being—or failing to be—strategic. *Structure* refers to those functions that become organized in certain defined arrangements (e.g., how children enter the system, how services and supports are individualized, how care is managed, how services are financed). Process breakdowns are arguably more harmful to building systems of care and more difficult to repair than are structural breakdowns. However, structure (i.e., how functions are organized) can undermine even the most effective system-building processes. This chapter discusses the role of process and structure in systems of care, identifies key elements of effective system-building processes, outlines the many functions that must be structured or restructured within systems of care, and discusses the impact of structure on the experience of stakeholders and the achievement of desired outcomes.

CORE ELEMENTS OF AN EFFECTIVE SYSTEM-BUILDING PROCESS

Process has to do with *how*, meaning the manner in which system builders proceed, whom they involve, the relationships they establish, how they conduct themselves, and so forth. Based on their experience analyzing local systems of care throughout the country, a number of observers have identified certain core elements essential to an effective system-building process (Lourie, 1994; Stroul, 1996). These elements tend to cluster into two areas—*leadership and constituency building* as the first and *strategic orientation* as the second. These two clusters are obviously related, as effective leaders are strategic, and strategizing effectively requires leadership across stakeholder groups at both the state and local levels.

Importance of Leadership and Constituency Building

Core Leadership Group   When it comes to system building, someone has to give the ball its first push and then keep it rolling. Core group leadership members come from the constituencies that are affected by and have a vested interest in system of care building (e.g., family members and youth, neighborhood and community representatives, state and local officials, agency heads, staff, providers, advocates, funding entities, professional organizations, university researchers, union representatives, legislative body representatives). The core leadership group may start out small and grow over time, or vice versa. To be significantly effective, a core group must have "the five *Cs*":

1. *Constituency* representativeness

2. *Credibility* within the community

3. *Capacity* to engage other stakeholders

4. *Commitment* to the difficult work of system building

5. *Consistency* in focus

Evolving Leadership   Successful system-building processes tend to draw on different leadership styles at different developmental periods. Initially, or during periods when system building becomes stalled, the charismatic, visionary leadership style often dominates. In a developing system, the facilitative leadership approach of "giving away power" (i.e., empowering others to share leadership responsibilities) may prevail. In a maturing system, the leader with strong management skills may hold sway. There are no right or wrong leadership styles among these in and of themselves. Only timing and task make them so, and all are necessary in the system building formula. Successful system builders pay attention to the types of leadership styles needed at different developmental stages throughout the process. As Magrab (1999) noted, leadership for systems of care requires a shift in the leadership paradigm from independence to interdependence and from competition to collaboration. Successful systems of care strive to develop leadership and share it across stakeholder groups. Parent and youth leaders, state leaders in both executive and legislative branches, local leaders, judicial leaders, provider leaders, community leaders, and leaders among natural helpers are all important to the growth of systems of care.

Effective Collaboration   Collaboration is at the heart of system building (Hodges, Nesman, & Hernandez, 1999). Children and youth with emotional and behavioral challenges and their families depend on multiple agencies, providers, community supports, and funding entities, as well as their own internal resources. When one hand does not know what the other is doing, inefficiencies, frustration, and ultimately poor outcomes result at both the system and service levels. Building systems of care requires resources that span across agencies and among partners. Without collaboration, effective system building cannot occur. Collaboration merely for the sake of collaboration, however, can be just as destructive to system building as no collaboration at all. Effective collaboration has a purpose and concrete objectives that will change over time.

Effective collaboration does not just occur because stakeholders are well-meaning. It takes time, energy, and attention to relationship building, trust building, capacity building, team building, conflict resolution, mediation, development of a common language, and communication (Stark, 1999). Table 4.1 offers guidance for collaboration.

Partnership with Families and Youth The family movement in the children's mental health arena has adopted the maxim "Nothing about us without us." The system-building process that fails to develop a meaningful partnership with the constituency that will depend on the system is inherently suspect and limited in its capacity to build an effective system. Meaningful partnerships with families and youth require concerted attention, dedicated resources, and capacity building among all parties (Osher, deFur, Nava, Spencer, & Toth-Dennis, 1999).

Culturally and Linguistically Competent Processes Systems of care typically serve children, youth, and families from diverse racial, ethnic, and socioeconomic backgrounds. Effective systems of care make every effort to respect, understand, and be responsive to cultural and linguistic differences. Effective system-building processes also acknowledge and proactively address the disparities in access and treatment that historically have been the experience of racially and culturally diverse families in traditional systems (U.S. Department of Health and Human Services, 2000). One would be hard pressed to find a state or locality in the country in which ethnically, racially, and linguistically diverse children and

Table 4.1. Principles to guide collaboration

Build and maintain trust so collaborative partners are able to share information, perceptions, and feedback and work as a cohesive team

Agree on core values that each partner can honor in spirit and practice

Focus on common goals that all partners will strive to achieve

Develop a common language so all partners can have a common understanding of terms such as "family involvement" and "culturally competent services"

Respect the knowledge and experience each person brings

Assume best intentions of all partners

Recognize strengths, limitations, and needs; and identify ways to maximize participation of each partner

Honor all voices by respectfully listening to each partner and attending to the issues they raise

Share decision making, risk taking, and accountability so that risks are taken as a team and the entire team is accountable for achieving the goals

From Stark, D. (1999). *Collaboration basics: Strategies from six communities engaged in collaborative efforts among families, child welfare, and children's mental health* (pp. 5–6). Washington, DC: Georgetown Child Development Center, National Technical Assistance Center for Children's Mental Health; reprinted by permission.

families are not overrepresented in the most restrictive, deep-end services and under-represented in quality community-based services. This tends to be the case even in states and communities with relatively few racial and ethnic minority families.

To be effective, system-building processes must pay attention to the impact of culture, ethnicity, race, gender, sexual orientation, and class within the process itself, as well as to the ways systems operate and the ability of families to obtain and use services. Achieving cultural competence in systems of care is developmental and thus does not simply happen overnight. It requires concerted attention over time and clear priority designation by system leaders. Successful system leaders draw on a variety of approaches and strategies employed on an ongoing basis to build cultural proficiency into the system of care.

Connections to Neighborhood Resources and Natural Helpers

Successful systems of care blend clinical services and natural supports, helping families gain access and make use of both. Natural supports are those found within the neighborhoods in which families live and within the affinity groups with which they associate or would associate if they existed. Natural supports include people such as natural helpers, organizations such as faith-based entities and parent associations, programs such as mentoring support, and activities such as parent support and education activities (Lazear et al., 2001).

Families and youth are the best definers of natural supports that could make a difference in their lives. They are a critical voice in defining the supports that must be systemically available and those that must be integrated within their own individualized plans of care. The use of natural supports is essential for achieving quality, efficacy, and cost outcomes, particularly for families who have children with serious disorders, as well as for impoverished, inner city, and rural families who often feel isolated and for whom clinical services are especially in short supply. A connection to neighborhood resources and natural helpers is also critical to incorporate cultural competence into service delivery. Successful system builders figure out ways to include natural supports within the financing, benefit design, provider network, and care planning arrangements of local systems of care. They also ensure that natural helpers and providers of neighborhood resources and supports are engaged in the system-building process. This requires leadership across stakeholder groups at neighborhood, local (e.g., city, county), and state levels.

Bottom-Up and Top-Down Approaches

Neither a bottom-up (i.e., local) nor a top-down (i.e., state) approach on its own can lead to sustainable systems of care. Engagement and buy-in from stakeholders at both local (i.e., neighborhood, community, city, and county) and state levels are needed. Working simultaneously at multiple levels requires leadership and strategic partnerships and alliances.

Obviously, the more compatible stakeholder objectives are across state, local, and community levels, the greater the likelihood of success, if for no other reason than that system building requires resources from all levels. Compatibility may not be entirely achievable, but it is necessary to recognize its importance and make the effort to create it as opportunities continually present themselves. In general, the greater degree of alignment of interests across stakeholder groups at all levels, the more effective and sustainable the system-building effort will be.

Effective Communication Vehicles   System building is a complex task involving multiple players at different levels. Effective communication, both internal and external, is critical for many reasons. Communication conveys information, and information is power. Lack of communication is guaranteed to leave certain groups of stakeholders (e.g., youth, parents, providers, county officials, state officials, judges) feeling powerless and disenfranchised, not to mention angry and hostile toward the system-building effort. Effective communication helps prevent the misinterpretation of system design and implementation intentions that so often characterizes complex reform efforts. Communication is also critical to quality improvement and for allowing participants to learn as they go. It can help build credibility, which in turn helps expand systems of care. Communication also is essential for increasing awareness of mental health issues and reducing the stigma that is often associated with it.

Conflict Resolution, Mediation, and Team-Building Mechanisms
In the world of complex systems, ever expanding knowledge bases, and intricate webs of human relationships, it is a challenge for diverse groups of people to come together to effectively make decisions and solve problems (Schwarz, 1995). Even when stakeholders share a common vision, cohesion and consensus among disparate stakeholder groups does not simply materialize and remain constant. To address the interests of all those at the table, as well as to reach decisions that will lead to mutually acceptable actions, the system-building process must ensure that the capabilities and strengths of all members of the group are brought to bear on the solutions and actions that emerge. Where there is clear purpose, open communication, active participation, respectful disagreement, and consensus decision making, there is greater likelihood of sustainable decisions and long-term effectiveness.

Positive Attitude   There is an abundance of research in the health field to suggest that a positive outlook is associated with emotional and physical well-being and longevity. This would seem to be the case in the system-building arena as well. System of care observers have noted that successful systems seem to be blessed with leaders across stakeholder groups who think positively, even in the face of daunting challenges and setbacks. It is easy to find the negatives and accentuate the problems in system building, but doing so is singularly unhelpful. This is not to suggest that effective system leaders are or must be unrealistic or naïve. Indeed, successful leaders typically have considerable experience across diverse arenas and constituencies. They know that a system-building effort can be derailed too easily by naysayers, both within its own ranks and from outside entities, and that there is typically much that can be attacked as the system of care challenges existing ways of doing business and suffers its own growing pains. On an ongoing basis, successful leaders identify and help others to see what is positive and worth their continuing efforts to achieve.

Strategic Orientation

Importance of Being Strategic   Effective system builders strategically plan and implement, meaning they are continually scanning the environment in search of opportunities to generate interest, build constituencies, create buy-in, reengineer financing streams, utilize existing structures, and so forth. Being strategic is both a science and an art. It requires knowing how to use data and having good political instincts. It also requires knowing the timing and nature of key legislative and budget decisions and capitalizing on relationships with policy makers. Being strategic necessitates an understanding of how traditional systems can change and the ability to figure out how to convince traditional agency directors to join system change efforts. It requires an understanding of the implications for systems of care of related reform efforts such as Medicaid managed care and child welfare privatization, as well as the ability to figure out ways to connect those reform efforts to the system of care building process. In system building, the list of potential strategic alliances and opportunities is quite literally endless. It is constrained only by limited vision and a failure to comprehend all the possible connections.

Shared Vision Based on Common Values and Principles   A first step in being strategic is to engage in a process to understand one another's values, lay a common foundation of principles, and develop a shared vision for the system of care. Without a unifying vision based on agreed-upon values and principles, it is difficult to move forward toward articulating goals, objectives, and desired outcomes, and it is impossible to analyze whether the structures created are anchored by a shared perspective on the future.

Clear Population Focus   Developing a population focus (i.e., clearly identifying the children, youth, and families for whom the system is being built) is an essential feature of effective system building. Strategically, clarity about the population becomes a unifying frame of reference for system builders who come from different categorical programs, state and local perspectives, and stakeholder group interests. It is also essential to inform the community mapping process that identifies assets and needs, as well as to clarify issues of governance, system design, and financing.

Developing a clear population focus does not mean that one must adopt either a narrow or a broad target population definition. A team can choose to do either or something in between. What it does mean is that system builders must agree on and articulate the general identities of the children, youth, and families for whom the system is being built from among or including all of the total population of children and families dependent on public systems for mental health services. This total population includes:

- Children, youth, and families eligible for Medicaid and the State Children's Health Insurance Program (SCHIP)

- Impoverished and uninsured children, youth, and families who do not qualify for Medicaid or SCHIP

- Children, youth, and families eligible for Tribal Authority programs

- Families who are not impoverished or uninsured but who have exhausted their private insurance, often because they have a child with a serious disorder

- Families who are not impoverished or uninsured and who may not yet have exhausted their private insurance but who need a particular type of service that is unavailable through their private insurer and only available from the public sector

Within this total population of families dependent on public systems for mental health services are numerous subpopulations of children, youth, and families who have particular service needs over and above those of the total population. These include:

- Children, youth, and families involved in child welfare, juvenile justice, special education, substance abuse, intellectual and developmental disabilities systems, and systems serving children with special physical health care needs

- Children, youth, and families who need only brief, short-term services, those who need intermediate term care, and those who require services over an extended period of time

- Children and youth who are in or at risk for out-of-home placement

- Children and youth who do not have serious disorders but need some type of mental health service, children who do have serious disorders, and those who are at risk for serious disorders; risk factors can be described in many ways (e.g., having a parent with a serious mental illness, having been exposed to abuse or neglect, being impoverished, being a member of a minority group). System builders must create some clarity about what they mean when they use the term *at risk*.

- Children and youth who have co-occurring disorders (e.g., an emotional disorder and substance abuse, an emotional disorder and developmental disability, an emotional disorder and a chronic physical illness)

- Children and adolescents who cover a broad age range—from infants and toddlers, to preschoolers, to latency age children, to adolescents, to young adults

- Children, youth, and families who come from diverse racial and ethnic groups

- Children, youth, and families who live in cities, suburbs, and rural and frontier areas

The various subpopulations described are not homogeneous. Every decision that system builders make about who is included carries implications for the types of strategies that must be developed. For example, inclusion of infants and toddlers requires specialized infant and early childhood mental health services; partnerships with Head Start, child care, prekindergarten, and similar early childhood programs; and linkages with Child Find and Part C (early intervention program of the Individuals with Disabilities Education Act Amendments of 1997, PL 105-17). Inclusion of rural families carries implications for such things as outreach and access, service capacity, and attention to issues of isolation. Inclusion of children involved in the child welfare system ensures an overrepresentation of children who have serious attachment and posttraumatic stress disorders, as well as those who require specialized services for traumas such as sexual abuse. Inclusion of children and youth involved in child welfare and juvenile justice systems raises unique child and community safety issues, and thus linkages with court systems are critical.

This is not an argument for systems of care to be all things to all people, which is a specious argument in any event. It is instead an argument for system builders to develop a clear population focus and to be thoughtful about the characteristics, strengths, and needs of subpopulations within the population(s) of focus so that relevant strategies will be pursued and responsive structures can be built.

In addition to defining *who* will be served by the system of care, system builders must also establish *how many* children and families will be served and over what period of time. To make this determination, system builders must examine both the need for services (i.e., prevalence) and the demand for services (i.e., utilization) (Pires, 1990). National prevalence data must be adapted to local realities, (e.g., a high incidence of risk factors in a locality may indicate a higher need for services) (Friedman, Kutash, & Duchnowski, 1996). Analysis of state and local utilization data must be approached with the understanding that data are often of poor quality and that demand for services is affected by such variables as accessibility, quality, affordability, stigma, appropriateness, and administrative barriers. There is typically a pent-up or unmet demand in every locality that is not reflected in utilization data.

Determining how many will be served is also is a capacity issue (i.e., determining the number of children and families the system of care can be reasonably expected to serve over a certain period of time period given its capacity). It is also a political question (i.e., the extent of pressure and interest expressed from advocates, legislators, and other concerned parties). Effective system builders articulate global expressions of need because it is important to create a larger picture for the community and its representatives in state and local legislatures. Effective system builders, however, also move beyond these global expressions of need, which seldom get translated into operational realities, and project realistic numbers of children to be served over a given time period. These projections are informed by prevalence and utilization data, system capacity, and political realities.

Shared Outcomes   The process of identifying shared outcomes provides another route to exploring the values, needs, and interests of various stakeholder groups. Clarity about the expected outcomes is essential to inform the types of system structures to be built (Schorr, Sylvester, & Dunkle, 1999). For example, if improvement in the clinical and functional status of children is an agreed-on outcome, structures must be in place to ensure that appropriate services are available; children and families can access them; clinicians, youth, families, and natural helpers are trained; and means for measuring clinical and functional status over time are developed. Strategically, the process of identifying shared outcomes helps to build consensus among stakeholders regarding the goals that the system is expected to accomplish on behalf of the children, youth, and families to be served (i.e., the population of focus). The outcomes desired by one constituency may be threatening to another. For example, a system-level outcome of reducing the use of residential treatment may be desirable to state and local officials but threatening to providers. The process of establishing shared outcomes is one of finding common ground and purpose across diverse stakeholder groups (Usher, 1998). It is a process guided by values and vision, as well as an understanding of the needs and strengths of the identified population.

Community Mapping—Understanding Strengths and Needs
Agreeing on what should be built without a common understanding of what already exists and what is still needed is difficult. Community mapping is a process in which stakeholders join together to explore the needs, challenges, strengths, and resources within the population to be served, the community, the existing service systems, and provider agencies while keeping the population's strengths and needs foremost in the process (McKnight, 1994). Community mapping is a strategic process in itself. Different stakeholder groups have varying perspectives on strengths, problems, and useful resources (Bruner et al., 1999). A mental health agency director might consider the mental health clinic a resource, whereas families may view it as inconsequential because it fails to provide culturally relevant, family-focused care. Youth might view the recreation center as a resource, something that might be overlooked by others. Families might consider natural helpers in their neighborhoods to be critical resources, whereas others are unaware of the role they play. Through community mapping, system builders can develop a more complete shared appreciation of what must be built on, built anew, or not built at all.

Understanding and Changing Traditional Systems
Successful system builders become very sophisticated in their understanding of how the traditional government systems at federal, state, and local levels operate, the extent of the dollars they control, and the potential of each to change. For systems of care to sustain themselves and grow, system builders must be successful in altering how the traditional systems utilize their dollars, staff, authority, and other resources. This is essential because: 1) the traditional systems control the lion's share of the resources critical to supporting systems of care and 2) traditional ways of operating too often contradict the values and goals of systems of care and can thus sabotage system building if left unaddressed.

Without achieving some fundamental changes in the traditional child-serving systems, system builders are unlikely to create local systems of care that can be sustained over time (Koyanagi & Feres-Merchant, 2000). In addition, they run the risk of creating yet another parallel delivery system. If system builders rely only on grant monies or discretionary state and local allocations without figuring out ways to tap into the major system financing streams (e.g., Medicaid, child welfare dollars), if they only hire new staff without encompassing and retraining existing system staff, if they create new care management processes that parallel the case management provided in the traditional systems, they are not really creating systems of care. They are instead creating demonstration programs or special projects that may never change "business as usual," except for the small number of families who were fortunate enough to have landed in the demonstration project. System builders must first educate themselves about the ways traditional systems operate and why they do so. The more knowledgeable they are about these systems, the more strategic they can be in advancing a change agenda.

Understanding the Importance of "De Facto" Mental Health Providers

Effective system builders recognize that, in most communities, schools, child care centers, pediatric practices, Head Start programs, and other similar programs are either playing a major role in the provision of mental health services—perhaps with appropriate training but perhaps not—or playing a major role in the early identification and referral for treatment of mental health problems. These are natural settings in which children and youth with and at risk for emotional and behavioral challenges are intimately involved, thus making them natural partners in early intervention, screening, and linkage to appropriate services. In this case, the term *early intervention* is used not just in the context of infants and young children, but as it pertains to all children and adolescents—identifying and addressing problems early, before they reach crisis or intractability stages. Linkages with "de facto" providers require targeted strategies and persistence. Sometimes system builders are successful in conveying to these providers how the system of care can be useful to them, resulting in the system being inundated with referrals. It is critical that system builders approach these providers in ways that engage them as partners in the system of care, creating an understanding that the capacity of the system is a collective one.

Understanding Major Financing Streams

System builders must understand *all* of the major financing streams that support service delivery for children and youth with emotional disorders and their families (Armstrong et al., 2006). These funding streams can be found in multiple systems and at all levels of government. Typically, they operate independently from one another, each supporting its own service delivery system and each contracting with providers, although often with the same providers, in its own particular way. The world of child mental health financing is one of categorical "boxes within boxes." Families who have a child or youth with a serious emotional disorder usually find themselves in the precarious position of having a foot in several boxes at once.

One of the challenges facing system builders is creating one big financing box, or at least fewer boxes with more navigable pathways among them. To do this, system builders must figure out who is paying for what, as well as who controls which dollars at which levels, and then gauge which dollars are feasible for redirection and use in systems of care. They must think strategically about ways to create win–win situations for those who control funding. For instance, the system of care could help a juvenile justice system achieve lower costs and better outcomes by diverting youth from detention. Even when dollars are left outside of systems of care, it is still vital that system builders determine the interface among financing streams to minimize cost shifting and confusion for families who rely on services supported by multiple funding streams.

Connection to Related Reform Initiatives   In virtually every state and community, there are reform initiatives underway that have or should have a major bearing on system building (e.g., Medicaid managed care reforms, child welfare privatization, juvenile justice deinstitutionalization, full service school reforms, special education inclusion efforts). Effective system builders recognize the strategic importance of connecting to related reform initiatives to minimize duplication of efforts, maximize resources, and reduce service fragmentation for families.

Clear Goals, Objectives, and Benchmarks   Successful system builders become concrete, meaning they iterate and over time reiterate clear objectives tied to goals with recognizable benchmarks of progress along the way. Objectives clearly state what is to be done, by whom, and by when. Successful system builders also know that when objectives address systemic or structural change, there is greater likelihood that the system of care will be sustainable (Pires, 1991).

A structural change objective is one that seeks to change existing structures (e.g., the Medicaid system, how providers are paid, how clinicians are trained, the ways families and youth are involved). Other objectives may be worthwhile, but they are unlikely to create fundamental change. For example, an objective to create a newsletter for parents (i.e., a nonstructural objective) is worthwhile, but it does not fundamentally change a system as would an objective to require involvement of and support for parents in service planning, monitoring, and governance processes. Similarly, an objective to change the state's Medicaid plan from the clinic to the rehabilitation services option addresses structural change that has a more institutionalized impact on system building than would an objective to create a one-time allocation of funding to create community-based services, although both are worthwhile objectives.

Structural change objectives concern themselves with those aspects of current operating procedures—usually the most entrenched—that seem most irrational in light of the values, vision, and goals of the system of care. In the world of public child mental health service delivery, the irrational aspects may include:

- The child mental health, child welfare, juvenile justice, education, health, and substance abuse systems do not collaborate, although they serve many of the same children, youth, and families.

- Most of the state's population of children and youth in out-of-state residential care have serious emotional challenges, but the mental health system plays no role in the placement or prevention of placement of these youth, the monitoring of their care, or the development of after-care plans.

- Seventy-five percent of the resources are spent on out-of-home placements.

- There is no requirement or mechanism to collect child-specific utilization data or to develop child-specific standards either within the mental health system or across child-serving agencies.

- Clinicians in the system view parents as part of the problem.

The irrational aspects of current systems may vary from one state and community to another; system builders must identify these fundamental barriers within their respective communities and develop clear structural change objectives.

Trigger Mechanisms—Being Opportunistic　In the system building process, something must initially launch the ball and then keep it rolling. A system-building trigger mechanism might be the opportunity to apply for a major systems change grant such as those provided by the Child, Adolescent, and Family Branch at the federal Center for Mental Health Services. It might be a critical legislative report or a lawsuit brought by families and advocates. It might be a change in administration. System-building efforts are launched and sustained by taking advantage of opportunities. It is therefore critical for system builders to constantly scan the environment to identify those opportunities. This is a key element of being strategic.

Opportunity for Reflection　The process of system building is both linear (i.e., moving toward goals and clearly stated objectives) and circular (i.e., constantly revisiting assumptions, progress, and opportunities). As a matter of strategy, successful system builders take time for reflection. They periodically ask, "Is our strategy working? Are there opportunities we are missing? Are we leaving someone out? What impact does our work have on the people we serve?" as well as other similarly reflective questions. Although some benchmarks are reached, objectives achieved, and outcomes realized, system building is not a finite activity. What is built today will be changed tomorrow. An important point to consider is whether changes are planned and purposeful or haphazard. That will depend on whether the system of care leaders value the need for reflection and whether evaluation, monitoring, and feedback loops (i.e., the structures that support reflection) are in place.

Adequate Time System building does not happen overnight. Systems of care address long-entrenched systemic problems. Because system building takes time, it is important for system builders to experience and celebrate achievements along the way and to recognize the developmental nature of the process. Successful system builders recognize and tolerate the tension inherent between the desire for immediate results and the recognition that meaningful change often takes time.

ROLE OF STRUCTURE

Structure is defined as "something arranged in a definite pattern of organization" (*Webster's Seventh New Collegiate Dictionary*, 1970). The important role that structure plays in systems of care is based on several premises.

Premises Regarding Structure

Premise 1: Certain functions must be organized to successfully implement systems of care. They cannot be left to happenstance. For example, if there is no structure, (i.e., no defined arrangement) for the way by which care is managed, it is unlikely that care will be managed.

Premise 2: The structures that are created send messages that either undermine or reinforce the values and principles that have been adopted. For example, individualized, flexible service provision is a key principle of systems of care; however, if the financing structure only attaches dollars to programs, the principle of individualizing care will be undermined. That does not mean to suggest that it is impossible to incorporate individualized service provision within this structure. It is simply more difficult to do so. The structure in this instance sends a message about how much the system truly values an individualized, wraparound approach.

Premise 3: The structures that are created are relative to how power and responsibility are distributed. One goal of systems of care is to invest families with shared decision-making power and responsibility at the service and system levels (i.e., policy, management, monitoring). A system-level structure that involves one parent on an advisory committee obviously distributes less power and responsibility than a structure that requires and strengthens the capacity of families to participate in all aspects of system-level decision making. In turn, the latter structure distributes less power and responsibility than that which mandates majority representation of families on decision-making or governance bodies and also provides funding and support to implement the mandate.

Premise 4: The structures that are created affect the subjective experiences of stakeholders (i.e., the ways families, youth, providers, staff, administrators, and others feel about the system). In the previous example of the lone parent on a system-level advisory committee, families are likely to feel that the system, no matter how innovative certain aspects of it may be, is being tokenistic.

Premise 5: Structure affects practice and outcomes. Even if structure merely affects how people feel, it will also affect practice and outcomes. For many reasons, the structures created can either support or hinder intended practice and attainment of desired outcomes to lesser or greater degrees. The previously noted financing structure that attaches dollars only to programs is likely to hinder—although not necessarily entirely defeat—the practice of individualizing services. This could, in turn, frustrate—although again, not necessarily defeat—attainment of the goal of improving clinical and functional outcomes. Another desired outcome may be the reduction in out-of-home placements. If the benefit structure (i.e., the allowable services and supports) and the provider network structure do not encompass an adequate array of home- and community-based services and supports, it is highly unlikely that out-of-home placements will be reduced, at least not without affecting other desired outcomes such as an improvement in the clinical and functional status of children or reduced recidivism.

Premise 6: Structures must be evaluated and modified, if necessary, over time. Because system building occurs in an ever-changing environment and is, by its nature, not a finite activity, structures that are created today may not encompass what will be needed tomorrow.

Premise 7: New structures replace existing ones; some existing ones may be worth keeping, and some are more difficult to replace than others. This is an admonition not to throw the baby out with the bathwater because there are existing structural strengths in every system worth preserving in whole or part. It is also an admonition to be strategic in regard to the amount of precious time and energy spent at each juncture because timing is (almost) everything when trying to replace intractable structures.

Premise 8: There are no perfect or correct structures. Sometimes the most desirable structures for the attainment of system goals are ones that for political, financial, technical, or other reasons cannot be created at the time. Sometimes there is no agreement among stakeholders or even clarity about what the most desirable structures would be. The most desirable structures in one community may be very different from those in another. What is important is that all stakeholders in a given community involved in system building take the time to analyze, acknowledge the strengths and weaknesses of, and plan contingencies in response to the structures that are either created or left standing. This reflection must consider how the created structures reflect values, distribute power and responsibility across different stakeholder groups, affect the subjective experiences of different stakeholder groups, and affect goal attainment. Box 4.1 provides an example of the role that structure plays.

System of Care Functions Requiring Structure

There are certain functions within systems of care that must be structured, (i.e., organized in some defined arrangement and not left to happenstance). Many functions require structure at both the state and local levels. Table 4.2 delineates the list of functions, providing a good starting point for system builders that they can adapt and expand on based on their own experiences.

This list of functions may seem daunting, but in reality, most of these functions already are structured; they may not, however, be structured in ways that

Box 4.1. Role of structure

Consider the example of the organizational structures of two different state departments of mental health. Both state departments have system of care–like mission statements and expressed values to create a comprehensive array of services and supports for children and youth with emotional and behavioral challenges, as well as their families.

In Department A, responsibility for children's services is fragmented across three divisions.

1. The Division of Institutions, which has budgetary and operational responsibility for child and adolescent inpatient and residential treatment facilities

2. The Division of Community Programs, which has jurisdiction over community mental health centers that provide adult, child, and adolescent outpatient services

3. The Division of Special Populations, which includes the children's director, who has responsibility for special projects related to children such as grant-funded programs and demonstration projects (e.g., home and community-based and wraparound services).

The children's director is relatively buried within this organizational structure and lacks line authority over most services and most dollars related to children. He or she must negotiate with three division directors, two of whom control the lion's share of the resources needed to create a continuum of care.

Although it is certainly possible to create a continuum of care within the structure of Department A, it is certainly more difficult than it is within a structure where there is a children's division with line budget and operational responsibility over the entire continuum of care. This is the structure of Department B, which has a director of adult services and a director of child, adolescent, and family services. The structure in Department A sends a message about the extent to which the state truly values an integrated continuum of care, will most likely create frustrations for the children's director and key stakeholders concerned about the system, and generates confusion for families and providers. In spite of both states having similar values and goals, the structure of Department A is less likely to support achievement of those goals than the structure of Department B.

Adapted from Pires, S.A. (2002) *Building systems of care: A primer* [p. 19]. Washington, DC: Georgetown University, National Technical Assistance Center for Children's Mental Health.

support system of care goals. A fundamental part of the system building process is examining existing structures in light of system of care objectives and strategically determining which lend themselves to restructuring if change is needed. Not every function that must be structured within systems of care can be tackled at once. System builders should consider the functions that require structure and weigh the pros and cons of different structural arrangements; they must also think operationally and strategically about which functions to address at which stage in the system-building process.

To be effective, system builders must ensure that every structure they build or rebuild encompasses three fundamental characteristics:

Table 4.2.   Functions requiring structure in systems of care

Planning: The planning process itself requires structure

Decision making and oversight at the policy level (i.e., governance)

System management (day-to-day management decisions)

Benefit design/service array (definition of the types of services and supports that are allowable and under what conditions within the system of care)

Evidence-based practice

Outreach and referral

System entry/access (i.e., intake—how children, youth, and their families enter the system and what happens when they get there)

Screening, assessment, and evaluation—three separate functions but are important to link

Decision making and oversight at the service delivery level, including the following:

- Care planning (i.e., *treatment* or *service planning*—planning of services and supports for individual children, youth, and their families)
- Care authorization
- Care monitoring and review

Care management or care coordination

Crisis management at the service delivery and system levels

Utilization management

Family involvement, support, and development at all levels (i.e., policy level, management level, service level)

Youth involvement, support, and development

Staffing structure (e.g., defining the staffing structure, determining how functions are staffed)

Staff involvement, support, and development

Orientation and training of key stakeholders (e.g., staff, providers, families)

External and internal communication

Provider network (network of services and supports)

Protecting privacy

Ensuring rights

Transportation

Financing

Purchasing/contracting

Provider payment rates

Revenue generation and reinvestment

Billing and claims processing

Information management

Quality improvement (monitoring, feedback loops, adjustment mechanisms)

Evaluation

System exit (how families leave the system; what happens when they leave)

Technical assistance and consultation

From Pires, S.A. (2002) *Building systems of care: A primer* (pp. 21–22). Washington, DC: Georgetown University, National Technical Assistance Center for Children's Mental Health.

1. Cultural and linguistic competence (i.e., structures that support the capacity to function effectively in cross-cultural/linguistic situations)

2. Meaningful partnership with families and youth in structural decision making, design, and implementation

3. A cross-agency perspective (i.e., structures that operate in a noncategorical fashion)

It is beyond the scope of this chapter to explore every system of care function. Several functions have been specifically selected to explore the role that structure plays, beginning with the planning structure, which is typically where system builders begin.

Structuring the Planning Process   Because system of care building is a dynamic process occurring in a volatile environment, *planning* is an ongoing process that requires structure. It may require different structures and more or less structure at different times, but it needs structure nonetheless. Staffing is an element of structure, and effective planning processes tend to be staffed. The time and place of meetings, the roles and responsibilities of those involved, the manner in which work gets done (e.g., through committees or work groups), the way information is communicated and to whom it is communicated all require structural considerations in planning processes. The location and time of meetings may discourage some stakeholders from attending or alternatively make it possible for them to participate. Whether meetings are organized sends signals about the importance of the process. The method by which information is imparted can value or devalue the work of participants.

Structures for planning may be initiated at the local level and then draw in state-level stakeholders. Alternately, the state may create a structure for planning and engage local-level stakeholders. The important point is that the structure must allow for the involvement of stakeholders at both levels.

An inappropriate structure can be as detrimental as no structure at all. For example, a structure that is highly rigid can stifle creativity and the inclusion of key stakeholder groups such as youth, who are often uncomfortable with highly-structured processes (Academy for Educational Development, 1996). By the same token, a very loose structure may be frustrating to those whose input is also crucial (e.g., agency directors). In reality, effective planning processes create a variety of different structures to support system building. This is also important for responding to the racial, ethnic, linguistic, and cultural diversity that exists across stakeholder groups.

Effective system builders typically structure planning processes in ways that create a variety of mechanisms for meaningful involvement of families and youth. In some communities with a strong family organization, families may structure their own planning process, which is formally linked to the system-building process. There may be a youth council that serves a similar purpose. These mechanisms allow for a broader family and youth voice to influence system-building planning than representation on only one planning body might allow.

Other communities may have one planning body with multiple subcommittees or workgroups to facilitate the involvement of a large number of people. The subcommittees or workgroups may be time-limited, and they typically establish their own guidelines for meeting schedules and places. The point is that meaningful involvement of families and youth requires a planning process structure that is flexible and informed by their needs. The strategies displayed on Table 4.3 were developed with parents in mind, but many are applicable to involving youth as well.

The planning process structure must encompass mechanisms to build capacity among all stakeholders, recognizing that different stakeholders have different

Table 4.3. Strategies for involving parents in planning

Provide special orientation and training, as well as ongoing assistance, to parents who need a better understanding of administrative, budgetary, and other issues that play a role in planning. This might also include consulting with parents prior to a meeting to highlight what they might expect to be covered.

Have more than token representation of parents at meetings.

Contract with community-based organizations or parent advocacy groups to develop and direct a process that ensures sustained and thoughtful parental participation in planning.

Working through Head Start parent advisory groups, Parents Anonymous, and other parent organizations (e.g., the Federation of Families for Children's Mental Health, the National Alliance for Mental Illness Child and Adolescent Network).

Ask agencies that work with parents (e.g., schools, child care centers) to recommend parents to participate in planning.

Pay a stipend to parents who participate in planning sessions and provide or pay for transportation and babysitting.

Hold planning meetings in the evenings or on weekends, in communities across the state, and in locations such as schools, community centers, and other settings that may be more familiar and comfortable to parents than state or local office buildings.

Conduct surveys to elicit the views of a wide range of parents.

Use parents or others who work regularly with parents to conduct focus groups that probe the views of selected groups of parents (e.g., teenage parents, single parents, grandparents raising children, foster parents, adoptive parents).

Work with family support programs to tap into informal networks (e.g., parent support groups, parents who routinely visit a neighborhood drop-in center).

Work with home-visiting programs and health clinics to involve parents who may be otherwise hard to reach.

Work with family preservation and family reunification programs to identify and involve families who have benefited from these services.

Conduct sessions for planning group members, administrators, and staff led by an experienced facilitator to explore attitudes and stereotypes toward different ethnic, racial, and religious groups, as well as toward parents.

Publicly acknowledge the contributions of parents and other family members.

From Emig, C., Farrow, F., & Allen, M. (1994). *A guide for planning: Making strategic use of the family preservation and support services program.* Washington, DC: Center for the Study of Social Policy and Children's Defense Fund; adapted by permission.

capacities for participation with respect to information, knowledge, and skills, as well as in regard to practicalities such as the availability of transportation and child care, the ability to leave work or school to attend meetings, and the ability to communicate in the English language when English is not one's primary language. This is true of all stakeholders, not just parents and youth, although other stakeholders often have more resources available to them to obtain necessary information or to accommodate a meeting schedule.

Governance Structure *Governance* (i.e., policy level decision making and oversight) should not be confused with system management, which is discussed later in this chapter. These are two distinct functions. While it is conceivable that system builders might utilize the same players to perform both functions, such as in rural communities where there are limited resources, the functions themselves are distinct.

Governance in systems of care is decision making at a policy level that has legitimacy, authority, and accountability. To embody these characteristics, governance structures for systems of care are by necessity interagency bodies, and they legitimize the voice of family and youth consumers by including them as equal partners in governance mechanisms.

Governing bodies for systems of care exist at the state level, at the local or neighborhood levels, and in some places, at all levels for the same system of care. Some are created by legislation, some by executive order, some by memoranda of agreement, and some by community will. Some are governmental or quasi-governmental bodies, and some are 501(c)(3) (private, not-for-profit) entities.

There are some basic questions to be considered about governance structures before deciding what forms they should take. The questions discussed below are far more important to answer initially with respect to governance structures than whether the structure should be a 501(c)(3), a governmental or quasi-governmental entity, or some other arrangement. There are pros and cons to each of these types of governance structures, depending very much on the particular circumstances in a given locality. Important questions to consider include the following:

From whom does the governance body get its authority to govern the system of care? From legislation? Executive order? Regulation? Contractual obligation? Interagency memorandum? Community will, as expressed through some defined, credible process? System of care governance structures must derive their authority from an entity that possesses the authority to give it or they risk being viewed as tangential.

Is there clarity about what the governance body is responsible for governing? In some states, there is more than one governance structure for the same system of care—one at the state level and one at the local level. Are the roles and responsibilities of each clear and nonredundant? Even where there is only one governance structure, system builders must be very clear about what the governance body is governing or there will be confusion, dashed expectations, and resentment among stakeholders.

Are those who sit on the governance body representative of the stakeholders that have an interest in the system of care? Does the body include families and youth, state, local, and community representatives, providers, and other representatives? If there is some stakeholder group that by consensus among system builders cannot sit on the governing body because of a potential conflict of interest, in what other more appropriate ways can this group have input into the governing body? This is an issue that has arisen with respect to providers, and in some communities, it has been resolved by the creation of a formalized *providers' forum* that meets periodically with the governance body to offer input and feedback. If the governance body is not representative, it will be viewed with skepticism, its decisions will be questioned, and its effectiveness will be compromised.

Does the governing body have the capacity to govern the system of care? Does it have the talent, time, staff, data management, and other resources to operate? Many times, system of care governance structures are created that are not staffed, have no dedicated resources for their own operations, and include members who have other full-time responsibilities. This is a recipe for failure. A lack of capacity to govern obviously affects outcomes, builds resentment among stakeholders, unfairly assigns responsibility without providing power, and sends a message that system of care governance is not valued. In some communities, the system management entity staffs the governance body because governance and system management are subsets of the same entity. In other localities, governance and system management may be lodged within two discrete entities. The governance body may be overseeing the system management structure in a contractual relationship, and in this instance, it needs its own staff and management information capability.

Does the governance structure have credibility among key stakeholder groups to govern the system of care? The answer to this question relates not only to the answers to the previous questions, but also to the effectiveness of the governance body in communicating its functions to key stakeholders. A governance body may be doing a terrific job, but if key stakeholders do not know about it, it might as well be doing no job at all.

Does the governance structure embrace the concept of shared liability among partners? Systems of care serve populations of children, youth, and families for whom different agencies have legal responsibilities (e.g., children and youth involved in the child welfare, juvenile justice, and special education systems). If the system of care governance structure does not assume shared liability to meet these legal responsibilities, system builders are creating a situation of double jeopardy for partner agencies that have legal mandates and that have committed resources for the population to be served by the system of care. The principle of unconditional care, which is so important to the integrity of the system of care, begins with the governing body's embracement of the concept of shared liability. Without it, governing bodies leave themselves "outs" that are inherently suspicious to partners with legal mandates and to families who are tired of having to navigate multiple systems.

Box 4.2 provides an example of a governance structure that evolved over time as system builders addressed these questions.

Box 4.2. Example of an evolving governance structure

Figure 4.1 describes the evolving governance structure in a county in an eastern state with state legislation mandating local systems of care to reduce the number of children and youth in out-of-home placements. In this particular county, the system-building effort is housed operationally within the Department of Mental Health (DMH), although it is envisioned as an interagency effort. In Figure 4.1, it is not clear from whom the governing body derives its authority. This structure also does not clarify what the local governing board actually governs because it appears as if the board simply oversees the DMH effort. Indeed, when asked to whom the system of care director reports and who is accountable for expenditures, both the DMH director and board members responded, "To me/us."

While the board includes representation from the statewide family organization, it does not include representation from families and youth actually served by the system of care. In addition, providers are not represented on the board. Figure 4.1 seems to suggest that the staff of the system-building effort work for the Department of Mental Health. No feedback loops or communication structures are indicated. Those closest to the frontline (i.e., families, youth, care managers), are those most removed from the governing body. It is not clear from Figure 4.1 that the board embraces the notion of shared liability; indeed, it would appear as if DMH has the liability.

Figure 4.2 indicates a restructuring of the board, achieved through a process of clarifying roles, responsibilities, vision, and so forth. Figure 4.2 makes it clear that the board derives its authority from the County Executive, who issued an executive order creating the board, citing the relevant state legislation. Figure 4.2 clarifies that the system-building staff are accountable directly to the board and not through the DMH director, whose position on the board is now the same as every other agency director, even though the project remains housed in DMH for operational purposes. The board changed its bylaws to increase family and youth membership and ensure representation from families and youth actually being served by the system of care, in addition to representation from the statewide family organization. The board decided against including providers on the board, citing concerns about potential conflicts of interest, but instead created a Providers' Forum, which meets regularly with the board.

Communication and feedback loops are shown in Figure 4.2 by two-way arrows, indicating that care managers now have direct input to the board on a periodic basis, in addition to providing input through the system of care director, who functions as staff to the board. Figure 4.2 shows more clearly the board's intent to assume shared liability for children and youth served through the system of care.

Adapted from Pires, S.A. (2002). *Building systems of care: A primer* (p. 33). Washington, DC: Georgetown University, National Technical Assistance Center for Children's Mental Health.

System Management Structure System management has to do with day-to-day operational decision making. System management may be lodged with a lead state or local agency, as in the previous example, an interagency body at either level, a quasi-governmental entity, a private, nonprofit lead agency, or a commercial company such as a managed care organization. System management might be lodged with one entity or shared between a family organization and a lead provider

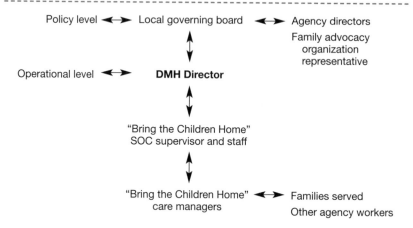

Figure 4.1. The original governance structure of an evolving system of care. (Adapted from Pires, S.A. [2002]. *Building systems of care: A primer* [p. 33]. Washington, DC: Georgetown University, National Technical Assistance Center for Children's Mental Health.) (*Key:* DMH, Department of Mental Health; SOC, system of care.)

agency, between a commercial company and a state agency, or between a commercial company and a coalition of nonprofit providers. When system management is shared, clarity of the roles and responsibilities of each party is critical.

Like governance structures, there are pros and cons to each type of management structure depending on the circumstances in the state or community. In some localities, particularly where there are many 501(c)(3) organizations, creation of a new 501(c)(3) may be viewed as creating yet another private nonprofit that will compete for funds. In other localities, designation of an existing private nonprofit agency to serve as the system manager might not be viable for political or technical reasons (i.e., there may simply be no existing organization with the capacity to perform system management functions). In some states or localities, due to long histories of contention and mistrust across child-serving agencies or because the internal management capability does not exist, it may be impossible to designate a lead government agency as a system manager. In still other circumstances, it may be impossible to use a commercial company because of stakeholder resistance to the use of profit-making entities or stakeholder beliefs that commercial companies lack adequate knowledge of the populations that rely on public systems of care.

As with governance structures, before determining the type of structure that makes sense, system builders must be able to answer a number of questions:

- Is the reporting relationship clear? Is it understandable to those to whom the system management structure reports?

- Are expectations clear as to what the system management structure is managing and what information it is expected to provide to the governing body?

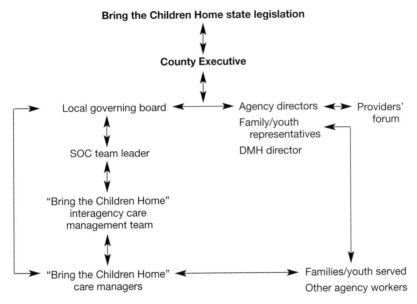

Figure 4.2. The modified governance structure of an evolving system of care. (Adapted from Pires, S.A. [2002]. *Building systems of care: A primer* [p. 33]. Washington, DC: Georgetown University, National Technical Assistance Center for Children's Mental Health.) (*Key:* DMH, Department of Mental Health; SOC, system of care.)

- Does the system management structure have the capacity to manage (e.g., qualified staff, data management capacity, leadership)?

- Does the system management structure have credibility with key stakeholders, or can it create such credibility?

For example, in one case, the system management function is being contracted to a commercial company that lacks credibility with certain key stakeholder groups because it is a profit-making entity or because it lacks familiarity with the population. With orientation, training, communication, targeted strategies to build relationships with stakeholders, and limits set on profits, in addition to effective performance, is it possible to create credibility? If not, no matter how effective the performance, there is likely to be a constant "energy drain" from system-building efforts caused by the negative perceptions and resistance of key stakeholders.

Different illustrations of system management structures that also show the relationship to the governance structure are shown in Box 4.3.

Structuring Care Management Depending on the population focus, a given system of care may encompass more than one care management approach (Evans & Armstrong, 2002). If, for example, the population includes both children with serious, complex needs and children with less intensive needs, the system may include both intensive care management (i.e., care managers work with

---

Box 4.3. Examples of system management structures and their relationship to the governance structure

In Figure 4.2, the governance structure is an interagency body created by executive order; the management structure is an in-house management team with system management and care management staff. In this example, the system of care team leader reports directly to the interagency board, even though the system of care is housed within the Department of Mental Health. The system of care team leader staffs the governing board, similar to an executive director in a nonprofit organization staffing a board of directors.

In Figure 4.3, the governing body is a countywide purchasing alliance or co-operative that has taken the form of a new quasi-governmental body. The system manager is a commercial managed care company that has partnered with a lead nonprofit provider in the county. The system manager is contractually accountable to the county purchasing alliance. The county purchasing alliance has its own monitoring and quality assurance staff.

Adapted from Pires, S.A. (2002). *Building systems of care: A primer* (pp. 37–38). Washington, DC: Georgetown University, National Technical Assistance Center for Children's Mental Health.

---

a very small number of families and play very active roles in care planning, monitoring, and service provision) as well as a more basic approach (i.e., care managers engage in more general advocacy, coordination, and monitoring of activities on behalf of larger numbers of children and families).

In the case of children and youth with serious or complex disorders and their families who are involved in multiple systems, much has been learned about the importance of creating a structure in which a family has one care manager who is accountable across systems. These care managers typically have very small caseloads (i.e., one care manager to eight families) and play a very active role in supporting and advocating for children and families to obtain and coordinate services. They may lead and have the authority to convene service planning teams (sometimes referred to as *child and family teams* or *wraparound teams*); they may control flexible dollars to authorize wraparound supports; they are typically available to families on a 24-hour, 7 day-a-week basis; and they also may play a therapeutic role with children, youth, and families (Goldman & Faw, 1999).

Many systems of care have moved to create or contract out for one care management entity statewide or within regions or localities that is accountable across systems for managing care for populations of children, youth, and families who are involved in multiple systems; this is particularly true for populations where states or localities are experiencing high costs or poor outcomes (e.g., youth in out-of-home placements). These care management entities employ, train, and supervise intensive care managers. The illustration of the New Jersey system of care design in Box 4.4 shows how care management entities fit within the overall system that serves a total population (i.e., all children and youth in the state with emotional and behavioral health challenges and their families).

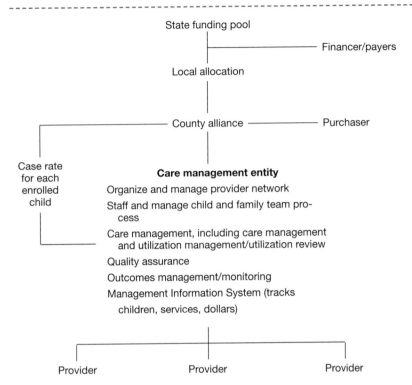

Figure 4.3. Example of a system management structure and its relationship to the governance structure. (Adapted from Pires, S.A. [2002]. *Building systems of care: A primer* [pp. 37–38]. Washington, DC: Georgetown University, National Technical Assistance Center for Children's Mental Health.)

Provider Network and Procurement Structures Effective systems of care structure provider networks that have certain characteristics:

- They are responsive to the population that is the focus of the system of care.

- They encompass both clinical treatment service providers and natural social support resources such as mentors, and they include both traditional and non-traditional indigenous providers.

- They include culturally and linguistically diverse providers.

- They include families and youth as providers of services and supports.

- They are flexible, allowing for additions to and deletions from the network as system needs change over time.

- They are accountable, as they have been organized to serve the needs of the system of care.

Systems of care must typically contend with larger state or county procurement structures. Even within this context, it is usually possible to make choices for structuring the procurement of services and supports for the system of care. Each

---

Box 4.4. New Jersey system of care structure showing care management organizations

New Jersey's locally based Care Management Organizations (CMOs) have the responsibility to serve as the "locus of accountability" for children and youth with complex, serious challenges who are involved in multiple systems, and they employ intensive care managers (see Figure 4.4). The CMOs partner contractually (as required by the state) with locally based Family Support Organizations (FSOs), which are family-run and provide family and youth peer mentors to the wraparound and care management process. The statewide Contracted Systems Administrator (CSA) is a managed care organization, acting as a statewide Administrative Services Organization, that helps families access services, including access to CMOs, and the CSA tracks utilization statewide.

From Pires, S.A. (2002). *Health Care Reform Tracking Project (HCRTP): Promising approaches for behavioral health services to children and adolescents and their families in managed care systems—1: Managed care design and financing.* Tampa: University of South Florida, Louis de la Parte Florida Mental Health Institute, Division of State and Local Support, Department of Child and Family Studies, Research and Training Center for Children's Mental Health; adapted by permission.

---

of these choices, however, has pros and cons associated with it, as the following discussion of four potential choices—preapproved provider lists, fixed price contracts, capitation or case rate contracts, and performance-based contracting—illustrates.

Preapproved Provider Lists Some systems of care prequalify providers as potential resources for the system of care and then draw on them as the need arises. These are cost-reimbursable structures in which providers get paid for services after the services are provided. Such an arrangement gives the system enormous flexibility to individualize services and supports for children and families, although it can create an overload on some providers. It may also be a disadvantage to small, indigenous providers who do not have the cash flow to exist viably within a cost-reimbursable structure. A possible tinkering with this structure would be to provide fixed price contracts for a certain amount of service for those providers whom the system absolutely wants and needs in the provider network but who cannot exist within a strictly cost-reimbursable structure.

Fixed Price Contracts Some systems of care have in place—either intentionally or inherited—fixed price or fixed service contracts in which providers make available a designated amount of service, usually stated as number of service units or days, at a rate per service unit up to a specified amount. This arrangement creates predictability and a certain funding stability for providers; alternately, it is not particularly flexible and poses the risk of families' having to fit what is available, rather than the other way around.

Capitation or Case Rate Contracts Capitation contracts provide prospective, preset funding assigned on the basis of the number of people in the target

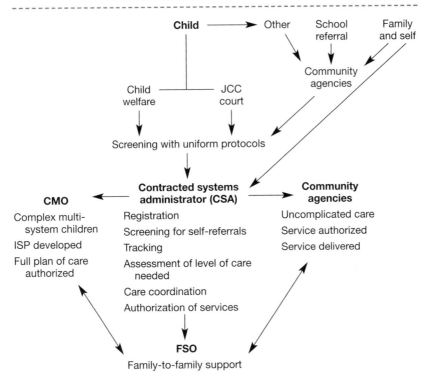

Figure 4.4. System of care structure showing care management organizations (CMOs). (From Pires, S.A. [2002]. *Health Care Reform Tracking Project [HCRTP]: Promising approaches for behavioral health services to children and adolescents and their families in managed care systems—1: Managed care design and financing.* Tampa: University of South Florida, Louis de la Parte Florida Mental Health Institute, Division of State and Local Support, Department of Child and Family Studies, Research and Training Center for Children's Mental Health; adapted by permission.) (*Key:* FSO, Family Support Organizations; ISP, individualized service plan; JCC, Juvenile Conference Committee.)

population (i.e., covered by the system of care's benefit plan). Providers receive per capita funding (i.e., funding for every person covered by and enrolled in the system regardless of whether every person uses services). In return, the provider assumes the risk of serving everyone in the population who shows up for services within the total payment allocation. The capitated (per person) rate is determined by estimating how many people can be expected to use services, as well as the amount and type of service they can be expected to use, and then translating that use to a cost. It spreads the cost of serving those who do use services over a larger population.

Arguably, capitation makes sense only for systems of care serving a total eligible population (all children in a given community) and not for those serving only deep-end populations or those at risk for deep-end services (children with or at risk for serious disorders), who can be expected to use services. For this latter population, case rate contracting structures may be more appropriate (Broskowski, 1996). Case rate contracts provide prospective, preset funding per actual user of service, as opposed to potential user, typically based on the child's meeting a certain diagnostic level of functioning or service profile (e.g., children with serious disorders). Rates are determined by estimating the amount and type of services that these children can be expected to use. In this arrangement, the contractor is not at risk for the number of people who use services but only for the amount and types of services that will be used. In contrast, the contractor with a capitation contract is at risk both for the number of children who use services and the types and amount of services used. Capitation is obviously a riskier arrangement for the provider than is case rate contracting, although case rate contracting carries risk as well.

Risk-based contracts using capitation or case rate financing have both advantages and disadvantages (Pires, 2002b). They allow contractors a great deal of flexibility, which can be used to individualize services and supports for families in a wraparound approach. They also allow systems of care as purchasers to integrate cost and quality of care considerations by tying flexibility at the provider level to accountability and adherence to system-of-care–determined outcomes and performance measures (Stroul, 2003). They also, by definition, pose a risk to both providers and purchasers, and thus to families. If the capitation rate paid to the contractor is too low, it creates an incentive for the contractor to underserve by not reaching out to families who may need services or by providing insufficient service to those who do seek services. A rate that is too high places the system of care in the position of overpaying for services.

Performance-Based Contracting   Performance-based contracting ties provider payment to performance and can be built into virtually any contracting structure. The advantages are that it creates greater control for the system of care as purchaser over the quality of services and supports provided, and it can create greater clarity of expectations for providers. On the downside, particularly if performance measures are unclear or beyond the provider's capacity, this structure can lead to tensions between purchasers and providers that will ultimately affect system goal attainment.

CONCLUSION

This chapter discussed the role that process and structure play in systems of care. It has identified key elements of an effective system-building process and outlined many of the functions that must be structured or restructured within these systems. The chapter discussed structural considerations with respect to a few of these functions (e.g., planning, governance, system management, care management, provider network and procurement) to illustrate the importance of system builders' thinking strategically about the importance of structure and its effect on outcomes. Since the 1980s, much has been learned about effective system of care processes and structures. As systems of care continue to develop and mature, and attention is paid to process and structural issues, this knowledge base will continue to grow.

REFERENCES

Academy for Educational Development. (1996). *A youth development structural perspective.* Washington, DC: Center for Youth Development and Policy Research.

Armstrong, M., Pires, S., McCarthy, J., Stroul, B., Woods, G., & Pizzigati, K. (2006). *A self-assessment and planning guide: Developing a comprehensive financing plan.* Tampa: University of South Florida, Louis de la Parte Florida Mental Health Institute, Research and Training Center for Children's Mental Health.

Broskowski, A. (1996). The role of risk sharing arrangements. In L. Scallet, C. Brach, & E. Steel (Eds.), *Managed care: Challenges for children and family services* (pp. 69–89). Baltimore: Annie E. Casey Foundation.

Bruner, C., Cahn, E., Gartner, A., Giloth, R., Herr, T., Kinney, J., et al. (1999). *Wise counsel: Redefining the role of consumers, professionals, and community workers in the helping process.* Des Moines, IA: Child and Family Policy Center.

Emig, C., Farrow, F., & Allen, M. (1994). *A guide for planning: Making strategic use of the family preservation and support services program.* Washington, DC: Center for the Study of Social Policy and Children's Defense Fund.

Evans, M.E., & Armstrong, M.I. (2002). What is case management? In B.J. Burns & K. Hoagwood (Eds.), *Community treatment for youth: Evidence-based interventions for severe emotional and behavioral disorders* (pp. 39–69). New York: Oxford University Press.

Friedman, R., Kutash, K., & Duchnowski, A. (1996). The population of concern: Defining the issues. In B.A. Stroul & R.M. Friedman (Series Eds.) & B.A. Stroul, (Vol. Ed.), *Systems of care for children's mental health: Children's mental health: Creating systems of care in a changing society* (pp. 69–99). Baltimore: Paul H. Brookes Publishing Co.

Goldman, S.K., & Faw, L. (1999). Three wraparound models as promising approaches. In B.J. Burns & S.K. Goldman (Eds.), *Systems of care: Promising practices in children's mental health, 1998 series: Vol. IV. Promising practices in wraparound for children with severe emotional disturbance and their families.* Washington, DC: American Institutes for Research, Center for Effective Collaboration and Practice.

Hodges, S., Nesman, T., & Hernandez, M. (1999). *Systems of care: Promising practices in children's mental health, 1998 series: Vol. VI. Promising practices: Building collaboration in systems of care.* Washington, DC: American Institutes for Research, Center for Effective Collaboration and Practice.

Individuals with Disabilities Education Act Amendments (IDEA) of 1997, PL 105-17, 20 U.S.C. §§ 1400 *et seq.*

Koyanagi, C., & Feres-Merchant, D. (2000). *Systems of care: Promising practices in children's mental health, 2000 series: Volume III. For the long haul: Maintaining systems of care beyond the federal investment.* Washington, DC: American Institutes for Research, Center for Effective Collaboration and Practice.

Lazear, K., Pires, S., Pizarro, M., Orrego, M., Lara, S., & Lavernia, A. (2001). *Natural helper and professional partnership in children's mental health: Lessons learned from the Equipo del Barrio at Abriendo Puertas, Inc.* Tampa: University of South Florida, Louis De La Parte Florida Mental Health Institute.

Lourie, I. (1994). *Principles of local system development.* Chicago: Kaleidoscope.

Magrab, P. (1999). The meaning of community. In R. Roberts & P. Magrab (Eds.), *Where children live: Solutions for serving young children and their families* (pp. 5–12). Stamford, CT: Ablex Publishing Corporation.

McKnight, J. (1994). *Mapping community capacity.* Evanston, IL: Northwestern University, Center for Urban Affairs and Policy Research.

Osher, T., deFur, E., Nava, C., Spencer, S., & Toth-Dennis, D. (1999). *Systems of care: Promising practices in children's mental health, 1998 series: Vol. I. New roles for families in systems of care.* Washington, DC: American Institutes for Research, Center for Effective Collaboration and Practice.

Pires, S. (1990). *Sizing components of care: An approach to determining the size and cost of service components in a system of care.* Washington, DC: Georgetown University Child Development Center, National Technical Assistance Center for Children's Mental Health.

Pires, S. (1991). *State child mental health planning.* Rockville, MD: National Institute of Mental Health.

Pires, S. (2002a). *Building systems of care: A primer.* Washington, DC: Georgetown University Center for Child and Human Development, National Technical Assistance Center for Children's Mental Health.

Pires, S.A. (2002b). *Health Care Reform Tracking Project (HCRTP): Promising approaches for behavioral health services to children and adolescents and their families in managed care systems—1: Managed care design and financing.* Tampa: University of South Florida, Louis de la Parte Florida Mental Health Institute, Division of State and Local Support, Department of Child and Family Studies, Research and Training Center for Children's Mental Health.

Schorr, L., Sylvester, K., & Dunkle, M. (1999). *Strategies to achieve a common purpose.* Washington, DC: Institute for Educational Leadership.

Schwarz, R.M. (1995). *Ground rules for effective groups.* (Rev. ed.). Chapel Hill: The University of North Carolina, Institute of Government.

Stark, D. (1999). *Collaboration basics: Strategies from six communities engaged in collaborative efforts among families, child welfare, and children's mental health.* Washington, DC: Georgetown University Center for Child and Human Development, National Technical Assistance Center for Children's Mental Health.

Stroul, B. (Vol. Ed.). (1996). *Systems of care for children's mental health: Children's mental health: Creating systems of care in a changing society.* Baltimore: Paul H. Brookes Publishing Co.

Stroul, B.A. (2003). *Health care reform tracking project (HCRTP): Promising approaches for behavioral health services to children and adolescents and their families in managed care system—5: Serving youth with serious and complex behavioral health needs in managed care systems.* Tampa, FL: University of South Florida, Louis de la Parte Florida Mental Health Institute, Division of State and Local Support, Department of Child and Family Studies, Research and Training Center for Children's Mental Health.

U.S. Department of Health and Human Services. (2000). *Mental health: Culture, race, and ethnicity.* [A supplement to *Mental Health: A Report of the Surgeon General*]. Washington, DC: Author.

Usher, C. (1998, May). Managing care across systems to improve outcomes for families and communities. *Journal of Behavioral Health Services and Research, 25*(2), 217–230.

5

Individualized Services in Systems of Care

The Wraparound Process

JANET S. WALKER, ERIC J. BRUNS, AND MARLENE PENN

Wraparound is the term used to describe a team-based, collaborative process for developing and implementing individualized care plans for children with complex needs and their families. Since the 1980s, the wraparound process has grown to become one of the most popular strategies for realizing the system of care philosophy while providing care to individual children, youth, and families with high levels of need (Stroul, 2002). Data from a recent national survey indicate that nearly half of all states have a statewide wraparound initiative and that there are more than 800 wraparound programs across the country providing care to approximately 100,000 children, youth, and families (Sather, Bruns, Stambaugh, & Burns, 2007). It is likely that this number will continue to rise, given that wraparound has been identified variously as an evidence-based, promising, emerging, or recommended practice (Walker & Bruns, 2006b).

Perhaps more accurately, wraparound has been described as an "evidence-based *process* . . . that cuts across a number of clinical interventions" (Stroul, 2002, p. 6). This process requires that family members, providers, and key members of the family's social support network collaborate to build a creative plan that responds to the particular needs of the child and family. The wraparound plan includes and coordinates the entire array of services and supports that the family receives within the system of care. Team members then implement the plan and continue to meet regularly to monitor progress and make adjustments to the plan

The writing of this chapter was supported in part by funding from the National Institute of Disability and Rehabilitation Research, U.S. Department of Education, and the Center for Mental Health Services, Substance Abuse and Mental Health Services Administration (NIDRR Grant H133B040038; CMHS Contract 280-03-4201). The content does not necessarily represent the views or policies of the funding agencies. Special thanks to "Elizabeth" and "Devon" for sharing their story and to the following people, who provided material for this chapter: Sue Ryan of Partners for Kids and Families, Mt. Holly, New Jersey, and Lynette Tolliver and Jane Kallal of the Family Involvement Center, Phoenix, Arizona.

as necessary. The team continues its work until members reach the consensus that a formal wraparound process is no longer needed (Walker et al., 2004).

But wraparound is far more than just a planning process. It is a value-based approach to providing care to children with the most complex needs and their families. The values of wraparound as expressed in its core principles (Table 5.1) are fully consistent with the system of care approach (Stroul & Friedman, 1986). Wraparound's philosophy of care begins from the principle of *voice and choice*, which stipulates that the perspectives of the family—including the child or youth—must be given primary importance during all phases and activities of service delivery. The values associated with wraparound further require that the planning process itself, as well as the services and supports provided, should be individualized, family driven, culturally competent, and community based. In addition,

Table 5.1. Ten principles of the wraparound process

1. *Family voice and choice*—Family and youth/child perspectives are intentionally elicited and prioritized during all phases of the wraparound process. Planning is grounded in family members' perspectives, and the team strives to provide options and choices such that the plan reflects family values and preferences.

2. *Team based*—The wraparound team consists of individuals agreed upon by the family and committed to them through informal, formal, and community support and service relationships.

3. *Natural supports*—The team actively seeks out and encourages the full participation of team members drawn from family members' networks of interpersonal and community relationships. The wraparound plan reflects activities and interventions that draw on sources of natural support.

4. *Collaboration*—Team members work cooperatively and share responsibility for developing, implementing, monitoring, and evaluating a single wraparound plan. The plan reflects a blending of team members' perspectives, mandates, and resources. The plan guides and coordinates each team member's work towards meeting the team's goals.

5. *Community based*—The wraparound team implements service and support strategies that take place in the most inclusive, most responsive, most accessible, and least restrictive settings possible; and that safely promote child and family integration into home and community life.

6. *Culturally competent*—The wraparound process demonstrates respect for and builds on the values, preferences, beliefs, culture, and identity of the child/youth and family, and their community.

7. *Individualized*—To achieve the goals laid out in the wraparound plan, the team develops and implements a customized set of strategies, supports, and services.

8. *Strengths based*—The wraparound process and the wraparound plan identify, build on, and enhance the capabilities, knowledge, skills, and assets of the child and family, their community, and other team members.

9. *Persistence*—Despite challenges, the team persists in working toward the goals included in the wraparound plan until the team reaches agreement that a formal wraparound process is no longer required.

10. *Outcome based*—The team ties the goals and strategies of the wraparound plan to observable or measurable indicators of success, monitors progress in terms of these indicators, and revises the plan accordingly.

Reprinted from Bruns, E.J., Walker, J.S., Adams, J., Miles, P., Osher, T.W., Rast, J., et al. (2004). *Ten principles of the wraparound process*. Portland, OR: Portland State University, National Wraparound Initiative, Research and Training Center on Family Supports and Children's Mental Health.

the wraparound process should increase the *natural support* available to a family by strengthening interpersonal relationships and utilizing other resources available in the family's network of social and community relationships. Finally, the wraparound process should be *strengths based*, including activities that purposefully help children and families recognize, utilize, and build talents, assets, and positive capacities.

The wraparound process stands in sharp contrast to traditional forms of service delivery, which have often been experienced by youth and families as professional driven, family blaming, deficit based, and lacking in respect for the family's needs, beliefs, and values (Friesen & Huff, 1996; Rosenblatt, 1996). Consider the true story of one youth, "Devon," and his mother, "Elizabeth," which is discussed at several points throughout this chapter.

Devon had a close family that always took great pride in his athletic abilities and his participation in the gifted and talented program in school. Elizabeth said, "Devon was always a great kid," and spoke with pride about how he was invited to take the SAT in seventh grade through a university program. "Then," Elizabeth cringed, "he shut down over night, not caring about anything . . . depressed. He wouldn't get up in the morning. Devon was a happy kid who was on top of the world and fell off of the Earth."

Devon attempted suicide, and Elizabeth began navigating through the complicated, uncoordinated child-serving systems. Devon was hospitalized five times one year with what Elizabeth stated were "poor discharge plans that made recommendations like, 'make an appointment with therapist.'" Unfortunately, Elizabeth was unable to get an appointment with a therapist because there were waiting lists. "School was a joke," she reported. "He missed his whole freshman year. It took me three months to get tutors for him. They didn't understand his needs." Elizabeth, who has four other children, one of whom has cerebral palsy and requires very intensive care, lamented, "Everything was on me."

HISTORY AND EARLY DEVELOPMENT OF WRAPAROUND

In the United States, calls for reforming children's mental health care date back to the 1960s. Over the decades, the themes remained the same, reflecting similar frustrations as those expressed by Elizabeth: Access to services and supports was limited, child-serving systems rarely worked together, and available services were ineffective or provided in overly restrictive settings (Joint Commission on the Mental Health of Children, 1969; President's Commission on Mental Health,

1978; U.S. Congress Office of Technology Assessment, 1986; U.S. Public Health Service, 2000). Although these problems were pervasive, several pioneering efforts in the 1970s and 1980s provided cause for optimism and the basis for enthusiasm about the wraparound concept. Led by Karl Dennis, the Kaleidoscope program in Chicago demonstrated the success that could result from doing whatever was necessary to keep youth in their homes and communities (Dennis & Lourie, 2006). Using a similar approach, the Alaska Youth Initiative (AYI), led by Robert Sewell and John VanDenBerg, brought almost all youth with serious and complex needs who had been placed in out-of-state residential facilities home to Alaska (Burchard, Burchard, Sewell, & VanDenBerg, 1993).

Eventually, the term *wraparound* was coined to describe such efforts to provide an array of community-based services as an alternative to institutionalization. Support for the wraparound concept was found in several psychosocial theories of child development and social ecology (e.g., Bandura, 1977; Bronfenbrenner, 1977), and support for wraparound principles was derived from studies on family engagement strategies, team-based decision making, and the importance of maintaining youth in community-based living. At its core, the basic premise underlying initial projects such as Kaleidoscope and AYI was straightforward: If a family's needs can be identified, and adequate community resources can be directed to meet them, it is likely that the family will be able to lead a better life and the youth or child will be able to remain with his or her family or community (VanDenBerg, Bruns, & Burchard, 2003). Implicit in these efforts was the notion that providing wraparound to families within a community would also help promote the understanding and adoption of system of care principles such as community based, collaborative, and family driven (Stroul & Friedman, 1986).

Before long, these hypotheses were being tested through more rigorous research, including Project Wraparound in Vermont (Burchard & Clarke, 1990) and the California Model System of Care Project, which showed dramatic reductions in group home and residential placement rates and expenditures, as well as positive outcomes for enrolled youth (Rosenblatt, Attkisson, & Fernandez, 1992). In the mid-1990s, Wraparound Milwaukee established itself as a preeminent example of taking the wraparound concept to scale, moving from a successful "25-Kid" pilot project to assuming responsibility for more than 700 young people who otherwise would be served in out-of-community or institutional placements. Within a few years, use of residential treatment in Milwaukee County declined 60%, use of psychiatric hospitalization fell 80%, and average overall care costs for target youth dropped by one third, from more than $5,000 per month to less than $3,300. Meanwhile, rates of offending behaviors for these youth were cut dramatically from pretreatment levels (Kamradt, 2000).

The 1990s also saw rapid expansion of the research base relevant to wraparound, including randomized studies of wraparound-like projects in the mental health system in upstate New York (Evans, Armstrong, & Kuppinger, 1996) and with a child welfare population in Florida (Clark, Lee, Prange, & McDonald, 1996). Both of these studies found more positive outcomes for the care management/wraparound–enrolled youth than for youth in control groups. In addition, four quasi-experimental studies and multiple pre–post evaluations of wraparound programs were published in the 1990s and early 2000s, the vast majority of which concluded that wraparound implementation promoted positive outcomes for communities and families (for a review, see Burchard, Bruns, & Burchard, 2002). In total, results of eight controlled studies of wraparound-like efforts (four experimental and four quasi-experimental) have been published as of 2007, with an estimated average effect size across the wide range of outcomes assessed of 0.32 (Suter & Bruns, 2007).

The emergence of an evidence base for wraparound in the 1990s continued to promote wraparound implementation efforts nationally, but even early on, there were warnings about defining the process and maintaining its integrity. As Clark and Clarke stated,

> The push to rapidly implement wraparound approaches has resulted in a plethora of service models that vary widely in their implementation, processes, structures, and theories. While this push has been an important part of . . . the shift to less restrictive, more integrated community-based service alternatives, it has also resulted in an unsystematic application of the wraparound process. (1996, p. 2)

As a result of such concerns, a group of stakeholders gathered in 1998 to specify essential elements of the wraparound philosophy, as well as examples of implementation requirements (Burns & Goldman, 1999). Although it was a major milestone, this foundational document did not provide a specific description of what policy makers, providers, or team members should do to ensure that the philosophy is translated into practice (Walker & Bruns, 2006b; Walker & Schutte, 2004). Consequently, concerns persisted about ways to promote replication, measure implementation quality, and compare delivery strategies.

In the early 2000s, several research studies highlighted the *fidelity problem* in wraparound. First, several multisite studies found great variation in wraparound quality (Bruns, Burchard, Suter, Leverentz-Brady, & Force, 2004; Walker & Schutte, 2005), with many so-called wraparound programs failing to build high-functioning teams, develop individualized plans, monitor outcomes, incorporate informal supports, or use family and community strengths to implement services. Second, Bickman, Smith, Lambert, and Andrade (2003) published an evaluation study that showed no consistent difference in outcomes between a wraparound site and a non-wraparound comparison site. However, the study failed to assess "wrapness," thus concluding that "there is no evidence that the content or quality of services were [sic] different for the wraparound children" (p. 151).

Shortly after the turn of the millennium, it was becoming clear to those interested in implementing and researching the wraparound process that two of the model's strengths—its grassroots development and its focus on flexibility and individualization—were also presenting challenges. Researchers were unable to characterize implementation quality, compare results across studies, or replicate positive outcomes. Program developers found it difficult to compare notes on implementation strategies and share resources. The most problematic aspect was that families were not sure whether they were going to get "wraparound or the runaround."

Devon was referred to a "care management" program. At last, Elizabeth had some help with finding and managing the basic services that Devon needed. This provided some relief to her and the rest of the family. Devon was able to receive therapy through a local agency once per week, and a nurse practitioner monitored his medication. Elizabeth, however, felt Devon was getting worse. He had gained 40 pounds and "hated the way he looked." The medication seemed to be causing some bizarre symptoms.

Elizabeth remembered that the care manager kept her informed and was a "good case manager," but she complained that the care manager had a huge caseload and that formal resources were limited. There was no real problem solving around the family's broader needs. Elizabeth continued to feel overwhelmed, and she was certain that she had no support. She stated, "Devon had no life, and my other children were getting pushed to the side."

The continuing story of Devon and his family reflects a problem in the children's services world. Although systems were beginning to recognize the need to provide care management for families with complex needs, few programs featured mechanisms for supporting creative, team-based planning processes. Adding to the problem was the fact that many of these programs were calling themselves "wraparound," further confusing the field about the expected outcomes for a high-quality wraparound process.

DEVELOPING A PRACTICE MODEL FOR WRAPAROUND

Recognizing the need for a more precise description of practice expectations, a group of stakeholders from across North America came together in 2003 to explore a collaborative approach to defining wraparound and laying the groundwork for research on its effectiveness. By the end of the meeting, participants had agreed to work collectively on several priority areas: refining the principles of wraparound, describing the essential activities that constitute the wraparound process, articulating a theory of change for wraparound, and clarifying necessary implementation support. Beyond clarifying practice expectations, achieving a broad-based consensus on these areas would provide the necessary foundation for rigorous research on the effectiveness of the wraparound process.

Defining Principles and Essential Activities

By the end of 2004, the group of stakeholders, now called the National Wraparound Initiative (NWI; Walker & Bruns, 2006a), had grown to more than 80 members, including family members, advocates, youth consumers, service providers, and administrators and policy makers from the agency level to the state and national levels. Membership in the NWI was open to anyone with a high level of experience with wraparound, and work was conducted largely via e-mail and the Internet, using a range of collaborative and consensus-building strategies. The first work of the NWI was to refine and clarify the principles of wraparound so that each principle was clearly described and distinct from the others and, when taken together, the principles expressed the complete philosophy for wraparound practice. On the basis of several rounds of NWI member feedback and ratings, a new version of the principles was created. The revised principles (see Table 5.1) were acceptable to a large majority of NWI members (Walker & Bruns, 2006b).

A similar consensus-building process was used to develop a description of the core activities of the wraparound process (Walker & Bruns, 2006a). The practice model that emerged from this process includes 32 activities grouped into four phases—engagement and team preparation, initial plan development, implementation, and transition (Table 5.2). The activities are defined in a manner that is

Table 5.2. Phases and activities of the wraparound process

Phase 1: Engagement and team preparation

1.1. Orient the family and youth to wraparound and address legal and ethical issues.

1.2. Stabilize crises: Elicit information from family members, agency representatives and potential team members about immediate crises or potential crises, and prepare a response.

1.3. Explore strengths, needs, culture, and vision during conversations with child/youth and family, and prepare summary document.

1.4. Engage and orient other team members.

1.5. Make necessary meeting arrangements.

Phase 2: Initial plan development

2.1. Develop an initial plan of care: Determine ground rules, describe and document strengths, create team mission, describe and prioritize needs/goals, determine outcomes and indicators for each goal, select strategies, and assign action steps.

2.2. Create a safety/crisis plan to ameliorate risk and respond to potential emergencies.

2.3. Complete necessary documentation and logistics.

Phase 3: Implementation

3.1. Implement action steps for each strategy of the wraparound plan, track progress on action steps, evaluate success of strategies, and celebrate successes.

3.2. Revisit and update the plan, considering new strategies as necessary.

3.3. Maintain/build team cohesiveness and trust by maintaining awareness of team members' satisfaction and "buy-in," and addressing disagreements or conflict.

3.4. Complete necessary documentation and logistics.

Phase 4: Transition

4.1. Plan for cessation of formal wraparound: Create a transition plan and a post-transition crisis management plan, and modify the wraparound process to reflect transition.

4.2. Create a "commencement" by documenting the team's work and celebrating success.

4.3. Follow up with the family.

Reprinted from Walker, J.S., et al. (2004). *Phases and activities of the wraparound process.* Portland, OR: Portland State University, Research and Training Center on Family Support and Children's Mental Health, National Wraparound Initiative.

sufficiently precise to permit fidelity measurement but also sufficiently flexible to allow for diversity in the methods by which a given activity might be accomplished. The intention is to provide a "skeleton" of essential activities that can be accomplished or "fleshed out" in ways that are appropriate for individual communities or even individual teams. For example, an important activity during the phase of initial plan development is the team's elicitation of a range of needs or goals on which they will work, then prioritization of a small number of these goals to pursue first. The practice model specifies that both of these steps must happen, but it does not specify the definite manner in which they must occur. Teams may use a variety of processes or procedures for eliciting needs or goals, and priority needs or goals can be selected using any of the many forms of decision making (e.g., voting, consensus building).

Developing a Theory of Change for Wraparound

Most, if not all, of the wraparound principles are well-supported by theory and research. For example, the principle of "family voice and choice," as well as the engagement phase that takes place early in the process, is supported by multiple studies (e.g., Heflinger, Bickman, Northrup, & Sonnichsen, 1997; McKay & Bannon, 2004; Spoth & Redmond, 2000) concerning the relationship between child and family engagement in services and outcomes. Similarly, the principle of services being "team based" is supported by positive outcomes for models using interdisciplinary teams, as well as more general organizational studies showing that well-functioning teams succeed in generating far more effective plans than individuals (see Walker & Schutte, 2004). However, while wraparound has always had implicit associations with various psychosocial theories (Burchard, Bruns, & Burchard, 2002), only preliminary efforts had been made to explain why practice undertaken in accordance with wraparound's principles should produce the desired outcome (Walker & Schutte, 2004).

Incorporating research findings from related fields, the theory of change developed collaboratively by the NWI (Figure 5.1) posits that participation in wraparound is expected to lead to desired outcomes via two main interacting routes. One route highlights the fact that increasing family and youth/child empowerment, optimism, and efficacy contributes to achieving team goals and mission and also leads directly to positive outcomes (i.e., independently of therapeutic services provided in the plan) for children and their families. These outcomes include increased resilience and developmental assets, better quality of life, improved coping, and increased ability to initiate and maintain heath-promoting behavior change. The other route highlights how building team collaboration and promoting family and youth empowerment and engagement in choosing services and supports increases the extent to which services and supports "fit" family and youth needs, goals, preferences, and values. This, in turn, leads to increased treatment engagement, retention, and effectiveness.

As Devon's story continued, it was not difficult to identify several of these pathways promoting positive family outcomes.

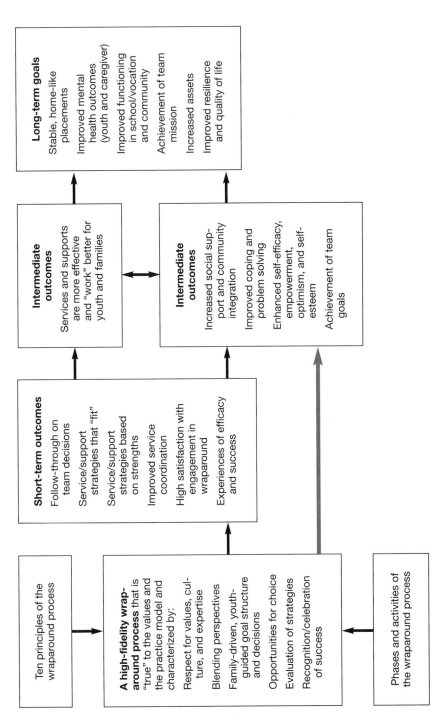

Figure 5.1. A theory of change for wraparound: Overview.

After several months of struggle, Devon was referred to an organization that provided care management via the wraparound process. The wraparound care manager began the process by visiting with Elizabeth and Devon several times and identifying the sources of formal and informal support from which the family might draw. At the first team meeting, held at Elizabeth and Devon's house, many new team members participated along with the care manager, Elizabeth, and Devon. These included Devon's father and stepfather, his Aunt Becky, his grandfather, his older brother, his older sister, his younger brother, his younger sister, one of his teachers whom he liked very much, a family support partner, his therapist, and a behavioral assistant who was also viewed as one of Devon's mentors.

"That meeting was incredible," Elizabeth said. "Even Daisy the dog was there. We started out with strength exercises, and we talked about everything good about my son. It was amazing. Everybody said good things about Devon, things he needed to hear. He had gone into his own shell, and he hadn't heard good things about himself in a long time.

"We put this plan together, and Devon drove his own plan. He figured out things that he wanted to do. He wanted to play baseball. It was like you could see the light in him. He talked about how much music meant to him. His team helped him start music lessons, and he went back to baseball. The team was able to work with this plan by having his dad coach. His teacher made a plan with him that every day she would check in with him because he was so behind in school. Some safety plans were also put into place, which included him being honest with me every day. He developed a close relationship with Jason, the behavioral assistant. Jason would come even when he didn't have to. The next behavioral assistant, Kevin, was the same way. If I had to call Kevin today, he would come."

Elizabeth continued, "The plan worked for a while, and we got through sophomore year of high school. My husband, Devon's stepfather, went to Iraq at this point. Devon did start to fall apart again. I can't pinpoint what happened. He was cutting himself and then cut someone else. Things with Devon were incredibly unsafe. He went to a residential facility for a period of time. We stayed in wraparound and held the meetings at the facility."

When Devon turned 18, representatives of the facility wanted him to go to a step-down unit at the same facility, but Devon desperately wanted to go home and be with his family and in his community. The wraparound team created a plan that enabled him to return home with safety plans. They were able to get the school to come to the facility to design an individualized education program that was in line with the wraparound plan. The school representative wanted to know "why is everyone jumping through hoops for this kid?" Devon now says that this mean-spirited remark challenged him to succeed.

With support from an ever-changing team, Devon caught up with his schoolwork and graduated. The child and family team ended its formal process after he graduated, having achieved its team mission of helping Devon stay safe and graduate high school. The process, however, did not end abruptly. Team members worked to find Devon a job, and other team members supported him in other ways. Devon now works and plays music in a garage band. Elizabeth said, "He's not perfect. He still gets in trouble sometimes, but he has found coping skills, and he is close to his family."

Supporting High-Fidelity Wraparound

Supporting high-quality wraparound such as that experienced by Devon and his family is not easy, and care managers and teams without access to needed resources can rapidly "burn out." Communities seeking to implement wraparound quickly encounter the need for many kinds of resources and materials, including orientation and training materials, job and role descriptions, forms, templates, tools, descriptions of practice elements, fidelity and quality assurance tools, interagency agreements, and so forth. In early implementation efforts, communities needed to create many of these materials from scratch. As wraparound became more widely implemented, sharing between programs became more common. This sharing, however, was informal, so communities in need of materials often did not know where resources might already exist and whom they should ask to acquire them. Furthermore, the lack of a base of common understanding about practice and implementation expectations made sharing or collaborating difficult. How could communities share job descriptions if there was no agreement about job titles, competencies, or responsibilities? How could communities share informational materials if each community had its own terminology for describing various aspects of wraparound? How could communities share quality assurance or fidelity tools if there was no common understanding of practice?

From the outset, one of the primary goals of the NWI was to facilitate collaboration and the sharing of data, resources, and innovations across communities implementing wraparound. Establishing a consensus about the wraparound principles, practice, and theory was a first step in building the foundation for this kind of sharing. In the sections that follow, examples are provided that illustrate how this foundation has enabled further collaboration and sharing, which has, in turn, offered many potential benefits to the "field" of wraparound.

Tools Compendium   The description of the phases and activities of the wraparound process does not prescribe procedures or techniques, nor does it require the use of specific forms or templates. Indeed, as previously mentioned, the descriptions of the phases and activities were written with the idea that, although there is a core set of activities essential for wraparound, many options exist for carrying out these activities. One early goal of the NWI was to collect and make generally available resources that proved helpful for actually accomplishing the various activities. This idea evolved into a vision for an online, searchable compendium of tools that would provide ideas and options for carrying out each activity.

Since its inception in 2005, the NWI has invited its members to submit materials for the compendium. Visitors to the NWI's web site (http://www.rtc.pdx .edu/nwi) can view an outline of the phases and activities, click on any activity, and receive a listing of various tools that may be helpful for that activity. Visitors can download and use any tool, although they are encouraged to cite the tool's contributor and developer. Visitors can also read comments and ratings for each tool and provide their own ratings or comments about when and why a tool is most or least useful.

For example, within the engagement phase, one activity requires that teams "explore strengths, needs, culture, and vision during conversations with child/youth and family, and prepare a summary document." Upon reading this description, it is natural to wonder exactly how these topics are to be explored and what sort of document is to be produced. Using the compendium, one can call up a list of tools that include variations of ecomaps and genograms for drawing out information about strengths and social support, lists of questions and topics for strengths/needs/culture exploration, and so forth. Sample summary documents are also available. Similarly, for the plan development phase, tools include sample lists of ground rules for team interactions, examples of team mission statements, techniques for eliciting and prioritizing needs for the plan, and crisis and wraparound templates and sample plans.

The tools compendium has also been extended to include resources helpful for other aspects of program implementation (e.g., job descriptions, skill sets and competencies, quality assurance tools).

User's Guide to Wraparound   One challenge that wraparound teams and programs typically encounter is the ongoing need to orient participants and stakeholders to the philosophy of wraparound and the activities of the wraparound process. Elizabeth's story demonstrates the importance of making such information available and readily accessible.

During her time attempting to find services and supports for Devon, Elizabeth was a founding member and then later President of the Board of Directors of a very new family support organization. This organization partnered with the care management organization that facilitated the wraparound process for Devon and other children and youth. Elizabeth was eager to learn everything that she could about wraparound, finding materials about the process and even attending care manager training sessions taught by Wraparound Milwaukee.

Orientation materials provided to families must be accessible, attractive, and accurate, giving families a clear overview of what they can expect from the wraparound process and what participation in wraparound will require of them. Many wraparound programs have created their own family guides to the process. Other programs have found this difficult because creating a high-quality guide consumes extensive time and effort. In the past, the lack of a clear, shared definition of the wraparound process made it difficult for one program to use a family guide developed by another program.

With the clarity provided by the NWI description of the wraparound process, it became possible to create a family guide that could be used in any community implementing the specified practice model. The vision was to create a guide that not only oriented families to the wraparound process but also empowered them by describing exactly what they should expect during each phase of the process and encouraging them to take action if these expectations are not met. With this as the goal, a group of NWI members consisting primarily of family members produced a booklet called *The Wraparound Process User's Guide: A Handbook for Families* (Miles, Bruns, Osher, Walker, & the National Wraparound Initiative Advisory Group, 2006). The guide has been translated into Spanish, and both versions are available to order or download at http://www.rtc.pdx.edu.

Communities that disseminate the guide have not restricted its distribution to parents and family members. The guide has also been found useful for orienting many other stakeholders (e.g., agency administrators, legislators, service providers such as probation officers, teachers, child welfare workers).

Role of the Family Partner

The first principle of wraparound is "family voice and choice." From the early days of wraparound, it became clear that realizing this principle in practice could be challenging. Family members involved with traditionally organized service systems often have little opportunity to think about family needs or goals for treatment, or to make choices about service and support strategies. Instead, many family members report that service providers typically make the choices and tell families what they need and what they must do. The experience often leaves families feeling blamed, ashamed, and powerless. Thus, when families enter wraparound, they may not have much experience with making meaningful choices or using their "voices," and they may not trust providers on their wraparound teams enough to reveal what they really think. Families in such a position may not fully benefit from the experience of participating on a wraparound team, even a well-resourced one composed of helpful team members.

To help ensure family voice and choice, many communities have adopted a peer-to-peer strategy with a family receiving support from another family member—a family partner—who has personally experienced both the stresses and the rewards of caring for a child with challenging emotional, behavioral, or mental health needs. Family partners know firsthand the frustrations that come from dealing with a service system that is complex and often unresponsive, as well as with providers who seem to see parents as barriers to rather than resources for their children's successful treatment. Family partners can offer relevant help and "often provide the type of practical advice that can only be imagined by one who has been in the situation" (Pumariega & Winters, 2003, p. 38).

Despite widespread acknowledgment of the importance of the family partner role and research demonstrating the potential for positive impact of incorporating family support mechanisms into service delivery, there has historically been little clarity about exactly how family partners are to provide support and advocacy as part of the wraparound process (Hoagwood, 2005; Vostanis, Anderson, & Window, 2006). In 2006, the NWI identified this as a high priority, and a task force, chaired by and composed primarily of family members, spearheaded efforts to describe more clearly how the parent partner role promotes the wraparound principles, as well as what the parent partner actually does to help the family and wraparound team move through the phases and activities of the wraparound process.

Products from this work describe how the family partner becomes a formal member of the wraparound team, with a unique role in promoting each of the wraparound principles. This unique role is particularly clear in the case of the principle of "voice and choice." The family partner endeavors to learn of the family's concerns, needs, and past experiences (good and bad), helps translate these needs to the team, and advocates for the family. Such activity helps ensure that the wraparound process is grounded first and foremost in the family's perspective. At the same time, other wraparound principles require that people involved in implementing wraparound, including family partners, work to promote collaboration between the family, professionals, and other wraparound team members. Performing both aspects of the role—supporting and advocating for families while also promoting collaboration—is a central challenge of the family partner role.

Another aspect of the family partner role involves promoting the principles of "natural support," "individualized," and "community based." Family partners are in a unique position to promote these principles because they have strong connections to the community and are knowledgeable about the resources, services, and supports that can be accessed by the family and the wraparound team. Family partners are also in a unique position to help the family and team successfully participate in the phases and activities of the wraparound process. The family partner often undertakes specific tasks focused on helping the family engage with team members and other providers of services and supports, participate actively on the team, and make informed decisions that drive the wraparound process.

Achieving greater clarity about the family partner's contributions within the wraparound process makes it easier to see what skills are needed and to hire the right people for each job. Serving as a family partner is a role best suited for individuals who are well into the "legacy stage of advocacy" (Donner, 2004, p. 4). They have worked through their own initial stages of understanding their children's issues and are able to help others who are taking the same journey. In addition, the family partner must develop strategies to assist families throughout the stages of the wraparound process. Members of the Family Task Force from the NWI took the lead in creating a document that details the role of the family partner within the wraparound process (Osher, Penn, & National Wraparound Initiative Family Task Force, 2007).

Monitoring Implementation Quality

During the 1980s and early 1990s, when wraparound was initially being developed, service researchers and program evaluators were focused almost exclusively on documenting whether programs achieved their proposed outcomes. More recently, however, evidence has grown about treatments, processes, and system activities that may lead to positive outcomes. As a result, there has been a surge of interest in measuring implementation "fidelity" (i.e., how well a specific program conforms to its defined program model or protocol).

Wraparound has certainly proven to be no exception to this trend. As noted, concerns about conformance to the philosophy and values of wraparound have been consistent and expressed for more than a decade (Clark & Clarke, 1996; Rosenblatt, 1996; Walker & Bruns, 2006b). When the core elements of wraparound were defined in 1998, they provided the first clearly defined expectations for calling a process *wraparound*, as well as the basis for the first wraparound implementation measures, including the Wraparound Fidelity Index (WFI), developed by John Burchard, and the Wraparound Observation Form (WOF), developed by Michael Epstein and colleagues (Bruns, Burchard, Suter, Leverentz-Brady, & Force, 2004; Nordness & Epstein, 2003). Over several years of pilot testing, both of these measures have been established as reliable. In the case of the WFI, validity has been established through a series of studies finding total scores to be associated with expert ratings of implementation quality and with child and family outcomes. WFI scores have also been found to differ significantly for wraparound versus non-wraparound comparison groups in controlled research studies, further establishing its construct validity (Bruns, Burchard, Suter, & Force, 2005).

The advent of fidelity measurement has provided a boost to high-quality wraparound implementation. The WFI, WOF, and other measures provide a template for providers to understand basic practice guidelines. Data can be fed back to providers, supervisors, and stakeholders to inform areas in which service delivery is not adequately conforming to the program model. Fidelity measures also provide a critical tool for researchers, allowing them to assess wraparound implementation in evaluation studies and thus better explain study results. For example, fidelity measurement using a version of the WFI in Nevada found that fidelity for the wraparound group was significantly greater than for a comparison group and that training and quality assurance helped improve this fidelity over time (Bruns, Rast, Walker, Bosworth, & Peterson, 2006; Rast, Brown, Bruns, Mears, & Peterson, in submission). Such results were important for explaining why outcomes were likely better for the wraparound group and for establishing the degree of implementation fidelity needed to produce these outcomes.

Fidelity data collection has also helped the field understand critical issues regarding wraparound implementation. For example, one study confirmed the hypothesis that system and organizational supports were critical to achieving wraparound fidelity for individual families (Bruns, Suter, & Leverentz-Brady, 2006). Data collection across many communities nationally using the WFI was able to illuminate areas in which implementation consistently veers away from the prescribed wraparound principles and thus set the stage for the NWI. Eventually, results of fidelity assessments across many studies hold the promise of explaining what factors are related to outcomes and why more positive outcomes may have occurred for certain communities and programs than others.

To date, the methods used by the WFI (interviews with parents, wraparound facilitators, youth, and team members) and the WOF (rating of practice quality during team meetings) still represent two of the most common approaches to assessing wraparound implementation quality. Initial versions of these measures, however, were not based on a clear practice model that described the specific activities that should take place during the wraparound team process. With the development of more specific descriptions of the phases and activities of wraparound, new versions of fidelity measures have been developed that are more directly aligned with the practice model for the wraparound process. It is expected that WFI Version 4, and other components of the Wraparound Fidelity Assessment System (e.g., a new Team Observation Measure and Document Review Measure) will be more useful to evaluators, supervisors, and program administrators. Fidelity assessment will be based on several sources of information, making assessment more comprehensive, valid, and capable of presenting more specific strengths and weaknesses in areas of implementation. Sample items from the various measures are provided in Table 5.3.

Importance of System Supports for Wraparound

Research and experience have shown that successfully implementing the wraparound process at the team level requires extensive support and collaboration from agencies and organizations that are part of the larger system of care. For example, these agencies and organizations must collaborate to develop and provide access to the services and supports included in wraparound plans, ensure that personnel are trained for their roles on teams, allow staff the time and flexibility required to carry out team-assigned tasks, and monitor the quality of wraparound provided and the outcomes for children and families. Typically, providing the necessary level of system support requires that collaborating agencies and organizations make many changes that involve the reallocation of resources and the creation of new policies. Furthermore, because wraparound is a collaborative effort that is not "owned" by a single agency, communities usually find it necessary to create some kind of collaborative system-level body or governance structure through which stakeholders act collectively to carry out key functions (e.g., strategic planning, risk management, oversight).

Experience has also shown that achieving the necessary level of collaboration and support is challenging due to entrenched organizational cultures and ways of doing business, interagency barriers, funding exigencies, and skepticism regarding the effectiveness of family-driven, strengths-based practices. It is also not easy to

Table 5.3. Sample items from measures included in the Wraparound Fidelity Assessment System (WFAS)

WFAS measure	Sample items	Wraparound principle assessed
Wraparound Fidelity Index, Version 4 (interviews with parents/caregivers, youth, facilitators, and team members)*	1.4 Did you select the people who would be on your youth and family team?	Family voice and choice
	3.7 Does your team evaluate progress toward the goals in the wraparound plan at every team meeting?	Outcome based
	4.5 After formal wraparound has ended, do you think the process will be able to be "re-started" if you or your family need it?	Persistence
Team Observation Measure	2a. Team meeting attendees are oriented to the wraparound process and understand the purpose of the meeting.	Team based
	6a. Planning includes action steps or goals for other family members, not just the identified child.	Individualized
	8a. Brainstorming of options and strategies include strategies to be implemented by natural and community supports.	Natural supports
Document Review Measure	3. Documentation includes detailed examples of youth, family, and team strengths.	Strengths based
	11. Services are coordinated through a single plan.	Collaboration
	19. The plan includes strategies for involving the youth in community activities.	Community based

*Sample items are from the Caregiver Version of the WFI-4 (Wraparound Evaluation and Research Team, 2007).

look at an existing system and see exactly what kinds of supports are lacking or where system development efforts should focus. What is more, when system development is underway, it can be difficult to assess whether meaningful progress is occurring.

Recognizing these difficulties, the NWI developed and tested the Community Supports for Wraparound Inventory (CSWI), an assessment of the system-level collaboration and support for wraparound. The CSWI is based on research that enumerated a series of "necessary conditions" that must be in place at the organization and system levels for wraparound implementation to be successful and sustainable (Walker & Koroloff, 2007; Walker, Koroloff, & Schutte, 2003). The CSWI contains 40 items grouped into six themes—community partnership, collaborative action, fiscal policies and sustainability, access to needed supports and services, human resource development and support, and accountability. As the sample CSWI items listed in Table 5.4 illustrate, the system-level supports re-

Table 5.4. Themes and sample items from the Community Supports for Wraparound Inventory

Item	Fully developed system support	Least developed system support

Theme 1: Community Partnership. *Collective community ownership of and responsibility for wraparound is built through collaborations among key stakeholder groups. (7 items)*

| Item 1.3 Influential family voice | Families are influential members of the community team and other decision-making entities, and they take active roles in wraparound program planning, implementation oversight, and evaluation. Families are provided with support and training so that they can participate fully and comfortably in these roles. | Family members are not actively involved in decision-making, or are uninfluential or "token" components of the community team, boards, and other collaborative bodies that plan programs and guide implementation and evaluation. |

Theme 2: Collaborative Action. *Stakeholders involved in the wraparound effort take concrete steps to translate the wraparound philosophy into concrete policies, practices and achievements. (8 items)*

| Item 2.3 Proactive planning | The wraparound effort is guided by a plan for joint action that describes the goals of the wraparound effort, the strategies that will be used to achieve the goals, and the roles of specific stakeholders in carrying out the strategies. | There is no plan for joint action that describes goals of the wraparound effort, strategies for achieving the goals, or roles of specific stakeholders. |

Theme 3: Fiscal Policies and Sustainability. *The community has developed fiscal strategies to meet the needs of children participating in wraparound and methods to collect and use data on expenditures for wraparound-eligible children. (6 items)*

| Item 3.3 Collective fiscal responsibility | Key decision-makers and relevant agencies assume collective fiscal responsibility for children and families participating in wraparound and do not attempt to shift costs to each other or to entities outside of the wraparound effort. | Each agency has its own cost controls and agencies do not collaborate to reduce cost shifting, either to each other or to entities outside of the wraparound effort. |

Theme 4: Access to Needed Supports and Services. *The community has developed mechanisms for ensuring access to the wraparound process and the services and supports that teams need to fully implement their plans. (6 items)*

| Item 4.6 Crisis response | Necessary support for managing crises and fully implementing teams' safety/crisis plans is available around the clock. The community's crisis response is integrated with and supportive of wraparound crisis and safety plans. | Support for managing crises is insufficient, inconsistently available, or uncoordinated with wraparound teams' crisis and safety plans. |

Theme 5: Human Resource Development and Support. *The community supports wraparound and partner agency staff to work in a manner that allows full implementation of the wraparound model. (6 items)*

Item 5.5 Supervision	People with primary roles for carrying out wraparound (e.g., wraparound facilitators, parent partners) receive regular individual and group supervision, and periodic "in-vivo" (observation) supervision from supervisors who are knowledgeable about wraparound and proficient in the skills needed to carry out the wraparound process.	People with primary roles for carrying out wraparound receive little or no regular individual, group, or observational supervision and/or supervisors are inexperienced with wraparound or unable to effectively teach needed skills.

Theme 6: Accountability. *The community has implemented mechanisms to monitor wraparound fidelity, service quality, and outcomes, and to assess the quality and development of the overall wraparound effort.*

Item 6.1 Outcomes monitoring	There is centralized monitoring of relevant outcomes for children, youth, and families in wraparound. This information is used as the basis for funding, policy discussions and strategic planning	There is no tracking of relevant outcomes for children and youth in wraparound, or different agencies and systems involved maintain separate tracking systems.

From Walker, J.S. (2007, June 1). *Community support for Wraparound Inventory: Results of the pilot study.* Conference presentation at the State of the Science Conference: Effective Strategies for All: Strategies to Promote Mental Health and Thriving for Underserved Children and Families, Portland, OR.

quired for successful, sustainable wraparound are extensive and varied. Furthermore, the system context described by the items of the CSWI is one that shares many key features with a system of care. In fact, although research in this area is still in its early stages, it is becoming increasingly clear that wraparound is not likely to be successful in the long run unless it is embedded in an organizational and system context that is transformed or transforming into a system of care.

Research using the CSWI has provided evidence of the measure's reliability and validity. Within communities, there is typically a fairly high level of agreement about the areas in which the greatest progress has been made and the areas in which most work remains to be done. Different communities show variation both in the overall level of implementation support, recognized by item grand means that are high relative to those in other communities, and in areas of strength and challenge. Moreover, previous studies of system and organizational support for wraparound implementation have shown that greater levels of such supports are associated with higher wraparound fidelity scores (Bruns, Suter, & Leverentz-Brady, 2006). Future research using the CSWI will attempt to determine just how important community supports are to both wraparound implementation and child and family outcomes.

FURTHER CHALLENGES AND STRATEGIES

The need for sufficient system and organizational support for wraparound is just one of many challenges to translating the wraparound philosophy into effective practice in the real world. This section describes three additional major challenges that have faced communities across the country and provides examples of effective strategies that can be used to address them.

Ensuring the Use of Natural Supports

Research and anecdotal evidence reveal that teams consistently have difficulty incorporating significant levels of "natural support" into wraparound plans. A promising strategy for addressing this challenge is the creation of new formal roles that focus on increasing natural support resources. One such role is the resource director (RD), a full-time position funded by each care management organization (CMO) in New Jersey. The emphasis of this role is to help the community create support resources needed by wraparound teams that are currently lacking.

Often, wraparound teams focus primarily on a child's emotional or behavioral needs and pay less attention to needs in other life domains. The RD's role emphasizes meeting needs in other life domains and creating community connections that anchor children in community life. For instance, one RD partnered with a local job development program to create a specialized program for youth in the CMO. This program helps teens explore their job interests, learn job skills, and acquire and keep jobs. The RD has also helped to create recreational opportunities for youth (e.g., basketball camps, youth-in-transition camps, respite camps). By working with wraparound facilitators, RDs can develop supports based on families' needs. The result is a support system that is need driven rather than provider driven.

A somewhat different approach to increasing natural support in wraparound plans provides teams with the necessary tools and training to help them more effectively identify and engage potential natural support providers. In Arizona, the state's Department of Health Services contracted with the Family Involvement Center, a family advocacy and support organization, to develop a toolkit to assist with building natural support on wraparound teams. The toolkit features a DVD in which families and youth are shown talking about their lives and their needs, as well as the role that natural support has played in meeting some of those needs and improving their quality of life.

Showing the DVD to people whom the family has identified as potential natural supports serves several important purposes. First, it can be used to help educate members of a family's natural support network about emotional and behavioral disorders, showing them that disorders are not just the result of poor parenting or willful bad behavior on the part of children and youth. Thus, potential natural supporters are encouraged to take a less blaming and more sympathetic stance toward the child and his or her family, which then elicits greater willingness to provide support. Second, the DVD provides examples of natural support that were valuable to children and families in real life. Exposure to the DVD helps friends, family, and community members understand that the support they offer can have a profound effect in the life of a child and his or her family. In addition to the DVD, the toolkit contains training materials that provide specific strategies that families and other team members can use to connect or reconnect with people who may be able to provide natural support, engage them in the wraparound process, and maintain an awareness of their morale to ensure that they will not feel overtaxed by their roles in the wraparound plan.

Increasing Youth Involvement

Ensuring meaningful youth participation in wraparound planning is another challenge that has been documented through both research and anecdotal evidence. Typically, youth are blamed equally, if not more, than their parents for the difficulties they experience, and they are even less encouraged to use their voices and make choices. The Research and Training Center on Family Support and Children's Mental Health in Portland, Oregon, is developing and testing two promising strategies for addressing this challenge. First, the Center has developed and validated two measures—one to assess youth participation in planning and another to assess youth empowerment in planning. These are the first measures that can be used to assess the extent to which wraparound, as well as other programs are successful in promoting youth voice in mental health treatment and planning.

Second, the Center has developed an intervention called Achieve My Plan (AMP). AMP works simultaneously to empower youth within a team planning process and to help youth-serving organizations undertake team planning in ways that encourage and support youth participation. To promote empowerment, AMP calls for training agency staff to facilitate an engagement and preparation process with youth before team meetings so that youth come to meetings ready to contribute goals and strategies to the team plan. The AMP process also teaches youth what to expect during meetings and strategies for positive communication. To promote a planning environment that encourages youth participation, AMP calls for a structured planning process that, among other things, includes time during each meeting to focus on personally meaningful goals identified by the youth. AMP also provides guidelines to which all meeting participants must adhere so as to create an environment in which the youth will feel comfortable participating. In addition, AMP provides DVD- and web-based video clips and other orientation and training materials so that all members of the planning team are educated about the importance and feasibility of youth participation.

Other sites, including one system of care in New York City, have explored using youth in roles parallel to the previously described role of the family partner. In this community, the youth advocate role includes four main functions—mentoring, advocating for, and supporting the youth and serving as a bridge and "translator" between the youth and the service providers. The system of care has developed guidelines for identifying, hiring, training, and supervising youth to serve in the advocate role.

Finally, many communities have encouraged and supported youth to participate in making decisions and creating policies at the program and system levels. An excellent guide that summarizes this work and provides strategies to empower youth is *Youth Involvement in Systems of Care: A Guide to Empowerment* (Matarese, McGinnis, & Mora, 2006).

Workforce Development in Wraparound

Among the challenges inherent to wraparound implementation, perhaps none is as fundamental as the challenge of workforce development. In essence, basic concerns facing the children's mental health field (e.g., the shortage of practitioners in child-serving disciplines, the mismatch between professional training programs and the demands of actual service delivery) are magnified for wraparound initiatives. Wraparound implementation requires practitioners who are prepared to undertake tasks that are extremely complex and outside the bounds of traditional practice models (e.g., facilitating interdisciplinary teams, employing strengths in assessment and treatment, partnering actively with families, using "systems thinking" to develop and implement effective plans of care). Moreover, wraparound requires development for staff across multiple systems (e.g., schools, juvenile justice, child welfare, mental health), all of whom may be asked to participate actively on youths' wraparound teams. Leaders of these systems must also be educated about wraparound implementation so that they will support the vision of the wraparound effort and support their staff to actively participate.

Because university-based training programs do not typically prepare the workforce for this "new way of doing things," the task falls to local agencies and systems, which must make careful decisions about how to invest the necessary resources. Historically, communities have met this need by employing national experts to train staff and stakeholders. Unfortunately, this has been found to have major shortcomings for two reasons. First, training alone has been found to be a poor approach to ensuring high-quality implementation, a hard lesson that is also consistently backed by research (Fixsen, Naoom, Blase, Friedman, & Wallace, 2005). Second, relying on external experts means that local capacity is not created to consistently and efficiently support workforce development.

To address these concerns, states and communities have become more likely to develop local capacity, often through partnerships between public agencies, universities, and family organizations. Maryland's Child and Adolescent Community Innovations Institute and the Eastern North Carolina Public-Academic Liaison are two such examples. In other communities, including Los Angeles County, provider agencies responsible for wraparound implementation have joined into training consortia, leveraging shared resources in partnership with national consultants who help devise workforce development plans.

Another advance has been that national training entities, as well as states and localities, are moving beyond reliance on training alone as the method for ensuring practitioner competence. Increasingly, staff development includes steps (e.g., training, shadowing, in-vivo coaching, demonstration of proficiency) that lead to the required credentialing before a staff person or supervisor can practice independently in his or her role. Data collection is increasingly being employed in these procedures, including the use of supervisor assessments, self-assessments, and consumer and family reports. In addition, when external training and technical assistance are employed to support a community's wraparound effort, workforce development procedures often include methods for credentialing local trainers and coaches, who can then operate independently in that state or community.

Creating local workforce development capacity has several additional benefits. First, as wraparound becomes the standard "way of doing business," a community with a systematic workforce development strategy can use it to create a career ladder (e.g., from wraparound facilitator to certified coach to supervisor). When parent and youth partners, resource development specialists, and other roles are also included, career mobility options increase even further. Wraparound Milwaukee is one initiative that has effectively created such a career ladder, increasing retention of skilled individuals who fill wraparound roles.

A second advantage to localized professional development is that communities can train and support professionals to fill roles specific to the needs of the local wraparound effort. This also can lead to significant innovation as new types of positions are created and traditional professional roles are reconfigured to better meet the needs of families served by wraparound teams. For example, in Los Angeles County, Hathaway-Sycamores trains and employs wraparound clinicians. Rather than traditional office-based services, activities of wraparound clinicians are specific to wraparound (e.g., supporting clinical decision making on teams, translating wraparound plans into Medicaid plans). Similarly, some local wraparound initiatives also train and employ behavioral support specialists, whose work is defined by the goals in wraparound plans and evaluated by indicators of youths' behavioral success as defined by the wraparound team.

A final benefit of innovating local workforce development is that it helps sustain community wraparound efforts. When professional development is effective, is conducted through multidisciplinary partnerships, engages many types of professional roles, and spans across levels from administrators to staff to family members, it serves as a means of reinforcing the initial vision of a wraparound initiative and the more fundamental system of care principles.

CONCLUSION

As described in this chapter, enthusiasm for implementing the wraparound process continues in the field of child and family services. This enthusiasm, however, has been mitigated by the need to better define the practice model and clarify the supports necessary for making it happen in the "real world." There is also concern that, although the evidence base on wraparound is largely positive, results of more rigorous evaluation are needed to justify its widespread use (Farmer, Dorsey, & Mustillo, 2004). The rush to establish wraparound as an "evidence-based practice" highlights unique challenges, including wraparound's status as a care management process as opposed to a treatment, its individualized nature, and its grounding in a value base.

At the same time, the research base on wraparound is rapidly expanding, and more recent controlled research (Carney & Buttell, 2003; Pullmann et al., 2006) and success stories from individual communities (Anderson, Wright, Kooreman, Mohr, & Russell, 2003; Bruns, Rast et al., 2006; Kamradt, 2000) have served to support the wraparound movement. In general, the story of wraparound's potential for impact for different types of families will not be decided by one or even several well-controlled studies but by multiple research efforts across many settings. In addition, the experiences of children and families continue to reinforce wraparound's expansion.

Elizabeth summed it up this way: "You are so emotionally involved, and this is your heart. Having someone to actually help you organize and find services and supports—that is the major key when it feels like every day is chaos. Having a child-family team when you're in the middle of this, you really see who is there for you. They were always there, I guess, but realizing it was everything."

REFERENCES

Anderson, J.A., Wright, E.R., Kooreman, H.E., Mohr, W.K., & Russell, L. (2003). The Dawn Project: A model for responding to the needs of young people with emotional and behavioral disabilities and their families. *Community Mental Health Journal, 39,* 63–74.

Bandura, A. (1977). *Social learning theory.* Englewood Cliffs, NJ: Prentice Hall.

Bickman, L., Smith, C.M., Lambert, E.W., & Andrade, A.R. (2003). Evaluation of a congressionally mandated wraparound demonstration. *Journal of Child and Family Studies, 12,* 135–156.

Bronfenbrenner, U. (1979). *The ecology of human development: Experiments by nature and design.* Cambridge, MA: Harvard University Press.

Bruns, E.J., Burchard, J.D., Suter, J.C., & Force, M.D. (2005). Measuring fidelity within community treatments for children and families. In M.H. Epstein, K. Kutash, & A.J. Duchnowski (Eds.), *Outcomes for children and youth with emotional and behavioral disorders and their families* (pp. 175–197). Austin, TX: PRO-ED.

Bruns, E.J., Burchard, J.D., Suter, J.C., Leverentz-Brady, K., & Force, M.M. (2004). Assessing fidelity to a community-based treatment for youth: The Wraparound Fidelity Index. *Journal of Emotional and Behavioral Disorders, 12,* 79–89.

Bruns, E.J., Rast, J., Walker, J.S., Bosworth, J., & Peterson, C. (2006). Spreadsheets, service providers, and the statehouse: Using data and the wraparound process to reform systems for children and families. *American Journal of Community Psychology, 38,* 201–212.

Bruns, E.J., Suter, J.C., & Leverentz-Brady, K.L. (2006). Relations between program and system variables and fidelity to the wraparound process for children and families. *Psychiatric Services, 57*(11), 1586–1593.

Bruns, E.J., Walker, J.S., Adams, J., Miles, P., Osher, T.W., Rast, J., et al. (2004). *Ten principles of the wraparound process.* Portland, OR: Portland State University, Research and Training Center on Family Supports and Children's Mental Health, National Wraparound Initiative.

Burchard, J.D., Bruns, E.J., & Burchard, S.N. (2002). The wraparound approach. In B.J. Burns & K. Hoagwood (Eds.), *Community treatment for youth: Evidence-based interventions for severe emotional and behavioral disorders* (pp. 69–90). New York: Oxford University Press.

Burchard, J.D., Burchard, S.N., Sewell, R., & VanDenBerg, J. (1993). *One kid at a time: Evaluative case studies of the Alaska Youth Initiative Demonstration Project.* Washington, DC: Georgetown University Child Development Center, CASSP Technical Assistance Center.

Burchard, J.D., & Clarke, R.T. (1990). The role of individualized care in a service delivery system for children and adolescents with severely maladjusted behavior. *Journal of Mental Health Administration, 17,* 48–60.

Burns, B.J., & Goldman, S.K. (1999). *Systems of care: Promising practices in children's mental health, 1998 series: Promising practices in wraparound for children with severe emotional disorders and their families* (Vol. 2). Washington, DC: American Institutes for Research, Center for Effective Collaboration and Practice.

Carney, M.M., & Buttell, F. (2003). Reducing juvenile recidivism: Evaluating the Wraparound services model. *Research on Social Work Practice, 13*(5), 551–568.

Clark, H.B., & Clarke, R.T. (1996). Research on the wraparound process and individualized services for children with multi-system needs. *Journal of Child and Family Studies, 5,* 1–5.

Clark, H.B., Lee, B., Prange, M.E., & McDonald, B.A. (1996). Children lost within the foster care system: Can wraparound service strategies improve placement outcomes? *Journal of Child and Family Studies, 5,* 39–54.

Dennis, K.W., & Lourie, I.S. (2006). *Everything is normal until proven otherwise.* Washington, DC: Child Welfare League of America.

Donner, R. (2004). *Putting the pieces together: Skills for family support partners.* Trenton, NJ: New Jersey Division of Child Behavioral Health.

Evans, M.E., Armstrong, M.I., & Kuppinger, A.D. (1996). Family-centered intensive case management: A step toward understanding individualized care. *Journal of Child and Family Studies, 5*(1), 55–65.

Farmer, E.M.Z., Dorsey, S., & Mustillo, S.A. (2004). Intensive home and community interventions. *Child and Adolescent Psychiatric Clinics of North America, 13*(1), 857–884.

Fixsen, D., Naoom, S.F., Blase, K.A., Friedman, R.M., & Wallace, F. (2005). *Implementation research: A synthesis of the literature.* Tampa: University of South Florida, Louis de la Parte Florida Mental Health Institute, National Implementation Research Network.

Friesen, B.J., & Huff, B. (1996). Family perspectives on systems of care. In B.A. Stroul & R.M. Friedman (Series Eds.) & B.A. Stroul (Ed.), *Systems of care for children's mental health: Children's mental health: Creating systems of care in a changing society* (pp. 41–67). Baltimore: Paul H. Brookes Publishing Co.

Heflinger, C.A., Bickman, L., Northrup, D., & Sonnichsen, S. (1997). A theory-driven intervention and evaluation to explore family caregiver empowerment. *Journal of Emotional and Behavioral Disorders, 5,* 184–191.

Hoagwood, K. (2005). Family-based services in children's mental health: A research review and synthesis. *Journal of Child Psychology and Psychiatry: Annual Research Review, 46,* 690–713.

Joint Commission on the Mental Health of Children. (1969). *Crisis in child mental health.* New York: Harper & Row.

Kamradt, B. (2000). Wraparound Milwaukee: Aiding youth with mental health needs. *Juvenile Justice, 7,* 14–23.

Matarese, M., McGinnis, L., & Mora, M. (2006). *Youth involvement in systems of care: A guide to empowerment.* Washington, DC: American Institutes for Research, Technical Assistance Partnership.

McKay, M.M., & Bannon, W. (2004). Engaging families in child mental health services. *Child and Adolescent Psychiatric Clinics of North America, 13,* 905–921.

Miles, P., Bruns, E.J., Osher, T.W., Walker, J.S., & the National Wraparound Initiative Advisory Group. (2006). *The wraparound process user's guide: A handbook for families.* Portland, OR: Portland State University, Research and Training Center on Family Support and Children's Mental Health, National Wraparound Initiative.

Nordness, P.D., & Epstein, M.H. (2003). Reliability of the Wraparound Observation Form (2nd version): An instrument designed to assess the fidelity of the wraparound approach. *Mental Health Services Research, 5,* 89–96.

Osher, T.W., Penn, M., & National Wraparound Initiative Family Task Force. (2007). *Phases and activities of the wraparound process: What the family partner contributes.* Portland, OR: Portland State University, Research and Training Center on Family Support and Children's Mental Health, National Wraparound Initiative.

President's Commission on Mental Health. (1978). *Report of the sub-task panel on infants, children, and adolescents.* Washington, DC: Author.

Pullmann, M.D., Kerbs, J., Koroloff, N., Veach-White, E., Gaylor, R., & Sieler, D. (2006). Juvenile offenders with mental health needs: Reducing recidivism using wraparound. *Crime and Delinquency, 52,* 375–397.

Pumariega, A.J., & Winters, N.C. (Eds.). (2003). *The handbook of child and adolescent systems of care: The new community psychiatry.* San Francisco: Jossey-Bass.

Rast, J., Brown, E.C., Bruns, E.J., Mears, S.L., & Peterson, C.R. (in submission). Impact of the wraparound process in a child welfare system: Results of a matched comparison study. *Social Work Research.*

Rosenblatt, A. (1996). Bows and ribbons, tape and twine: Wrapping the wraparound process for children with multisystem needs. *Journal of Child and Family Studies, 5*(1), 101–117.

Rosenblatt, A., Attkisson, C.C., & Fernandez, A.J. (1992). Integrating systems of care in California for youth with severe emotional disturbance: II. Initial group home expenditure and utilization findings from the California AB377 Evaluation Project. *Journal of Child and Family Studies, 1,* 263–286.

Sather, A., Bruns, E.J., Stambaugh, L.F., & Burns, B.J. (2007, June). *The state wraparound survey.* Paper presented at the Building on Family Strengths Conference: Research and Services in Support of Children and their Families, Portland, OR.

Spoth, R., & Redmond, C. (2000). Research on family engagement in preventive interventions: Toward improved use of scientific findings in primary prevention practice. *Journal of Primary Prevention, 21,* 267–284.

Stroul, B.A. (2002). *Systems of care: A framework for system reform in children's mental health* (Issue brief). Washington, DC: Georgetown University Child Development Center, National Technical Assistance Center for Children's Mental Health.

Stroul, B.A., & Friedman, R.M. (1986). *A system of care for seriously emotionally disturbed children and youth.* Washington, DC: Georgetown University Child Development Center.

Suter, J.C., & Bruns, E.J. (2007, June). *A critical review of the evidence base for wraparound.* Paper presented at the Building on Family Strengths Conference: Research and Services in Support of Children and their Families, Portland, OR.

U.S. Congress Office of Technology Assessment. (1986). *Children's mental health: Problems and services—A background paper.* Washington, DC: Author.

U.S. Public Health Service. (2000). *Report of the Surgeon General's Conference on Children's Mental Health: A national action agenda.* Washington, DC: Department of Health and Human Services.

VanDenBerg, J., Bruns, E., & Burchard, J. (2003). The history of the wraparound process. *Focal Point, 17*(2), 4–7.

Vostanis, P., Anderson, L., & Window, S. (2006). Evaluation of a family support service: Short term outcomes. *Clinical Child Psychology and Psychiatry, 11*, 513–528.

Walker, J.S. (2007, June 1). *Community support for Wraparound Inventory: Results of the pilot study.* Conference presentation at the State of the Science Conference: Effective Strategies for All: Strategies to Promote Mental Health and Thriving for Underserved Children and Families, Portland, OR.

Walker, J.S., & Bruns, E.J. (2006a). Building on practice-based evidence: Using expert perspectives to define the wraparound process. *Psychiatric Services, 57*, 1597–1585.

Walker, J.S., & Bruns, E.J. (2006b). The wraparound process: Individualized, community-based care for children and adolescents with intensive needs. In J. Rosenberg & S. Rosenberg (Eds.), *Community mental health: Challenges for the 21st century* (pp. 47–57). New York: Routledge Press.

Walker, J.S., Bruns, E.J., Rast, J., VanDenBerg, J.D., Osher, T.W., Koroloff, N., et al. (2004). *Phases and activities of the wraparound process.* Portland, OR: Portland State University, Research and Training Center on Family Support and Children's Mental Health, National Wraparound Initiative.

Walker, J.S., & Koroloff, N. (2007). Grounded theory and backward mapping: Exploring the implementation context for wraparound. *Journal of Behavioral Health Services and Research, 32*(4), 443–458.

Walker, J.S., Koroloff, N., & Schutte, K. (2003). *Implementing high-quality collaborative individualized service/support planning: Necessary conditions.* Portland OR: Portland State University, Research and Training Center on Family Support and Children's Mental Health.

Walker, J.S., & Schutte, K.M. (2004). Practice and process in wraparound teamwork. *Journal of Emotional and Behavioral Disorders, 2*, 182–192.

Walker, J.S., & Schutte, K.M. (2005). Quality and individualization in wraparound planning. *Journal of Child and Family Studies, 14*, 251–267.

Wraparound Evaluation and Research Team. (2007). *Overview of the Wraparound Fidelity Assessment System.* Available online at http://depts.washington.edu/wrapeval

6

Implementing Evidence-Based Practices within Systems of Care

CHRISTINE WALRATH, KAREN A. BLASE, AND PATRICK J. KANARY

An important strategy for improving services within systems of care involves the implementation of evidence-based programs and practices. This chapter outlines key issues that should be considered as evidence-based practices (EBPs) and programs are integrated into a system of care framework. A theory-driven, step-by-step approach to the integration of EBPs into a system of care environment is presented, as well as examples and lessons learned from communities that employ the practice.

DEFINING EVIDENCE-BASED AND IMPLEMENTATION

A common lexicon is essential to advance and facilitate the implementation of evidence-based practices and programs. While seemingly fundamental in nature, points of synergy, discrepancy, and divergent opinions related to terminology and definition must be recognized and understood if appropriate evidence-based programs and practices are to be selected and successfully implemented.

What is Evidence-Based?

Communities and partners need a common frame of reference to discuss evidence-based practices and programs. The Institute of Medicine (2001) defined EBPs as the integration of best research evidence with clinical expertise and patient values. Oregon's Addiction and Mental Health Division (2006) defined EBPs as those "that effectively integrate the best research evidence with clinical expertise, cultural competence and the values of the persons receiving services" (p. 1). The California Evidence-Based Clearinghouse for Child Welfare similarly defined EBPs as incorporating best research evidence, best clinical expertise, and interventions consistent with family/client values (Advisory Committee and Scientific Panel, n.d.).

The inclusion of *values* in several of the definitions is consistent with implementing EBPs within a system of care framework. The values and principles of systems of care are well-articulated and serve as key elements of system change. Thus, the intersection of an evidence-based program or practice with the values and principles of systems of care must be taken into account from the outset (Box 6.1).

Despite the similarity in definitions, there are different opinions among stakeholders as to the level of evidence required to be considered evidence-based and the meaning of the evidence. A variety of terms are used to describe programs and practices based on various degrees of scientific evidence, including *evidence-based practices and programs, promising practices, emerging practices*, and *practice-based evidence*. These terms are embedded in a number of publications (Hoagwood, Burns, Kiser, Ringeisen, & Schoenwald, 2001; Huang, Hepburn, & Espiritu, 2003; President's New Freedom Commission on Mental Health, 2003; Walker & Bruns, 2006) and in registries that list evidence-based programs and practices, along with a variety of definitions for various levels of evidence. There is no definitive listing or source for such information, and the research and knowledge base related to effective programs and practices continues to grow and develop. The web-based resources shown on Table 6.1 can help communities explore evidence-based interventions, as well as the range of definitions and criteria.

It is appropriate and educational for community partners to struggle with the task of sorting through the registries of EBPs and assessing each registry's criteria and process for evaluating evidence. The discussions that occur among system partners during this process can be used to further strengthen partnerships, build consensus, and refine a shared mission and vision (Box. 6.2).

Box 6.1.   Highlights from the field: Provider awareness
                  of evidence-based practices

As part of the National Evaluation of the Comprehensive Community Mental Health Services for Children and Their Families Program (Walrath, Sheehan, Holden, Hernandez, & Blau, 2006), providers affiliated with two waves of federally funded system of care communities have been surveyed about their knowledge, use, perception, organizational supports, and attitudes about evidence-based treatments and practices.

Nearly two thirds (65.4%) of providers responding (*N* = 766) indicated that they were familiar with the terms *evidence-based treatments* and *evidence-based practices*. When asked more in-depth questions, the providers familiar with the term(s) endorsed that researched effectiveness was a critical element of the definition.

In response to being asked to define *evidence-based treatment*, one respondent wrote, "A treatment that has been developed through research protocol, is supported by results of controlled treatment studies, and has guidelines and procedures for its implementation."

Source: Walrath, Sheehan, Holden, Hernandez, & Blau (2006).

Table 6.1. Web-based resources and registries

NREPP—The National Registry of Evidence-based Programs and Practices— http://nrepp.samhsa.gov/

Center for the Study and Prevention of Violence, Blueprints for Violence Prevention— http://www.colorado.edu/cspv/blueprints/index.html

*Strengthening America's Families: Effective Family Programs for Prevention of Delinquency—*http://www.strengtheningfamilies.org/

*National Institute on Drug Abuse—*http://www.nida.nih.gov/prevention/examples.html

*Office of Juvenile Justice and Delinquency Prevention (OJJDP) Model Programs Guide—*http://www.dsgonline.com/mpg2.5/mpg_index.htm

Promising Practices Network on Children, Families and Communities— http://www.promisingpractices.net/programs.asp

Office of Justice Programs, Community-based Programs— http://www.ojp.usdoj.gov/commprograms/field_tested_programs.htm

Surgeon General's Report on Youth Violence— http://www.surgeongeneral.gov/library/youthviolence/chapter5/sec3.html

The Collaborative for Academic, Social, and Emotional Learning— http://www.casel.org/about_sel/SELprograms.php

Department of Education, Safe and Drug Free Schools— http://www.ed.gov/admins/lead/safety/exemplary01/index.html

*Johns Hopkins Bloomberg School of Public Health—*http://www.jhsph.edu/ PreventYouthViolence/Resources/Model-Promising%20Programs.html

Making good choices about which EBPs to implement not only requires an understanding of the levels of evidence promulgated by the various registries but also involves a number of additional planning steps for systems of care. These include assessing needs, identifying gaps, assessing provider and community capacity, and ultimately, identifying EBPs that fit the needs of the population of concern. These decisions must be aligned with system of care values and principles, fit with the cultural and linguistic characteristics of the community, and bring sufficient value over practice as usual to warrant the effort and expense; however, both effective intervention practices *and* effective implementation practices are needed to produce benefits for children, youth, and families.

Box 6.2. Highlights from the field: Beware the lists

Although using a reliable registry from one or more of the sources in Table 6.1 is a viable strategy for determining what or if a specific evidence-based practice (EBP) is right for a specific situation, there is no replacement for direct contact with either the developer of the EBP or interviews with a good cross-section of sites currently implementing the program or practice. Systems of care or others with expectations from funders interested in employing an EBP must resist taking the short cut of picking from the lists and should instead follow a due diligence process. This will make all the difference in implementation.

What is Implementation?

Choosing which program or practice to implement is only half of the equation. A wise choice must be accompanied by careful implementation. *Implementation* is defined as "a specified set of activities designed to put into practice an activity or program" (Fixsen, Naoom, Blase, Friedman, & Wallace, 2005, p. 5). Evidence-based programs and practices will be ineffective and impossible to sustain unless they are fully and sufficiently implemented with fidelity (Box 6.3).

Systems of care must be vigilant to ensure that *performance* implementation, in contrast to *paper* or *process* implementation, occurs as desired. Performance implementation ensures that procedures and processes are put into place in such a way that the identified functional components of the intervention are actually used as intended by practitioners (e.g., clinicians, care managers, teachers) to benefit children, youth, and families (i.e., the integrated theory of change) (Hernandez & Hodges, 2003; Paine, Bellamy, & Wilcox, 1984). Many programs stall at the paper or process implementation levels (Fixsen et al., 2005):

Box 6.3.   Highlights from the field: Provider implementation
of evidence-based practices

A recent survey of providers affiliated with federally funded system of care communities conducted as part of the national evaluation of the Comprehensive Community Mental Health Services for Children and Their Families Program indicates a high degree of familiarity with a variety of evidence-based treatments and practices and a reasonably high level of perceived effectiveness and utilization (Walrath, Sheehan, Holden, Hernandez, & Blau, 2006).

For practices such as Cognitive-Behavioral Therapy, 97.7% of the sample indicated they were familiar, 89.5% indicated they believed it resulted in positive outcomes, and 62.1% indicated that they used Cognitive-Behavioral Therapy in the course of their work. In contrast, although a similar 97% of the sample indicated familiarity with therapeutic foster care, 66.7% indicated that they felt it resulted in positive outcomes, and only 2.6% reported that they used this practice in the course of their work.

After reporting use of a practice, providers in this same survey were asked about the extent to which they implemented the practice's full protocol. A similarly wide range of full protocol implementation was reported, suggesting some important implications for fidelity maintenance and monitoring. Among the large number of providers reporting the use of Cognitive-Behavioral Therapy in their work, only 36.2% indicated implementing the full protocol. Alternatively, among the small number of providers reporting the use of therapeutic foster care, 83.3% reported full protocol implementation. This variation suggests that evidence-based practice fidelity maintenance may present a serious and pervasive implementation challenge among system of care affiliated providers that must be addressed at the local level through supports and monitoring.

Source: Walrath, Sheehan, Holden, Hernandez, & Blau (2006).

- *Paper implementation* creates policies and procedures that can be tracked on paper but have no impact on service performance and outcomes (i.e., the recorded theory of change) (Hernandez & Hodges, 2003)

- *Process implementation* focuses on training events, changes in procedures, and provider and system language that pay lip service to implementation but do not create actual changes in practice that can produce outcomes that will benefit children, youth, and families. For example, clinicians may attend an intensive training event (i.e., process) but do not change their practice as a result, and still the organization will claim to be implementing the new way of work (Box 6.4).

Another important concept related to implementation is that of a *purveyor group*. This term refers to a group of professionals affiliated with or including the original program developers and researchers who actively work to assist others in implementing their practice or program with fidelity and good outcomes (Fixsen et al., 2005). A purveyor group has special expertise in the EBP itself, along with experience utilizing the methods for implementing the EBP successfully in the community (e.g., Nurse-Family Partnership National Service Office, Incredible Years, MST [Multisystemic Therapy] Services, Inc.). Implementation in the absence of a knowledgeable purveyor group appears to be much more challenging than installing and implementing the innovation with the assistance of such a group, but not all purveyor groups are equally knowledgeable about effective implementation strategies. Systems of care should interview representatives of the purveyor group to understand their range of experience and success in helping others. It makes a difference if you are the first community the group has tried to help or the 50th (Box 6.5).

Whereas implementation efforts that have the benefit of an experienced purveyor group benefit greatly from this expertise, it should be noted that many EBPs are "orphans" in that they do not have a designated or established purveyor

---

Box 6.4. Highlights from the field: Results of inadequate readiness and implementation

In one community, when faced with an opportunity to implement an emerging evidence-based practice as part of a randomized clinical trial, the selection of the intervention was not embedded within the community or provider's framework, but was instead recommended from several layers above. While the providers were positive about the opportunity, the fit of the intervention within their organizational cultures and the greater system of care was not adequately assessed. When implementation moved forward, the site was confronted with major unresolved issues such as the financing of the service, the lengthy start-up training period, a high level of staff frustration with what felt like open-ended training with unclear indicators for successful completion, and several bureaucratic layers and factors that impeded communication.

Box 6.5. Highlights from the field: Purveyor perspective

The role of Intermediary Purveyor Organizations (IPO) as a technical assistance resource for the implementation of evidence-based practices (EBPs) appears to be
growing. There are several such organizations and IPO models across the country;
however, like EBPs, IPOs are not of the one size fits all variety. They all come with
their own set of experiences, depending to some degree on the EBPs with which
they are associated. One community contracted with an IPO to assist it in implementing a practice. Although the practice was not part of the experience base of
the IPO, the IPO itself was very experienced in implementing EBPs. Although the
IPO assisted with many helpful strategies, the lack of specific experience and
knowledge related to the practice (e.g., its training methods, its infrastructure, relationship with the developers) was evident in the implementation phase. The general
lesson learned is that while some implementation tenets are fairly universal, there
are EBP-specific nuances that can affect the implementation process. To be sure,
there were many factors that affected implementation in this example, but experience and depth of understanding of the actual practice is clearly an added value for
any IPO. Communities looking for technical assistance may want to consider not
only the breadth and depth of the IPO's experience generally related to EBP implementation but also its specific EBP experience and current and past working
relationship with the original developer/purveyors.

---

group to actively support implementation. Resources for systems of care may be
limited to researchers or program developers willing to consult by phone, modest support or advice from other communities that have successfully implemented EBPs, or one-time training events with manuals for future use. These
conditions appear to be more challenging than working with an active purveyor
group.

Implementation of Evidence-Based
Practices in the Context of a System of Care

There are many goals and activities involved in establishing and sustaining a functional system of care. The goals, strategies, and desired outcomes are best articulated through the careful development of a *logic model* that articulates the intended *theory of change* (Hernandez & Hodges, 2003). Implementing an EBP in
the context of a system of care is a complicated strategy designed to achieve outcomes for a specific population. When strategies chosen by a system of care are
complicated and require considerable planning, coordination, and resources to
implement, it is often helpful to move certain strategies into the outcome column
of the logic model and then consider the strategies needed to operationalize the
initiative. Figure 6.1 provides an example of this cascading logic model that involves moving the intervention strategy to the implementation outcome column
and then developing implementation strategies related to the desired implementation outcome. Thus, the implementation of the EBP becomes an outcome for
which articulated strategies have been designated.

Population of concern	Intervention strategies	Desired intervention outcomes
Children age 7–12 experiencing extreme anxiety and avoidance	Develop a cadre of school- and clinic-based therapists able to implement Cognitive-Behavioral Therapy with fidelity	Improved school attendance Improved peer relationships Improved family relationships
Population of concern	**Intervention strategies**	**Desired intervention outcomes**
Outpatient and school-based behavioral health professionals	Form implementation team Identify key stakeholders Develop plan to get "buy-in" Recruit agencies and clinicians for initial discussions and much more!	Develop a cadre of school- and clinic-based therapists able to implement Cognitive-Behavioral Therapy with fidelity

Figure 6.1.   An example system of care cascading logic model.

IMPLEMENTATION PROCESS

The implementation process is a complex series of interrelated prerequisites, preparations, steps, and stages—all of which must be carefully considered and addressed.

Getting Started—Prerequisites

There are a number of essential questions to be answered before considering an EBP as a key strategy:

- For whom are we not doing well?

- For whom must we do better?

- Who defines the concept of *doing well*?

- How is the concept of *doing well* defined and measured in our community?

How well the community is doing with regard to accessible and effective service provision should be addressed through current data sources. At a minimum, the community must understand the prevalence of behavioral health concerns in child, adolescent, and young adult populations and the degree to which current services are accessible and effective in addressing these needs. In large part, desired outcomes must be defined by the goals of the families, youth, and children who are unable to access services or for whom effective services are not yet available. Answering these questions will help focus the discussion regarding the availability and viability of evidence-based approaches to meet the specific needs of specific populations.

Getting Started: The EBP Implementation Team

Forming an EBP implementation team can greatly enhance the likelihood of successfully selecting and implementing an EBP (Box 6.6.). The effectiveness of the implementation team can be enhanced if written terms of reference (TOR) are developed and approved by the governing body of the system of care to detail the scope, objectives, and guiding principles for EBP implementation (United Way of Canada, n.d.). Articulating the TOR increases the likelihood that expectations are clear to all stakeholders, reduces conflict, and improves communication. TOR components for the EBP implementation team might include:

- Scope, objectives, and expected outcomes

- Term, either time- or outcome-based

- Membership inclusive of family members, youth, system partners, and providers, with attention paid to cultural diversity

- Leadership roles and functions

- Boundaries and limitations (i.e., what is *not* authorized)

- Authority, accountability, and reporting requirements

- Decision-making processes (e.g., majority, consensus)

Box 6.6.   Highlights from the field: Implementation teams

The California Institute for Mental Health (CIMH) is a nonprofit, statewide organization supported by county mental health stakeholders. Part of its mission is to provide technical assistance to communities implementing evidence-based practices (EBPs). The CIMH model uses a team approach that partners them with the developer of the EBP, as well as with designated implementing communities. The CIMH serves as the connector on virtually all aspects of implementation from the selection of sites, to readiness, to financing, to evaluation. A unique strategy of the CIMH is its bundling of implementing sites into a learning community, thus creating a peer network and support system around the implementation of a specific intervention. The CIMH has community development teams for implementing Multidimensional Treatment Foster Care and Functional Family Therapy.

- Values and principles that are to be evident during the term of work (e.g., no meetings without family members and youth present)

In general, the EBP implementation team may be charged with three overarching responsibilities:

1. Moving the project through the *stages of implementation*

2. Ensuring that the *implementation drivers* needed for fidelity and sustainability are integrated and successfully embedded in the overall effort

3. Examining the *fit* of the EBP or program with system of care values and principles throughout the implementation process

Stages of Implementation

In 2005, a review of implementation research and evaluation literature revealed six stages in the implementation process (Fixsen et al., 2005):

1. Exploration and adoption

2. Program installation

3. Initial implementation

4. Full implementation or operation

5. Innovation

6. Sustainability

The stages overlap, and activities from more than one stage may be occurring simultaneously. It should also be noted that moving from exploration and adoption to full implementation can take 2–4 years, and the process is characterized by progress, setbacks, and ongoing problem solving.

Stage 1: Exploration and Making the Decision to Adopt an Evidence-Based Practice   Through the work of the EBP implementation team and community consultations, the system of care goes through a process to arrive at a final decision whether to adopt a particular EBP. Key activities during this stage include:

- Documenting the need, identifying possible evidence-based approaches to meet the need, and determining which EBP(s) will be explored in more depth

- Fact-finding regarding the identified EBP(s), including the availability of qualified purveyors, experiences of others who have successfully implemented the EBP, start-up and ongoing costs, and changes required of systems and organizations

- Assessing the fit with other EBP implementation efforts in the local area, county, region, or state; there may be advantages or disadvantages to selecting an EBP that already has a strong infrastructure presence in the state (e.g., systems for recruiting staff, training, and coaching).

- Creating opportunities for informed community choice, stakeholder buy-in, and community consensus building; such consensus and cross-system buy-in and ownership may be more likely to occur when there is a population of concern that all systems see as needing attention. For example, transition-age youth might be seen as poorly served by behavioral/mental health, child welfare, education, and juvenile justice systems.

- Engaging and assessing providers' interest and ability in participating as host agencies for the EBP initiative; this may involve identifying and consulting with agencies that have a history of being innovative and are comfortable managing the inherent risks that accompany any new venture. There are some implementation research findings indicating that organizations that feel they can manage risk are more likely to make the decision to adopt a new practice or program (Panzano & Roth, 2006).

- Evaluating the fit of the EBP under consideration with the system of care's values and principles, as well as with the continuum of services in the community; this fit is important for the eventual successful implementation, integration, and sustainability of the new way of work. For example, the degree to which the EBP will fit with current wraparound approaches, with a strengths-based approach, and with family and youth involvement should be taken into consideration (Box 6.7).

- Evaluating the fit of the EBP under consideration with the cultural and linguistic characteristics of the community and the populations to be served; another key for successful implementation is the EBP's degree of cultural and linguistic competence (Box 6.8).

Typical challenges during this phase include:

- Choosing an EBP for reasons other than needs, thereby not obtaining developing community ownership and creating resistance and resentment from

---

Box 6.7.   Highlights from the field: Evidence-based practices (EBPs) and community structure

Some EBPs have highly defined protocols, approved approaches, record keeping/reporting formats, and evaluation requirements such as a lead clinical authority model (i.e., the EBP service provider takes the primary and most active role in determining and delivering intervention and support services). If the entity does not first possess an understanding of the very specific requirements (deal breakers) of the model and the ways in which those do or do not fit into the community culture or system, there are likely to be significant surprises during the implementation stage. The strategy is to determine at the front end, during the exploration stage, the exact means by which the components of the system will work together. It must not be assumed that direct care providers or individual staff will work it out at a later point.

Box 6.8. Highlights from the field: Consideration of culture in implementation of evidence-based practices (EBPs)

One county uses *cultural responsiveness* as a criterion to judge each EBP in which it is involved. The EBP combined with initiatives to improve cultural and linguistic competence has led to Latino involvement in each of its EBPs.

Another community noted that in considering EBPs for implementation, it looked for data on the use of the EBP with a variety of culturally diverse groups. Ultimately, an EBP was selected with study results indicating its effectiveness for various major ethnicities and cultures. Given this evidence, system of care leaders were satisfied that the EBP would be appropriate for the demographic range of families in their community.

---

providers and families who may already feel well-served by current services or have different views about what is needed to fill service gaps (Box 6.9)

- Rushing the process and failing to obtain buy-in from key stakeholders or without understanding what will be required for successful, high-fidelity implementation; data from business indicate that when adoption decisions are mandated or driven by funding and occur without adequate time for exploration, fewer organizations choose to adopt. Those that do make the adoption decision take longer to implement under such conditions (Nutt, 2002) (Box 6.10).

- A lack of commitment to fidelity and early discussion of modifying the EBP to fit the community; research data, while correlating, are generally clear that higher fidelity leads to better outcomes (Felner et al., 2001; Henggeler, Melton, Brondino, Scherer, & Hanley, 1997; Washington State Institute for Public Policy, 2002). Some EBPs are more clear than others about the core elements of the intervention that are theory-driven and open to modifications in form (e.g., language, incorporation of culturally compatible strategies) as long as the core functional elements continue to be maintained (e.g., skill-building in real world settings, size of groups, number of sessions, parental involvement). Unfortunately, a community decision that involves changing the

---

Box 6.9. Highlights from the field: Selection and funding before need and buy-in

One key community member became very determined to bring a specific evidence-based practice (EBP) to the community, and had, in fact, gone as far as to secure funding for the practice. Although the need and general interest from stakeholders was present, the engagement process was not fully implemented. Eventually, the community moved forward with its decision to endorse the model, but only after a strategic regrouping to the buy-in phase. Although champions are often needed to initiate the discussion and decision making related to EBPs, getting too far ahead of the other necessary partners can lead to negative outcomes on multiple levels.

Box 6.10. Highlights from the field: Family and consumer involvement

In one community, a county funding board had to approve the adoption of a promising practice for the treatment of youth sex offenders. Two consumers were in attendance at the meeting. Their feedback was persuasive to the board as to the need and appropriateness of this model. These consumers were not likely recipients of this type of model; however, they resonated with the family-centered nature of this intervention and could make useful comments to the board. In another locale, the family organization is involved in the development and decision-making process for evidence-based practices. This has proven to be helpful because the involvement rounds out the perspective. Involvement has been helpful in meeting the needs of families and identifying the most beneficial locations for implementation of the practice.

EBP in response to implementation barriers can result in modifying the intervention in ways that make it no longer evidence-based and therefore no longer effective (Box 6.11).

• An inability to identify and ensure the availability of three types of funding: 1) start-up funding to pay for program developers (purveyors) to visit the community and conduct their own readiness assessment, to host community meetings to build consensus, and to acquire necessary materials and equipment; 2) funding for the service itself (federal, state, local, foundation); and 3) funding for the ongoing infrastructure or core implementation components (e.g., staff training, coaching, fidelity measurement, data collection) (Box 6.12)

Box 6.11. Highlights from the field: Adapting before adopting

Increasingly, evidence-based practices are introduced into communities as a result of a requirement of state or federal funders. When applying for a grant, a community-based behavioral health care provider identified a specific need for the treatment of youth with alcohol and drug addictions as well as mental health conditions. The applicant located developers of a promising model that seemed appropriate to meet these needs and had an initial discussion regarding the overall fit of the intervention. When the developers read the first draft of the grant application, it was clear that significant adaptations had been made to the model for which there was no evidence of effectiveness. The adaptations were related to addressing organizational issues and structural challenges (e.g., methods for serving rural areas, ways to maximize human resources). A candid discussion took place between the developers and the applicant to address these concerns and to clarify the parameters of the intervention. Subsequently, the application was rewritten to accurately reflect the model and to plan for its implementation in the manner required. Had the application been approved as it was originally written without the additional input from the developers, it could have resulted in a funded proposal that might have been difficult or impossible to implement.

> **Box 6.12.** Highlights from the field: Where buy-in means financial survival
>
> In one community, an evidence-based practice had been adopted largely through the advocacy and resources of a single community entity. Although there was no argument that the need for the service was present, the processes related to exploration (e.g., community consensus building, buy-in) did not occur prior to implementing the new program. Fortunately, the consensus building and buy-in activities occurred even as the program was being installed and implemented, albeit out of order in terms of implementation stages. This ongoing attention to buy-in during implementation proved to be crucial. When the community was confronted with an unexpected and significant cut in funding for the program, the ongoing development of community ownership for the intervention was the single reason the program was continued through financial investments by each community stakeholder. The program was beginning to show promise in its early phase, but the decision to continue funding was predicated on the understanding by stakeholders that a longer term of operation, experience, and evaluation were necessary before any consideration of reduced funding was entertained. This example demonstrates the risk of not fully engaging stakeholders at the front end, as well as the critical value of engaging them in a meaningful manner during implementation and ongoing operation of the program. Therefore, despite the fact that the young program had yet to fully demonstrate its effectiveness, community ownership and engagement activities continued and the program funding was sustained.

Stage 2: Program Installation This stage involves identifying and accomplishing tasks needed to launch the new practice or program, including preparing the organizational home(s) for the EBP. During this stage, the system of care must develop a strong working relationship with the provider agencies that have agreed to come on board to deliver the EBP. These providers will find themselves engaged in organizational change, and they are often surprised at the degree to which the new practice affects the organization as a whole or the other services it provides. To facilitate the new way of work, the agencies and practitioners must provide feedback at the organizational and system levels regarding readiness challenges and implementation barriers. The role of the system of care and the EBP implementation team is to facilitate the readiness work of the providers, negotiate and eliminate systemic barriers, and promote integration of the EBP within the overall system of care effort. System of care leaders and the EBP implementation team also play a bridging role in working with the purveyor of the program or practice. Because the system of care and the associated implementation team members know the state, community, provider, and consumer context better than the external purveyor, they can help the purveyor group understand the context and facilitate the policy and practice changes required at practice and system levels.

During this stage, providers will be involved in developing new policies; obtaining necessary resources and equipment; recruiting, interviewing, and hiring new staff; and coming to grips with the impact of the new way of work on their organizational structure and culture. In addition, if there is a formal purveyor or purveying organization, providers will be developing a working relationship and any necessary agreements with that entity. The system of care and EBP implementation team can play a role in ensuring that the provider–purveyor relationship gets off to a good start, with frequent communication, mutual understanding of constraints and facilitators, and attention to broader system issues. The need for attaining solutions to the funding stressors may appear at this stage, as well as in the initial implementation stage because, although funds are being expended, billing for services is not yet occurring or is not occurring at a sufficient rate.

Stage 3: Initial Implementation   Implementation begins during this stage, but the program or practice is not yet fully operational. During this stage, many implementation attempts end because they are overwhelmed by inertia or by implementation challenges. Such challenges include coping with unanticipated system impacts (e.g., insufficient referrals) or a lack of acceptance by partners who seemed to be on board during the exploration stage.

The role of the system of care during this stage is to help analyze challenges, arrive at solutions, and codify or institutionalize facilitative ways of work. The EBP implementation team or other relevant system of care committee must hear about barriers and challenges directly from the provider agencies and practitioners, and it must be committed to addressing barriers to implementation that lie within the system's realm of influence. This stage can be characterized by a higher than normal turnover in staff due to inexperienced trainers, coaches, and supervisors, as well as the compounding effect of destabilizing the old service system while making room for the new program or practice. Provider organizations and practitioners will need support and encouragement to continue their efforts, along with advice and strategies for overcoming practical challenges. In turn, they will be able to offer advice to the system of care that is relevant for future EBP implementation efforts.

Stage 4: Full Implementation   Full implementation is characterized by a program or practice that is fully operational, with full staffing complements, full case loads, and the ability to deal with the realities of providing a new service in settings and systems that are often not designed to accommodate or support EBPs. At this point, the EBP is ready for rigorous outcome evaluation. Outcome evaluations that come too early are really an evaluation of partially implemented programs and practices, and thus they may not reflect the value of a fully implemented program. In addition, the system of care should remain vigilant to ensure the integration of the program or practice with the system of care framework, values, and principles. Provider partners must continue to have avenues for problem solving and for celebrating successes.

Stage 5: Innovation   At this stage, agency administrators and staff members have enough experience with the EBP to refine and expand its implementation based on community needs and the growing skill of the practitioners. Key to any innovation is to first conduct the program or practice as intended to evaluate the effectiveness under high-fidelity conditions. Winter and Szulanski (2001) found that adaptations made after a business innovation is implemented with fidelity are more successful than modifications made before full implementation.

Changes to structure, dosage, the population of concern, or the active ingredients should be carefully justified, grounded in theory, discussed with the developers, documented, and evaluated to ensure that the innovation is, in fact, desirable. Desirable changes that generate data indicating improved program effectiveness are innovations and can become part of the standard practice of the program; however, some changes represent program drift and are therefore a threat to fidelity and outcomes. Drift often occurs in response to barriers to high-fidelity implementation or a mistaken belief that the effective program or practice can be extended to new populations. It may be appropriate to adopt the mantra of "quality insistence, not the path of least resistance" for the system of care.

Stage 6: Sustainability   Sustainability is not a stage in the sense of a bounded beginning and end point. Instead, it is a key issue addressed at each of the previous stages. The goal, of course, is the long-term survival, continued fidelity, and ongoing effectiveness of the EBP. As noted, sustainability may be facilitated when EBPs are selected that not only meet the community's needs, but are also being more broadly promulgated in the state or region. Sustainability issues are also more likely to be successfully addressed when multiple systems have been bought into the need for the EBP and experience the benefits of the new way of providing services. Joining with others helps ensure that there is an infrastructure to house and monitor the quality of the implementation drivers (e.g., staff selection, staff training, coaching and supervision, staff evaluation, fidelity monitoring, data collection) and that this may present economies of scale with regard to funding this crucial infrastructure. Funding for start-up, expansion, the implementation infrastructure, and the service itself must all receive attention from exploration through innovation (Box 6.13).

IMPLEMENTATION DRIVERS

The goal of implementation is to have practitioners (e.g., clinicians, counselors, care managers, teachers) use the EBP effectively. High-fidelity practitioner behavior is developed and supported by core implementation components or drivers. Another task for the EBP implementation team and the system of care initiative as a whole is to gain an understanding of the implementation drivers needed to install and maintain the EBP with fidelity (Fixsen et al., 2005).

Shown in Figure 6.2, implementation drivers include staff recruitment and selection, preservice and in-service training, supervision and coaching, staff performance evaluation, decision support data systems, facilitative administrative support, and system interventions. These interactive processes are integrated to maximize their influence on practitioner behavior and on the organizational culture as a whole. They can also compensate for one another to bolster high-fidelity and effective practices. For example, if practitioners do not initially have all the skills and abilities needed (i.e., selection), they can begin to acquire those in train-

---

Box 6.13. Highlights from the field: Implementation of Common Sense Parenting

In an effort to better understand difficulties associated with engaging families in an evidence-based intervention, a retrospective implementation study of Common Sense Parenting (CSP) was conducted as a part of the national evaluation of the Comprehensive Community Mental Health Services for Children and Their Families Program. CSP is a skill-based parent training program adapted from the Teaching Family Model (TFM) of group home care and the Boys Town Family Home (BTFH) program.

CSP consists of six weekly 2-hour group sessions, with each session building on techniques learned in previous sessions. Communities attempting to engage families for participation in CSP struggled with low attendance at the intervention sessions despite families agreeing to participate. Exit interviews were conducted with families to gain a better sense of the mitigating factors associated with the lower-than-anticipated attendance. Specifically, the interviews were conducted with 38 caregivers—11 who attended CSP and 27 who did not attend—to identify implementation factors that affected participation, assess motivations for participation or the lack thereof, and identify organizational or community supports for evidence-based practice (EBP) implementation.

Findings indicated a number of factors that had an impact on family engagement in the CSP intervention, including the strategies for reaching out and engaging families, the accessibility of the intervention, the supports provided to facilitate participation, family life situations, and the perceived need for this type of help. Specifically, just over one third of nonattendees did not remember being contacted and indicated they would have attended had they remembered. In addition, 50% of attendees had scheduling problems with days and times, location, and child care related to attending the intervention sessions, and approximately one third of nonattendees would have attended if times and locations had been more flexible.

Furthermore, family life situations (e.g., health problems, mental health issues, children running away or placed in alternate care) were also reported as being strong mitigating factors associated with participation in the intervention. In addition, just over one third of caregivers indicated not needing the intervention and reported having all the help they needed.

These findings, albeit retrospective, suggest that successful EBP implementation requires consideration of community, provider, and consumer characteristics and motivations to ensure that the EBP selection is the right match for all community stakeholders. It also highlights some of the types of issues that require attention during exploration and indicates the need for active, frequent problem solving as the EBP moves throughout the stages of implementation.

---

ing. Training compensates for skill deficiencies present at hiring, and similarly, coaching can compensate for that which is missed in training.

The implementation drivers are important to explore because there will be infrastructure and funding implications to be considered by the system of care. Structures, functions, and processes related to the implementation drivers may be quite clearly specified by the purveyor of the program or practice; however, when there is no purveyor group, or when the purveyor has not yet thought through the role of the implementation drivers in ensuring implementation and sustainability, the system of care must determine which of these drivers are crucial, where these

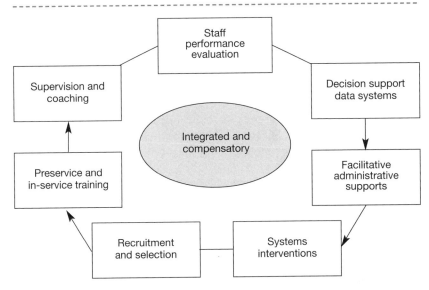

Figure 6.2. Implementation drivers. (From Fixsen, D.L., Naoom, S.F., Blase, K.A., Friedman, R.M., & Wallace, F. [2005]. *Implementation research: A synthesis of the literature* [FMHI Publication #231] [p. 29]. Tampa: University of South Florida, Louis de la Parte Florida Mental Health Institute, National Implementation Research Network. Copyright © 2005, The National Implementation Research Network, Louis de la Parte Florida Mental Health Institute, University of South Florida—All rights reserved.) (*Note:* Implementation drivers are mechanisms that help to develop, improve, and sustain the practitioners' ability to implement an evidence-based practice to benefit children, youth, and their families and to help ensure fidelity, sustainability, and a continuous quality improvement process.)

functions will be lodged (e.g., in individual provider agencies, in a local, regional, or state training body), how the skills needed for high-quality implementation drivers will be acquired (e.g., how trainers will be trained, how coaching will be learned), and how the costs associated with this infrastructure will be met. The system of care must consider the organizational, financial, and delivery issues related to each implementation driver in relation to the particular EBP being considered or implemented.

Recruitment and Selection

What baseline knowledge, skills, and attitudes are needed to implement the EBP? What are the methods for recruiting and selecting practitioners with those characteristics? Beyond experience and academic qualifications, certain practitioner characteristics may be difficult to teach or acquire through the other implementation drivers (e.g., training, coaching), so they must be part of the selection criteria. In particular, an affinity for and understanding of system of care values and principles may be important. A practitioner may find it difficult to take a strengths-based approach. If this is a basic tenet of the EBP and key for system of care implementation, this selection factor must be embedded in the interview process for potential EBP practitioners. Some programs are purposefully designed to minimize the need for careful selection (Baker, Gersten, & Keating, 2000). Others have more specific and complex requirements for practitioner qualifications (e.g., Chamberlain, 2003; Phillips, Burns, & Edgar, 2001; Schoenwald, Brown, & Henggeler, 2000) and methods for assessing competencies (e.g., Blase, Fixsen, & Phillips, 1984; Maloney, Phillips, Fixsen, & Wolf, 1975; Reiter-Lavery, 2004). In a recent qualitative study of the capacity of EBP developers, many program developers and purveyor groups stated that selection of staff was critical to the delivery of their model, but very few program developers had established staff selection criteria or interview protocols to guide provider organizations in the selection of staff (Box. 6.14) (Naoom, Fixsen, Blase, Gilbert, & Wallace, 2007).

Staff selection also represents the intersection with a variety of larger system variables. General workforce development issues, the overall economy, organizational financing, salaries and benefits, and the demands of the innovation in terms of time and skill all affect the availability of staff for human service programs. The move toward EBPs in human services has prompted concerns about advanced education, the availability of a suitable workforce, and sources of funding for highly skilled practitioners (Blase & Fixsen, 1981; O'Connell, Morris, & Hoge, 2004). Workforce issues comprise a challenge for systems of care that must be addressed at local, state, and national levels.

Preservice and In-Service Training

It seems obvious that practitioners must acquire knowledge and develop skills related to the EBP, and skill-based training (e.g., behavior rehearsals, practice sessions) is a key to acquiring such skills. Training alone is an ineffective implementation strategy regardless of how skillfully the training is done (Azocar, Cuffel, Goldman, & McCarter, 2003; Stokes & Baer, 1977; Schectman, Schroth, Verme,

---

Box 6.14. Highlights from the field: From selection to staffing

One of the challenges of implementing a highly structured evidence-based practice is finding the right fit of staff to model. Although many well-trained clinicians can deliver effective treatment, doing so within the structure of a highly researched model with strict fidelity standards is an important consideration in hiring staff. Multisystemic Therapy (MST) has developed a specific hiring toolbox for organizations that are implementing this model. Screening protocols have been developed for both clinicians and supervisors. Clinical competency is an important factor, but so, too, is the ability to implement a model with fidelity and to work within the required organizational and coaching environment. One agency executive who was ready to hire someone for the MST supervisor position was encouraged to use the supervisor hiring protocol, and much to his delight, he found the protocol a useful tool and hired the right person. He enthusiastically stated, "This was the best experience I've ever had in all my years of hiring staff." Conversely, a team of interviewers using the therapist hiring protocol decided not to go with the candidate that emerged from that process and instead hired the person about whom they had the best gut feelings. That person left the program within a month.

& Voss, 2003). Preservice and in-service training, however, are efficient ways to provide knowledge about the theory, philosophy, and values of the EBP, as well as to provide opportunities for practitioners to try out new skills and receive feedback in the safety of a supportive training environment. The system of care and the involved providers must determine how quality, up-to-date training can be provided to all new employees who are expected to implement the EBP in a timely fashion.

Supervision and Coaching

Although key skills related to the EBP can be introduced to practitioners during training, proficient use of the new knowledge is best learned on the job through skillful coaching. A coach who can identify, demonstrate, and provide feedback on use of the EBP components while also providing encouragement and support can help move a practitioner through the awkward stage and on to skillful clinical use of the EBP. Training and coaching are the principal ways in which practitioner behavior change occurs in the initial stages of implementation and over time. Systems of care must determine who will serve as the coach for new practitioners, how the coach will acquire the skills and competencies needed, and how coaching and supervision will be funded, monitored, and evaluated.

Staff Performance Evaluation

Staff evaluation procedures are put in place to assess the use and outcomes of the skills needed to implement the EBP—skills that are reflected in the selection criteria, taught in preservice and in-service training, and reinforced and fully developed through coaching. Assessments of practitioner performance include measures of fidelity to help ensure that the EBP is being implemented as intended. Typically, these measures include observational data and data reported by the consumers of the services. In addition to ensuring fidelity at the practitioner level, these measures provide feedback useful to interviewers, trainers, coaches, administrators, and the purveyor group regarding the progress of implementation efforts. The cumulative results of fidelity measures across a number of practitioners can help assess the impact of recruitment and selection processes, skill-based training efforts, and coaching procedures on practitioner fidelity. The system of care must determine who will define these staff evaluation processes, who will perform this function, how the evaluator(s) will learn protocols and acquire needed skills, and how the staff evaluation and fidelity monitoring function will be funded.

Decision Support Data Systems

Other measures (e.g., quality improvement information; organizational fidelity measures; child, youth, and family satisfaction; outcomes) assess key aspects of the overall performance of the organization and the EBP. Data systems provide information to support and inform decision making designed to assure effective implementation of the EBP over time. An important task for systems of care involves determining which data should be collected; how often it will be collected; whether the data are meaningful to families, youth, and children; the entity that will review the data; the ways the data will be used for program and organizational improvement; and how funding for this function will be secured.

Facilitative Administrative Supports

Facilitative administration includes steady, determined, and supportive leadership that makes use of data to inform decision making and ensures that staff have the resources and supports necessary for the high-fidelity implementation needed to achieve the desired outcomes. In organizations with a facilitative administration, careful attention is given to policies, procedures, structures, culture, and climate to ensure alignment of these aspects of an organization to support practitioners in achieving high-fidelity and positive outcomes for those they serve. Leaders must decide how agency administrative personnel will come to understand their roles as facilitators of the EBP, how administrators will ensure that they have a direct line of communication with practitioners to identify and remove barriers and to sustain facilitative administrative practices, and how the administration will monitor the overall quality and integration of the other implementation drivers (e.g., selection, training, coaching, fidelity, data).

System Interventions

The descriptions of the implementation drivers provide systems of care with a template for analyzing and attending to implementation. A survey of providers affiliated with the national evaluation of the federal Comprehensive Community Mental Health Services for Children and Their Families Program provides some interesting insights into a subset of implementation drivers and the relationship of these drivers to behavioral health service provider attitudes about EBPs (Walrath, Sheehan, Holden, Hernandez, & Blau, 2006). Although the survey was not designed to assess implementation drivers, it suggests the overall importance of a community-based understanding of the various implementation drivers, their compensatory relationship, and their potential impact on provider knowledge, use, and attitudes toward EBPs (Box 6.15).

The exploration stage is the most opportune time to gain knowledge about the implementation driver requirements of the EBP. A particular EBP may require more or less attention to any given implementation driver for the practice or program to be implemented successfully, and some practices may be designed specifically to eliminate or minimize the need for one or more of the implementation drivers. For example, in the Start Making a Reader Today (SMART) program, business leaders were recruited as volunteers to tutor children in reading twice per week, but they were not given training on tutoring, nor was their adherence to the program evaluated. Heavy reliance was placed on selection, and the training was

---

Box 6.15. Highlights from the field: Community understanding of
implementation drivers

An evidence-based practice (EBP) survey was administered in 2005 as a part of the
congressionally mandated national evaluation of the federal Comprehensive Community Mental Health Services for Children and Their Families Program (Walrath,
Sheehan, Holden, Hernandez, & Blau, 2006). The survey was completed by 255
mental health service providers affiliated with the 22 communities that received
federal funding in 1999 and 2000 to implement a system of care. The survey domains and questions were retrospectively evaluated as potential implementation
driver proxies, and a subset of variables were identified for investigation
(see Table 6.2).

These implementation drivers were investigated in relation to provider attributes such as knowledge of evidence-based practices (EBPs; i.e., number of EBPs
known to respondent of a possible 31), use of EBPs (i.e., number of EBPs used by
respondent of a possible 31), and attitudes toward EBP implementation as measured by the Evidence-Based Practice Attitude Scale (EBPAS) total score (Aarons,
2004).

Overall, the respondents on average indicated that they were familiar with approximately 22 EBPs and that they had used 10 on average in the last year. Furthermore, the average attitudes toward EBPs was 3.38 (SD = .43), indicating moderate
to positive attitudes toward EBPs.

Primary findings include:

- Staff-related implementation drivers were found to be largely nonpredictive of
  provider EBP knowledge, use, and attitudes.

- Agency/system-related drivers, specifically requirements by the employer to
  provide EBPs and the staff's feeling that they were supported by the agency to
  implement EBPs, were predictive of both the number of EBPs known to the respondent and the respondents' total score on the EBPAS.

- The existence of an agency formal training program was not predictive of EBP
  knowledge, use, and attitude.

Although additional planned investigation into the implementation drivers and their
relationship to provider attitudes and attributes is warranted, these findings collectively indicate the importance having a community understanding of implementation drivers and their compensatory relationship.

Source: Walrath, Sheehan, Holden, Hernandez, & Blau (2006).

---

minimized due to turnover in volunteers. In this case, there was a heavy reliance
on the selection implementation driver for the required skill set (i.e., the ability
to read and the willingness to tutor twice per week) (Baker, Gersten, & Keating, 2000).

In addition, the compensatory nature of these drivers helps to ensure that
there are multiple systems, procedures, and opportunities to support high-fidelity
implementation. For example, in an implementation infrastructure that has minimal training opportunities for practitioners, intensive coaching with frequent
feedback loops may compensate for the lack of training. Alternately, careful selec-

Table 6.2.   Implementation drivers: Survey variables of interest

Implementation drivers	Variables
Staff-related practitioner selection	Demographic characteristics (gender, age, race)
	Licensure
	Level of education
	Years of work experience with children
	Years with current employer
Agency/system-related facilitative administration	Required by agency to use evidence-based practice
	Supported by agency to implement evidence-based practice
	Agency-sponsored training program for clinical staff

tion and very well-designed staff performance evaluations may compensate for less training and coaching. The implementation drivers also compensate for the fact that practitioners acquire skills and abilities at different rates over time. For example, one practitioner may significantly benefit from the skill-based training driver and require less intensive coaching, whereas another practitioner may leave the preservice training somewhat overwhelmed and require significant and immediate coaching. The integrated and compensatory nature of the implementation drivers helps to ensure a robust and flexible approach to promoting high fidelity of the EBP. Efforts to make use of an EBP on a significant scale require careful consideration of each implementation driver and its role in supporting skillful implementation of the EBP, as well as adequate organizational attention and alignment to support both fidelity and sustainability.

Sources of Implementation Drivers

As noted, the system of care may be able to receive considerable advice, training, and support in installing these implementation drivers when working with an experienced purveyor group. Alternatively, it may be largely up to the system of care, the provider organization, and the community partners to figure it out. The essential questions to address include

- Who provides the selection, training, coaching, staff evaluation, program evaluation, and administrative support services at an implementation site?

- Who intervenes with larger systems when needed?

Systems of care must determine if this will be the responsibility of people inside the organization, contracted to individuals or groups outside the implementation site (e.g., purveyor groups, other qualified technical assistance providers), or if it will be some combination (e.g., the organization recruits, selects, and coaches at which time a separate entity trains and monitors fidelity). Another approach is to develop regional or statewide entities that have the full capacity to provide all of the implementation drivers within their own organization (e.g., the MST Partners Network) or that join collectively with other organizations to establish a center or other structure that can provide reliable and up-to-date access to both the functions of the implementation drivers and the latest material and training related to the drivers (e.g., new fidelity instruments, training protocols for supervisors or trainers, evaluation routines) either independently or by remaining connected to the program developers. Examples of such entities created to support the implementation of EBPs include Colorado's, nonprofit group Invest in Kids, which has been promoting Incredible Years and Nurse Family Partnership programs throughout the state; Ohio's Center for Innovative Practices, funded in part by the state mental health authority; and the California Institute for Mental Health, funded in part by the county mental health associations.

CONCLUSION

The journey from identifying needs for specific populations to effective and sustainable implementation of EBPs is a protracted and challenging one; however, providing necessary services that work for families and their children and youth is not an afterthought in a system of care. It is central to making a difference. By engaging in a thoughtful process and carefully making adjustments throughout the process, systems of care can ensure that the values and principles are alive and well as EBPs are chosen, implemented, evaluated, and sustained.

Attention to developing community ownership; creating, using, and frequently revisiting a sound theory of change; wisely selecting needed EBPs; matching strategies and activities with the stages of implementation; attending to the installation of implementation drivers; and measuring both fidelity and outcomes can help systems of care as they ensure that effective services are available for children, youth, and families. Throughout the process, the system of care can safeguard, integrate, and further bolster its living values and principles by continuing to ensure that families and youth are taking their rightful place at decision-making tables and that they are acquiring networking and advocacy skills. Service providers are learning to work together in more seamless ways. Care managers are learning to let families drive and youth guide planning, as well as coordinate and evaluate service plans. System partners are learning ways to communicate with one another and to find common ground for improving and funding services. Data systems are being developed to inform decision making, and cultural and linguistic competence is being infused into each goal and activity. Services for the population of concern are improved in terms of accessibility and effectiveness. This careful attention to implementation strategies in the context of a system of care builds the bridge from science to services.

REFERENCES

Aarons, G. (2004). Mental health provider attitudes toward adoption of EBPs: The EBPAS. *Mental Health Services Research, 6*(2), 61–74.

Advisory Committee and Scientific Panel. (n.d.). *Importance of evidence-based practice.* San Diego: California Evidence-Based Clearinghouse for Child Welfare (CEBC). Retrieved March 21, 2007, from http://www.cachildwelfareclearinghouse.org/importance-of-evidence-based-practice#explain

Azocar, F., Cuffel, B., Goldman, W., & McCarter, L. (2003). The impact of evidence-based guideline dissemination for the assessment and treatment of major depression in a managed behavioral health care organization. *Journal of Behavioral Health Services & Research, 30*(1), 109-118.

Baker, S., Gersten, R., & Keating, T. (2000). When less is more: A 2-year longitudinal evaluation of a volunteer tutoring program requiring minimal training. *Reading Research Quarterly, 35*(4), 494–519

Blase, K.A., & Fixsen, D.L. (1981). Structure of child care education: Issues and implications for educators and practitioners. *Child Care Quarterly Special Issue: Emerging Issues in Child and Youth Care Education, 10,* 210–225.

Blase, K.A., Fixsen, D.L., & Phillips, E.L. (1984). Residential treatment for troubled children: Developing service delivery systems. In S.C. Paine, G.T. Bellamy & B. Wilcox (Eds.), *Human services that work: From innovation to standard practice* (pp. 149–165). Baltimore: Paul H. Brookes Publishing Co.

Chamberlain, P. (2003). The Oregon Multidimensional Treatment Foster Care Model: Features, outcomes, and progress in dissemination. *Cognitive and Behavioral Practice, 10,* 303–312.

Felner, R.D., Favazza, A., Shim, M., Brand, S., Gu, K., & Noonan, N. (2001). Whole school improvement and restructuring as prevention and promotion: Lessons from STEP and the project on high performance learning communities. *Journal of School Psychology, 39*(2), 177–202.

Fixsen, D.L., Naoom, S.F., Blase, K.A., Friedman, R.M., & Wallace, F. (2005). *Implementation research: A synthesis of the literature* (FMHI Publication #231). Tampa: University of South Florida, Louis de la Parte Florida Mental Health Institute, The National Implementation Research Network.

Henggeler, S.W., Melton, G.B., Brondino, M.J., Scherer, D.G., & Hanley, J.H. (1997). Multisystemic therapy with violent and chronic juvenile offenders and their families: The role of treatment fidelity in successful dissemination. *Journal of Consulting and Clinical Psychology, 65*(5), 821–833.

Hernandez, M., & Hodges, S. (2003). *Crafting logic models for systems of care: Ideas into action.* Tampa: University of South Florida, Department of Child and Family Studies, Louis de la Parte Florida Mental Health Institute.

Hoagwood, K., Burns, B.J., Kiser, L., Ringeisen, H., & Schoenwald, S.K. (2001). Evidence-based practice in child and adolescent mental health services. *Psychiatric Services, 52,* 1179–1189.

Huang, L.N., Hepburn, K.S., & Espiritu, R.C. (2003). To be or not to be . . . evidence-based? [Electronic version]. *Data Matters: An Evaluation Newsletter, 6,* 2–3.

Institute of Medicine Committee on Quality of Health Care in America. (2001). *Crossing the quality chasm: A new health system for the 21st century* [Electronic version]. Washington, DC: National Academies Press. Retrieved March 22, 2007, from http://www.iom.edu/CMS/8089/5432.aspx

Maloney, D.M., Phillips, E.L., Fixsen, D.L., & Wolf, M.M. (1975). Training techniques for staff in group homes for juvenile offenders. *Journal of Criminal Justice and Behavior, 2,* 195–216.

Naoom, S.F., Fixsen, D.L., Blase, K.B, Gilbert, T., & Wallace, F. (2007). *Lessons learned from program developers and purveyors of child welfare and violence prevention evidence-*

based programs (Final report for Grant No 9211973-2513-2005). Unpublished manuscript.

Nutt, P.C. (2002). *Why decisions fail.* San Francisco: Berrett-Koehler.

O'Connell, M.J., Morris, J.A., & Hoge, M.A. (2004). Innovation in behavioral health workforce education. *Administration and Policy in Mental Health, 32*(2), 131–165.

Oregon Addictions and Mental Health Division. (2006). *Operational definition for evidence-based practices.* Retrieved March 21, 2007, from http://www.oregon.gov/DHS/mentalhealth/ebp/ebp-definition.pdf

Paine, S.C., Bellamy, G.T., & Wilcox, B. (Eds.). (1984). *Human services that work: From innovation to standard practice.* Baltimore: Paul H. Brookes Publishing Co.

Panzano, P.C., & Roth D. (2006). The decision to adopt evidence-based and other innovative mental health practices: Risky business? *Psychiatric Services, 57,* 1153–1161.

Phillips, S.D., Burns, B.J., & Edgar, E.R. (2001). Moving assertive community treatment into standard practice. *Psychiatric Services, 52,* 771–779.

President's New Freedom Commission on Mental Health. (2003). *Achieving the promise: Transforming mental health in America. Final report.* DHHS Pub. No. SMA-03-3832. Rockville, MD: 2003.

Reiter-Lavery, L. (2004). *Finding great MST therapists: New and improved hiring guidelines.* Paper presented at the Third International MST Conference, MST Services, Charleston, SC.

Schectman, J.M., Schroth, W.S., Verme, D., & Voss, J.D. (2003). Randomized controlled trial of education and feedback for implementation of guidelines for acute low back pain. *Journal of General Internal Medicine, 18*(10), 773–780.

Schoenwald, S.K., Brown, T.L., & Henggeler, S.W. (2000). Inside multisystemic therapy: Therapist, supervisory, and program practices. *Journal of Emotional and Behavioral Disorders, 8*(2), 113–127.

Stokes, T.F., & Baer, D.M. (1977). An implicit technology of generalization. *Journal of Applied Behavior Analysis, 10,* 349–367.

Stroul, B.A., & Friedman, R.M. (1986). *A system of care for severely emotionally disturbed children and youth.* Washington, DC: Georgetown University Child Development Center.

Stroul, B.A., & Friedman, R.M. (1996). The system of care concept and philosophy. In B.A. Stroul & R.M. Friedman (Series Eds.) & B.A. Stroul (Vol. Ed.), *Systems of care for children's mental health: Children's mental health: Creating systems of care in a changing society* (pp. 3–21). Baltimore: Paul H. Brookes Publishing Co.

United Way of Canada. (n.d.) *Standard committee terms of reference.* Retrieved March 22, 2007, from http://www.boarddevelopment.org/display_document.cfm?document_id=50

Walker, J.S., & Bruns, E.J. (2006). Building on practice-based evidence: Using expert perspectives to define the wraparound process. *Psychiatric Services, 57,* 1579–1585.

Walrath, C., Sheehan, A., Holden, E.W., Hernandez, M., & Blau, G. (2006). Evidence-based treatment: Provider knowledge, training, and practice. A brief report. *Journal of Behavioral Health Services Research, 33*(1), 1–10.

Washington State Institute for Public Policy. (2002). *Washington State's implementation of functional family therapy for juvenile offenders: Preliminary findings* (No. 02-08-1201). Olympia, WA: Washington State Institute for Public Policy.

Winter, S.G., & Szulanski, G. (2001). Replication as strategy. *Organization Science, 12*(6), 730–743.

7

Financing Strategies for Systems of Care

Sheila A. Pires, Beth A. Stroul, Mary Armstrong, Jan McCarthy,
Karabelle A. Pizzigati, Ginny Wood, and Holly Echo-Hawk

inancing systems of care is a strategic endeavor that involves determining what funds will be used, how they will be used, and how they will be managed. As shown in Figure 7.1, there are numerous funding streams across various systems that are potential sources of financing for systems of care. Some are controlled at the state level, some at the local level, and some jointly. There are pros and cons to utilizing each type of funding, which can vary based on state and local circumstances. Both state and local stakeholders must play a role in determining the types of dollars that can be utilized and the purposes for which they can be allotted within systems of care.

Effective systems of care strive to achieve several goals related to financing through restructuring financing systems (Pires, 2002a):

- *Maximizing federal reimbursement,* principally through Medicaid and Title IV-E (child welfare), to generate new dollars for the system of care (Bazelon Center for Mental Health Law, 1999)

- *Redirecting dollars* from costly *deep-end* services (e.g., inpatient hospitalization, residential treatment, other out-of-home care) to home and community-based services and supports by reducing deep-end expenditures and reinvesting savings in the system of care; systems of care experiment with incentive-based financing structures (e.g., capitation, case rate financing) in which the state may capitate the county, or the state and/or county may capitate a care management entity or entities, to reduce reliance on high-cost services with a history of poor outcomes (Pires, 2002b).

- *Realigning and reallocating* resources away from traditional categorical funding silos to the system of care, for example, pooling or braiding dollars from multiple systems (Edelman, 1994). Some systems of care promise savings to traditional systems in return for gaining access to those systems' dollars.

- *Generating new dollars* for systems of care through advocacy, particularly through family and youth advocacy, as well as through the presentation of data documenting good outcomes and cost benefits, and social marketing campaigns

There are advantages and disadvantages related to each of these financing strategies. Capitation financing provides flexibility to the capitated entity, but it also poses risk (Stroul, Pires, & Armstrong, 2004). A structure that maximizes federal reimbursement can generate new dollars for the system of care, but it also presents specific administrative and technical challenges, has implications for the types of services that can be provided, and requires that state or local dollars are available for match. A structure that redirects dollars from deep-end services to home and community-based services and supports through reinvestment strategies provides an important means of funding a system of care, but it requires front door spending (i.e., creation of some home and community-based service capacity) before back door (i.e., deep-end) dollars can be redirected (Ireys, Pires, & Lee, 2006).

Figure 7.2 illustrates a framework for financing strategies that can be used in systems of care. Adapted from the work of Mark Friedman (1995), the framework begins with a principle that states, "System design drives financing," meaning that financing structures should support system design requirements rather than dictate system practices.

Medicaid
- Medicaid Inpatient
- Medicaid Outpatient
- Medicaid Rehabilitation Services Option
- Medicaid Early Periodic Screening Diagnosis and Treatment (EPSDT)
- Targeted Case Management
- Medicaid Waivers
- TEFRA Option

Substance Abuce
- SA General Revenue
- SA Medicaid Match
- SA Block Grant

Mental Health
- MH General Revenue
- MH Medicaid Match
- MH Block Grant

Child Welfare
- CW General Revenue
- CW Medicaid Match
- IV-E (Foster Care and Adoption Assistance)
- IV-B (Child Welfare Services)
- Family Preservation/ Family Support

Juvenile Justice
- JJ General Revenue
- JJ Medicaid Match
- JJ Federal Grants

Education
- ED General Revenue
- ED Medicaid Match
- Student Services

Other
- WAGES
- Children's Medical Services/Title V— Maternal and Child Health
- Mental Retardation/ Developmental Disabilities
- Title XXI—State Children's Health Insurance Program (SCHIP)
- Vocational Rehabilitation
- Supplemental Security Income (SSI)
- Local Funds

Figure 7.1. Sources of financing for child and adolescent behavioral health services in the public sector. (Adapted from Pires, S. [2002]. *Building systems of care: A primer.* Washington, DC: Georgetown University Center for Child and Human Development, National Technical Assistance Center for Children's Mental Health.)

FIRST PRINCIPLE: System design drives financing

REDEPLOYMENT Using the money we already have The cost of doing nothing Shifting funds from treatment to prevention Moving funds across fiscal years	**REFINANCING** Generating new money by increasing federal claims The commitment to reinvest funds for families and children Foster Care and Adoption Assistance (Title IV-E) Medicaid (Title XIX)
RAISING OTHER REVENUE TO SUPPORT FAMILIES AND CHILDREN Donations Special taxes and taxing districts for children Fees and third party collection including child support Trust funds	**FINANCING STRUCTURES THAT SUPPORT GOALS** *Seamless services:* Financial claiming invisible to families *Funding pools:* Breaking the lock of agency ownership of funds *Flexible dollars:* Removing the barriers to meeting the unique needs of families *Incentives:* Rewarding good practice

Figure 7.2. A financing framework for systems of care. (From Friedman, M. [1995]. *Financing strategies to support improved outcomes for children.* Washington, DC: Center for the Study of Social Policy; adapted by permission.)

Virtually all systems of care rely on discretionary grant dollars (e.g., federal and foundation grants, demonstration grants, one-time legislative allocations). These dollars provide critical start-up and leverage funds, and they are important sources of flexible dollars. Systems of care that rely solely on discretionary dollars, however, will not sustain themselves over time. Such systems are not truly systems of care in that they are not fundamentally altering traditional delivery systems by changing how they spend their dollars. They are instead creating delivery systems that are alternatives to—but not reformations of—traditional systems.

As part of the financing structure, systems of care must designate the entity that will control and manage dollars. In some systems of care, dollars are lodged with a lead government agency (e.g., the state or county mental health agency) even though they include dollars from many agencies across traditional systems. In other systems of care, dollars are lodged with a new quasi-governmental agency or contracted out to a commercial or nonprofit care management entity. In still other systems, dollars are placed with an interagency body at the state or local level, and in still others, dollars may remain with their home (categorical) agencies, which agree to reimburse the system of care for expenditures affecting their respective populations.

There are obviously pros and cons to these financial management structures, many of which concern control, accountability, and flexibility. When dollars remain with home agencies, the system of care has less control and flexibility—and, arguably, less accountability—than when cross-system dollars are placed with the system of care itself. Structures that accord the system of care greater control, flexibility, and accountability facilitate attainment of system of care goals and help to alleviate some of the frustrations that are typically associated with financing.

The financial management structure must concern itself not only with who controls dollars, but also with who makes decisions about how dollars are spent and who has authority to spend within the system of care itself. In some systems of care, care managers are allocated a budget that they control, enabling them to be flexible in their purchase of services and supports in a wraparound approach. Similarly, systems of care may allocate budgets to interagency service planning teams or give teams the authority to approve the expenditure of resources on services and supports. These approaches help to integrate financial and service delivery considerations at the service level, which is highly desirable in systems of care that are trying to meet both cost and quality of care goals. On the other hand, such a structure requires the training of frontline workers and excellent communication between fiscal, clinical, and care coordination staff and families to ensure the efficient use of dollars. Other systems of care may require greater top-down approval of decisions made at the service planning and care management level in the interest of exercising more control over spending. Unless there is a shared commitment to values and goals, this structure presents the risk of inciting a constant sense of tension between those concerned about meeting cost goals and those concerned about maintaining the quality of care.

STRATEGIC APPROACH TO FINANCING

A strategic approach to financing begins with system of care stakeholders answering two key questions: 1) financing for whom? and 2) financing for what? To answer these questions, system of care planners must:

- Identify the population(s) of focus, including the demographics, size, strengths and needs, current utilization patterns, and disparities and disproportionality in service use among the identified population(s)

- Agree on underlying values and intended outcomes

- Identify the services and supports and the desired practice model (e.g., a strengths-based, individualized, culturally competent, family-driven and youth-guided wraparound approach) to achieve outcomes, including identification of evidence-based and promising practices

- Determine how services and supports will be organized into a coherent system design

- Identify the administrative infrastructure needed to support the delivery system

- Cost out the system of care

Once these issues are addressed, system builders can then undertake a strategic financing analysis (Armstrong et al., 2006). Steps in undertaking such an analysis include the following:

- **Identify the state and local agencies that spend dollars on behavioral health services and supports for the populations of focus.**

Often the largest purchasers or payers of behavioral health services are not state or local mental health systems but other child-serving systems (e.g., education, child welfare, Medicaid). Medicaid is estimated to be the largest funder of behavioral health services for adults and children (Buck, 2003). Similarly, education systems are reported to be the largest providers of mental health services for children (Rones & Hoagwood, 2002), and both child welfare and juvenile justice systems spend significant amounts in purchasing or directly providing behavioral health care (Burns & Hoagwood, 2002).

- **Identify how much each agency spends and the types of dollars spent (e.g., federal, state, local, tribal, discretionary, entitlement, formula grant, block grant dollars), as well as utilization patterns.**

The identification of current spending and utilization patterns is an important first step in the development of a strategic financing plan for systems of care. This process enables a state, tribe, or community to understand how funds across all child-serving systems are spent and which children and families utilize services. It also assists in projecting expected utilization and costs, identifying potential resources, and planning accordingly. This type of cross-system expenditure analysis can be difficult and time consuming because various systems track expenditures and utilization differently, systems may not track mental health spending or utilization per se, service definitions vary, dollars are controlled at both state and local levels, and so forth (Pires, 2002c). It is, however, an analysis well worth undertaking as it can begin to tell a story about where dollars are going, who is controlling them, what services they are supporting, who is being served, and where spending and utilization seem inconsistent with system of care goals. Such an analysis creates cross-system awareness of spending and utilization issues and areas that should be considered for reform.

- **Identify resources that are untapped or underutilized, such as Medicaid.**

If child-serving systems are spending general revenue dollars for Medicaid-eligible populations on services that could be covered by Medicaid, it makes sense to look at revenue maximization strategies. By utilizing Medicaid where possible, states can bring in the federal financing share and offset state- or local-only expenditures (Bazelon Center for Mental Health Law, 2003).

- **Identify utilization patterns and expenditures that are associated with high costs or poor outcomes.**

Dollars for child and adolescent services tend to be finite and are often limited. It makes little sense for states or localities to continue spending scarce resources to purchase or provide poor outcomes at high costs. A goal of systems of care is to move from a mentality of funding programs to that of purchasing or providing quality care. This requires a redirection of expenditures from high costs/poor outcomes to more effective practices. For example, there is a growing body of research indicating that out-of-home placements are associated with poor outcomes and high costs (Burns & Hoagwood, 2002). Redirection of spending to support home and community-based alternatives, particularly those that are evidence based or show clear promise, is a major goal of systems of care.

- **Identify disparities and disproportionality in service access and utilization.**

Expenditure and utilization analyses can yield important information about areas in which there are disparities based on race, ethnicity, gender, and geography (e.g., low utilization of home-based services) and disproportionality (e.g., an overrepresentation of racial and ethnic minority youth in restrictive levels of care such as residential treatment or juvenile detention).

- **Determine the funding structures that will best support the system design, (e.g., blended funding, risk-based financing).**

A number of factors must be weighed to determine which funding structures are feasible (i.e., the capacity, technology, and political will to support various approaches).

- **Identify short- and long-term financing strategies (e.g., federal revenue maximization, redirection of spending from restrictive levels of care, taxpayer referenda).**

Not all strategies can be undertaken at once, and some lend themselves to a more immediate versus long-term timeframe. For example, developing political support for a taxpayer referendum to generate new revenue for the system may take time and thus be a long-term strategy. Amending the state Medicaid plan to cover new types of home and community-based services may take time. Better coordinating financing through blending or braiding approaches or through cost-sharing arrangements may be incorporated into upcoming budget cycles within a shorter timeframe.

FINANCING STRATEGIES IN SYSTEMS OF CARE

National research has found that effective systems of care use a variety of financing strategies (Stroul et al., 2008). These strategies cluster into a number of areas:

1. Identifying spending and utilization patterns

2. Realigning funding streams and structures

3. Financing appropriate services and supports

4. Financing to support family and youth partnerships

5. Financing to improve cultural and linguistic competence and reduce disparities in care

6. Financing to improve the workforce and provider network

7. Financing for accountability

Each of these areas is addressed below, with examples of effective strategies drawn from selected states and communities studied, as well as from federally funded system of care sites. This is not intended to be an exhaustive listing of all state and local financing innovations, but rather a sampling to illustrate particular strategies.

Identifying Spending and Utilization

As noted, a strategic approach to financing begins with system leaders supporting an analysis of child behavioral health expenditures and utilization across systems. Such an analysis sheds light on spending that supports or thwarts system of care goals and on utilization patterns that may be problematic, often because they are associated with high costs and poor outcomes. In Arizona, the mental health and child welfare systems worked to identify utilization and costs associated with behavioral health services financed by the child welfare system that were being provided to children eligible for Medicaid coverage and which could be covered by Medicaid instead of using all state general revenue dollars. These analyses also led to a revision upward in the capitation rate for children involved in child welfare services (i.e., development of a risk-adjusted rate). Following these analyses, system leaders also expanded the definition of the term *urgent* as it relates to the provision of crisis services. In the new definition, children removed from their homes by the child welfare system are considered to have urgent behavioral health needs, requiring a 24-hour response by the behavioral health system to conduct an initial assessment. This expansion was made both to ensure timely response to children removed from their homes and to intervene early to prevent the need for out-of-home therapeutic placements further down the road. While most of these children become state wards and thus eligible for Medicaid, at the time of the urgent care response, financial eligibility verification is not required. The state develops a yearly utilization management report that looks at units of service and financial expenditures, and that can be broken down by race/ethnicity, system involvement (e.g., child welfare involvement) and so forth.

Realigning Funding Streams and Structures

Using Diverse Funding Streams from Multiple Agencies   As noted, a multitude of funding streams at federal, state, and local levels can be drawn on to support systems of care, but the maze of funding streams that finance children's mental health services must be better aligned, better coordinated, and often redirected to provide individualized, flexible, home and community-based services

and supports. Table 7.1 illustrates the diversity of funding streams at federal, state, and local levels drawn on by federally funded system of care sites (Koyanagi & Feres-Merchant, 2000).

Blending or Braiding of Funds   Wraparound Milwaukee in Milwaukee County, Wisconsin, provides one example of a blended funding approach. It blends several funding streams, including Medicaid dollars through a capitation from the state Medicaid agency of $1,589 per member per month (pmpm), which was based primarily on Medicaid historical expenditures for hospital and clinic services; child welfare dollars through a case rate of $3,900 pmpm based on child welfare expenditures for residential treatment; mental health block grant dollars; and both contract and case rate dollars from the juvenile justice system. The blending of funds for youth deemed delinquent is based on two target populations: 1) youth whom the delinquency program would otherwise place and fund in residential treatment centers (about 350 youth) for whom Wraparound Milwaukee receives $8.2 million in fixed funds from the budget that the juvenile justice system would otherwise use to pay for this level of care, and 2) youth who would otherwise be committed to the state Department for Corrections for placement in a locked correctional facility and who have serious emotional disorders for whom Wraparound Milwaukee receives a case rate from juvenile justice of $3,500 per youth per month. If these youth were placed in a state correctional facility, Milwaukee County would be charged about $7,000 per youth per month for the cost of these placements under the state's charge-back mechanism to counties.

Prior to the establishment of Wraparound Milwaukee, both the child welfare and juvenile justice systems paid for residential treatment. Thus, both systems have incentives to utilize Wraparound Milwaukee, which delivers lower pmpm costs and better outcomes. The child welfare and juvenile justice systems each pay 50% of the cost of youth with dual delinquency and dependency court orders.

Operated by Choices, Inc., the Dawn Project in Marion County, Indiana, provides an example of a braided funding approach. Each system (e.g., child welfare, juvenile justice, special education) pays the case rate for each child it refers for care, and the Dawn Project also bills Medicaid for covered services for eligible youth. The case rate dollars can be used to purchase any services included in the individualized service plan developed by the child and family team that are not covered by Medicaid. The care plan drives the service delivery process, and any type of service or support included in the service plan is considered authorized.

Cost-Sharing for Specific Services and Supports   A number of states and localities have implemented cost-sharing across child-serving systems for specific services. In Arizona, funding for therapeutic foster care is shared among the Medicaid, mental health, and child welfare systems. Specifically, the Medicaid behavioral health managed care system uses only therapeutic foster homes licensed by child welfare for the managed care provider networks, with the exception that tribes may license homes, thus enabling Title IV-E funds to be used for room and board costs for eligible children. The mental health system in Hawaii shares costs with the child welfare, juvenile justice, and education systems for specific services

Table 7.1. Diversity of funds used in system of care grant sites

Source	System	Description
State	Mental Health	General fund, Medicaid (include FFS/managed care/waivers), federal mental health block grant, redirected institutional funds, funds allocated as a result of court decrees
	Child Welfare	Title IV-B (family preservation), Title IV-B (foster care services), Title IV-E (adoption assistance, training, administration), technical assistance, in-kind staff resources
	Juvenile Justice	Federal formula grant funds to states for juvenile justice prevention, state juvenile justice appropriations, and juvenile courts
	Education	Special education, general education, training, technical assistance, in-kind staff resources
	Governor's Office/ Cabinet	Special children's initiatives, often including interagency blended funding
	Social Services	Title XX funds and realigned welfare funds (TANF)
	Bureau of Children with Special Needs	Title V federal funds and state resources
	Health Dept.	State funds
	Public Universities	In-kind support, partner in activities
	Dept. of Children	In states where child mental health services are the responsibility of child agency, not mental health, sources of funds similar to above
	Voc. Rehab.	Federal- and state-supported employment funds
Local	County, City, or Local Township	General fund
	Juvenile Justice	Locally controlled funds
	Education	Courts, probation department, and community corrections
	County	May levy tax for specific purposes (mental health)
	Food Programs	In-kind donations of time and food
	Health	Local health authority-controlled resources
	Public Universities/ Community Colleges	
	Substance Abuse	In-kind support
Private	Third Party Reimbursement	Private insurance and family fees
	Local Businesses	Donations and in-kind support
	Foundations	Robert Wood Johnson, Annie E. Casey, Soros Foundation, and various local foundations
	Charitable	Lutheran Social Services, Catholic Charities, faith organizations, homeless programs, food programs (in-kind)
	Family Organizations	In-kind support
	Housing	Various sources

Reprinted from Koyangi, C., & Feres-Merchant, D. (2000). For the long haul: Maintaining systems of care beyond the federal investment. In *Systems of care: Promising practices in children's mental health* (Vol. 3, p. 12). Washington, DC: American Institute for Research, Center for Effective Collaboration and Practice.

Key: Dept., Department; FFS, fee for service; TANF, Temporary Assistance for Needy Families; Voc. Rehab., Vocational Rehabilitation.

(e.g., therapeutic foster care, mental health services in the juvenile detention facility). Vermont, Central Nebraska, and Wraparound Milwaukee also demonstrate cost sharing among partner agencies for a range of services including care coordination, Multisystemic Therapy (MST), school wraparound teams, family support, and mobile response services. In Central Nebraska, the development of MST was funded by a federal system of care grant. A variety of funding sources cover the actual service costs. MST providers are paid a case rate based on outcomes achieved with each youth/family. Medicaid reimburses a significant portion of the case rate as intensive outpatient services.

Maximizing Federal Entitlement Funding   Strategies used by systems of care to maximize federal entitlement funding include maximizing eligibility or enrollment for Medicaid and the State Children's Health Insurance Program (S-CHIP); covering a broad array of services and supports under Medicaid; using the multiple Medicaid options allowable under federal law; using Medicaid in lieu of state-only general funds; generating Medicaid match; maximizing Title IV-E funds; and maximizing special education funds. Hawaii and Vermont have worked to maximize eligibility and enrollment for the state Medicaid and S-CHIP programs by establishing high eligibility levels for these programs to increase the number of children who benefit.

Arizona, Hawaii, New Jersey, Vermont, and Alaska have all included an extensive list of services in their state Medicaid plans, including services such as respite, family and peer support, supported employment, therapeutic foster care, one-to-one personal care, skills training, and intensive in-home services. Hawaii, Vermont, and Nebraska have maximized Medicaid financing of behavioral health services for children by taking advantage of the multiple options available to states under the Medicaid program, including the clinic and rehabilitation options, targeted case management, the Early Periodic Screening, Diagnosis and Treatment (EPSDT) program, the Katie Beckett (i.e., Tax Equity and Fiscal Responsibility Act of 1982, PL 97-248) option, and several different types of waivers (e.g., Home and Community-Based Services, managed care).

Wraparound Milwaukee illustrates use of other systems' funds as Medicaid match to expand service capacity. Milwaukee Public Schools and child welfare general revenue provide match for the expansion of Milwaukee's Mobile Urgent Treatment Team (MUTT), a dedicated mobile crisis team providing crisis intervention and ongoing (30-day) follow-up. Each system provides funding of $450,000 to support this enhanced capacity. Since Wraparound Milwaukee can recover a percentage of its costs by billing Medicaid for children eligible for Medicaid coverage, it is able to add about $180,000 to the Milwaukee Public Schools capacity and about $200,000 to the child welfare capacity through federal Medicaid match dollars.

An example of maximizing special education funds is provided by the Dawn Project where the education system pays a case rate to obtain home and community-based wraparound services and supports to avert the need for an out-of-school or residential placement.

Redirecting Spending from Deep-End Placements to Home and Community-Based Services Strategies utilized by systems of care include redirecting dollars from deep-end placements to home and community-based services and supports, investing funds (e.g., savings generated by returning or diverting youth from out-of-home placements and reducing lengths of stay) to build home and community-based service capacity, and promoting the diversification of residential treatment providers to offer a range of home and community-based services.

Arizona provides one example of redirection with its use of an 1115 Medicaid (managed care) waiver, which has a central goal of fostering home and community-based alternatives to out-of-home services. The behavioral health system, in partnership with the state Medicaid agency, significantly expanded the array of covered home and community services and supports by adding new service types to the Medicaid benefit and expanding service definitions of already covered services. In addition, rates were restructured to better correspond to the system goals of encouraging the provision of home and community-based services and reduced reliance on residential treatment. Rates for residential treatment decline as lengths of stay increase. The state specifically included family-based therapeutic foster care (TFC) as a covered service as an alternative to congregate settings.

Wraparound Milwaukee has achieved significant reductions in use of deep-end placements, namely in use of inpatient hospitalization, residential treatment, and juvenile corrections facilities. Previously, Milwaukee County's child mental health system operated a 120-bed inpatient unit with an average length of stay (ALOS) of 70 days. As Wraparound Milwaukee developed over a period of approximately 15 years, the children's system closed beds. The state Medicaid agency provided *bridge* money to close inpatient beds by giving the children's system 40% of the Diagnosis Related Group (DRG) rate for every child diverted from inpatient care. These dollars helped to build home and community-based service capacity. Today, the ALOS is 1.7 days, and inpatient utilization has declined from 5,000 days a year to 200.

Wraparound Milwaukee also has reduced the use of residential treatment centers (RTCs) from an average daily population of 375 to 50 youth. It is estimated that if the child welfare system had not invested in Wraparound Milwaukee, the $18 million that child welfare was spending 10 years ago on residential treatment would be $46 million today. Instead, Wraparound Milwaukee is essentially using the same monies that were in the system 10 years ago—without new state or county revenues—to serve more children in home and community-based services with better outcomes.

By diverting youth to Wraparound Milwaukee, the county juvenile justice system can also save dollars and obtain better outcomes. Wraparound Milwaukee's average monthly costs for youth referred by juvenile justice are about $3,500 pmpm, compared with $6,000 pmpm for juvenile detention. Wraparound Milwaukee has reduced recidivism rates for youth in juvenile justice by 60% from 1 year prior to enrollment to 1 year postenrollment. Use of group homes dropped 75%. In place of congregate care, Wraparound Milwaukee provides crisis one-to-one stabilization, parent assistance, therapeutic foster care, offense-specific doctoral-level individual therapy, in-home therapy, parent education and support, safety plans, and a range of other individualized services to this population.

In addition to the use of the wraparound approach to reduce the use of deep-end services, Wraparound Milwaukee also operates MUTT, which is supported by Wisconsin's Medicaid crisis benefit as another means to divert children from high-cost services. The county provides 40% of the Medicaid match and receives 60% of federal Medicaid reimbursement from the state. Milwaukee's mobile crisis capacity can be utilized in a flexible manner by both the crisis team and the Wraparound Milwaukee care coordinators, who can use the benefit for time spent on crisis planning and crisis stabilization activities. The benefit can also be used to cover crisis group homes and crisis foster homes for up to $88 per day in non–room and board costs. This crisis benefit is a key factor in reducing the use of deep-end services such as hospitals, and it has also helped to prevent placement disruption of children in child welfare, which has been reduced from 65% to 38%.

Investing in New Home and Community-Based Service Capacity

Effective systems of care invest funds to develop home and community-based service capacity. In Arizona, the behavioral health and Medicaid agencies worked in partnership to expand the availability of home and community-based services by spending increased dollars, adding new service types, restructuring rates, and creating new types of providers. In Hawaii and New Jersey, state funds have been used for capacity building and start-up resources, and in Vermont, multiple sources of funding (e.g., state general revenue, federal grants, foundation grants) have been used to create new service capacity, particularly for early childhood mental health services. In both Central Nebraska and Wraparound Milwaukee, savings generated by avoiding deep-end services are reinvested in the system of care to expand service capacity. In Nebraska, the Integrated Care Coordination Unit (ICCU) approach, supported by case rate financing, achieved an initial cost savings of $500,000, which later grew to $900,000, allowing the target population to be expanded to include youth at risk.

Reengineering Residential Treatment

Effective systems of care work with residential treatment providers to encourage them to adopt the system of care philosophy and diversify by providing new types of services and supports. In Arizona, the state has established a work group to examine the use of residential treatment and has collaborated with RTCs to encourage them to deliver home and community-based services such as MST, Functional Family Therapy, and therapeutic foster care. Wraparound Milwaukee has used a market-driven approach to encourage changes in RTCs, promoting changes based on the services that it procures. Virtually all of the RTCs in Milwaukee diversified in response to what Wraparound Milwaukee indicated it was willing to purchase. While few RTCs actually closed, beds were reduced, campus facilities were sold or leased, and new home and community-based products were developed.

Financing a Locus of Accountability for Service, Cost, and Care Management for Children with Intensive Needs   Systems of care recognize that children and youth with serious behavioral health challenges and their families are involved in multiple systems. When many entities are responsible for financing, providing, and managing care, the opportunity arises for no one entity to be held accountable because the various systems can shift responsibility and costs among one another. Effective systems of care recognize the importance of financing one *locus of accountability and care management* for children with serious and complex challenges involved in or at risk for involvement in multiple systems.

The locus of management responsibility for children and youth with serious behavioral health challenges and their families may be a lead government entity, a private nonprofit entity, or even a commercial managed care entity. In Central Nebraska, the regional behavioral health and child welfare authorities created an in-house locus of accountability through their development of care management teams nested within integrated care coordination units. A local government agency is the locus of accountability for Wraparound Milwaukee. New Jersey contracts with nonprofit care management organizations in every region of the state to create this locus of accountability for children with complex issues.

Many systems of care that create a locus of accountability for populations of youth and families who are involved in multiple systems use some type of risk-based financing and various risk adjustment strategies. Hawaii's system of care, operated by the public Child and Adolescent Mental Health Division, receives a case rate from Medicaid for each child with a serious emotional disorder deemed eligible for services. Central Nebraska uses case rate financing to support its Integrated Care Coordination Units, with differential case rates based on the target population and a risk pool to protect against higher than anticipated expenses. Choices in Indiana has a case rate structure with four tiers based on youth with different levels of need, and Wraparound Milwaukee receives risk-adjusted capitation rates from Medicaid and case rates from the child welfare and juvenile justice systems.

Increasing the Flexibility of State and Local Funding Streams and Budget Structures   Flexible use of resources is an important element in financing systems of care and services. In Hawaii, local lead agencies (i.e., family guidance centers) have significant flexibility in the use of resources, and the child and family teams determine how resources will be used for each individual child and family. Similarly, Vermont incorporates local flexibility in the use of resources for local lead agencies and child and family teams. Arizona, Central Nebraska, Choices, and Wraparound Milwaukee use managed care approaches and managed care financing mechanisms (capitation and case rates), which allow for the flexible use of resources to meet individual needs. Many systems of care also have flex funds, meaning dollars specifically designated for flexible use, often for one-time purchases.

Coordinating Cross-System Funding   Systems of care utilize a variety of strategies to coordinate funding across systems, including controlling and monitoring cost shifting, coordinating funding across child-serving systems at the system level, and coordinating the procurement of services and supports across agencies, in addition to structural reforms that pool or braid dollars. In Hawaii, memoranda of understanding have been negotiated between the mental health system and the Medicaid agency, as well as with the child welfare, education, and juvenile justice systems. Vermont enacted legislation mandating interagency coordination and established local and state interagency teams that address the coordination of resources and services.

Incorporating Mechanisms to Finance Services for Uninsured and Underinsured Children and Their Families

Systems of care address the issue of financing services and supports for uninsured and underinsured families, incorporating strategies that enable families to obtain services without custody relinquishment, and encouraging private insurers to cover a broader array of services and supports. In Hawaii, general fund dollars are used to finance services to uninsured and underinsured children who are determined to be in need of mental health services. In addition, families above the eligibility level can buy into the state Medicaid program. New Jersey's system of care, by combining Medicaid and general funds, enables children who are not eligible for Medicaid to obtain services as a *system of care child*. Both Arizona and Central Nebraska have sliding fee scales for services and use state funds to cover services to children who are not covered by Medicaid or S-CHIP. Vermont has enacted legislation that prohibits custody relinquishment for the purpose of obtaining needed mental health care and can serve families that are not eligible for Medicaid through its 1915(c) Home and Community-Based Services Waiver.

Hawaii attempts to bill private insurers for covered services, and in addition, has had preliminary talks with Blue Cross about allowing their insured population access to the Child and Adolescent Mental Health Division's service array. Vermont enacted a parity law requiring health plans to cover mental health and substance abuse services to the same extent as other health services. Minnesota is working collaboratively with the private sector to develop a model behavioral health benefit that would be applicable to both publicly and privately insured populations.

Financing a Broad Array of Services and Supports

By definition, systems of care include a comprehensive array of services and supports. Financing mechanisms must also support individualized, flexible service delivery; the incorporation of evidence-based and promising practices; mental health services to young children, their families, and transition-age youth; early identification and intervention; and the coordination of services across child-serving agencies.

Types of Services and Supports Financed

Table 7.2 provides a representative listing of the types of services and supports financed by systems of care. Particular systems may also cover additional services, such as supported employ-

Table 7.2. Array of services and supports

Nonresidential services	Residential services
Assessment and diagnostic evaluation	Therapeutic foster care
Outpatient therapy (individual, family, group)	Therapeutic group homes
Medication management	Residential treatment center services
Home-based services	Inpatient hospital services
School-based services	**Supportive services**
Day treatment/partial hospitalization	Care management
Crisis services	Respite services
Mobile crisis response	Wraparound process
Behavioral aide services	Family support/education
Behavior management skills training	Family and youth peer mentors
Therapeutic nursery/preschool	Transportation
	Mental health consultation

ment, peer support, traditional healing, flexible one-time funds, respite homes, respite therapeutic foster care, supported independent living services, intensive outpatient services, treatment/service planning, parent skills training, ancillary support services, family and individual education, consultation, emergency/hospital diversion beds, after school and summer programs, substance abuse prevention, youth development, and mentor services. These services and supports are typically covered using Medicaid and a variety of other financing streams from child-serving systems.

Financing Individualized, Flexible Service Delivery   Systems of care utilize financing strategies to support individualized, flexible service delivery that include incorporating flexible funds for individualized services and supports; financing staff participation in individualized service planning processes; and incorporating care authorization mechanisms that support individualized, flexible service delivery. A number of states and localities use flexible funds. Typically, child and family teams can gain access to these flex funds to provide ancillary services and supports as needed. Managed care financing approaches can make the resources within the system inherently flexible and available to meet individualized needs. In Indiana, the Dawn Project uses its case rate financing to provide flexible funds. Eleven categories of flexible funds have been established that allow child and family teams to finance supports, including transportation (e.g., bus, car repairs), housing, utilities, clothing, food, summer camps for youth and their siblings, home repairs, and so forth.

Financing and Providing Incentives for Evidence-Based and Promising Practices   As knowledge about evidence-based and effective services has grown since the 1990s in the child behavioral health arena, systems of care have developed financing strategies for the development, training, fidelity monitoring, and ongoing costs associated with effective practices. Strategies range from establishing Medicaid billing codes for specific evidence-based practices to providing financial support for the initial training and start-up or developmental costs involved in adopting evidence-based practices, and in some cases, providing resources for ongoing training and fidelity monitoring. Arizona provides MST, Functional Family Therapy, Multidimensional Treatment Foster Care, and Dialectical Behavior Therapy. Hawaii's approach has been to identify the specific practice components that comprise clinical approaches supported by research evidence and then promote their use among providers. In Central Nebraska, the use of MST is integral to the system of care. In Indiana, the technical assistance center operated by Choices is charged with helping to build a culture in the state that is supportive of implementation of evidence-based practices, and there are billing codes for MST and Functional Family Therapy under Indiana's current Medicaid plan. In California, the state finances the California Institute of Mental Health to support counties in the development and implementation of evidence-based practices.

Financing Early Childhood Mental Health Services   As research has continued to shed light on the importance of early childhood mental health services (Knitzer, 1998), systems of care have developed financing strategies particularly focused on young children, including maximizing Part C of the Individuals with Disabilities Education Act Amendments of 1997 (PL 105-17) and Child Find financing; financing a broad array of services and supports for young children and their families; using multiple sources of financing for early childhood mental health services; financing early childhood mental health consultation to natural settings such as Head Start programs; and financing services to families of young children. In Arizona, the behavioral health system has collaborated with Part C to develop workshops in early childhood mental health to create an assessment tool for the birth to 5-year-old population and accompanying training for providers, as well as to build provider capacity for working with young children.

Both Arizona and Vermont finance a broad array of services and supports for young children and their families, using multiple sources of funding, including Medicaid, general revenue, Part C, Head Start, and a variety of other federal, state, and local funding streams. To support the use of Medicaid for early childhood mental health services, the Arizona Department of Human Services/Behavioral Health Services conducted a cross-walk of DC 0-3 and ICD 9-CM services with Medicaid-covered services to provide guidance to providers on the procedure for billing Medicaid for services for the birth to 3-year-old population (see http://www.azdhs.gov/bhs/provider/icd.pdf). Many covered services in Arizona can be provided in natural settings. The system can cover mental health consultation services to child care and Head Start providers, among others, even if the child is not present as long as the consultation pertains to an identified child. The system can also provide consultation to families even when the child is not present, again, as long as the consultation pertains to the identified child, and also covers family education and support services.

Vermont received a federal children's services mental health grant in 1997 to create the Children's UPstream Services project (CUPS), a comprehensive early childhood mental health initiative to expand community-based mental health services for young children experiencing serious emotional disturbances and their families and to strengthen local interagency coordination to increase the number of children who enter kindergarten with the emotional and social skills necessary to be active learners in schools. The initiative served as the foundation for the development of a strategic approach to maximizing the impact of federal grant dollars with the utilization of Medicaid and EPSDT funds, as well as state match funds.

Financing Early Identification and Intervention   A core principle of systems of care is providing early identification and intervention, rather than waiting until problems reach a crisis stage when interventions may be less effective and more costly. Financing strategies to support early identification and intervention include financing behavioral health screening of high-risk populations and linkages, incorporating behavioral health screening in EPSDT-funded screens, financing early intervention services for at-risk populations, and incorporating financing and incentives for linkages with and training of primary care practitioners.

Systems of care finance strategies for screening high-risk populations for behavioral health problems and linking youth to needed services. In Arizona, an urgent response system ensures that all children entering the child welfare system are referred to the behavioral health managed care system for assessment, and the Massachusetts Youth Screening Instrument Version 2 (MAYSI-2) is used to screen youth entering the juvenile justice system. In Vermont, Medicaid resources finance the screening of children entering both the child welfare and juvenile justice systems, and Medicaid resources finance assessment of youth entering the juvenile justice system in Central Nebraska. In New Jersey, common screening and assessment tools based on the Child and Adolescent Needs and Strengths (CANS) are used across systems to screen and evaluate children for risk and mental health treatment needs. In Vermont, EPSDT screens, paid for by Medicaid, incorporate behavioral health screening components. In Hawaii, behavioral health services are provided in the schools to identify children at risk for special education involvement and intervene before students must become eligible for services through an individualized education program.

Systems of care are increasingly implementing strategies to finance linkages with primary care practices. Vermont has financed a pediatric collaborative approach, largely using Medicaid dollars, whereby community mental health professionals are colocated at pediatric and family practice offices to provide screening, consultation, and short-term interventions. Wraparound Milwaukee conducts weekly reviews with primary care practitioners at the city's federally qualified health center.

Supporting Cross-Agency Service Coordination   A core principle of systems of care is the coordination of services and supports across systems. Financing for dedicated care managers (i.e., full-time care managers responsible for care coordination across systems) is an essential element of financing in systems of care. In New Jersey, cross-agency care management is provided through New Jersey's locally based Care Management Organizations (CMOs), which are private nonprofit entities. The CMOs are funded through performance-based contracts with the state utilizing Medicaid and state dollars. In Central Nebraska, funding supports several care coordination programs that offer care coordination to certain targeted populations of children and families (e.g., the Professional Partners Program [PPP], the ICCU, the School Wraparound Program, the care management team). A case rate comprised of child welfare and mental health dollars funds the care coordinators in the PPP and the ICCU, and these two systems also co-fund the care management team. The mental health and school systems share the costs of employing the facilitators in the School Wraparound Program. Wraparound Milwaukee funds care coordinators who work with small numbers of children and their families (1:8) and are responsible for outcomes across systems. Care coordinators are financed through Wraparound Milwaukee's blended funding pool, comprised of child welfare, juvenile justice, Medicaid, and mental health dollars.

Financing to Support Family and Youth Partnerships

A central tenet of the system of care philosophy is that families and youth are full partners in all aspects of the planning and delivery of services and at the system policy and management levels. The concept of family and youth involvement has been strengthened over time, and the new concept of *family-driven, youth-guided* care is achieving broad acceptance, specifying that families and youth have decision-making roles in their own services, as well as in the policies and procedures governing care for all children and families in their community, state, tribe, and nation. Thus, financing strategies are needed to support partnerships with families and youth at the service delivery level in planning and delivering their own care, as well as at the system level in designing, implementing, and evaluating systems of care. In addition, partnering with families and youth requires financing for services and supports not only for the identified children but also for family members to support them in their caregiving roles. Financing to fund family- and youth-run organizations, as well as programs and staff roles for family members and youth, also reflects a system of care that is committed to partnerships (Pires & Wood, 2007).

Supporting Family and Youth Involvement and Choice in Service Planning and Delivery   Financing strategies to support family and youth partnership at the service level include financing supports for families and youth to participate in service planning meetings (e.g., transportation, child care), financing of family and youth peer advocates, enabling families to have choices of services or providers, and paying for training for providers on ways to partner with families and youth.

In Arizona, the behavioral health managed care system pays for child care, transportation, food, and interpreters as needed. In Hawaii, child care may be provided if the family member has to fly to another island to participate in a child and family team meeting. Transportation and food are funded out of ancillary funds. In Vermont, local teams determine the appropriate funding resources for supports (e.g., child care, interpretation services, transportation) necessary to facilitate family participation. The funding resources depend on the supports required (e.g., interpretation services would be covered by Medicaid; others by state mental health, other partner agency funding, or available flexible funds.) In Indiana, flexible funds are used by Choices for such supports as bus passes, reimbursement for gas, and child care. Wraparound Milwaukee pays for child care, transportation, food, and interpreters to ensure that families can participate, using dollars from its blended funds pool.

Financing Family and Youth Peer Advocates   Systems of care typically provide financing for family and youth peer advocates. These peer advocates work with families and youth to support them through the service planning and delivery process and provide various types of direct assistance. Arizona requires its core service agencies to hire family support partners, and family and youth peer support is a covered service under Medicaid. Similarly, Hawaii finances parent partners through its contract with the statewide family organization. New Jersey funds family support organizations in every region, which are required to hire family support partners to provide peer support and advocacy for families served by care management organizations. Family support partners are funded with a combination of state general revenue, Medicaid administrative case management dollars, and federal discretionary grants. Central Nebraska finances family partners who are employed by the family organization and a youth group. Both Choices and Wraparound Milwaukee purchase family and youth peer advocacy services on a fee-for-service basis. In Indiana, family advocates are employed by Rainbows, the family organization, and they are available on an as-needed basis. In Milwaukee, family and youth peer support is provided through individuals and agencies that are part of Milwaukee Wraparound's extensive provider network.

Incorporating Financing to Provide Families and Youth with Choice of Services and Providers   Systems of care typically use an individualized care planning process with child and family teams in which the youth and family are integral to decision making about the services and supports that will be provided. They may also offer choices of providers to families and youth if they have been able to develop an extensive provider network, as in Wraparound Milwaukee and the Dawn Project in Indiana. In Milwaukee, the child and family team, on which the family and youth are key players, determines the array of services and supports for a child and family, drawing from a very broad provider network of more than 200 providers and 85 services and supports and access to flexible, individualized (e.g., one-time) supports. The plan of care developed by the team details the specific services and supports that will be provided but not the specific provider. The family itself may choose the provider. In Arizona, the system can enter into individual contracts with a provider outside the managed care network (i.e., *single-case agreements*) if there is a need for the service. Also, the system uses flex funds to support family choice.

Incorporating Financing to Train Providers on How to Partner with Families and Youth
Systems of care use various approaches to finance training for providers on how to partner with families and youth. Arizona has spent tobacco settlement monies, discretionary and formula grants, and managed care organization investments to pay for the training and coaching of families, providers, and others to develop a statewide practice approach designed to actualize Arizona's vision of family-centered practice and its system of care principles. The family organization in Maricopa County partnered with the behavioral health managed care organization's training department, core service agencies in the provider network, and others to design a curriculum on how to partner with families and youth. Hawaii incorporates a focus on family and youth partnerships in all training, employs family members as trainers, and contracts with the family organization to train providers.

Financing Family and Youth Involvement in Policy Making and Service Provision Through Contracts with Family Organizations
Although systems of care use a variety of financing strategies to support family and youth involvement at the policy and system management levels, contracting with family organizations is a primary one. Contracts with family organizations specify a wide variety of roles, including serving on committees and advisory bodies; participating in evaluation activities; providing training; providing family advocates, peer mentors, and ombudspersons; developing and disseminating information; and organizing and facilitating youth groups and youth councils. Arizona uses both discretionary and formula grant dollars to contract with two family organizations—MIKID, a statewide family organization, and the Family Involvement Center (FIC) in Maricopa County. The family organizations hold both miniconferences and a statewide conference to reach more families. They support families to serve on committees, participate in practice evaluation, and conduct trainings for providers and others. Arizona also paid the first year's dues of these family organizations in the Arizona Council of Providers.

In Maricopa County, Arizona, the behavioral health managed care organization has funded the FIC for several years for system transformation activities, including staffing and participating on the Children's Advisory Committee for the managed care organization, recruiting and training families, organizing open education opportunities for families, providing information and referral, co-facilitating meetings, recruiting and training family support partners who are outstationed with each of the core service agencies in the provider network, training and supervising family members who participate in performance improvement reviews, paying stipends to families, and providing technical assistance to providers and others on family partnership. Every family enrolled with the managed care organization receives a family handbook developed by the FIC and is invited to attend the orientation it conducts. The behavioral health managed care organization has several full-time family members on staff. The family organization also is a Medicaid provider in the managed care network, providing direct services such as respite services, behavioral coaching, skills training, peer support, personal care services, and care management.

In Hawaii, Medicaid, block grant, and general funds finance parent partners, parent skills training, peer mentoring services for youth, and parent-to-parent supports. State general fund dollars and federal block grant funds are used to fund the policy-level activities of the family organization Hawaii Families as Allies (HFAA) to serve on a range of committees and participate in other policy-level activities through the contract resources. Parent partners are employees of HFAA; they attend meetings such as individualized education program meetings and court proceedings with families, conduct workshops and support groups for families, and support families in numerous other ways. Parent partners are tied to the various family guidance centers, and they serve on family guidance center committees and management teams representing the interests of and advocating for families.

In Central Nebraska, federal system-of-care grant funds were initially used to fund the family organization Families CARE. Now the regional behavioral health system contracts with Families CARE using funds saved from the ICCU program case rate. This began as a cost reimbursement contract and then moved to 8% of the case rate based on actual costs. In Indiana, Rainbows provides services such as mentoring. In this role, it is treated like any other service provider and is paid on a fee-for-service basis, with financing coming from the case rates. In New Jersey, Family Support Organizations (FSOs) are funded via contract with the state in every region. They are family-run, not-for-profit organizations designed to ensure that the family voice is incorporated at the system and service levels. The care management organizations are required to utilize the services of the FSOs, which provide advocacy, information, referral, education, and peer mentorship. The FSOs are financed with a combination of Medicaid administrative case management dollars and state general revenue.

Incorporating Strategies Under Medicaid and Other Financing Mechanisms that Allow Services and Supports to Families

Effective systems of care have incorporated strategies to ensure that services and supports can be provided to families and are not limited to the identified child. In Arizona, Medicaid can pay for family education and peer support, respite, behavioral management skills training, and other supports to families if these supports are geared toward improving outcomes for the identified child. Medicaid can also be used to pay for transportation and interpretation services for families. Non-Medicaid allowable services (e.g., certain cultural supports such as Native healers) can be paid for with non-Medicaid dollars in the managed care capitation. Arizona uses a broad definition of the term *family* (see http://www.azdhs.gov/bhs /bhs_guide .pdf). In Wraparound Milwaukee, services to family members are financed through its blended funding approach. The system also pays for substance abuse services for parents, if necessary, and has partnered with the adult substance abuse system to adopt a wraparound approach.

Financing to Improve Cultural and Linguistic Competence and Address Disparities

A core value of systems of care is that they be culturally and linguistically competent, with agencies, programs, and services that respect, understand, and are responsive to the cultural, racial, ethnic, and linguistic differences of the populations they serve. Financing strategies are needed to incorporate specialized services, culturally and linguistically competent providers, and translation and interpretation. Financing strategies also are needed to support leadership capacity for cultural and linguistic competence at the system level and to allow for analysis of utilization and expenditure data by culturally and linguistically diverse populations. Effective systems of care also incorporate strategies to proactively address the disparities in access to care and in the quality of care experienced by culturally and linguistically diverse groups, as well as in underserved geographical areas.

Financing of Specialized Services   Effective systems of care incorporate financing for specialized services that are specifically designed to respond to the ethnic and cultural characteristics of the children and families served. In Arizona, many covered services within the managed care system (e.g., counseling) can be provided in any location, including locations that may be more culturally appropriate such as a sweat lodge. Translation and interpretation is a service covered by Medicaid. Certain cultural activities such as traditional Native healing can be paid for by the managed care system using the non-Medicaid dollars in the system. The managed care system also uses *promotores*, outreach workers and counselors for the Latino community, which it covers in a number of ways under Medicaid (e.g., as health promotion, family support, peer support).

In Hawaii, interpretative services are provided through flexible funding for ancillary services and supports, as well as other nontraditional services and supports such as martial arts provided as a therapeutic service for children. Traditional healer services and other Eastern approaches to treatment (e.g., Asian healer services) are funded under Medicaid or with mental health general fund resources. The state is attempting to integrate Eastern and Western approaches to medicine to meet the needs of the diverse cultural and ethnic groups served.

Incorporating Financing and Incentives for Culturally and Linguistically Competent Providers, Nontraditional Providers, and Natural Helpers   Effective systems of care incorporate financing and various types of incentives for culturally and linguistically competent providers, including natural helpers and traditional healers, to participate as service providers. In Arizona, there are clear expectations in managed care contracts related to serving culturally diverse populations, and fiscal penalties may be attached to serving an inadequate number of culturally diverse members. There also are requirements for recruitment and retention of Latino providers, and managed care organizations are contractually required to have specialized Native American providers in their networks. Nontraditional providers, paraprofessionals, and natural helpers can be included in managed care networks as community service agencies, a new type of Medicaid provider created by the state as a means to involve more nontraditional providers. Informal incentives also are used; the behavioral health managed care organization in Maricopa County loaned a staff person for a year to the People of Color Network in Maricopa to help them develop the infrastructure needed to join the Medicaid provider network.

Hawaii's system of care pays higher rates for clinicians who are fluent in various languages, and providers under contract with the system are required to have cultural competence policies and training. Central Nebraska provides Spanish language classes for providers. There are more than 40 racially and ethnically diverse providers in Milwaukee Wraparound's provider network. The system will also pay for interpretation and translation services and uses nontraditional providers. It also tracks use of informal helping supports through its management information system.

Analyzing Utilization, Expenditures, and Outcomes by Culturally and Linguistically Diverse Populations

Analysis of utilization, expenditure, and outcome data by culturally and linguistically diverse populations allows systems of care to identify disparities or disproportional circumstances in access to services, in service utilization, and in the quality and outcomes of care (Cuellar, Libby, & Snowden, 2003). Arizona uses special studies to examine data in this way (e.g., determining the underutilization of services by the Latino community). Hawaii and Wraparound Milwaukee also analyze data by cultural groups, and Wraparound Milwaukee has been able to tap into federal Disproportionate Minority Confinement (DMC) dollars through its partnership with the juvenile justice system. Specifically, Wraparound Milwaukee has reduced placement of African American youth in corrections facilities, which enables the juvenile justice system to draw down DMC monies, which it, in turn, uses to pay Wraparound Milwaukee.

Financing Cultural Competence Coordinators and Leadership Capacity at State or Local Levels

Systems of care also finance leadership for cultural and linguistic competence by employing cultural competence coordinators at the state and local levels or various types of cultural competence advisory committees or teams. Arizona has a cultural competence advisory committee at the state level, and the Regional Behavioral Health Authorities are required to have cultural experts and cultural competency plans. Hawaii's provider agencies are required to have a cultural coordinator. Wraparound Milwaukee has a cultural competence committee.

Incorporating Financing Strategies to Reduce Geographic Disparities

Systems of care also pay attention to geographic disparities. In Hawaii, incentive pay that is 10% above the standard pay scale is offered as an incentive to work in underserved areas. In addition, transportation is paid for providers to fly to the islands, and travel time is considered billable time. Service utilization patterns and expenditures are analyzed by geographic areas. Arizona pays higher rates for clinicians to provide out-of-office services to achieve several goals, one of which is to increase access to services in rural areas. Also, there is flexibility in the capitation paid to the behavioral health managed care organizations, which allows them to pay more to attract providers to rural areas. Arizona pays for transportation under its Medicaid managed care system. In addition, the state established a telemedicine system serving remote areas using federal grant dollars. Medicaid can then be used to pay for certain services provided through the telemedicine system (e.g., medication management, psychological evaluation, health promotion and education).

Financing to Improve the Workforce and Provider Network

Financing strategies are needed to support a broad, diversified network of providers that is capable of supplying a wide range of services and supports and is committed to the system of care philosophy. Workforce development strategies are needed to address preservice training programs to prepare individuals for work within community-based systems of care and to implement in-service training strategies to help the existing workforce to infuse the new values, approaches, and evidence-based practices into their work. The payment rates established for providers must allow systems of care to attract and retain qualified providers and create incentives for providers to develop and provide home and community-based services.

Supporting a Broad, Diversified, Qualified Workforce and Provider Network   Systems of care use various strategies to finance a broad array of providers. In Arizona, development of a *community service agency*, a new Medicaid provider type, within the managed care system opened up the provider network to nontraditional entities, including family organizations and community agencies that do not have to be licensed as outpatient mental health clinics to provide certain Medicaid services. These services include respite, peer support, habilitation, skills training, and crisis services. There is also a category of outpatient provider called a *paraprofessional*, whose services can be reimbursed under Medicaid, as well as a category called *habilitation worker* that was derived from the developmental disabilities long-term care system.

Wraparound Milwaukee has a very large provider network of more than 200 providers, including both individuals and agencies, and more than 40 racially and ethnically diverse providers. The network includes clinical treatment providers, as well as providers of supports such as respite and mentoring. No formal contracting with providers is used. Instead, Wraparound Milwaukee develops service definitions, rates, and standards for 85 different services and supports. Community agencies and individual practitioners are invited during the first 90 days of each calendar year to apply to provide one or more of the services. Wraparound Milwaukee then credentials providers to be part of a qualified provider pool. The broad provider network is overseen by Wraparound Milwaukee's Quality Assurance Office.

Financing of Workforce Development Activities   Systems of care recognize that providers, staff, family and youth partners, and other stakeholders do not necessarily have the requisite knowledge, attitudes, and skills to function effectively within systems of care, and they incorporate financing strategies geared to workforce development. Arizona has used general revenue, block grants, tobacco funds, and federal State Infrastructure Grant discretionary dollars to pay for training and coaching. In Hawaii, general fund and Title IV-E resources are used to finance workforce development activities. A practice development section of the child mental health system's clinical services office oversees a range of activities on evidence-based clinical practice and care coordination practice for state child mental health staff, contracted providers, staff of other state agencies, and families of children and youth with special needs. In New Jersey, using Title IV-E and general revenue, the state contracted with the University of Medicine and Dentistry of New Jersey to be the fiscal agent for all training and technical assistance activities through a new Behavioral Research and Training Institute. All new system of care staff must go through training or orientation on the system of care, and the state also mandates work-specific training (e.g., all care management organizations are trained to use the assessment and screening tools relevant to their roles in the system). The state finances a web-based certification program in use of the CANS tools.

Financing Appropriate Provider Payment Rates and Payment Methods   Effective systems of care incorporate financing strategies that allow for sufficient rates to attract and retain providers and that offer incentives for providers to supply the types of home and community-based services and supports needed in the system. In Arizona, the state established higher rates for out-of-office than for in-office services to encourage therapists to provide services in homes and schools. It also pays a tiered system of rates for out-of-home care, with rates decreasing with longer stays. Wraparound Milwaukee pays its providers very quickly, which is another incentive for providers to participate that can also help to offset concerns about rate sufficiency. Providers bill every week for services rendered, and they are paid within 5 days.

Financing for Accountability

Systems of care need reliable, practical data and accountability mechanisms to guide decision making and quality improvement in service delivery (Hernandez, 1998). The development of strong accountability and continuous quality improvement (CQI) procedures requires investment in good information systems, as well as financing to support the collection, analysis, and use of data by administrators and other stakeholders. Accountability and CQI procedures require data on the population being served, service utilization, service quality, cost, and outcomes at multiple levels (the system, program, and child and family levels). Use of performance-based or outcomes-based contracting allows systems of care to incorporate accountability procedures in contracts with providers. In addition, financing is required for a focal point of accountability for systems of care—that is, an agency, office, or entity that is responsible for system of care policy and overall system management. Accountability procedures must also involve periodic assessment of financing policies and strategies to ensure their consistency and support for system of care goals.

Incorporating Utilization, Quality, Cost, and Outcomes Management Mechanisms

Effective systems of care finance mechanisms to track and manage utilization, quality, cost, and outcomes and to use data to guide financing and service delivery policies. In Arizona, there is a quality management children's subcommittee and a quality system tied to Arizona's system of care principles, which includes both process and outcomes monitoring. Each regional behavioral health authority (i.e., behavioral health managed care organization) undergoes an intensive review of the child and family team processes throughout its provider network through chart reviews and interviews with families conducted by independent teams of family members and wraparound specialists. For every child in the system, behavioral health managed care organizations are required to report outcomes in several areas (success in school, safety, preparation for adulthood, decreased criminal justice involvement, lives with family, increased stability in family and living conditions). There is a different set of outcomes for the birth to 5-year-old population, which include emotional regulation, readiness to learn, safety, and stability. Outcomes are reported by child and family teams at enrollment and at 6 months.

The system also tracks cost by funding source and cost by rate group (e.g., child welfare population). There are 22 different funding categories, and these cost data are part of managed care organization deliverables. Arizona uses independent quality monitoring teams that include family members; there is also a quality monitoring process mandated by Medicaid that involves independent case reviews of 1,500 adult and child cases per year. The system has access to 16,000 sets of data representing more than 50,000 children and youth, and the data can be cut by age, ethnicity, region, and the child's access to a child and family team to support special analyses. In addition, Arizona utilizes financial incentives related to quality in its contracts with the behavioral health managed care organizations. The incentive pool represents 1% of the entire capitation pool. If managed care organizations meet performance standards, they may receive funding from the incentive pool.

In Hawaii, the system has utilization, cost, quality, and outcome data managed by the Child and Adolescent Mental Health Management Information System. The state Child and Adolescent Mental Health Division (CAMHD) has a quality assurance and improvement program operated by its central office and guided by a performance improvement steering committee. Each family guidance center (i.e., core service agency) has an internal interdisciplinary quality assurance team for reviewing performance data and managing performance improvement initiatives, as well as a quality assurance specialist to manage these efforts. In addition, each provider agency with which CAMHD contracts is required to have a CQI system and to submit quality data to CAMHD on a quarterly basis. Outcome data are collected on each child served by CAMHD.

The state also routinely collects system performance information such as financial information about the cost of services. The statewide performance improvement committee reviews data and provides the data along with recommendations to the governing body. In addition, data are provided to the quality assurance teams at each of the family guidance centers for review, and care managers receive data reports on their practice, comparing their service utilization patterns with those of other care managers and with statewide patterns. Data are used for system improvement. Data from the Fiscal Year 2005 Annual Evaluation Report showed that disruptive behavior disorders comprised the most common problem among youth registered in the CAMHD system. In response to the data, two evidence-based interventions for youth with disruptive behaviors—MST and Multidimensional Treatment Foster Care—have been increased in the system.

Hawaii also uses cost–benefit analysis, referred to as *data envelope analysis* (DEA), for accountability. DEA is a linear programming methodology that examines the relative efficiencies of the family guidance centers. The method involves examining multiple resource inputs (e.g., costs of operating expenses, staffing patterns) along with multiple quality outputs (e.g., youth outcomes, quantity of services). These multiple input and output (i.e., cost and quality) measures are converted to a single comprehensive measure of efficiency. Results from one application of this methodology showed that five of the family guidance centers could be considered efficient, but one had the lowest percentage of clients showing improvement on the Child and Adolescent Functional Assessment Scale or Achenbach System for Empirically Based Assessment, as well as the highest input of resources per client day for three of the five resource inputs. Use of the methodology allowed managers to compare themselves with those with the lowest costs and highest outputs and undertake improvement strategies.

In Central Nebraska, the contract with Families CARE includes monitoring fidelity to the wraparound model. Families CARE staff collect information from parents, youth, and care coordinators to measure fidelity and to assess satisfaction. The results are aggregated and distributed to the various wraparound-based programs. This feedback allows for continual improvements in the programs and builds capacity for parent-to-parent support by using family members as evaluators. To track utilization and case rate expenditures, Region 3 Behavioral Health Services (BHS) prepares a monthly report that identifies direct service costs by child (e.g., services provided, flex funds spent, concrete expenditures such as transportation or rent) and nondirect service costs. This monthly report shows the extent to which the case rate was under- or overspent for each child. From these reports on individual children/families, Region 3 BHS is able to track trends over time, including the average cost per family and the average monthly costs for different types of placements.

In Indiana, an integrated management information system called *The Clinical Manager* (TCM) was developed by Choices as a tool for system management in both the clinical and fiscal arenas to support the Dawn Project and its other systems of care. TCM includes clinical information and plan of care, claims adjudication, service authorization, service utilization, progress, outcomes, costs tracking, medication management, historical information, and contract management data. Clinical and fiscal records for a child and family can be viewed together, affording team members prompt access to both types of data and resulting in more efficient care management. Data are analyzed by payers, the team, and the individual care coordinators.

Wraparound Milwaukee is also a data-driven system supported by a web-based management information system called *Synthesis* that allows the system to capture both real-time and retrospective data. *Synthesis* captures all care planning, crisis plans, safety plans, and progress notes. It tracks all services and supports provided, the youngsters for whom they were provided, and the cost that was incurred, as well as demographic data and outcome data. It also is used for billing and claims adjudication and links to a system for automatic check writing. More than 300 people use *Synthesis*; Milwaukee uses a "train the trainers" approach to build capacity to use *Synthesis*. The system has an incentive to pay attention to cost and quality issues because the bulk of its funding is risk-based (i.e., either capitation or case rates). Providers are paid on a fee-for-service basis; Wraparound Milwaukee closely monitors performance and stops using providers that do not meet quality standards.

Supporting Leadership, Policy, and Management Infrastructure for Systems of Care   Effective systems of care finance some type of focal point for policy and overall management of the system of care. In most cases, this involves a state-level focal point of responsibility, as well as a local entity for local system management. Effective systems also finance leadership development and training for system of care leaders. In Arizona, tobacco monies, formula grants, and discretionary grants are used to support leadership development across stakeholder groups. In Hawaii, a 10-week leadership development program was financed by the state agency. Nebraska has used its Central Nebraska system of care to provide technical assistance and leadership development to other areas of the state. In Indiana, Choices has been funded by the state to create a technical assistance center for systems of care that provides assistance and leadership development to other areas of the state.

Financing Strategies for Tribal Systems of Care

Financing systems of care and their component services is particularly challenging in tribal communities, which operate as sovereign nations or urban Indian communities and have their own unique financing streams and service systems in addition to involvement with state and local systems. Also, system of care development in tribal communities occurs in the context of historical trauma and in the context of a non-Western view of mental heath problems and treatment. A study of financing for systems of care in tribal communities identified a number of issues that impact the financing of children's mental health services (Echo Hawk & Lichtenstein, 2008):

- *Tribal sovereignty*—A federally recognized tribe has a unique status as a nation-within-a-nation (i.e., a tribal nation within the nation of the United States). Tribal status results in the ability to leverage Medicaid payments with no general fund match requirement by the state. However, state policy makers often do not understand the financial advantage of partnering with tribes under the Medicaid program. Furthermore, states often count tribal populations within their federal block grant formulas, but they do not provide funding for services as they erroneously assume that the Indian Health Service and other tribal-specific services are adequately funded to address health care and mental health needs.

- *Medicaid partnership*—Federal and state Medicaid support for tribal behavioral health services can be a win–win for both state and tribal governments. Partnership in financing culturally competent behavioral health care results in a reduction of the high human and financial cost of out-of-home placement, hospitalization, and correctional facility utilization. Although not extensively implemented, examples of such partnerships include state–tribal workgroups on Medicaid policy, colocation of Medicaid enrollment staff at tribal locations, inclusion of tribal services in state Medicaid plans, Medicaid administrative match payments to tribes, and Medicaid access training for tribes.

- *Lack of organizational infrastructure*—Reflecting the economic challenges of rural and frontier communities, many smaller tribes may lack basic infrastructure, which impedes their ability to develop and manage financing plans for systems of care. They often lack current computer technology, dependable Internet access, advanced billing systems and supports, credentialed workforce, and other infrastructure elements, resulting in the perpetuation of short-term, underfunded services and a crisis management approach to financing.

- *Understanding state funding streams*—Gaining access to state funding streams involves a complex learning curve and full understanding of current and upcoming state initiatives, state funding cycles, and state billing and reporting requirements. Tribes have demonstrated success partnering with a champion within a state system who is willing to guide the tribe through the state process, but dwindling state resources creates significant challenges in nurturing these tribal–state relationships.

- *Impact of tribal leadership elections*—Elections for leaders of tribal governments can occur as often as every 2 years, thus adding another layer of complexity to long-term financing of tribal systems of care. Although new leadership creates opportunities for creative partnerships or unexplored avenues for behavioral health care financing, turnover in leadership can be disruptive and requires continual training of elected leadership on behavioral health issues and systems of care.

Effective financing strategies in tribal communities involve collaboration among states, localities, and tribes, as well as coordination of federal, state, local, and tribal financing streams. As noted, health and behavioral health services provided by tribal-run facilities are eligible for 100% federal Medicaid contribution, known as the *federal pass-through program*. Arizona illustrates the complexity of the system. Arizona tribes must deal with a bifurcated Medicaid system—the 1115 waiver in the state and the federal pass-through for tribes. The federal pass-through benefit is more traditional than the array of services covered under the 1115 waiver, but the federal pass-through rate is higher than state rates, with the additional bonus of 100% federal funding. For example, case management is not a covered service by the pass-through, but it can be paid for through the 1115 waiver.

In Arizona, Tribal Behavioral Health Authorities (TRBHA) were created, and they can pick and choose whether or not to bill the federal pass-through or the 1115 waiver. The federal pass-through can only be used for services directly provided by the tribe. There are more than 60 providers serving adults and children in the overall Gila River TRBHA network, which is composed of both on-reservation and off-reservation providers. Only those that are Gila River tribal community providers can be billed through the federal pass-through process; the off-reservation providers are billed through the 1115 waiver. As part of its strategic financing approach, the Gila River TRBHA has moved more to a staff model of owning its own services and clinical staff, rather than exclusively contracting out for services. Most of this new service and infrastructure capacity has been made possible with funding from the state behavioral health system through federal discretionary State Infrastructure Grant monies, state general revenue, or Medicaid. The TRBHA believes that its staff model approach will accomplish several goals—a higher degree of culturally relevant care, easier access to care, greater continuity and coordination of care between therapists and care managers employed by the TRBHA, and generation of Medicaid revenue from the staff model that can be used to build tribal infrastructure capacity and expand services. The TRBHA example illustrates the complexity and range of financing strategies that can be available through tribal–state partnerships.

CONCLUSION

This chapter has offered a strategic approach to financing and described an array of financing strategies in selected systems of care, drawing on national research (Stroul et al., 2008). It argues for the importance of system of care leaders to analyze and utilize financing across child-serving systems for child and adolescent behavioral health services and supports. As illustrated in Figure 7.3, an underlying principle of strategic financing for systems of care is to create win–win scenarios for those that control resources.

The process of identifying and implementing win–win financing scenarios is inherently a strategic one, supported by an understanding of the populations of focus, the systems that control resources, the constraints and opportunities associated with particular funding streams, and the technologies for utilizing dollars in a more coordinated manner.

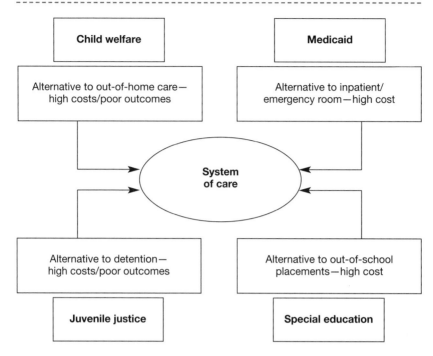

Figure 7.3. Win–win scenarios for systems of care. (Reprinted from Pires, S. [2006]. *Primer Hands On–Child Welfare* [p. 64]. Washington, DC: Human Service Collaborative.)

REFERENCES

Armstrong, M., Pires, S., McCarthy, J., Stroul, B., Wood., G., & Pizzigati, K. (2006). A self-assessment and planning guide: Developing a comprehensive financing plan. In *RTC Study 3: Financing structures and strategies to support effective systems of care* (FMHI Pub. No. 235–01). Tampa: University of South Florida, Louis de la Parte Florida Mental Health Institute, Research and Training Center for Children's Mental Health.

Bazelon Center for Mental Health Law. (1999). *Making sense of Medicaid for children with serious emotional disturbance.* Washington, DC: Author.

Bazelon Center for Mental Health Law. (2003). *Covering intensive community-based child mental health services under Medicaid.* Washington, DC: Author.

Buck, J. (2003). Public financing of mental health services. *Psychiatric Services, 54,* 969–975.

Burns, B., & Hoagwood, K. (Eds.). (2002). *Community treatment for youth: Evidence-based interventions for severe emotional and behavioral disorders.* New York: Oxford University Press.

Cuellar, A., Libby, A., & Snowden, L. (2003). Minority youth in foster care: Managed care and access to mental health treatment. *MedCare, 41*(2), 264–274.

Echo Hawk, H., & Lichtenstein, C. (2008). *Exploratory description of financing and sustainability in American Indian and Alaska Native systems of care.* [Draft report.] Rockville, MD: Substance Abuse and Mental Health Services Administration, Center for Mental Health Services.

Edelman, S. (1994). *Developing blended funding programs for children's mental health care systems.* Sacramento, CA: Cathie Wright Center for Technical Assistance to Children's System of Care.

Friedman, M. (1995). *Financing strategies to support improved outcomes for children.* Washington, DC: Center for the Study of Social Policy.

Hernandez, M. (Ed.). (1998). System accountability in children's mental health [Special Issue]. *Journal of Behavioral Health Services and Research, 25*(2).

Individuals with Disabilities Education Act Amendments of 1997, PL 105-17, 20 U.S.C. §§ 1400 *et seq.*

Ireys, H., Pires, S., & Lee, M. (2006). *Public financing of home and community services for children and youth with serious emotional disturbances: Selected state strategies.* Washington, DC: U.S. Department of Health and Human Services, Office of the Assistant Secretary for Planning and Evaluation.

Knitzer, J. (1998). Early childhood mental health services through a policy and systems development perspective. In S.J. Meisels & J.P. Shonkoff (Eds.), *Handbook of early childhood interventions* (2nd ed.). New York: Cambridge University Press.

Koyanagi, C., & Feres-Merchant, D. (2000). For the long haul: Maintaining systems of care beyond the federal investment. In *Systems of care: Promising practices in children's mental health* (Vol. 3). Washington, DC: American Institutes for Research, Center for Effective Collaboration and Practice.

Pires, S. (2002a). *Building systems of care: A primer.* Washington, DC: Georgetown University Center for Child and Human Development, National Technical Assistance Center for Children's Mental Health.

Pires, S. (2002b). *Health Care Reform Tracking Project (HCRTP): Promising approaches for behavioral health services to children and adolescents and their families in managed care systems–1: Managed care design and financing.* Tampa: University of South Florida, Louis de la Parte Florida Mental Health Institute, Research and Training Center for Children's Mental Health.

Pires, S. (2002c). *Report on children's mental health spending in Hennepin County.* Washington, DC: Human Service Collaborative.

Pires, S., (2006). *Primer Hands On—Child Welfare.* Washington, DC:. Human Service Collaborative.

Pires, S.A., & Wood, G. (2007). *Issue brief #2: Effective strategies to finance family and youth partnerships.* Tampa: University of South Florida, Louis de la Parte Florida Mental Health Institute, Research and Training Center for Children's Mental Health.

Rones, M., & Hoagwood, K. (2002). School-based mental health services: A research review. *Clinical Child and Family Psychology Review, 3*(4), 223–241.

Stroul, B., Pires, S., & Armstrong, M. (2004). *Using research to move forward: A consensus conference on publicly funded managed care for children and adolescents with behavioral health disorders and their families.* Tampa: University of South Florida, Louis de la Parte Florida Mental Health Institute, Research and Training Center for Children's Mental Health.

Stroul, B., Pires, S., Armstrong, M., McCarthy, J., Wood. G., & Pizzigati, K. (2008). *Effective financing strategies for systems of care: Examples from the field.* Tampa: University of South Florida, Louis de la Parte Florida Mental Health Institute, Research and Training Center for Children's Mental Health.

Tax Equity and Fiscal Responsibility Act of 1982, PL 97-248, 96 Stat. 324.

8

Sustaining
Systems of Care

BETH A. STROUL AND BRIGITTE MANTEUFFEL

The Comprehensive Community Mental Health Services for Children and Their Families Program (CMHS Program) was initiated by the Center for Mental Health Services (CMHS) of the Substance Abuse and Mental Health Services Administration (SAMHSA) in 1992 to assist communities in developing comprehensive, community-based systems of care for children and adolescents with or at risk for serious emotional disturbances and their families. Since the program's inception, a national evaluation conducted by Macro International has documented both the process and outcomes of system development efforts. As part of the national evaluation, a study was undertaken to assess the ability of funded sites to sustain their systems of care beyond the federal grant period. The study involved examining the extent to which key components of systems of care were maintained during the period in which federal funds were phasing out and during the postgrant period, factors that contribute to or impede the ability to sustain systems of care, and the effectiveness of various strategies for sustainability. This chapter summarizes the results of the study and identifies lessons learned that will assist states and communities in maximizing the likelihood that their systems of care will be maintained over time. It is important to note that although the study focused on federally funded communities, the findings yielded important lessons that are applicable to all communities regardless of whether they received federal funding or other special funding to initiate their systems of care. Thus, the concept of sustainability is applicable to a variety of efforts designed to create comprehensive mental health services for children and families.

BACKGROUND

Application of the findings of the study on sustainability to enhance state and local efforts to maintain systems of care over time requires an understanding of the origins and philosophical underpinnings of the CMHS Program and of the purposes and methodology of the sustainability study.

Comprehensive Community Mental Health Services for Children and Their Families Program

In response to widespread criticisms and systemic problems associated with service delivery to children and adolescents with mental health needs and their families, the concept of a *system of care* was developed as a framework for reform (Stroul, 2002; Stroul & Friedman, 1986, 1996). A *system of care* was defined as "a comprehensive spectrum of mental health and other necessary services and supports which are organized into a coordinated network to meet the multiple and changing needs of children with serious emotional disturbances and their families" (Stroul & Friedman, 1986, p. 3). A distinct philosophy was also defined to guide service delivery. This philosophy comprised the core values of community-based, child-centered, family-focused, and culturally competent services. Its principles included a broad array of services and supports, individualized care, services provided in the least restrictive setting, coordination across child-serving systems, early intervention, and partnerships with families and youth. This system of care approach has formed the basis for numerous federal, state, and foundation initiatives geared toward developing more comprehensive integrated systems of community-based services for children.

The CMHS Program, the largest of these initiatives, was authorized by Congress in 1992 and has provided grants to states, communities, territories, and Indian tribes to develop the infrastructure and services that comprise systems of care (U.S. Department of Health and Human Services, 2002). Under the leadership of the Child, Adolescent, and Family Branch of CMHS/ SAMHSA, system of care sites initially received grants for 5-year periods; in 2002, the grant period was extended to 6 years by amending the authorizing legislation, a decision based on the observation that building system of care infrastructure and services is a developmental process that requires a significant investment of time and effort. The CMHS Program has been supported by federally funded technical assistance to system of care communities and has been reviewed via a national evaluation, including system-level and practice-level assessments, as well as the measurement of outcomes for children and their families (Center for Mental Health Services, 2001).

A key issue for systems of care is the ability to sustain the infrastructure and services over time, along with the capacity to continue to develop and evolve the system after the federal funding cycle is completed. Observations during system-level site visits conducted as part of the national evaluation suggested significant variation among sites in their expectations and experiences regarding the ability to maintain the services and infrastructure when federal funding ends. System leaders alluded to many factors that affect the sustainability of the systems of care, some related to the approach used to develop and finance the systems and others related to the larger policy context and environment in which the systems operate (Stroul, 2004). To better understand these issues, it was determined that sustainability would be studied through the national evaluation.

Study on the Sustainability of Systems of Care

In 2002, a study on sustainability was initiated to (Stroul, 2006; Stroul & Manteuffel, 2007):

1. Evaluate the extent to which system of care services, infrastructure, goal achievement, and principles have been maintained at the end of the grant period when federal funding is phasing down and at a point in time approximately 5 years after federal funding has been terminated

2. Identify and elucidate factors that contribute to or impede the ability of communities to sustain systems of care

3. Identify and assess the effectiveness of specific strategies used by sites to maintain their systems of care beyond the federal grant period

4. Explore the perspectives and roles of state mental health agencies on the sustainability of local systems of care

5. Provide information and guidance to federally funded system of care communities and to nonfunded communities engaged in system of care development to enhance their ability to sustain systems of care over time

6. Provide information that will assist federal, state, and local policy makers, technical assistance providers, family members, advocates, and other key groups to more effectively support the development of viable, sustainable systems of care

The first task in this study involved defining the term *sustainability*. Definitions found in the literature emphasized the long-term survival of services and programs initiated with grants or other specialized funding. Ager (1990) defined *sustainability* as the maintenance of programs through mechanisms that serve to support changes brought about by the formal introduction of interventions. Holder and Moore (2000) discussed *sustainability* as the long-term maintenance or the "institutionalization" of services that outlive their original funding, including policy and structural changes that support desired outcomes. They assert that these types of changes suggest sustainability, even if all of the specific elements developed with the original funding are ultimately not maintained. Johnson, Hays, Center, and Daley (2004) cited a number of different terms used for *sustainability* (e.g., *continuation, durability, institutionalization, maintenance*) and noted that decision makers involved in implementing an innovation must face the ultimate challenge of planning for the time when the implementation phase is completed and continuation of the innovation becomes the primary goal. They defined sustainability as ensuring that an innovation is fully integrated into ongoing, normal system operations, and they viewed sustainability as an ongoing "change process with specific action steps to strengthen system infrastructure and innovation attributes that are necessary to sustain a particular innovation" (p. 137).

In a volume on promising practices for the sustainability of systems of care, Koyanagi and Feres-Merchant (2000) noted that sustainability may be defined differently by different stakeholders. Policy makers may focus on sustaining the vision and philosophy, state-level administrators may emphasize maintaining an approach that is consistent with other state policy goals, and local stakeholders typically work toward keeping the services and staff in place. Regardless of which aspect of sustainability is emphasized, all stakeholders acknowledge that adopting a long-term system of care approach requires a sea change in policy, clinical practice, administration of children's mental health systems, and maintenance of all of these elements of systems of care in the face of budgetary challenges and changing political environments. A similar conceptualization of sustainability is reflected in a sustainability toolkit that includes a sustainability self-assessment and strategic planning template developed by CMHS to provide assistance to the federally funded system of care sites (CMHS, 2004). Thus, for purposes of the study, *sustainability* was defined as the maintenance of systems of care over time, including the services, infrastructure, goals, and philosophy.

Methodology

The study methodology involved a web survey for completion by key informants at each site and telephone interviews with key informants at the local and state levels. The major study tasks included gathering information, selecting the sample of sites, identifying respondents, developing and administering the web survey, conducting telephone interviews with site-level and state-level key informants, analyzing data, and preparing reports.

Information Gathering   A thorough review of the published and unpublished literature was conducted on the sustainability of federal and other grant programs, including journal articles, reports, promising practices manuscripts, and a variety of documents pertinent to the CMHS Program. In addition, site visit reports generated as part of the national evaluation were reviewed to extract material related to sustainability. The information review focused on issues including the definition of sustainability, factors that affect sustainability, strategies for sustainability, and the experience of states and communities in maintaining the infrastructure and services developed with grant funds over time in a range of health and human service programs. A focus group of representatives of communities funded by the federal CMHS Program was conducted at a national system of care community meeting, and informal conversations with individuals with expertise in sustainability were also used to gather information. The information generated through these strategies provided the basis for developing the survey instrument and telephone interview protocols.

Sample Selection and Identification of Respondents   The study sample was composed of the first 37 communities funded to develop and improve systems of care through the federal CMHS Program. The sample included all sites whose federal grant periods had terminated at the time of survey. These sites are referred to as *Phase I* or *graduated* communities, those with grants awarded in 1993 ($N = 4$) and in 1994 ($N = 22$). The federal funds in these communities had been terminated for at least 4 years at the time of the survey. In addition, sites funded in 1997 that were approaching the end of their federal grant period were included in the study sample ($N = 11$). These sites are *Phase II* or *nearly graduated* communities; most were in their final year of federal funding at the time of the survey or were operating with small amounts of carry-forward funding, and were dependent on state and local match funds or financing from other sources to continue system of care activities and services. Some CMHS Program grants were awarded to multisite areas or to state agencies for statewide system development initiatives, as in Vermont and Rhode Island. In these instances, the study team purposively selected one or two representative communities to include in the sample. Table 8.1 delineates the communities included in the study sample and denotes sites that represent a selected locality in a multisite or statewide grant.

A site contact person was identified for each site included in the sample. Study team members telephoned each contact person to apprise them of the study, enlist their cooperation, identify appropriate respondents for each site based on defined criteria, and obtain contact information for the respondents. Four key informants were identified for each site included in the sample: 1) a current or former project director of the system of care, 2) a representative of the mental health system at a mid-level or high-level position in the children's mental health system, 3) a family member who was involved at the system level, either as a representative of a family organization or independently, and 4) a representative of a partner child-serving agency who was involved in system of care activities, and in most cases, was in a mid-level or high-level position in the child welfare, education, or juvenile justice system. With some variance particular to each respondent, the criteria generally required that the respondents be involved with the system of care during the last year of funding and that they remained involved in the community in any capacity at the time of the survey to enable them to have sufficient information to respond. The family member was required to be affiliated with the family organization that participated in the national evaluation's system-level assessment, was a member of the governing body for the system of care, or had a child receiving services from the system of care, and at the time of the survey, was affiliated with a family organization or was a member of a community task force or coalition to enable him or her to have sufficient information to respond.

Web Survey Development and Administration
The survey instrument was developed for data collection from the sites based on information gathered during the first phase of the study. The survey was designed to compare the status of elements of systems of care—services, philosophy, goal achievement, and infrastructure—during the *grant-funded period* (i.e., any time during the grant period prior to the previous 12 months) and during the *current period* (i.e., the previous 12 months). Scaled items of the status of each element during the grant period and during the current period were rated on Likert scales. In addition, the

Table 8.1. Sites included in the study sample

Phase I—graduated sites (N = 26)

Funded in October 1993	East Baltimore Mental Health Partnership, East Baltimore, MD
	Stark County Family Council, Stark County, OH*
	The Village Project, Charleston/Dorchester Counties, SC
	ACCESS (Statewide), Burlington, VT*
Funded in February 1994	Children's System of Care, Riverside County, CA
	Children's System of Care, San Mateo County, CA
	Children's System of Care, Santa Cruz County, CA
	Children's System of Care, Solano, CA
	Children's System of Care, Ventura, CA
	COMCARE, Sedgwick County, KS
	Wings for Children and Families, Piscatquis, Hancock, Pebnobscto, and Washington Counties, ME
	Olympia, Doña Ana County, NM
	PEN-PAL (Pitt-Edgecombe-Nash Public-Academic Liaison Project), Pitt, Edgecombe, and Nash Counties, NC
	Project Reach, RI (Statewide), Washington County, RI*
	Wraparound Milwaukee, Milwaukee County, WI
Funded in September and November 1994	Multiagency Integrated System of Care (MISC), Santa Barbara, CA
	Sonoma-Napa Comprehensive System of Care, Sonoma and Napa Counties, CA
	Hawaii Ohana Project, Wai'anee Coast and Leeward, Oahu, HI
	Community Wraparound Initiative, Lyons, Riverside, and Proviso Townships, IL
	KanFocus, Parsons, KS*
	K'e Project, Navajo Nation, AZ, CO, NM, and UT
	FRIENDS (Families Reaching in Ever New Directions), Mott Haven, NY
	Partnerships Project, Bismark, ND*
	New Opportunities, Lane County, OR
	South Philadelphia Family Partnerships Project, South Philadelphia, PA
	City of Alexandria System of Care, Alexandria, VA

Phase II—nearly graduated sites (N = 11)

Funded in October 1997	The Jefferson County Community Partnership, Jefferson County, AL
	Children's Mental Health Services Initiative, San Diego, CA
	Kmihqitahasultipon (We Remember) Project, Passama-quoddy Tribe Indian Township, ME
	Southwest Community Partnership, Detroit, MI
	Nebraska Family Central, 22 Central Counties, NE
	North Carolina FACES (Families and Communities with Equal Success), Blue Ridge, NC*

North Carolina FACES (Families and Communities with Equal Success), Sand Hills, NC*

Sacred Child Project, Fort Berthold, Standing Rock, Spirit Lake, and Turtle Mountain Indian Reservation, ND

Children's Upstream Services (Statewide), Washington County, VT*

Children's Upstream Services (Statewide), Franklin/Grand Isle, VT*

Northwood Alliance for Children and Families, Langlade, Lincoln, and Marathon Counties, WI*

Reprinted from Stroul, B. (2006). *The sustainability of systems of care: Lessons learned. A report on the special study on the sustainability of systems of care* (p. 8). Atlanta, GA: Macro International.

*One selected locality in a statewide or multisite grant.

survey was designed to explore factors that either positively or negatively affected the sustainability of systems of care and to assess the effectiveness of a range of strategies for maintaining systems of care over time. The survey included the following sections:

1. Demographic information

2. The availability of an extensive list of system of care services and supports, rating each on a 1–5 scale during the grant period and current period, plus ratings of the extent of availability

3. The implementation of system of care principles, rating each on a 1–5 scale during the grant period and during the current period, plus ratings of the extent of implementation (Each principle was defined operationally to be consistent with definitions in the national evaluation's system-level assessment site visit protocol, and respondents rated each element, with ratings aggregated to derive composite scores for each principle.)

4. Goal achievement (including infrastructure goals) rated on a 1–5 scale during the grant period and during the current period, plus ratings of extent of goal achievement

5. Factors affecting sustainability, with specification of the presence of factors rated on a 1–4 scale and the degree of positive or negative impact of various factors on a 1–5 scale

6. Sustainability strategies (general strategies and financing strategies), with specification of the use of various strategies and ratings of the effectiveness of each strategy used on a 1–5 scale

Extensive follow-up procedures were implemented using repeated e-mail and telephone contacts in order to obtain the highest possible response rate. Of

148 total respondents, completed surveys were received from 140, a 94.6% response rate. One community was ultimately dropped from the analysis because responses from at least three of the four respondents could not be obtained despite repeated follow-up attempts, leaving 36 communities in the sample for data analysis. A data report was produced for each community that provided aggregate data across all respondents for each individual site and showed average ratings for each item. These site-specific data reports were used as a basis for discussion during follow-up telephone interviews with site-level respondents. In addition, an aggregate data report was generated across all sites in the sample.

Site-Level and State-Level Telephone Interviews Two of the respondents from the web survey were selected to be interviewed by telephone to obtain explanatory information about the community's survey responses. Using a structured protocol, telephone interviews were conducted with the current or former project director or the representative of the mental health system and the family member survey respondent. Telephone interviews also were conducted with the state children's mental health director in each state that had one or more system of care communities included in the sample. A structured interview protocol was used to explore actions, circumstances, policies, or factors in the state that might have had an impact on the maintenance of systems of care over time in the grant communities in the state and on children's mental health services in general, as well as the role of the state in facilitating the maintenance of systems of care.

Data Analysis and Preparation of Study Products A mixed methods model was used to collect data on the maintenance of systems of care over time in grant communities. The data from the web-based sustainability survey was analyzed using a paired samples *t*-test to compare the average ratings for each item on the survey about the status of systems of care during the grant period and during the current period. Frequency data for appropriate items were also generated. For qualitative data, telephone interview reports for each site and for each state were prepared, and content analyses of information generated through the telephone interviews were conducted. These content analyses provided the basis for the interpretation and explanation of survey results. To assist in data analysis, a meeting was held to review both quantitative and qualitative data, as well as to assist in the interpretation of results involving all members of the study team plus additional evaluation staff from Macro International and consultants with expertise in developing and sustaining systems of care. Several products from the sustainability study were prepared, including a full report detailing the methodology and results and evaluation briefs.

SUSTAINABILITY OF SYSTEMS OF CARE

The results of the study on sustainability have revealed some of the challenges involved in sustaining systems of care and have important implications for the continuing system-building work of states and communities—again, regardless of whether they have received federal funding. The results of the study are summarized next, including: 1) sustainability of services, 2) sustainability of the system of care philosophy, 3) sustainability of goal achievement, 4) factors affecting sustainability, 5) strategies for sustainability, and 6) state perspectives.

Sustainability of Services

Across all sites in the sample, some services increased in availability from the grant period (i.e., for sites not yet graduated, defined as any time before the 12 months prior to survey administration) to the current period (i.e., the 12 months prior to survey administration) based on differences in ratings of availability for each of the time periods on the five-point scale. As shown on Table 8.2, the largest increases were shown for behavioral aide services in homes, schools, and other settings; transition from residential treatment settings to community-based service settings; transition to adult services from services within the children's mental health system of care; medication monitoring; and substance abuse treatment; however, only increases in behavioral aide services achieved statistical significance. Although these increases in availability were relatively small, they indicate a process of increasing service capacity during the period of federal funding for these services with continued progress in the phase-out or postgrant period for many communities, resulting in even greater availability.

Table 8.2 also shows decreases in the availability of some services from the grant period to the current period across all sites in the sample. The differences in reported availability were also relatively small and reached statistical significance for flexible funds and transportation, which showed the largest reduction in availability with the loss of federal funding. Despite the small differences the pattern suggested by the data indicates that many of the services that decreased in availability may be characterized as *supportive* services, including flexible funds, respite care, family preservation or home-based services, family support services, recreation, transportation, tutoring, professional consultation, vocational services, and mentoring. Study findings suggest that the federal grant provided resources for flexible funds and other supportive services that sites have had difficulty replacing with other financing streams to support ongoing service delivery postgrant.

Comparison of the graduated with the nearly graduated communities revealed that decreases in the availability of services are attributable to the graduated communities, which were 4–5 years postgrant. The sites with continued federal funding, albeit greatly reduced and approaching termination, were still in the process of building service capacity and thereby increasing the availability of most services; the average increase in availability for all services as a group was +.11 from the height of grant period to the current period for the nearly graduated sites. In contrast, graduated communities reported an average decrease of –.05 in the availability of all services as a group from the grant period to the current period. Results suggested that the challenges involved in maintaining services that were developed with federal grant funds over time at the same level of availability, especially supportive services, are often difficult for some communities to overcome.

Table 8.2. Sustainability of services

	All sites n = 139 respondents in 36 sites	Phase I graduated sites (funded in 1993 or 1994) n = 97 respondents in 25 sites	Phase II nearly graduated sites (funded in 1997) n = 42 respondents in 11 sites
Increased availability from grant period to current period across all sites			
Behavioral/therapeutic aide services	+.17	+.16	+.19*
Transition from residential to community	+.16	+.17	+.15
Transition to adult services	+.11	+.06	+.22
Medication treatment/ monitoring	+.10	+.04	+.21
Substance abuse treatment	+.10	+.08	+.14
Therapeutic group homes	+.09	+.09	+.09
Independent living services	+.08	+.05	+.14
After-school and/or summer programs	+.08	+.03	+.17
Care management/service coordination	+.05	−.02	+.21
Diagnostic and evaluation	+.04	−.04	+.20
Residential treatment	+.04	+.03	+.04
Neurological/psychological testing	+.03	+.03	+.01
Emergency/crisis services	+.03	−.01	+.08
Therapeutic foster care	+.01	−.05	+.15
Decreased availability from grant period to current period across all sites			
Flexible funds	−.59*	−.80*	−.04
Transportation services	−.18*	−.28*	+.06
Respite care	−.12	−.19	+.07
Caregiver/family support services	−.11	−.22	+.20
Inpatient hospitalization	−.10	−.14	−.01
Recreational services	−.08	−.17	+.13
Outpatient family counseling	−.06	−.08	−.01
Outpatient group counseling	−.06	−.08	−.01
Outpatient individual counseling	−.04	−.08	+.06
Family preservation/ home-based services	−.04	−.08	+.07
Tutoring	−.04	−.05	0.00
Professional consultation	−.03	−.08	+.08
Intensive day treatment	−.02	−.06	+.11
Vocational services	−.01	−.01	+.02
Mentoring services	−.01	−.07	+.13
Average	**−.02**	**−.05**	**+.11**

Adapted from Stroul, B. (2006). *The sustainability of systems of care: Lessons learned. A report on the special study on the sustainability of systems of care* (pp. 18–19). Atlanta, GA: Macro International.

Note: The scale ranged from 1 (Not At All Available) to 5 (Extensively Available).

*Significance was found at $p < .05$ level using paired samples t test analysis.

Despite the increased availability of some services during and even after the receipt of federal CMHS Program grants, none of the services in the service array were judged to be extensively available (a rating of 5 on the five-point scale) in either time period. In fact, only care management and outpatient individual counseling were found to be very available (a rating of 4). Most other services were characterized as either somewhat available or moderately available (ratings from 2–3). These data suggest that, even with the investment of federal funds, communities have struggled to build capacity in a comprehensive array of services commensurate with the need. The explanations provided through telephone interviews for changes in the availability of services from the grant to the postgrant period are summarized in Table 8.3.

Sustainability of the System of Care Philosophy

The success of communities in sustaining the various elements or features of the system of care philosophy was assessed by comparing the implementation of these features at any point during the grant period and during the current period. As shown on Table 8.4, changes in the implementation of system of care principles were small, yet the implementation of most of these features across all sites in the sample decreased from the grant to the current period; the implementation of individualized care and family involvement at the system level showed the largest declines, reaching statistical significance for graduated sites.

Although the communities in the sample lost ground on some principles, the implementation of several principles increased across all sites from the grant

Table 8.3.   Reasons for changes in availability of services

Most frequent explanations for declines in the availability of services included the following:

Loss of grant funds that had been used to support specific services within the service array

Lack of providers and provider agencies to deliver specific services

Fiscal crises and budget cuts that have dramatically curtailed potential sources of financing to replace federal resources

Inability to obtain Medicaid reimbursement for some of the services included in the array that are not included in state Medicaid plans and therefore are not billable under this program

Most frequent explanations for increases in the availability of services included the following:

Formation of partnerships among child-serving systems that provide both the mechanism and the resources for the continuation of services and expansion of their availability

The ability to bill Medicaid for services, often the result of successful work with state Medicaid and mental health agencies to add new service definitions and billing codes to state Medicaid plans

New state funds that have enabled services to be sustained and enhanced as grant funds are phased out and terminated

---

Source: Stroul (2006).

Table 8.4.   Sustainability of philosophy

Principle	All sites n = 139 respondents in 36 sites	Phase I graduated sites (funded in 1993 or 1994) n = 97 respondents in 25 sites	Phase II nearly graduated sites (funded in 1997) n = 42 respondents in 11 sites
Increased implementation from grant period to current period across all sites			
Family involvement in the service planning and delivery process (services level)	+.09	−.09	+.19
Cultural competence of services (services level)	+.07	−.07	+.23
Cultural competence of system policy and management (system level)	+.01	−.06	+.15
Decreased implementation from grant period to current period across all sites			
Individualized care approach	−.21*	−.27*	−.01
Interagency planning and coordination in system policy and management (system level)	−.23	−.21	+.06
Interagency coordination in planning and delivering services (services level)	−.13*	−.33*	+.03
Family involvement in system policy and management (system level)	−.10	−.20*	+.19
Services accessibility (e.g., times, locations)	−.04	−.13	+.20
Shared administrative processes among agencies	−.02	−.04	−.02
Average	**−.08**	**−.16**	**+.11**

Adapted from Stroul, B. (2006). *The sustainability of systems of care: Lessons learned. A report on the special study on the sustainability of systems of care* (pp. 28–29). Atlanta, GA: Macro International.

Note. The scale ranged from 1 (Not At All Used) to 5 (Extensively Used)

* Significance was found at $p < .05$ level using paired samples t test analysis.

to the current period—family involvement at the service delivery level and cultural competence at both the system and service delivery levels—although these increases did not achieve statistical significance.

Similar to findings on the sustainability of services, graduated sites reported declines in the implementation of system of care principles (an average decline of −.16 for all principles), whereas implementation of these principles increased in the communities that were nearing graduation but still retained some level of federal funds and grant-related activities (an average increase of +.11). These data suggest that with the termination of federal funding and without the visible presence of system of care development requirements and activities, communities have encountered challenges in maintaining the implementation of system of care principles over time at the same level as during the grant funded period.

Despite small overall declines in the implementation of system of care principles from the grant to the current period across all sites, several of the system of care principles were rated by respondents as being close to the *very much implemented* category, with average ratings higher than 3.5 in both time periods (i.e., *family involvement at the system* and *service delivery levels and individualized care*). These principles represent some of the key recommendations of the President's New Freedom Commission on Mental Health (2003) and the subsequent Federal Action Agenda (Substance Abuse and Mental Heath Services Administration, 2005), as well as being central tenets of the system of care philosophy. Although two of these were among the principles with the largest declines from the grant period to the current period, they were still rated as the most highly implemented principles in both time periods. Most other principles were rated as moderately implemented in both time periods. Thus, moderate levels of implementation of system of care principles were maintained in the communities over time, even with positive or negative changes from the grant period to the current period.

Table 8.5 details the explanations offered during telephone interviews for changes in the implementation of system of care principles from the grant period to the postgrant period.

Sustainability of Goal Achievement

Table 8.6 shows that for half of the system of care goals, communities reported greater success in goal achievement during the current period than they did during the grant period, although changes were small. Changes in goals examined across all sites did not achieve statistical significance, but some trends are worth noting. Goals with increased achievement across all sites included key system of care goals, including *minimizing the need for children to leave the community for services* (i.e., providing community-based care), *reducing the number of children in restrictive service settings* (i.e., care in the least restrictive setting), and *achieving general acceptance of the system of care philosophy among both service providers and among system managers and leaders* (i.e., community-based, family-focused, individualized, least restrictive, coordinated, accessible, and culturally competent care). For the other goals, sites reported less success in goal achievement during the current period as compared with the height of the grant-funded period, again with small differences between periods. Less success was found in *ensuring sufficient service capacity, using evaluation data to inform policy and program decisions, maintaining a designated focal point* (e.g., an agency, office, entity) *to manage the system of care,* and *supporting and maintaining an active family organization*. All of these can be characterized as parts of a system of care's infrastructure, and the accomplishment of these goals requires targeted resources. The data suggested that these infrastructure goals pose more challenges to achieve without federal grant funding and accompanying mandates. The largest decline in goal achievement

Table 8.5.   Reasons for changes in implementation of system of care principles

Most frequent explanations for declines in the implementation of principles included the following:

The loss of grant funds coupled with budget cuts resulted in cuts in staff and services or structural changes that have not been supportive of the system of care philosophy and approach.

Changes in administrators and leadership at the highest levels of some states or communities resulted in policy changes, with new leaders shifting systems from the system of care philosophy to a greater emphasis on traditional services and on the "bottom line."

The loss of grant funds led to the loss of key system of care leaders at the community level, leaving a leadership void and no one to carry the mantle of the system of care philosophy and convene structures and processes critical to the operation of systems of care.

The loss of federal requirements and mandates connected to the grant program and loss of the meetings, technical assistance, resource materials, and monitoring that served to bombard communities with the philosophy reduced public awareness.

Training related to system of care principles and approaches was discontinued in some states and communities because these activities had been supported by grant resources.

Sufficient buy-in to the system of care philosophy by system leaders, staff, and providers was not available to maintain the momentum as federal funds were reduced or eliminated.

Grant-related activities never became fully integrated into the overall system and did not result in substantial changes in the existing system.

Most frequent explanations for increases in the implementation of principles included the following:

Elements of the system of care philosophy became well institutionalized within the children's mental health system and shaped the way the entire system operated.

Institutionalization of the system of care philosophy by legislation, plans, regulations, and other policy instruments formed the basis for state policy and resultant maintenance and enhancement of the principles in local systems of care.

Continued emphasis was placed on the principles, coupled with continued funding and activities to support their enhancement.

A continuity of leadership was maintained at the state and community levels.

Advocacy of a family organization was sustained.

Source: Stroul (2006).

across all sites was in *maintaining an active family organization,* a goal that other findings reveal is an important key to sustainability.

Consistent with findings on services and the philosophy, comparison of ratings of goal achievement among graduated sites and nearly graduated sites reveals that the decreases in goal achievement from the grant period to the current period are entirely attributable to the graduated sites, with an average decline of −.08. Goal achievement from the height of the grant period to the current period increased for the sites retaining some federal funding and grant-related activity (average increase of +.16). Increased achievement shown by reductions in the use of restrictive settings achieved statistical significance when scores for the prior period and the current period were compared among sites in their final year of funding (nearly graduated sites). Decreased achievement shown by reductions in *main-*

Table 8.6. Sustainability of goal achievement

Principle	All sites $n = 139$ respondents in 36 sites	Phase I graduated sites (funded in 1993 or 1994) $n = 97$ respondents in 25 sites	Phase II nearly graduated sites (funded in 1997) $n = 42$ respondents in 11 sites
Increased achievement from grant period to current period across all sites			
Minimizing need for children to leave the community for services	+.06	+.03	+.15
Reducing the number of children in settings more restrictive than necessary	+.09	+.05	+.21*
Achieving general acceptance of the system of care philosophy among service providers	+.12	+.07	+.24
Achieving general acceptance of the system of care philosophy among system managers and leaders	+.06	+.02	+.16
Decreased achievement from grant period to current period across all sites			
Ensuring that services in the service array have sufficient capacity	−.09	−.16*	+.06
Using evaluation data to inform policy and program decisions	−.05	−.16	+.19
Maintaining a designated focal point (i.e., agency, office) for the system of care	−.09	−.15	+02
Supporting and maintaining an active family organization	−.16	−.35*	+.23
Average	**−.01**	**−.08**	**+.16**

Adapted from Stroul, B. (2006). *The sustainability of systems of care: Lessons learned. A report on the special study on the sustainability of systems of care* (pp. 38–39). Atlanta, GA: Macro International.

Note: The scale ranged from 1 (No Success) to 5 (Complete Success)

*Significance was found at $p < .05$ level using paired samples *t*-test analysis.

taining sufficient service capacity and *supporting family organizations* only reached statistical significance for graduated sites.

In addition, no goals were rated by respondents as having been achieved with substantial success or complete success across all sites (4–5 rating on a five-point scale), but the achievement of most goals approached the level of *substantial success* with ratings higher than 3.5. Across all sites, *achieving general acceptance of the system of care philosophy among system managers/leaders and among service providers, maintaining a designated focal point for system of care management, reducing the use of unnecessarily restrictive service settings,* and *minimizing the need to leave the community for services* were goals that were reportedly achieved with near substantial success in both time periods. The remaining goals (*maintaining an active family organization, ensuring sufficient service capacity, using evaluation data*) were reportedly achieved with moderate success in both time periods, regardless of positive or negative changes. Explanations for changes in goal achievement over time derived from telephone interviews are shown on Table 8.7.

Factors Affecting Sustainability

Many factors affect the ability to maintain systems of care over time. Some of these are controlled by communities whereas others are controlled by the political and economic environments in which they exist. Two of the factors reportedly had a *somewhat negative* impact on sustainability (a rating of 2 on the five-point scale)—*changes in the larger economic climate,* which generally have resulted in fewer resources, and *changes in elected or appointed officials,* which often change policy and programmatic directions in a state or community. No factors were rated as having a *very negative impact.* The implementation of managed care in behavioral health service systems, which has occurred in most states, was judged by respondents across all sites as having little or no impact at all on the maintenance of systems of care over time. All of the other factors assessed reportedly had a positive influence on sustainability to the extent that they were present in sites, either a *somewhat positive impact* (a rating of 4 on the five-point scale) or close to that with average ratings higher than 3.5. Reports on the impact of the various factors were consistent for the two groups of sites (Phase I graduated sites and Phase II

Table 8.7. Reasons for changes in goal achievement

Most frequent explanations for declines in goal achievement included the following:

Loss of grant funds and budget cuts

Loss of grant emphasis and mandates, resulting in insufficient commitment or foundation to maintain activities directed at goal achievement in the postgrant era

Changes in state and community leadership, resulting in shifting goals and emphasis, as well as a loss of focus on the achievement of system of care goals

Most frequent explanations for increases in goal achievement included the following:

Continued commitment to system of care goals among system leaders, staff, and providers, who conceptualized system of care goals as goals for the larger service system

Creation of an infrastructure and capacity for goal achievement that could be maintained with the reduction or termination of federal funding, ensuring resources to maintain the capacity to achieve goals over time; for example, sustaining an active family organization by creating funding structures and mechanisms for their ongoing support, including contracting for a wide range of services and products, which enable family organizations to advocate for services and continued adherence to the system of care philosophy; or sustaining the staff and infrastructure needed to collect, interpret, and use data to demonstrate outcomes and advocate additional support, often with cross-agency funding.

Source: Stroul (2006).

nearly graduated sites). For all sites, the factors rated as having the most positive impact on sustainability are shown on Table 8.8. Nearly all of the factors found to have the most positive impact on sustainability were those subjected to influence through strategic activities. System of care communities should take advantage of opportunities to maximize the potential positive impact of these factors by developing a strategic plan with specific action steps delineated to influence as many of these factors as possible.

Strategies for Sustainability

A range of strategies for sustainability were examined to assess the extent to which they were used by communities and the extent to which they were considered by key informants to be effective for maintaining their systems of care over time. All of the strategies assessed were used by the vast majority of sites included in the sample, but none were rated by respondents as being *completely effective* (a rating of 5 on a five-point scale) or *very effective* (a rating of 4). A number of strategies, however, approached the *very effective* level, with a mean rating higher than 3.5 across all sites. These included *cultivating strong interagency relationships, involving stakeholders, establishing a strong family organization, using evaluation results,* and *creating an ongoing focal point for managing the system of care.*

All of the other strategies were rated as *moderately effective,* including *making policy or regulatory changes supportive of systems of care, infusing the system of care into the broader service system, providing training, creating an advocacy base, mobilizing resources,* and *generating political support.*

Table 8.8. Factors with most positive impact on sustainability

Inclusion of key stakeholders
Interagency partnerships
Local commitment to the system of care approach
Existence of ongoing leadership
Provision of training
Existence of a constituency to advocate systems of care
Presence of a champion with the power to focus energy and resources
Infusion of the system of care into the larger service system
Existence of positive evaluation data on system effectiveness
State commitment and involvement
Existence of formal policies supportive of systems of care
Engagement of political and policy leaders
State financial support
Increased utilization of Medicaid for financing services

Adapted from Stroul, B. (2006). *The sustainability of systems of care: Lessons learned. A report on the special study on the sustainability of systems of care* (pp. 48–49). Atlanta, GA: Macro International.

Interestingly, two strategies—*making policy or regulatory changes* and *infusing the system of care into the broader system*—were rated closer to the *very effective* category for Phase I (graduated) communities. This may suggest greater recognition of the importance of these systemic changes for maintaining systems of care over time—4–5 years postgrant—in the absence of federal funding, requirements, and grant-related activities.

At least two of the sustainability strategies—*creating an ongoing focal point for system of care management* and *establishing a strong family organization*—were less successfully achieved during the current period, yet they were considered by sites to be two of the most effective strategies for maintaining systems of care over time. In addition, all sites attempted to mobilize resources as a strategy for sustaining their systems of care, but this was rated as only a *moderately effective* strategy, confirming the difficulty in securing ongoing funding to support systems of care and their component services.

Interesting contrasts were noted for strategies judged to be effective in some communities and ineffective in others, confirming that ratings of effectiveness were closely tied to each site's ability to implement the strategy well. For example, while some sites judged *generating political and policy level support* to be one of the most effective strategies, others were unable to mobilize state and local officials and decision makers in support of the system of care philosophy and approach due to changes in officials over time, the reluctance of officials to create new policies supportive of systems of care, fiscal crises, or the lack of political will to adopt this approach. As a result, these sites judged this strategy to be less effective. Similarly, many sites found that the *use of evaluation data to document the effectiveness of the system of care and to advocate policy and financial support for its maintenance* to be among the most successful strategies. On the negative side, a number of sites were unable to effectively translate evaluation data into a form that was helpful in making the case for sustainability, or they lost the staff and resources to continue evaluation activities with the reduction or termination of the federal grant. As a result, they had no access to evaluation information. A number of sites indicated that *establishing a strong family organization to provide a vocal and effective constituency to advocate continuation of the system of care* was a highly effective strategy for sustainability. An equal number of sites reported that they were unable to establish a viable family organization in the community or were unable to continue financial support for a fledgling organization because grant funds were reduced or terminated, leading them to consider this to be an ineffective strategy for sustaining their systems of care. *Mobilizing resources,* a strategy critical for sustaining systems of care, was also a strategy identified as among the most effective in sites that were able to garner resources and among the least effective for sites that were unsuccessful in obtaining the resources needed to continue their work.

Financing mechanisms to maintain the infrastructure and services comprising systems of care are critical aspects of sustainability. Sites reported using a range of financing strategies to maintain their systems of care. The strategy used across all sites most frequently was *increasing the ability to obtain Medicaid reimbursement for services,* suggesting the importance of Medicaid as a source of support. In addition, *operating more efficiently* (typically meaning cutting costs), *creating partnerships with other nonmental health child-serving systems, obtaining grants, coordinating categorical funds, obtaining new or increased state funds,* and *leveraging funding sources* were among the most frequently used strategies across all sites. Other financing strategies were used less frequently.

Examination of the effectiveness of the various financing strategies confirms the challenges faced by sites with respect to maintaining financing for systems of care. None of the strategies were rated as *completely effective* or *very effective,* nor did any approach the *very effective* level (i.e., a mean score across all sites higher than 3.5). Only two financing strategies—*increasing the ability to obtain Medicaid reimbursement* and *obtaining new or increased state funding*—received mean ratings higher than 3.4. Although ratings were in the *moderately effective* range, the strategies receiving the highest effectiveness ratings across all sites included *Medicaid funding, state mental health system funding, obtaining and coordinating funds with other systems,* and *redeploying funds to lower cost service alternatives.*

Increasing the ability to obtain Medicaid reimbursement was by far the strategy seen as most effective for sustaining systems of care and their component services as reported by key informants during telephone interviews. Use of this strategy has involved close collaboration with the state Medicaid agency to include the array of services and supports provided through systems of care in the state Medicaid plan, and in many cases, adding new service definitions and billing codes. Given some of the nontraditional and flexible services offered through systems of care, this work has been challenging in many states, but using mechanisms such as Medicaid waivers, the rehabilitation option, and the Early Periodic Screening, Diagnosis, and Treatment (EPSDT) Program have proven to be viable approaches to implementing the policy and regulatory changes needed to maximize Medicaid reimbursement for services. Phase II (nearly graduated) sites have reportedly had less success in increasing the ability to obtain Medicaid reimbursement than the Phase I graduated communities. This may be due to recent changes in the Medicaid program, making this strategy more challenging, or to the sites' earlier stages of development and the possibility that these policy changes were not yet solidified.

Obtaining new or increased state funding and *obtaining funds from partner child-serving agencies to support services* were also considered by interview respondents to be effective financing strategies. Second to Medicaid, obtaining state funds, typically from mental health general revenue and block grant funds, is reportedly critical for the continuation of systems of care. These funds have taken the form of legislative appropriations or administrative allocations targeted not only at continuing services in the grant community, but at providing system of care services on a statewide basis. Respondents from many sites noted that obtaining new or increased state funding has become more difficult in the current economic climate of fiscal crises and budget cuts; however, state funds have provided a major source of support for the continuation of systems of care and for the adoption of similar approaches throughout the state. State funds for sustaining systems of care also have come from child-serving agencies other than those concentrating on mental health. Interview respondents emphasized that partnerships with other systems provided highly effective vehicles for sustaining systems of care because they often resulted in a commitment to the philosophy and service approaches and a willingness to provide ongoing funding to sustain and enhance the services provided to children and families involved in their respective systems. The child welfare and juvenile justice agencies were most frequently mentioned as partners in the delivery of services and as sources of funding to maintain systems of care, although several sites reported such partnerships with the education and health systems as well.

State Perspectives

Interviews with state children's mental health directors yielded information about the sustainability of systems of care from a broader system perspective. The crucial role of state agencies in providing both leadership and resources was apparent in the many roles ascribed to state agencies and in the difficulty in sustaining systems of care over time without the policy and financial support of the state. Specifically, respondents related the multitude of ways in which the support of state agencies in partnership with communities is a necessary condition for sustainability. The roles that state agencies play in sustaining systems of care and in spreading the philosophy and approach statewide include the following:

- Working at the state level with the Medicaid agency to amend state Medicaid plans and rules to finance the services within systems of care

- Providing funds from state mental health agencies to finance systems of care and their component services

- Negotiating agreements with other child-serving systems (e.g., child welfare, juvenile justice, education, health, substance abuse) to support the system of care approach, to enhance interagency coordination at the system and service delivery levels, and to provide funding for services

- Implementing statewide programs (e.g., wraparound programs, crisis programs) that provide mechanisms for sustaining systems of care and individualized services

- Building on the system development work in funded communities by using these communities as pilots or models and as sources of experience, information, and training for system of care development statewide

- Enacting legislation that supports the statewide implementation of the system of care philosophy and approach

- Implementing mechanisms to provide technical assistance and training regarding the system of care philosophy and approach and evidence-based and promising service delivery approaches

- Creating entities at state, regional, and local levels to provide leadership, coordination, and support for systems of care

- Incorporating the system of care philosophy and approach in policy documents, plans, licensing requirements for provider agencies, and contracts with provider agencies and managed care organizations

- Removing barriers in policy, regulations, and financing identified by local communities in sustaining systems of care

- Monitoring compliance with the system of care philosophy and approach in communities and evaluating the outcomes of systems of care and services

Because of their critical role in sustaining systems of care and supporting the adoption of this approach in areas beyond those that received federal grant funds, respondents emphasized the importance of their involvement with system of care communities. They asserted that without state involvement, the likelihood of sustaining systems of care beyond the grant period is significantly diminished and that federal grants are reduced to projects that disappear when federal funding is terminated. With state involvement, the policies and financing mechanisms necessary to sustain systems of care with the phasing out and termination of federal funding are more likely to be implemented, enabling both the maintenance of funded systems of care and the application of the approach statewide to include areas that did not have the benefit of federal funding.

LESSONS LEARNED FROM SYSTEMS OF CARE

Interviews with both state and local respondents offered valuable insights about how to sustain systems of care and about unique challenges faced by certain communities in their efforts to maintain system of care elements over time.

Lessons and Advice

Interview data yielded a wealth of information about lessons learned from early systems of care and advice that those involved in these systems would offer to states and communities engaged in system building efforts.

Establish a Strong Link Between Local Systems of Care and State Agencies   As noted, state mental health and other agencies play crucial roles in establishing the policy and financing framework for sustaining systems of care and for expanding the application of this approach to other areas of the state. Given the essential role of states in sustainability, the establishment of a state–local partnership from the outset of system development is imperative, along with a joint focus on how the infrastructure, philosophy, and services will be maintained as federal funding declines and is eventually terminated. According to respondents, state involvement should be required for all CMHS Program grantees. Several suggested that an official from the state mental health agency should serve as coprincipal investigator for any grant given to a community within that state to firmly establish this linkage and to maximize the long-term vi-

ability of the systems of care. State agencies should feel ownership of systems of care along with communities to enhance long-term viability, as well as statewide impact of federal CMHS Program grants through state policy changes. In addition, respondents noted that sustainability is hindered by focusing federal resources and technical assistance solely on individually funded communities and not focusing sufficient resources on state agencies to provide incentives and support state system development strategies. It was noted that federal strategies should not bypass state agencies, but should instead be directed at affecting state planning and policy development processes, including incorporating system of care development as an explicit goal and requirement under the federal mental health block grant program.

Engage Top Policy Makers and System Administrators   According to respondents, to set the stage for sustainability, policy makers and system leaders at the highest levels must understand the system of care philosophy and approach. The support and commitment of legislators, state agency administrators, governors, local officials, and others is necessary to create the policy, regulatory and financing structures, and processes needed to maintain systems of care and their services over the long haul. The development of strategies to present information on the approach and its outcomes should be a priority for systems of care to maximize sustainability.

Respondents indicated that policy makers are engaged most effectively if systems of care can demonstrate that they are achieving results in solving specific problems. For example, compelling arguments for sustaining systems of care have been made in several states by demonstrating the amount of dollars saved by keeping youth out of state custody, inpatient care, and residential treatment settings. Both the executive and legislative branches of government must be engaged and committed to the system of care approach to ensure the system's sustainability. Intensive targeted activities to engage policy makers should be seen as an investment in the long-term sustainability of systems of care; one respondent stated that it often takes "dogged determination" to cultivate the support of policy makers. Many respondents noted that politics play an important role in any system reform and should not be overlooked in sustainability planning.

Incorporate System of Care Approach into Written Plans and Policies   Respondents maintained that written plans and policies that reflect the philosophy, approach, and goals of systems of care are needed to establish these as the basis for children's mental health service delivery. Codifying systems of care and then infusing this approach into the broader service system are ways to ensure that this approach becomes the way the entire system does business and guards against changes in system administration that might otherwise result in reversals of progress or changes in direction. Creating a separate project in one neighborhood, county, or region that does not become infused into the larger service system sets the stage for loss of the services that have been developed when federal funding is terminated. Thus, interviews suggested that philosophical support is not sufficient and that policy, regulatory, and financing changes are needed to ensure the long-term viability of systems of care.

Understand and Create Partnerships with Other Child-Serving Systems

Other child-serving systems have resources for mental health services within their budgets to provide care for youth with emotional and behavioral disorders within their systems. Respondents emphasized the importance of understanding the goals and cultures of other child-serving systems, engaging them in working toward joint goals, establishing partnerships from the outset of the system development process, and creating an array of services and supports that meet the unique needs of youth in other systems. To the extent that systems of care address the goals and meet the needs of youth in other systems, these partnerships will ultimately provide resources to sustain services after the federal grant period. Systems of care should learn how to present information to partner agencies, how to work toward the establishment of shared goals, and how to engage them effectively in building and sustaining systems of care. Several respondents commented that it is important for the system of care not to supplant what other systems are supposed to do. Instead, partnerships should be designed to enhance the services that all partner agencies are providing and share costs to achieve shared goals. One respondent counseled that agreements with partner agencies should specify that each assumes the cost for system of care services in annually increasing increments.

Involve and Strengthen Family Advocates and Family Organizations

Respondents at both community and state levels underscored the importance of targeted and ongoing activities to support the development of strong family organizations and family advocates and to involve them in system of care activities. The power of family organizations to advocate for sustaining systems of care and services is substantial, and this resource remains untapped in many states and communities. The capacity for family advocacy should be a focus of system of care communities from the earliest stages of their system-building work, not only to ensure that systems of care are family driven and responsive to their needs, but to cultivate a powerful advocacy constituency. Respondents commented that it is important to involve many family members and to create a sustainable structure for family advocacy rather than to rely on a few individuals for family input and involvement in system of care activities. Underlying the development of a strong family advocacy voice is the premise that systems of care must be driven by the needs of families and youth and that they value the services and supports provided through such systems; evaluation activities should be directed at assessing families' experiences with systems of care and services to ensure that their needs are being met, that they are achieving their desired outcomes, and that they have a positive view of their service experience.

Use Outcome Data and Personal Stories to Advocate Sustaining Systems of Care

Positive, understandable data demonstrating the outcomes of systems of care and their component services are essential tools for making the case to policy makers and system administrators across agencies for sustaining systems of care. According to respondents, the most powerful arguments for sustainability comprise both outcome data and the personal experiences and stories of families and youth who have benefited from systems of care. Thus, data collection to track service delivery and outcomes, which allows systems of care to clearly demonstrate results, should be a high-priority activity. At the same time, it was noted that systems of care take time to mature, and thus sufficient implementation time should be allowed prior to evaluating results. One respondent noted that valuable outcome data were not generated until the third year of system development activity, when data demonstrated positive outcomes such as improved school performance, reduced substance abuse, and reduced involvement with the juvenile justice system. The need for systematic efforts to improve the quality of services based on evaluation results was also noted as an important lesson learned.

Conceptualize Grants as Part of a Larger State Strategy for System of Care Development
Interviewees from both the community and state levels noted that CMHS Program grants should not be viewed as isolated projects in particular communities, but instead as components of a larger strategy for statewide system of care development and maintenance. Funded system of care communities can be used as pilot programs, models, learning labs to test approaches, and technical assistance and training resources to export approaches to other communities in support of an overall plan to implement and maintain systems of care on a larger scale. Both communities and states should identify and capitalize on opportunities to incorporate the system of care philosophy and approach into state plans, policies, regulations, financing streams, and other structures and processes, as well as to utilize federally funded system of care communities in ways that support the broader application of this approach. According to respondents, the sustainability of a system of care hinges on whether it becomes part of a long-term vision for the state and community.

Refinance System of Care Grants from the Outset with Multiple Funding Streams
Respondents suggested that federal funds might be considered *bridge funds* for system development and the development of service capacity and that states and communities maintain the perspective that grant funding is temporary. Due to the short-term nature of such funding, it was suggested that a plan for long-term financing should be part of the process of implementing any service within the array that is created or initially supported with federal funds. Failure to develop a sustainable financing stream for services at the earliest stages of development will result in an array of services that cannot be continued after federal funding is phased out, as well as the demand for services and supports among families and youth that can no longer be met. A thorough understanding of the financing streams in the state and community are essential to the creation of a strategic financing plan to support services over time based on the use of funding streams that are not time limited. Some respondents asserted that no service or support should be initiated without a concrete plan and approach for its

maintenance postgrant. Furthermore, respondents advised that multiple funding streams be used in a coordinated (i.e., *braided*) fashion to finance services and supports to maximize the likelihood of financial support for services postgrant.

Collaborate with the State Medicaid Agency More than any other financing stream, Medicaid has provided the means to sustain system of care services over the long term. Respondents emphasized the importance of establishing and maintaining a collaborative relationship with the state Medicaid agency to implement the changes needed to ensure coverage for the array of services and supports provided through systems of care. Demonstrating the cost-effectiveness of these approaches to state Medicaid agencies will help to establish a firm basis for covering these services and supports, and thus ideally create a viable financing stream for sustaining them.

Cultivate Leaders and Champions to Carry the Mantle over Time From the start of system of care development activities, attention should be devoted to developing and cultivating a cadre of leaders and champions who will be able to continue to provide leadership, advocacy, and support for systems of care beyond the grant period. Although some grant-funded positions might not be continued postgrant, the systematic development of leaders is an investment in the long-term maintenance of the approaches and services implemented during the grant period.

Incorporate Key Elements of Systems of Care into Contracts with Providers Respondents suggested that incorporating key system of care elements into contracts with provider agencies provides a mechanism to ensure both their implementation and maintenance over time. Elements such as using child and family teams for individualized service planning, care coordination across agencies, family and youth involvement, cultural competence, and others can be required of providers through the contracting mechanism.

Implement Mechanisms to Pay Providers for Interagency Coordination and Individualized Service Planning Processes Individualized services planning processes (the wraparound process) and coordination of service delivery across child-serving agencies are key elements of systems of care. Respondents noted that mechanisms to reimburse providers for the time spent in these activities are often not in place, and providers struggle to participate in these processes in the context of pressure for billable hours. The implementation of long-term financing mechanisms for individualized care and interagency coordination is critical to sustainability.

Use Effective Social Marketing Approaches to Disseminate Information and Garner Support for Systems of Care According to respondents, social marketing approaches are needed to effectively disseminate the system of care philosophy and approaches, as well as to generate support for their continuation among a wide range of stakeholders and constituencies. One respondent noted the need for both strength and passion in educating key stakeholders and the general public about children with mental health treatment needs and about the system of care philosophy and approach. Visibility and understanding of children's mental health issues in the community at large are necessary to generate support for services and for generating the commitment and resources for sustaining systems of care.

Use the First Year of Federal Grants for Implementation and Sustainability Planning   According to multiple respondents, the first year of federal system of care grants should be used for strategic planning. Planning should encompass not only what will be accomplished during the grant period, but also how system of care elements will be sustained after federal funding is terminated. Systematic strategies detailing how grant-funded activities and services will be maintained over time should be developed at the beginning of the grant period, and no activity should be undertaken without early attention to how it will be sustained.

Use Multiple Strategies for Sustainability   The importance of using multiple sustainability strategies was noted by respondents. It is likely that a range of strategies is needed to maximize the likelihood that systems of care will be sustained over time and will continue to evolve and improve.

Provide Extensive Training on Systems of Care and Service Delivery   The importance of training on the system of care philosophy and on specific service delivery approaches was highlighted by many respondents. Training was seen as a critical vehicle for achieving commitment to this approach among system leaders and providers across agencies and for building expertise in its implementation.

Adapt to Changing Circumstances   The need to adapt state and community goals to changing circumstances was noted by a number of respondents. Political or economic changes may require a shift in goals or priorities, or may offer opportunities to achieve progress in particular aspects of system development. As this vision is kept constant, adaptation consistent with environmental changes and with new information that emerges from evaluation results and accumulating experience is critical for maintaining and evolving systems of care over time.

Learn from the Experience of Graduated System of Care Communities   Respondents from numerous sites proposed that the lessons regarding sustainability in communities funded early in the history of the CMHS Program be used systematically to assist more recently funded communities. Technical assistance documents, training programs, and consultants from graduated sites were suggested for this purpose.

Unique Challenges for Sustainability

The communities reporting unique challenges related to maintaining their systems of care over time were most frequently those sites serving racially and ethnically diverse populations. For example, respondents from several sites noted that their target populations comprised Spanish-speaking children and families. The services provided during the grant period resulted in increased demand for Spanish-speaking providers and culturally appropriate service delivery modalities. In the context of diminishing resources, it has been particularly challenging to recruit and retain a sufficient number of Spanish-speaking providers to meet this demand, as well as to maintain an array of culturally competent services and supports. Challenges are also presented by the high degree of stigma associated with mental health services among Latino and Hispanic families.

The most significant challenges for sustaining systems of care were noted among respondents for tribal communities. The complications that arise when attempting to coordinate across multiple jurisdictions (e.g., multiple states, tribal governments, the Indian Health Service) are complex and difficult to navigate. Respondents asserted that systems of care in tribal communities may differ significantly from other systems of care in that they must fit within the reality of the multiple jurisdictions and bureaucracies that affect them. Strong leadership, political and policy support, and skilled diplomacy were highlighted as factors critical to achieving and sustaining system change in tribal environments.

In addition, system of care development in tribal communities occurs in the context of historical trauma and a non-Western view of mental heath problems and treatment. Thus, application of the system of care approach must be adapted to consider the conceptualization of illness and traditional healing approaches found in Native American communities. The application of the system of care approach without such cultural adaptations has resulted in an inability to sustain the services and supports after federal funding is terminated.

CONCLUSION

As noted, the study on sustainability was undertaken to provide information that will assist states and communities to enhance the maintenance of their systems of care and component services over time. In this context, the results are most useful when they are interpreted as focusing attention on those areas that may be at risk for not being fully sustained over time. Ideally, these results will serve as an alert to systems of care that specific attention and strategies should be targeted to ensure that these elements of systems of care do not lose ground with the loss of federal funds and accompanying mandates. The study provides valuable lessons learned, strategies to avoid some of the pitfalls, and methods for addressing some of the challenges experienced by the communities included in this study sample. Targeted attention to these areas should be directed toward avoiding some of these difficulties in maintaining progress. Table 8.9 shows some of the potential challenges in sustaining systems of care and the strategies suggested by the study that could be used to address them.

Table 8.9. Sustainability challenges and effective strategies

Challenges to sustainability	Effective strategies
Sustaining supportive services	Cultivating interagency partnerships to develop strategies and proposals to braid or pool funds, and for partner agencies to purchase specific services or packages of services through case rates
	Increasing the ability to obtain Medicaid reimbursement by amending the state Medicaid plan to add new service definitions and billing codes; implementing behavioral health carve outs with capitated or case rates; expanding the rehabilitation option; obtaining waivers; or using the Early Periodic Screening, Diagnosis, and Treatment (EPSDT) Program
	Obtaining new or increased state funds to obtain legislative appropriations for treatment and supportive services not covered by any other source; providing outcome data and a rationale for such appropriations (e.g., diverting children from out-of-home placements)
	Enlisting a strong family organization to advocate for the need to maintain supportive services and the important role these services play in their lives to local and state government agencies, state legislatures, state Medicaid agencies, and others
	Using evaluation results and outcome data to document the effectiveness of an individualized approach to care that involves treatment interventions as well as supportive services
Sustaining philosophical elements (e.g., individualized care, interagency coordination at the system level, interagency coordination at the service delivery level, family involvement at the system level)	Cultivating leaders committed to the philosophy among policy makers, provider agencies, families, and youth such that changes in leadership will not impede sustainability; integrally involving key stakeholders in policy and governing bodies; providing outcome data documenting positive results; and using social marketing approaches to generate support and commitment
	Incorporating requirements for individualized care, interagency coordination, and family involvement into state and local policy including legislation, state plans, regulations, licensing requirements, contracts, managed care systems, monitoring protocols, financing streams, and other policies; establishing the philosophy as a fundamental expectation of the system and endemic to the way the system operates as dictated by policy
	Providing ongoing training to strengthen the commitment to the philosophy and approach and to infuse these philosophical elements into the larger service system, for example, creating training structures such as a wraparound training academy that offers regularly scheduled training on individualized service planning and delivery
	Creating mechanisms for provider reimbursement for individualized service planning and delivery and for interagency service coordination by working in partnership with state mental health, state Medicaid, and other child-serving agencies to create mechanism to reimburse providers for time spent in child and family team meetings for individualized service planning and delivery and cross-agency care coordination

Challenges to sustainability	Effective strategies
	Continuing an emphasis on and activities geared toward these elements, including continuing to operate interagency collaboration entities after the termination of federal grant funds; working with state and local mental health and partner agencies to ensure continued support for a family organization over time; continuing to involve families at the system level in policy making, planning, system oversight, evaluation, and other activities; continuing to support cultural competence staff and committees; continuing to maintain these principles and others as priorities, even in the absence of federal funds and mandates
Sustaining the achievement of goals, including infrastructure goals of service capacity, evaluation capacity, a focal point for system management, and an active family organization	**Overall goal achievement** Cultivating commitment to system of care goals and philosophy by providing ongoing training in the philosophy for continued exposure and reinforcement and to reach new staff and leaders as a result of staff turnover; providing positive outcome data and family experience; creating effective social marketing approaches; cultivating commitment among policy makers and system leaders; developing leaders beyond grant-funded staff; infusing goals into the broader children's mental health system such that they become part of the culture Incorporating infrastructure elements of state and local policy, plans, regulations, legislation, and other policy instruments **Ensuring that services in the service array have sufficient capacity** Cultivating strong interagency partnerships by establishing joint goals, meeting the service needs of youth involved in other systems, and developing financing strategies involving funds from partner agencies to finance services (e.g., by purchasing services, braiding funds, pooling funds) Increasing the ability to obtain Medicaid reimbursement by amending the state Medicaid plan to add new service definitions and billing codes; implementing a behavioral health carve out with capitated or case rates, expanding the rehabilitation option, obtaining waivers, or using the EPSDT Program Obtaining new or increased state funds by obtaining legislative appropriations for services not covered by any other source, and providing outcome data and a rationale for such appropriations (e.g., diverting children from out-of-home placements) Considering grant funds as bridge funds with the expectation that they are start-up funds to develop service capacity and ensuring that new services are implemented in conjunction with a long-term financing strategy

(continued)

Table 8.9. *(continued)*

Challenges to sustainability	Effective strategies
	Redeploying funds across child-serving systems from high-cost inpatient and residential placements to lower cost home and community-based service approaches
	Expanding provider networks to increase the range of providers and provider agencies with the capacity and skills to provide the broad array of services offered by systems of care
	Providing ongoing training to providers on evidence-based/promising practices to strengthen the skills, expertise, and capacity of providers to offer evidence-based and promising services and supports through systems of care (e.g., creating training structures that offer regularly scheduled training on evidence-based and promising interventions)

Using evaluation data to inform policy and program decisions

Continuing evaluation capacity within system infrastructure when federal funding is terminated because data can be used as a highly effective tool to demonstrate outcomes and advocate continued funding

Cultivating strong interagency relationships with buy-in from partner agencies to continue evaluation activities by providing policy-relevant, useful information regarding outcomes of all partner agencies; developing strategies for joint financial support for data collection, interpretation, and dissemination

Maintaining a focal point for the system of care

Creating a sustainable focal point for system management by building on the existing system infrastructure rather than creating something separate, enabling this focal point to become ingrained in the system; integrally involving high-level system administrators and leaders so that they can carry the mantle postgrant and continue the commitment to achieving system of care goals; continuing the interagency entity and continuing to provide staff support for its operation

Incorporating a focal point of responsibility for systems of care in state policy, plans, regulations, legislation, and other policy instruments

Supporting and maintaining an active family organization

Continuing financial support for the family organization through direct appropriations from mental health or other agencies, grants, contracts that purchase specific services from family organizations (e.g., family advocates, parent training, family support, representation on policy making bodies, participation in evaluation activities)

Challenges to sustainability	Effective strategies
Changes in larger economic climate	Using economic crises strategically as opportunities to offer more cost-effective service delivery approaches (e.g., creating interagency partnerships, offering cost-effective approaches) documented with positive outcome data and family stories; in difficult economic times, agencies may be receptive to purchasing care viewed as more cost-effective than the more expensive, often residential, services that they have been providing.
Changes in elected/ appointed officials	Involving new elected and appointed officials in system of care policy and activities; informing and educating new officials through targeted social marketing approaches to generate their involvement and support; using outcome data coupled with family stories to provide a basis for new officials to support the system of care approach; and developing new leaders for systems of care among new officials

Source: Stroul (2006).
Key: EPSDT, Early Periodic Screening, Diagnosis, and Treatment Program.

Caution is recommended, however, to avoid focusing on these areas to the exclusion of other areas in which communities in the study sample experienced greater success in sustaining progress postgrant. Instead, it is imperative that communities, in close collaboration with state agencies, develop a strategic plan for sustaining systems of care that encompass all of the essential elements, that is based on multiple sustainability strategies, and that is systematically implemented from the earliest phases of system of care implementation.

A strategic planning framework is suggested by the study results, including systematic attention to those strategies that emerged from the web survey and telephone interviews as being most effective. This is the first guidance for sustainability planning that is based on research evidence derived from the experience of communities (Table 8.10).

It is important to note that this study was conducted on Phase I and Phase II sites, the first communities funded through the federal system of care initiative. As the federal program has evolved, so too have efforts to increase sustainability, and it will be an interesting empirical question as to whether there are differences in experience for more recent sites. Early sites were essentially expected to sustain their efforts because "it was the right thing to do," and limited attention was initially paid to the topic. Over time, however, as these lessons were learned, more attention has been focused on strategies for sustainability. For example, since financing was identified as one of the most significant obstacles to maintaining services, especially those considered more supportive than medical, CMHS commis-

Table 8.10.   Strategic framework for sustainability planning

Sustainability Strategies

1. Ongoing Locus of Accountability
   - Create a viable, ongoing focal point for system management

2. Family Organization and Advocacy Base
   - Establish a strong family organization
   - Create an effective advocacy base

3. Evaluation/Accountability Data
   - Use evaluation/accountability results to "make the case" for sustaining the system and care and services

4. Interagency Partnerships
   - Cultivate strong interagency relationships and partnerships for service delivery and coordination
   - Cultivate strong interagency partnerships for ongoing financing of services

5. Infusion of System of Care Approach into Larger System
   - Make state-level and local-level policy and regulatory changes that support the system of care approach
   - Make the system of care philosophy and approach the way the community's larger service system operates

6. Training
   - Provide ongoing training and coaching regarding system of care philosophy and approach
   - Provide ongoing training and coaching regarding effective services (evidence-based and promising interventions)

7. Commitment and Support for System of Care Approach
   - Generate political and policy level support for the system of care approach
   - Generate state involvement and commitment
   - Generate local involvement and commitment
   - Cultivate ongoing leaders and champions for system of care philosophy and approach

Financing Strategies for Sustainability

1. Medicaid
   - Increase ability to obtain Medicaid reimbursement for services

2. State Mental Health Funds
   - Obtain new or increased state mental health funds

3. Other Child Service Systems Funds
   - Obtain new or increased funds from other child-serving agencies
   - Coordinate, blend, or braid funds with other child-serving agencies

4. Redeployed Funds
   - Redeploy/shift funds from higher to lower cost services

5. Local Funds
   - Obtain new or increased local funds (e.g., taxing authorities)

From Stroul, B., & Manteuffel, B. (2007). The sustainability of systems of care for children's mental health: Lessons learned. *Journal of Behavioral Health Services and Research, 34*(3), 237–259; reprinted with kind permission from Springer Science and Business Media.

sioned the development of the Match Guide to Sustainability (Bazelon Center for Mental Health Law, 2004). This document identifies strategies that communities can use to meet their financial match requirements and ways that these activities can be sustained.

More recently, CMHS has emphasized sustainability from the very early stages of federal funding for systems of care. In fact, the development and identification of sustainability mechanisms has become part of the Request for Application (RFA) process. Furthermore, to jump start community planning and long-range thinking, CMHS supports a technical assistance start-up visit to each newly funded community. These visits, which occur within the first 6 months of program operation, are specifically designed to assist communities in thinking strategically about the development and sustainability of the system of care philosophy, including family-driven, youth-guided care and cultural and linguistic competency, and in thinking strategically about the financing and sustainability of services. Beyond these enhancements, for sites funded in fiscal years 2005 and 2006, and in the RFA issued in fiscal year 2008, there are increased requirements to connect the funded system of care to broader state systems (e.g., mental health, child welfare, juvenile justice, education) and to other activities in the state that are working to reform and transform mental health service delivery. Such thinking and planning must be a focus within any reform effort, particularly as budgets and organizational capacities continue to experience significant challenges.

Involvement of key state and local stakeholders in sustainability planning from the earliest phases of system of care development offers an opportunity for strategic thinking about the ways in which system of care elements will be maintained over time. This type of strategic approach is applicable to communities and their state partners regardless of whether they have received federal funding for systems of care.

REFERENCES

Ager, A. (1990). The importance of sustainability in the design of culturally appropriate programmes of early intervention. *International Disability Studies, 12*(2), 89–92.

Bazelon Center for Mental Health Law. (2004). *Matching for sustainability: A guide for communities sponsoring systems of care for children with serious mental disorders and their families.* Washington, DC: Bazelon Center for Mental Health Law.

Center for Mental Health Services. (2001). *Annual report to Congress on the Evaluation of the Comprehensive Community Mental Health Services for Children and Their Families Program.* Atlanta, GA: ORC Macro.

Center for Mental Health Services. (2004). *Sustainability Assessment Toolkit.* Rockville, MD: Author.

Holder, H.D., & Moore, R.S. (2000). Institutionalization of community action projects to reduce alcohol use related problems: Systematic facilitators. *Substance Use and Misuse, 35*(1–2), 75–86.

Johnson, K., Hays, C., Center, H., & Daley. (2004). Building capacity and sustainable prevention innovations: A sustainability planning model. *Evaluation and Program Planning, 27*, 135–149.

Koyanagi, C., & Feres-Merchant, D. (2000). *Systems of care: Promising practices in children's mental health. For the long haul: Maintaining systems of care beyond the federal investment* (2000 Series, Vol. III). Washington, DC: American Institutes for Research, Center for Effective Collaboration and Practice.

President's New Freedom Commission on Mental Health. (2003). *Achieving the promise: Transforming mental health care in America. Final report* (DHHS Pub No. SMA-03-3832). Rockville, MD: Author.

Stroul, B. (2002). *Issue brief. Systems of care: A framework for system reform in children's mental health.* Washington, DC: Georgetown University Center for Child and Human Development, National Technical Assistance Center for Children's Mental Health.

Stroul, B. (2004, January). *Sustainability of systems of care: What have we learned?* Keynote presentation at System of Care Community Meeting of the Technical Assistance Partnership for Child and Family Mental Health, San Antonio, TX.

Stroul, B. (2006). *The sustainability of systems of care: Lessons learned. A report on the special study on the sustainability of systems of care.* Atlanta, GA: Macro International.

Stroul, B.A., & Friedman, R.M. (1986). *A system of care for seriously emotionally disturbed children and youth* (Rev. ed.). Washington, DC: Georgetown University Center for Child and Human Development.

Stroul, B.A., & Friedman, R.M. (1996). The system of care concept and philosophy. In B.A. Stroul & R.M. Friedman (Series Eds.) & B.A. Stroul (Vol. Ed.), *Systems of care for children's mental health series: Children's mental health: Creating systems of care in a changing society* (pp. 3–21). Baltimore: Paul H. Brookes Publishing Co.

Stroul, B., & Manteuffel, B. (2007). The sustainability of systems of care for children's mental health: Lessons learned. *Journal of Behavioral Health Services and Research, 34*(3), 237–259.

Substance Abuse and Mental Health Services Administration. (2005). *Transforming mental health care in America. Federal action agenda: First steps* (DHHS Pub. No. SMA-05-4060). Rockville, MD: Author.

U.S. Department of Health and Human Services. (2002). *Cooperative Agreements for the Comprehensive Community Mental Health Services for Children and their Families Program* (No. SM-02-002). Rockville, MD: Center for Mental Health Services, Substance Abuse and Mental Health Services Administration.

III

Recommended Practice Examples

The System Level

9

Partnerships with Families for Family-Driven Systems of Care

Trina W. Osher, Marlene Penn, and Sandra A. Spencer

Partnerships are a core element of systems of care. This chapter focuses on building and strengthening partnerships with families. It reviews the history of the family movement and the evolution of family involvement and family organizations in systems of care. It draws heavily on examples from systems of care to describe lessons learned about family involvement identifying the key pitfalls and offering safety net strategies to avoid them. The chapter closes with a case study of the development of family partnerships in New Jersey.

MOVEMENT TOWARD
FAMILY-DRIVEN CARE IN SYSTEMS OF CARE

The first core principle of systems of care, as originally articulated in 1986, was that they should be *child centered* and *family focused,* with the needs of the child and family dictating the types of services providers would offer. In addition, a guiding principle for systems of care declared that families of children with emotional disturbances should be full participants in all aspects of the planning and delivery of services, as well as in the making of system policy (Stroul & Friedman, 1986). The commitment to change practice from provider-driven to family-driven service delivery systems, however, was neither explicitly nor fully addressed in many of the early materials describing approaches to building systems of care (Osher & Osher, 2002). The development of a vigorous family movement in children's mental health, along with the more widespread use of wraparound approaches for service planning in the 1990s, have stimulated shifts in systems of care, service delivery, and agency culture toward the philosophy of family-driven care.

Being a parent raising a child with an emotional, behavioral, or mental health challenge is a full-time job without pay, vacations, or nights or weekends off. In spite of the stress and strain in their lives, individual families have persistently tried to be involved in their children's mental health care. The family movement, led by the national Federation of Families for Children's Mental Health, has capitalized on the resilience and creativity of families and their determination to obtain effective help for their children. In its brief 18-year existence, the federation has focused on strengthening *family voice* by supporting, training, and especially nurturing family-run organizations. The federation has become the center of a national network that links family-run organizations and families with each other, as well as with policy makers in every state and the U.S. capital. Using their collective voice, families have advocated for family-driven services and systems and influenced the policies and practices that govern systems of care.

Defining Family-Driven Care

With the growth and increasing influence of family-run organizations around the country, there has been an evolution in how systems of care are expected to involve families in their program design, implementation, and evaluation. Although the vision was previously espoused by family advocates, the term *family-driven* care was catapulted into widespread public use in 2003 by the President's New Freedom Commission on Mental Health, which called for "consumer- and family-driven care." Moving beyond the original values and principles of systems of care, commissioners insisted that families "must stand at the center of the system of care" and that the needs of children, youth, and families must "drive the care and services that are provided" (President's New Freedom Commission, 2003, p. 35). The commission, however, did not further define the term.

> "After working out the route with the family driver, the provider can hold the map and act as a guide and support. The provider certainly may help make the trip a safe and satisfying one." (Tannen, 1996)

In partnership with the federal Center for Mental Health Services (CMHS) of the Substance Abuse and Mental Health Administration (SAMHSA), the Federation of Families for Children's Mental Health initiated a 2-year inclusive developmental process to define this concept. The process culminated in the issuance of a working definition of the term *family-driven care*, along with a set of guiding principles and characteristics (Box 9.1). This definition provides a map for building and strengthening partnerships between family-run organizations and systems of care, as well as for transforming the relationship between families and providers.

> Providing family-driven care requires a major change in how people think and act. There must be administrative support to change behaviors and relationships. Developing, promoting, and supporting a commonly accepted definition of family-driven care is a necessary step in helping people change how they think and act. (Blau, Osher, & Osher, 2005, p. 3)

Role of Family Organizations

Family-run organizations have served as a highly effective vehicle for creating family partnerships in systems of care and for moving systems of care to adopt a

Box 9.1 Working definition of family-driven care

DEFINITION

The term *family-driven care* means families have a primary decision making role in the care of their own children as well as the policies and procedures governing care for all children in their community, state, tribe, territory and nation. This includes:

1. Choosing supports, services, and providers

2. Setting goals

3. Designing and implementing programs

4. Monitoring outcomes

5. Partnering in funding decisions

6. Determining the effectiveness of all efforts to promote the mental health and well being of children and youth

GUIDING PRINCIPLES OF FAMILY-DRIVEN CARE

1. Families and youth are given accurate, understandable, and complete information necessary to set goals and to make choices for improved planning for individual children and their families.

2. Families and youth, providers and administrators embrace the concept of sharing decision-making and responsibility for outcomes with providers.

3. Families and youth are organized to collectively use their knowledge and skills as a force for system transformation.

4. Families and family-run organizations engage in peer support activities to reduce isolation, gather and disseminate accurate information, and strengthen the family voice.

5. Families and family-run organizations provide direction for decisions that impact funding for services, treatments, and supports.

6. Providers take the initiative to change practice from provider driven to family driven.

7. Administrators allocate staff, training, support, and resources to make family-driven practice work at the point where services and supports are delivered to children, youth, and families.

8. Community attitude change efforts focus on removing barriers and discrimination created by stigma.

9. Communities embrace, value, and celebrate the diverse cultures of their children, youth, and families.

10. Everyone who connects with children, youth, and families continually advances their own cultural and linguistic responsiveness as the population served changes.

(continued)

Box 9.1 *(continued)*

CHARACTERISTICS OF FAMILY-DRIVEN CARE

1. Family and youth experiences, their visions and goals, their perceptions of strengths and needs, and their guidance about what will make them comfortable steer decision making about all aspects of service and system design, operation, and evaluation.

2. Family-run organizations receive resources and funds to support and sustain the infrastructure that is essential to insure an independent family voice in their communities, states, tribes, territories, and the nation.

3. Meetings and service provision happen in culturally and linguistically competent environments where family and youth voices are heard and valued, everyone is respected and trusted, and it is safe for everyone to speak honestly.

4. Administrators and staff actively demonstrate their partnerships with all families and youth by sharing power, resources, authority, responsibility, and control with them.

5. Families and youth have access to useful, usable, and understandable information and data, as well as sound professional expertise so they have good information to make decisions.

6. Funding mechanisms allow families and youth to have choices.

7. All children, youth, and families have a biological, adoptive, foster, or surrogate family voice advocating on their behalf.

Adapted from the Federation of Families for Children's Mental Health web site, http://www.ffcmh.org/systems_whatis.htm

---

family-driven approach. Few of these organizations existed prior to the 1980s, when a national family movement began to evolve (Bryant-Comstock, Huff, & VanDenBerg, 1996). In 1986, the first Families As Allies Conference was held with the sponsorship of the federal Child and Adolescent Service System Program (CASSP). This conference convened leaders of family-run organizations and family advocates, and ultimately resulted in the formation of the Federation of Families for Children's Mental Health. Most of these early family organizations had informal beginnings, consisting of a few families that had banded together for mutual support. Formal organizations began to coalesce when the group discovered a common cause or became involved in responding to a specific community crisis or issue related to mental health service delivery. At the beginning, they worked passionately on system change, rarely planning for the future of their organization. Because of their focus on system change and their informal, volunteer, and grassroots origins, emerging family-run organizations found it challenging to develop a sustainable organizational infrastructure.

In 1988, CASSP funds were used to provide grants to support the development of five statewide family networks. By 2007, the federal CMHS was funding 42 statewide family networks and a national technical assistance center to provide training, technical assistance, networking, and data collection. Thus, in addition to a strong national family organization focusing on children's mental health, statewide family organizations are now active in most states advocating for improved systems of care and services.

In addition, the federal Comprehensive Community Mental Health Services for Children and Their Families Program, generally known as the federal system of care program, has gradually increased its requirements for active family involvement in systems of care, which include the establishment of a partnership with a local family organization. Starting in 1993, communities that received funds to build systems of care began to actively seek out family members to help them implement these requirements. A new crop of family-run organizations emerged, largely supported with funds from system of care grantees, resulting in increasing numbers of local family organizations focusing on systems of care for children and youth with mental health needs.

When they are full partners in systems of care, family-run organizations make critical contributions, particularly with respect to advocacy. *Advocacy* is defined as "active support, as of a cause, idea or policy" (American Heritage Dictionary, 1957); all family-run organizations engage in some type of advocacy. In a family-driven system of care, advocacy focused on individual children, youth, or families is realized when families have the primary role in making decisions about services and supports for their children and share responsibility with providers for the implementation of their service plans and the realization of anticipated outcomes. Families seeking services for their children find family-run organizations to be reliable and trusted sources of information about how systems of care work, safe places for finding their own advocacy voices, and environments where they can develop the skills they need to drive the system. Family-run organizations and systems of care have increasingly employed family partners to help individual family members navigate the system of care and the wraparound process.

Advocacy also is focused on systems and aims to achieve broader goals such as a better quality of life for children with mental health needs. Family-run organizations play critical roles by bringing advocacy issues to the forefront, working in coalitions with other groups to frame issues and possible policy solutions, and supporting family members as they engage in advocacy activities. Family-run organizations have been instrumental in both national and state policy initiatives that create systems of care and sustain support for them. The advocacy efforts of independent family-run organizations can also be critically important in bringing attention to gaps and flaws in services and systems that are ineffective or inadequate.

In some cases, advocacy on the part of family-run organizations has resulted in active opposition from others. When powerful entities have insisted on the termination or resignation of specific family leaders or staff, or threatened to withdraw funding, family-run organizations have had to decide whether they should compromise their values, mission, or principles to maintain the good will and financial support from these external sources. When family-run organizations have diverse funding streams, are guided by their vision and mission, and have sound infrastructures and strong boards, they are more likely to be successful in withstanding this kind of outside pressure.

"Diversified funding is the key to independence."
—Jane Adams, Executive Director Keys for Networking,
  Topeka, Kansas (August 1999)

Despite the essential role of family organizations in systems of care, funding remains a significant challenge. Family-run organizations, like recent college graduates, must build a portfolio detailing their experience to establish themselves in the marketplace of human services. The crucial task of continually raising funds is exhausting and time consuming. It diverts energy and resources from the support and advocacy work that is the mission of most family-run organizations.

As family-run organizations mature to the more advanced stages of development, funding sources tend to shift from contributions, membership, sponsorship, and state mental health agency support to fees collected for providing services and government contracts. At some point, every family-run organization faces the temptation to follow the funding by contracting to provide services or engage in activities that are not necessarily congruent with its mission and values. Organizations must protect their missions to keep them from becoming sidetracked by their funding sources. For example, a family-run organization should not hesitate to advocate for the expansion of Medicaid services—even if it receives Medicaid payments for services that the organization provides to families. Family-run organizations typically do three things to avoid conflicts that may arise between the work of providing services and the efforts of advocacy:

1. Keep the functions of service provision and advocacy separate.

2. Maintain a clear audit trail of expenditures for all funding sources.

3. Make a point of providing services that are totally consistent with the organization's mission.

Family-run organizations have diversified their funding bases beyond support from a statewide family network grant or a system of care community by becoming vendors for Medicaid services, contracting as evaluators and trainers, seeking other grant and foundation funds, optimizing community resources, and engaging in mission-focused entrepreneurial ventures.

FAMILY INVOLVEMENT IN SYSTEM OF CARE COMMUNITIES

As noted, the federal system of care program requires funded communities to involve families. These requirements are reviewed below, along with ways in which systems of care approach family involvement and examples of effective strategies for partnerships between family organizations and systems of care.

Requirements for Family Involvement in Systems of Care

Beginning in 1993, and in keeping with the values and principles of systems of care, the federal CMHS has required that the systems of care it funds make a commitment to meaningful family involvement such as collaboration with family-run organizations. The specific requirements have evolved and expanded with each subsequent cycle of grants. Originally, applicants for federal funds were asked to explain: 1) how there would be full involvement and family–professional partnerships in the planning, implementation, management, delivery, and evaluation of the system of care, as well as in the planning and delivery of care for individual children and families; and 2) how they would ensure the existence of and collaboration with local family support organizations or a statewide family network organization that has the potential to rapidly create such an organization in the community served by the system of care.

By 2005, applicants were required to demonstrate the full participation of families and youth in service planning and in the development of local services and supports (Substance Abuse and Mental Health Services Administration, 2005). Applicants were required to articulate the means by which they would adhere to the definition of family-driven care and incorporate its values and principles, as well as provide greater detail on partnerships with families, including describing the following (reprinted from Substance Abuse and Mental Health Services Administration, 2005):

- How family partnerships will occur and will be demonstrated in planning, implementing, and evaluating the project.

- How a local parent support organization will be created or how an existing parent support organization will be included to complement the initiative (such as a statewide family network).

- Identify a full-time equivalent position for a family member to serve as the key family contact with responsibility for advocacy for other family members of children receiving services; outreach to family members of children not receiving services; and serving as one of the family member representatives on the governance body.

- How the project will provide financial support to sustain family involvement in the system of care throughout the duration of the project and beyond the federal funding period.

- How the project will create a strong partnership between professionals and family members that enables family members to participate in the planning, management, and evaluation of the system of care.

- How compensation and fiscal support will be provided for families whose children are eligible for services, as well as the existing family organizations whose focus is on these children and families.

The aim of such support is to enable family members and family organizations to participate in activities related to the development, implementation, and evaluation of systems of care. Support should also be provided for families and family organizations representing the racial or ethnic minority groups in the community.

The lead family member plays a pivotal role in a system of care. Typically, this position is filled by a parent or other family member of a child or adolescent with a serious emotional disturbance who has received or is receiving services from the mental health service system. This lead family contact is responsible for either creating or working with an existing family-run organization that represents the cultural and linguistic background of the target population. Responsibilities include working in partnership with the community in all aspects of developing, implementing, and evaluating the system of care, as well as providing support for families receiving services. This role is critical for systems of care regardless of whether they are recipients of federal grant funding with the accompanying family involvement requirements.

Approach to Family Involvement

Within this framework, systems of care have considerable latitude in determining how these requirements will be fulfilled. Each system of care community determines what human and financial resources will be devoted to accomplishing family involvement goals, taking an approach suited to its own community's mission, values, and needs. Technical assistance on family involvement is provided to federally funded system of care communities through the Federation of Families for Children's Mental Health and the Technical Assistance Partnership for Child and Family Mental Health. Systems of care generally take one of three pathways to involving families:

1. Use what is already there.

A number of systems of care build relationships with and provide financial support to existing local or statewide family-run organizations. They negotiate contracts or other forms of purchase-of-services agreements that clearly delineate the expectations and obligations of the systems of care and the family-run organizations. Channels of communication, authority, supervision, and control are clear and mutually understood.

2. Start from scratch.

When there is no preexisting family-run organization with which to work, some systems of care identify, recruit, and support grassroots family leadership. They hire family members from within the community and provide training and support to build a family-run organization from scratch. The resulting organizations tend to be different from family-run organizations that were independently established in the community prior to the establishment of the system of care in two respects. First, family groups initiated by systems of care must function at a very high level of partnership right from the start, yet they have little time to develop trust and unity inside their own organization or to create a strong infrastructure. Second, the drive for development of an organization is rooted in the needs of the system of care rather than in the needs of the families, who are on a mission of their own. Thus, these family groups appear to have greater difficulty reaching an agreement on their organizational mission, and they often rely heavily on the system of care for direction.

3. Support an emerging effort.

A third option is to contract with another family-run organization, advocacy agency, or a provider (e.g., the mental health association) to build and nurture a new local family-run organization. This model requires that there be a clearly written agreement listing the responsibilities and roles for all involved parties. It is important to provide adequate training and support for the new family leaders. In this approach, it is clear from the beginning that independence for the family-run organization is the ultimate goal. The sponsor embraces this goal by encouraging and supporting the new family-run organization's ability to take charge of its own affairs as quickly as possible.

Partnerships Between Family-Run Organizations and Systems of Care: What Works

Building family-run organizations has not been the primary focus of the federal system of care program, but it has been an important result. System of care communities have supported the development of family-run organizations and have fostered strong partnerships with them in many ways. These strategies have included building relationships, mentoring new leadership and organizations, encouraging autonomy in decision making, communicating over long distances, sharing power, providing in-kind services, and colocation of office space and activities.

Building Relationships Strong and viable family organizations are more likely to be established when the family group has a history of relationships with policy makers and providers in the community. Rhode Island's Parent Support Network had been in existence as a statewide organization for approximately 10 years before partnering with Rhode Island's system of care, REACH. Independent and nonprofit at the time that federal system of care funding was awarded, the organization had already been providing family supports, information, referral, and advocacy. The Rhode Island Parent Support Network was ready and able to work collaboratively with the recipient of the grant and the state mental health authority. The statewide nature of the family-run organization was especially appropriate because the system of care in Rhode Island was implemented in all eight regions of the state. Even with these advantages, it was critical to take the time—much more time than anyone anticipated—to work through the process of building sustainable relationships.

> "It took 2 years to develop trust and a shared vision, to work through our differences and gain respect for each other's roles."
> —Kathy Nicodemus, Former Children's Mental Health Director
> for Rhode Island (1998, as cited in Osher & Bestgen, 2005)

Family-run organizations without the lengthy history enjoyed by the Rhode Island Parent Support Network have been creative in building relationships with their system of care community partners. Recognizing conflict as a natural part of any relationship, the Burlington County System of Care, along with its local Family Support Organization, instituted formal and spontaneous fix-it meetings to address potential or real conflicts up front in a respectful manner. The family organization had full input in planning the agenda and shared responsibility for its facilitation. Although these meetings were held more frequently in the beginning of the relationship, they continued to be a viable tool for resolving conflict and building partnerships. Subsequently, other New Jersey Family Support Organizations and their local professional partners engaged in similar strategy sessions.

Mentoring   Anticipating that newly recruited family members may lack administrative experience, system of care leaders have sometimes been reluctant to give them sufficient authority to make decisions and manage even modest budgets. The supervision of family members by system of care personnel should be skillfully managed. The goal should be to guide, mentor, and support rather than direct and control. The relationships and feelings of all parties in this kind of arrangement are intense and complex, and the power at the core of it all must be handled with diplomacy, grace, and respect. System of care leaders have had years of experience developing relationships where power is concerned. When their own behavior toward families models the kinds of behavior and performance they expect from families, families have learned ways to harness their passion and become constructive, collaborative, and assertive partners.

Autonomy   Systems of care have sought family members to serve on an assortment of governing bodies, committees, and workgroups to participate in policy and decision making. However, when the same few individuals are called on to simultaneously serve on governance bodies, organize family activities, and develop new family organizations, no task gets the attention it needs to be accomplished well. These are all demanding jobs, and they each require different skills. Family expertise is more efficiently used when family member skills and interests are matched to specific tasks or roles. This means recruiting, training, and supporting a substantial number and a diverse group of family members. Giving family members a forum of their own and recognizing that they have the right to decide for and amongst themselves how these roles and resources should be distributed, demonstrates trust and confidence on the part of system of care leaders. It also encourages the family group to develop the unity and identity needed to start a viable family-run organization and to take responsibility for making decisions.

Geographic Proximity   Sponsorship of start-up family-run organizations, whether by local or state mental health associations, service providers, the lead agency for a system of care, or another family-run organization, tends to work better when sponsors are in close proximity to the organizations. Being nearby enables mentoring through daily interaction and facilitates familiarity with and acceptance by local stakeholders.

"Local people need to be responsible for local survival."
—Tevina Benedict, Former Director of Oregon Family
Support Network, Lane County, Oregon (1999)

Statewide family-run organizations, especially those that sit at the center of a network of local chapters, have developed strategies for overcoming the challenges of social, economic, cultural, and linguistic diversity, as well as those imposed by geography. With careful planning, a statewide family-run organization located far from system of care communities can successfully support the development of new local organizations. The best results are achieved when the individuals hired to do this organizational work have roots in the local community. Families Together in New York State has staff housed in local communities throughout the state. Technology (e.g., conference calls, web-based training, telecommuting) facilitates the process of supervising staff in remote locations and keeping in close touch with emerging family groups that are far away.

Sharing Power Perhaps the biggest challenge in any partnership is developing the trust necessary to actually share decision-making power. Partnerships between family-run organizations and systems of care are strongest when all parties attend to the inherent conflict associated with advocating for change, as they depend on the system of care for infrastructure support (e.g., fiscal management, space, training, supervision, fund raising). Family and system of care leaders who can manage and share power and responsibility and apply the principles of family-driven care to guide their decisions and actions become good partners.

"We were constantly fine tuning this delicate and evolving balance. This took time and a lot of energy and a determination to make it work. When we said build the infrastructure, no one knew what that meant. We [the community] had to learn to trust the parent organization."
—Tim Gawron, Former Project Director, Community
Wraparound Initiative, LaGrange, Illinois (1998)

In-Kind Supports and Colocation A number of family-run organizations receive direct benefits from a system of care in the form of in-kind supports (Table 9.1). In addition to their cash value, these supports help strengthen the relationship between family-run organizations and system of care communities in various ways.

For many organizations, simply having a home in the early stages of development is an invaluable asset. Sharing space and resources offers opportunities for mentoring with respect to the administrative responsibilities of running an organization and also helps families gain an insider's perspective about the service sys-

Table 9.1.   Examples of in-kind support for family organizations

Office equipment, office space, supplies, meeting places, telephone, utilities, postage, fax machine, furniture, voice mail, and photocopying

Training in a variety of specialized topic areas

Expenses incurred for trips, food, child care, and stipends for parents and board members to attend local system of care meetings

Support for registration and travel expenses for family members to attend national and regional conferences

Expertise in media presentation, public relations, grant writing, legal matters, and public speaking

tem. It also fosters positive relationships on which sustainable collaborations are built. Reaching for Rainbows in Indiana, G.I.F.T.S. (Guam Identifies Families Terrific Strengths, Inc.) in Guam, and Families United of Milwaukee are just of few of the many examples of family-run organizations that shared space with their system of care at the beginning.

There are, however, challenges associated with colocation related to the issue of dependence versus independence. Eventually, any family-run organization colocated with a system of care must consider whether it should get its own space. Regardless of how this issue is resolved, the process of discussing it raises issues of loyalty or gratitude that threaten shaky relationships and cause anxiety. Agencies and programs that serve as fiscal agents lose control over resources and activities when family-run organizations incorporate, gain a not-for-profit tax status of their own, and move out.

Overdependence on sponsor support leaves family-run organizations vulnerable to changes in its sponsor's status, situation, and commitment. For example, successful family organizations are likely to receive some ongoing funding from their system of care community, but as systems of care graduate from the federal program and lose their federal funds, or if they suffer other funding cuts, the family-run organization is likely to suffer funding cuts as well.

MAJOR LESSONS LEARNED: PITFALLS AND SAFETY NETS

Years of experience across the country have revealed practices that can divert or completely derail otherwise well-intentioned efforts to work with individual families or to develop and nurture partnerships between family-run organizations and systems of care. The following section describes lessons learned about common pitfalls and some safety net strategies for avoiding them.

Partnerships with Individual Family Members

Partnerships start with individuals. Partnering with family members who serve in various capacities is the foundation on which partnerships with family organizations can be built. Strong foundations support sturdy organizational structures and relationships.

Governance

• **The Pitfall**

The system of care approach gives family members a prominent role in governance. In early systems of care, family members served on advisory and governance boards in token roles. System of care administrators often selected one family member to serve on a governance structure or on multiple committees. The lone voice of that family member was often ignored or simply outvoted in the decision-making process. In some systems of care, one family member was unrealistically expected to be the voice of *all* families in that community. The strain of being the token family voice resulted in frustration and burnout. Some early family leaders just dropped out. Others were pushed out, and still others were co-opted and became routine agency employees, thus losing their family voice.

• **The Safety Net**

A system of care should adopt policies related to membership on governance boards so that a minimum of three family members must serve at the same time. This prevents the burnout of one person, broadens the family voice, and eliminates tokenism.

Family Members as Employees of Systems of Care

• **The Pitfall**

Many systems of care hire family members to do various jobs for the overall system or for specific partner agencies. Like all other employees, they are expected to support and protect their employer's interests. However, a family's interests may not always be the same as the employing agency's. Consequently, family members hired to promote family involvement may feel that their jobs are being threatened if, as advocates on behalf of an enrolled family, they find fault with their employer's policies, practices, or services.

The first family members hired by systems of care are often chosen because they surface as individuals who play active roles in advocating for their children and others to receive more or better services. These family members wear two hats—one as agency employees and one as advocates for their children and possibly others. As these families continue in their advocacy roles, it may appear as if they are "biting the hand that feeds them." Family members often work in isolation without a family organization or other family members as a support system.

• **The Safety Net**

Having a clear and shared understanding of the family members' job descriptions, expectations, responsibilities, and boundaries of their roles as employees helps to avoid this common pitfall. It is also critical to have a clear and shared understanding of when it is necessary and desirable to allow a family member who is an employee to temporarily step outside of the employee role so that he or she can take on an advocacy role. Contracting with a family-run organization to hire and outstation family staff in system of care positions in the community is another strategy used to overcome the isolation and advocacy issues. This works well when authority and strategies for ongoing support and supervision are clear and practical.

Balancing Parenting and System of Care Work

- **The Pitfall**

Some supervisors and administrators, particularly in the early stages of development of a system of care, fail to recognize the great demands faced by family members who serve on committees or who are system of care employees while they are in the thick of raising a child with a mental health challenge. System or agency personnel policies may place severe hardship on families who often need flexible working hours or time off to take care of the complex needs of their children (e.g., responding to emergency calls from their children's schools that require them to leave a meeting or their jobs to address the issues at hand). In addition, family members serving in advisory or governance roles often cannot afford to pay for the transportation, travel, child care, and other expenses incurred by their participation. They may be forced to miss work and forfeit pay to participate in system of care activities. Hardship is also created for many family members who are expected to pay work-related or travel expenses up front and wait for agency reimbursement.

- **The Safety Net**

Revising personnel policies, streamlining travel reimbursement processing, offering some petty cash up front, and establishing standards for compensating family members for their time, travel, and child care are all viable solutions. Anticipating these issues and addressing them at the earliest stages of system of care development helps to avoid these problems all together.

Vulnerability and Exposure

- **The Pitfall**

Whether they are paid staff or volunteers, family members being served by the system of care feel vulnerable because many of the partners sitting around the table or their colleagues at work know many intimate details about their families—the good, the bad, and the ugly. Even when confidential information regarding their lives is carefully protected, these family members feel an imbalance. They also feel exposed because they know nothing about the lives of their professional partners or coworkers. This creates a very unequal partnership.

- **The Safety Net**

Vulnerability and exposure are avoided by carefully assigning parent and professional teams so that families are not working directly with the providers serving their own children and families. Confidentiality is reinforced by creating formal agreements stating that no personal information about the families can be discussed at committee meetings or outside of staffing with other agency partners.

The Invisible Ceiling

- ## The Pitfall

There seems to be an invisible ceiling, meaning a point in the process when family partnership is no longer welcome. As family members work in and with systems of care, their knowledge and understanding of system issues are deepened. When they begin to see flaws or gaps and suggest changes, they may be viewed as a threat to the system, and as a result, they could be disciplined, reassigned to other work, or even fired. Agencies do not always welcome change, and they sometimes stand by a mantra that says, "This is the way we have always done it." Family members have no idea when they will reach the invisible ceiling, making it a risky business for one to be both an advocate and an employee.

- ## The Safety Net

Partnership between family staff, family volunteers in governance, and the system of care flourishes when information is equally shared, conversations are honest and held out in the open, as opposed to behind closed doors, and decisions are based on data or documented facts. All parties learn to avoid finger pointing and blaming, as well as to accompany criticism with constructive suggestions.

Partnerships with Family-Run Organizations

Family involvement in all aspects of system of care development and operations has been most successful when the system of care has contracted with a local family-run organization to facilitate and support family involvement. These contracts give family-run organizations resources and responsibility for recruiting, supporting, training, and providing supervision and technical assistance to family members working within the system, as well as to those serving on governance, advisory, and policy groups. This is a highly successful strategy, but it also has pitfalls. The relationship between a contractor and a client is not the same as a relationship between equal partners.

Family-run organizations focus on making life better for children and families. To be successful, they must have a broad perspective on what makes the system and its components work for children and families, as well as the areas and the means through which things must improve or change. A system of care may choose to work with an existing family-run organization in the community that has some infrastructure and experience or it may choose to start one. New organizations that start out as a component of a system of care face two daunting challenges from the outset—building their organization quickly and working immediately to diversify their funding. Often, family members identified to start a family-run organization have no business experience, yet they are expected to start and run the organization with great fiscal responsibility.

Balancing Competing Interests
While Building a Family-Run Organization

- **The Pitfall**

It has proven difficult to identify a new family leader in a community and hire that person to both build a local family-run organization and serve as the lead family partner in building the system of care. These endeavors simply require too much work for one person to do single-handedly. Reliance on the system of care for their continued employment—until the family-run organization is established and can pay salaries for its staff—creates a special vulnerability for a newly hired family leader.

Furthermore, systems of care, sometimes unreasonably, expect family-run organizations to *always* serve as their cheerleaders. When family-run organizations are co-opted by the system, they lose their credibility with grass roots families and with other system of care partners. Newly forming family-run organizations under the umbrella of a system of care must follow system mandates. Having only this one funding stream often dictates their mission. These family-run organizations struggle to be responsive to both their agency partners and to the families they serve. They also reach that same invisible ceiling when advocating for the best interests of families in the community is viewed as opposing the agency that provides their funding. There have been a few cases in which contracts with family-run organizations have been terminated when conflicts between the system of care or its leaders and the family-run organization or its leaders could not be resolved. New family-run organizations must find a balance between being strong and independent family voices and supporting the system of care's mission and policy positions.

- **The Safety Net**

There can only be a partnership when there is honest and open conversation and when criticism among all parties is based on documented facts. To fully appreciate this partnership, such criticism must be accompanied by constructive suggestions for system change aimed at achieving better outcomes for children, youth, and families.

Sustaining Funding

- **The Pitfall**

Funding from a system of care, although essential, must not be the sole source of funding for a family-run organization. Regardless of the stage of development, both the federally funded system of care communities and the family-run organizations typically face major challenges as the federal share of funding begins to decrease. Loss of federal funds may make it difficult for a system of care to sustain family-run organization activities and services that depended entirely on these resources (Stroul, 2006). Funding for family-run organizations and activities is often the first to be cut unless meaningful family involvement has really taken root in the system of care and all the partners have started to value and rely on a strong family presence. Regardless of federal funding, changes in the funding structure or budget cuts for a local system of care may jeopardize contracts with family organizations.

• **The Safety Net**

Some community partners have taken active roles in seeking funding to sustain the family organization. Shared responsibility for sustaining funding for a family organization must start at the earliest stages of the development of a system of care. Because the entire community benefits from the work of the family organizations, all partner agencies should contribute cash, in-kind, and other resources to sustain them.

FAMILY PARTNERSHIPS IN NEW JERSEY

"Family voice has significantly increased on all levels of care and is meaningful, ranging from representation on numerous state and county/area workgroups, to full engagement in individual treatment and support activities of new child behavioral health system services." (Armstrong et al., 2006, p. 13)

Family Support Organizations (FSOs) in New Jersey are effectively applying the definition and principles of family-driven care to systems of care statewide. This was not always the case. This section highlights the journey of FSOs as successful examples of strong family voices and partnerships in policy development and system management. It also describes how New Jersey's FSOs help individual families develop their own voices and strengthen their own partnerships with their service planning teams and with service providers in their communities.

Implementation of Family Support Organizations

Prior to 1999, formal involvement of families in state policy or system design, implementation, management, and evaluation was minimal in New Jersey. Programs made attempts to incorporate the system of care principle of family involvement by inviting family members to participate at state or local planning meetings, but there was no funding or structure designated for this activity. Kathy Wagner (2001), a family member who pioneered early efforts to build a better children's system of care that incorporated full family involvement, worked with a collaborative of family organizations, advocacy groups, and professional organizations to develop this concept. Comprised of groups such as the New Jersey Parents Caucus, the Statewide Parents Advocacy Network, the Association for Children in New Jersey, and the New Jersey Mental Health Association among others, the collaborative brought parents and professionals together to advocate for comprehensive, coordinated, culturally competent services for children and families across agencies. In 2000, this group developed a 10-point position paper (Box 9.2) that stressed full family involvement as a central guiding principle.

Box 9.2. The New Jersey Children and Family Initiative

Children and families face many obstacles in today's world. In these times of limited resources, it is essential that federal, state, and local services be delivered efficiently, effectively, without duplication or bureaucratic barriers to maximize funding for children and families. The Children and Family Initiative recognizes that this goal can only be attained if:

1. Children and families can access a fully unified and integrated system of supports and services. Children and families need a seamless process making available a comprehensive continuum of services in their communities. The establishment of a common point of entry for services to children and families will help reduce duplication of effort. Through a common point of entry, children and families can access the same basic assessment, a team approach to planning, case coordination/management, information and referral, and supports and services to both children and families. A system that allows children and families to move between levels of care on an as-needed basis without disruption to or loss of continuity of necessary services saves the expense of "recertification" for services and avoids the deterioration of family circumstances that often arises when services are disrupted. A new "tracking and payment" system, with pooled funding and funding attached to the child/family rather than to specific programs, would be a more efficient and effective way to address children/family needs.

2. Children and family services are planned and implemented with agency collaboration, coordination, and leadership at all levels (state, county, and local). Children and families need leadership and commitment from cabinet officers, division directors, and other senior officials toward parent/family empowerment and systems change. This leadership and commitment will be clear if the principles of the Children and Family Initiative are enforced from the top down and across systems. Services will be more effective and efficient if all agencies that impact children and families (education, health, human services, labor, community affairs, juvenile justice, etc.) collaborate in planning and service delivery, jointly funding and/or pooling funding to the maximum extent appropriate. While responsible oversight and enforcement is important, overregulation or rigidity can interfere with the most effective service delivery.

3. Parents/family members are full partners in all aspects of the process. Families need to be informed, effective participants in state, regional, and local policy planning, governance, and decision-making, and in decision-making for their own children. Families possess information that is crucial for effective service delivery; in addition, most families have the life-long commitment to their children that is necessary to ensure that services have the desired impact.

4. Children and families receive services from service providers and other professionals who are fully prepared to work as partners with families. Effective service providers are fully competent in working in partnership and mutual respect with diverse families; they recognize that valuing the hopes, dreams, and priorities of families and building on family and community strengths improves the impact of services. Higher education agencies and professional continuing education must incorporate this philosophy and relevant skill building into their programs.

5. Children and families can access "family-friendly," culturally competent service delivery. Effective professionals across systems work with and provide services in ways that are appropriate for diverse families, including foster parents, other relatives and nontraditional family constellations, and families from varying

racial/ethnic/socio-economic and linguistic backgrounds. When the focus is on the level and type of need rather than deficits, dysfunctions, negative labels, or blame, families are more receptive to services and change.

6. Children and families can access a full continuum of prevention services and models that promote healthy development and self-sufficiency. Preventive measures, such as pre- and post-natal medical care, nutrition, quality education, and access to decent housing and employment, have well-documented positive impacts on children and families. Schools that utilize their resources to become havens of emotional wellness allow children to learn and develop to their fullest potential. When social development/social problem-solving is part of the core curriculum, taught consistently in grades pre-K through 12, and made available to families, children, families, and communities all benefit. Positive Behavior Support in schools and families can reduce the need for more expensive services.

7. Children and families can access a full continuum of intervention services, as early as needed, in the least restrictive, most natural environments. Services are most effective when they are flexible, customized, comprehensive, and accessible, and are designed to offer supports and services in the most independent, normal manner and the least restrictive, most normal settings, as close to home as possible. Children and families also respond to incentives to maintain, develop or achieve maximum social and economic self-sufficiency. For those children who need more intensive services, planning and service delivery must avoid/minimize the potential for multiple placements/multiple failures, ensure a range of options and services for children and families, and provide appropriate education, mental health, and other services in all settings.

8. The needs of children and families are addressed by systems that engage in ongoing assessment of individual needs as well as overall needs of children and families throughout the state. Comprehensive, coordinated assessments of the strengths and needs of families and children must be available across systems to avoid duplication of effort and maximize efficiency and effectiveness. Assessment must include the hopes, dreams, and priorities of families. To measure effectiveness, the satisfaction of families and children must be periodically determined, outcomes and performance objectives must be reviewed on an ongoing basis, and periodic status updates or "report cards" must be provided to stakeholders for review and comment.

9. Children and families can readily access information regarding their own services, as well as the overall performance of systems of services. To ensure effectiveness and efficiency, services must be organized in a way that ensures ongoing performance outcomes that will drive system changes, funding directions, resource utilization, and planning.

10. Children and families receive efficient, sufficient, effective, and fully funded services. "An ounce of prevention is worth a pound of cure." When children and families receive sufficient appropriate services at the earliest stages, the need for more expensive services can be ameliorated or eliminated, and the health and well-being of children, families, and communities are most easily maintained.

Developed by Diana Autin, Executive Co-Director, Statewide Parent Advocacy Network on behalf of the Children and Family Initiative, a collaboration of SPAN, the NJ Parents' Caucus, Association for Children of New Jersey, and the Mental Health Association of New Jersey.

The parent leaders met with state planning bodies, established rapport with sympathetic state planners, and approached Governor Christine Whitman's office with their vision for an improved system. Concurrently, Burlington County was awarded a federal grant from CMHS/SAMHSA to implement a local system of care for children with mental health needs, providing a local example of a system of care that could inform statewide system improvement efforts.

Ultimately, the New Jersey Children's Initiative was implemented, putting into motion a sweeping reform of children's mental health services by establishing a system of care in each of the state's 15 regions, covering 21 counties. Family involvement and partnerships were conceived as an integral part of the new system. Replicating the model for family involvement developed in the Burlington County system of care, each region was mandated to fully fund a FSO as a component of its system of care.

> "That period was very rich, and full of learning about the potential value and challenges of empowering and funding families as an integral component of a state initiative that was quite radical in its efforts to transform the system."
> —Harry Shallcross, Consultant (2007)

There have been significant stops, starts, and revisions, as well as seven changes in leadership at the state governance level during the implementation period since the *Children's Initiative Paper* was written in 2000. The name of the initiative also changed several times. However, families and the system of care movement have been undaunted by these changes and have continued to move forward with the implementation of systems of care and FSOs.

New Jersey FSOs are family-led, community-based, nonprofit agencies, each with an executive director and a local board of directors. Their mission is to provide support, advocacy, and education to families and caregivers of children with emotional, behavioral, and mental health needs while working in a strategic partnership with the professional organizations that serve children and families. Family members who have navigated supports and services for their own children serve on the board of directors, making up at least 80% of its membership. FSOs are staffed by parents or caregivers. It is expected that the board and staff reflect and represent the cultural demographics of the local community, particularly those families whom the organizations are serving.

Three FSOs were established in January 2001, and the last of the 15 began its work in early 2006. There was much concern that due to state budget deficits and the resulting cuts in funding that occurred during that time, both existing and planned FSOs would be the first to suffer. This did not occur, although implementation and roll-out timeframes were drastically altered. A number of organizations, agencies, and advocates joined the FSOs in a successful effort to preserve the funding for systems of care and the family organizations. In a personal communication in 2007, Madeline Lozowski, one of the family leaders on the statewide management team, recalled, "During the process of statewide implementation, families connected to the Family Support Organizations already in existence were strong advocates for the continuation of the model and the proposed expansion. Family members spoke at budget forums, testified before the New Jersey Legislature, and visited their state senators and representatives in their local offices. Their message was clear—finally, families have a voice in the planning for their children's care, and they were not going to lose that. . . . At the same time, even with changes in state governance, there was a core group of dedicated state leaders who believed in the principles of system of care and valued meaningful family involvement. They did not give up on the effort to bring local systems of care, including Family Support Organizations, fully statewide."

> "The family movement is the essential ingredient in sustaining the change to New Jersey's system of care."
> —Carolyn Beauchamp, President of the Mental
>   Health Association of New Jersey (2007)

In early 2006, Governor John Corzine established the Department of Children and Families, which quickly embraced the role of families in its work. By the year's end, the Commissioner of the Department of Children and Families affirmed that the FSOs were one of the most successful elements of the system (Livio, 2006). In reflection during a personal communication in 2007, Nadezhda Robinson, the Director of Child Behavioral Health Services commented, "It is remarkable that this system of care has been through too many governors and changes in leadership, yet through it all, it has been the families who give the strength to system advocates and families who carry forward the integrity of the system as conceived."

Effective Strategies for Family Involvement in Policy and System Management

Family leaders in New Jersey are members of statewide and local children's behavioral health system design workgroups, committees, and advisory boards. A high standard for family involvement was established early in the development of these policy- and governance-level committees. Modeled after the approach implemented at the state's first system of care site in Burlington County, a state-level Family Professional Partnership Committee was created and is:

> Responsible for assuring that the children and families of Child Behavioral Health Services are properly integrated in the system as partners. The primary goal of the committee is to continuously increase and improve family/caregiver participation in care and services, and to promote families as leaders in their children's treatment and in system/community procedures and services. (New Jersey Division of Child Behavioral Health Services, 2002)

The Family Professional Partnership Committee promotes the following:

- Recognition and respect for family perspectives
- Keeping children within their home communities

- Outcomes that have a child, family, and community focus

- Collaboration between families, caregivers, and service agencies

- Strength-based treatment planning

- Family involvement in the treatment of the child

- Identification of needed enhancements to services

- One third participation of family and caregivers on all committees

The committee created a chart that lists all critical decision-making committees at the state level and in each of the 21 counties. As family members are recruited to serve on these bodies, their names are added to the chart. The strategy for statewide family involvement at the system level is to ensure that each committee has parents, family members who are primary caregivers, and youth representatives. All of the FSOs are represented on the Family Professional Partnership Committee, and they continuously link their volunteers and paid staff with opportunities for membership on various committees.

FSO staff and interested family members participate in system of care trainings and serve as trainers for all stakeholders in the system of care through the Behavioral Research and Training Institute of University Behavioral Healthcare, located at the University of Medicine and Dentistry of New Jersey. To sustain this level of statewide family involvement, stipends for families who are not employed in the system have been made available through the FSOs, governmental entities, the training institute, and various grants.

Evidence of the success of this approach to system-level family involvement is cited in many ways:

- FSOs are located in every geographic sector of the state, and they have the ability to share family voice and insight as they interact with management and frontline workers throughout local and state systems.

- Families are present in increasing numbers in key positions on all decision-making committees in New Jersey.

- There are family leaders on state-level policy and advisory bodies (i.e., the leadership group within the State's Division of Child Behavioral Health) representing the family-as-consumer point of view.

- There is a Family Ombudsperson on the staff of the state contracted Systems Administrator, Value Options.

- FSOs have partnered with Parents Anonymous and the Statewide Parents Advocacy Network to create a Parent Advisory Council to the Commissioner of the Department of Children and Families.

- Families representing the behavioral health, child welfare, and juvenile justice systems provide cultural and experiential diversity of perspective as they express the family voice.

Effective Family Involvement in Services

FSOs located in every geographic region of the state serve as the primary vehicles for ensuring family involvement at the service delivery level by providing a range of peer support and advocacy services. FSO services are based on a comprehensive model of community development and peer support and are contractually responsible for such functions as (New Jersey Division of Child Behavioral Health Services, 2004):

- Active recruitment and organization of community volunteers

- Development of peer support and education groups

- Ongoing outreach and training to all system partners to promote the role of the family in the children's behavioral health system and encourage family involvement and partnership in services and policy development

- Strategic partnership with care management organizations to ensure family voice on wraparound child–family teams

- Peer support for families during the initial engagement and service planning process, with intensity of support matched to family need

- Trained family support partners for individualized, face-to-face support for families requiring this level of intensity

- Support and housing for a youth partnership in every county, giving youth their own voice

The ability to build a supportive relationship with a peer who has "walked in your shoes" has proven helpful to parents who have felt isolated in the past. FSOs typically have two full-time equivalent family support partners and a family coordinator. These positions are filled by local family members who know the community and who have navigated supports and services for their own children and for other families.

In addition to peer-to-peer support, another role for family partners is to educate parents on the operation of the system and on the wraparound process. Families participating on their own wraparound teams are able to access a family support partner who is trained to provide support, education, and advocacy. A training curriculum was developed specifically to prepare family support partners for these roles (Donner, 2004).

Every FSO employs a community outreach coordinator who facilitates the development of support groups and educational forums as gathering places for families in the community. These coordinators also produce newsletters and educational materials for the community about the family organization and the system of care. *Warm lines* for reassurance and information are maintained at every FSO. Although these are not 24-hour crisis lines, the warm lines have proven effective in reaching out to the community and bringing parents into the larger family movement.

Progress in Family Partnership

In a mere 7 years, the family movement has gone statewide in New Jersey. Every community has as its strength homegrown leaders who recognized a need and developed a strategy to become formidable resources as advocates, educators, and supports for families. In this short span of time, FSOs and the families they represent have gained status and respect. They have learned how the system works and are teaching others how it needs to work.

> "Family Support Organizations throughout New Jersey are the family voice. We speak with and for families; we are listened to and heard by the professional community."
> —Rosemarie LoBretto, Executive Director of the Bergen County Family Support Organization and Founding Board President of the New Jersey Alliance of Family Support Organizations (2007)

CONCLUSION

Partnerships and collaborations between family-run organizations and systems of care support Goal 2 of the President's New Freedom Commission—mental health care will be consumer and family driven. Successful partnerships adhere to the definition of *family-driven care*, apply the principles, and display the characteristics in their everyday practice in service delivery to children and youth with behavioral health needs and their families. The path to genuine and effective collaboration and partnership has been blazed by pioneering family-run organizations and systems of care that have shared their successes and challenges in this chapter, leaving guidance for the next generation of systems of care. The key is sharing responsibility for making decisions about setting system goals; allocating funds and other resources; designing and implementing programs, supports, and services; choosing providers; monitoring outcomes; and determining the effectiveness of efforts to promote the mental health and well-being of all children and youth in the community.

REFERENCES

American Heritage Dictionary. (1957). Random House.

Armstrong, M.I., Blase, K.A., Caldwell, B., Holt, W., King-Miller, T., Kuppinger, A., et al. (2006, October). *Final Report: Independent Assessment of New Jersey's Children's Behavioral Health Care System.* Manuscript submitted to the New Jersey Division of Child Behavioral Health Services by the Louis de la Parte Florida Mental Health Institute.

Blau, G., Osher, T.W., & Osher, D. (2005). Need for a definition of family-driven care. *Family Ties*, 3–4.

Bryant-Comstock, S., Huff, B. & VanDenBerg, J. (1996). The evolution of the family advocacy movement. In B.A. Stroul & R.M. Friedman (Series Eds.) & B.A. Stroul (Vol. Ed.), *Systems of care for children's mental health: Children's mental health: Creating systems of care in a changing society* (pp. 359–374). Baltimore: Paul H. Brookes Publishing Co.

Dababnah, S., & Cooper, J. (2006). Strengthening family support in the context of services. In *Unclaimed Children Revisited working paper no. 1: Challenges and opportunities in children's mental health: A view from families and youth* (pp. 11–16). New York: Columbia University Mailman School of Public Health, National Center for Children in Poverty.

Donner, R. (2004) *Putting the pieces together: Skills for family support partners.* Trenton, NJ: New Jersey Division of Child Behavioral Health.

Livio, S.K. (2006, December 26). Troubled kids to get more help from state. *The Star Ledger*, p. 27.

New Jersey Division of Child Behavioral Health Services (2002). *Family/Professional Partnership Sub-Committee of the Quality Assessment and Performance Improvement Steering Committee.* Trenton, NJ: Author.

New Jersey Division of Child Behavioral Health Services. (2004). *Family support organization roles and responsibilities and contract deliverables.* Trenton, NJ: Author.

Osher, T., & Bestgen, Y. *Building sustainable family-run organizations in systems of care* (p. 59). Unpublished manuscript.

Osher, T.W., & Osher, D.M. (2002). The paradigm shift to true collaboration with families journal of child and family studies. *Journal of Child and Family Studies, 11*(1), 47–60.

Pires, S. (2002). *Building systems of care: A primer.* Washington, DC: Georgetown University Child Development Center, Children's Mental Health Center for Child Health and Mental Health Policy, National Technical Assistance Center.

President's New Freedom Commission on Mental Health. (2003). *Achieving the promise: Transforming mental health care in America. Final report* (DHHS Pub. No. SMA-03-3832). Rockville, MD: Author

Stroul, B. (2006, June) *Executive summary: The sustainability of systems of care: Lessons learned.* From the Report on the Special Study on the Sustainability of Systems of Care National Evaluation of the Comprehensive Community Mental Health Services for Children and Their Families Program prepared by ORC Macro, Atlanta.

Stroul, B., & Friedman, R. (1986). *A system of care for children and youth with severe emotional disturbances.* Washington, DC: Georgetown University Child Development Center.

Substance Abuse and Mental Health Services Administration. (2005). *Cooperative agreements for the Comprehensive, Community Mental Health Services for Children and Their Families Program* (SM-05-010). (2006). Retrieved February 15, 2005, from http://www .grants.gov

Tannen, N. (1996). A family-designed system of care: Families first in Essex County, New York. In B.A. Stroul & R.M. Friedman (Series Eds.) & B.A. Stroul (Vol. Ed.), *Systems of care for children's mental health: Children's mental health: Creating systems of care in a changing society* (pp. 359–374). Baltimore: Paul H. Brookes Publishing Co.

Wagner, K. (2001, Spring). The children's system of care initiative. *Reaching Today's Youth,* 31–34.

Ronnie —

My heart is filled with hope for our next generation. I will be grateful when System of Care is the norm and not a unique "quaint = intervention." From one warrior to another

Love your friend

[signature]

10

Partnerships with Youth for Youth-Guided Systems of Care

Marlene Matarese, Myrna Carpenter,
Charles Huffine, Stephanie Lane, and Kayla Paulson

Although systems of care have increasingly involved families, there is a growing realization of the need to fully involve youth as well. Research has shown that family engagement is a critical factor in the effectiveness of service delivery. It is important for consumers and families to direct their own recovery and feel committed to their own well-being. According to Burns, Hoagwood, and Mrazek,

> The effectiveness of services, no matter what they are, may hinge less on the particular type of service than on how, when and why families or caregivers are engaged in the delivery of care . . . It is becoming increasingly clear that family engagement is a key component not only to participation in care, but also in the effective implementation of it. (1999, p. 238)

Thomlison (2003) also stated that, "Not all the studies show that improvements resulted from the intervention specifically. Family engagement may play a stronger role in the outcomes than the actual intervention program" (p. 584). In addition, consumers and families reported to the President's New Freedom Commission on Mental Health (2003) that having hope and the opportunity to regain control of their lives was vital to their recovery. The commission noted that emerging research has validated that "hope and self-determination are important factors contributing to recovery" (p. 27).

Though evaluation of the involvement of youth consumers in systems of care is in early stages, anecdotal evidence supports the benefits of youth involvement. Emerging research findings confirm that youth involvement helps young people achieve positive development, assists in their successful transition to adulthood, and helps them develop deeper connections to their peers and their communities. In addition, youth involvement helps young people feel more confident about controlling their own lives in a positive way and avoiding risky behaviors, as well as enhancing the effectiveness of services (Fischhoff, Crowell, & Kipke, 1999; Lewis, 2003).

This chapter outlines the rationale for involving youth in every level of systems of care, from guiding their own services to system policy and management. The Positive Youth Development (PYD) approach is reviewed, and emerging roles for youth advocacy organizations in systems of care are discussed. The challenges and strategies for initiating, operating, and sustaining youth movements at local and national levels are examined, with an example provided by Youth 'N Action!, the statewide youth organization in Washington.

FRAMEWORK FOR YOUTH ENGAGEMENT: POSITIVE YOUTH DEVELOPMENT

The PYD approach has been evident in the literature on adolescent development since the 1980s. During this time, the concept of youth development has shifted from prevention (i.e., programs created to combat the problems of high-risk youth), to preparation (i.e., developing skills and encouraging broader development for all young people), to participation and empowerment (i.e., utilizing young people as partners in decision making). The Youth Development and Delinquency Prevention Administration described four components of positive youth development: 1) a sense of competence, 2) a sense of usefulness, 3) a sense of belonging, and 4) a sense of power (National Clearinghouse on Families and Youth [NCFY], 1996). When young people are not given opportunities to grow and develop in a positive way, they are more likely to find harmful alternatives. Some youth may consider joining gangs as a way to belong, find support, and make decisions; however, when young people have access to appropriate supports and opportunities, they are likely to avoid self-destructive lifestyles, as well as achieve a healthy sense of identity and the competencies necessary to become successful adults (Zeldin, 1995).

Fostering a PYD approach in a system of care requires a shift in beliefs related to young people. It is the responsibility of youth leaders and adult supports to serve as change agents and advocates to practitioners, policy makers, and community members to promote the importance of valuing youth as equal partners in creating system change and the benefits of authentic youth involvement.

Often, young people involved in systems of care are disconnected from their communities due to out-of-home placements and isolation as a result of stigma. Young people who have mental illnesses may be faced with reintegrating back into the community after stays in psychiatric hospitals, juvenile detention centers, foster homes, group homes, or residential facilities. Many experience poverty, school failure, family crises, and challenging behaviors (Roach, Yu, & Lewis-Charp, 2001). These factors have profound effects on their development, and many react to the loss of belonging by engaging in high-risk behaviors to lessen feelings of seclusion and isolation (Kirshner, O'Donoghue, & McLaughlin, 2003).

Resiliency is an important component in the positive development of young people, and it is particularly relevant for those involved in systems of care. Why do some youth make it and become successful? Care and support, high expectations, and opportunities to participate help young people become more resilient when faced with challenging life experiences. Young people who develop problem-solving skills and have positive relationships with adults, as well as a sense of social competence, safety, identity, autonomy, purpose, respect, and hope for the future, often have the ability to bounce back from adversity (Bernard, 1996). Resilience is a product of trusting relationships, internal strengths, skills in interpersonal relationships, and the ability to problem solve. Faith and self-esteem are also crucial in building resiliency in young people (Institute for Mental Health Initiatives, 1999). Having a sense of belonging and purpose, as well as resiliency, often allows young people to overcome the barriers they face due to mental illness.

The PYD approach provides a framework for youth involvement in system of care communities by emphasizing and developing strengths and resiliency, as well as by providing a variety of vehicles through which youth can contribute to their communities and become more connected (NCFY, 1996). For example, one young person may be able to advocate for youth through public speaking, whereas another may express him- or herself more effectively through art or writing. Consistent with the PYD framework, the development of youth groups in systems of care foster a sense of connectedness and provide opportunities for youth to move forward in positive ways.

YOUTH CONSUMER MOVEMENT IN SYSTEMS OF CARE

The Surgeon General's Conference on Children's Mental Health in 2000 was an important milestone in fostering a national youth consumer movement in mental health. For the first time, young people were invited to sit at the tables with families and professionals. Although the participating adults were well-intentioned, youth voice was largely lost in the jargon, competition for time, and other variables that made the youth feel unwelcome and tokenized. At that conference, the youth participants made a decision that would change the shape of youth voice in public policy—they unanimously decided not to attend the conference on the second day due to what they felt was a lack of respect. Their absence was keenly noted. The youth rejoined the group and presented a written manifesto requesting that professionals and family members treat them with respect and dignity. Among the requests they made were for professionals to stop using acronyms, labels, and/or diagnoses to describe youth in meetings, to fund and support youth organizations at the same level as family organizations, and to make room for youth to participate meaningfully in policy discussions. Following this presentation, the conference became more youth friendly, and the youth movement began to develop at a rapid pace.

Following the Surgeon General's Conference on Children's Mental Health, youth were significantly involved in the biannual system of care community meetings sponsored by the federal Comprehensive Community Mental Health Services for Children and Their Families Program (i.e., the Children's Mental Health Initiative) of the Center for Mental Health Services (CMHS). Each year, youth involvement at national system of care community meetings and related conferences has increased, with more than 100 youth attending each of these conferences. Youth participate in youth-driven leadership tracks at these conferences and serve as presenters in sessions. Starting in 2002, the Request for Applicants for the Children's Mental Health Initiative has required youth involvement in federally funded systems of care, including hiring local youth coordinators and ensuring youth involvement at every level of system of care development. To support these efforts, the Technical Assistance Partnership for Child and Family Mental Health (TAP), which provides technical assistance to the funded systems of care, hired a full-time national youth involvement resource specialist dedicated to supporting the various youth groups across the nation. There are currently more than 60 youth groups dedicated to youth voice in mental health policy.

In December 2003, a group of youth and youth coordinators came together with the support of TAP and CMHS and developed the National Youth Development Board (NYDB), specifying its structure, mission, vision, and policies. Funding was received from TAP and CMHS to hire 12 youth consumers and 3 youth coordinators to support the growth and work of the board. NYDB ultimately decided to transition to become a national youth organization called Youth Motivating Others through Voices of Empowerment (Youth M.O.V.E.).

Youth M.O.V.E. is composed of a diverse group of youth coordinators and young people from system of care communities who have had extensive experience in mental health and other youth-serving systems. The purpose of the organization is to unite the voices and causes of youth; to act as consultants to youth, professionals, families, and other adults; and to be involved in the politics and legislation of mental health policies. To support a national youth movement, Youth M.O.V.E. also assists in developing the youth leadership programs at conferences; creating youth movement principles and policies; and developing training tools, guides, and other documents. Youth M.O.V.E. staff are also national consultants who travel across the country to coach others in the area of authentic youth involvement. Youth M.O.V.E. is working toward a longer-term goal of becoming a 501(c)(3) organization, and it continues to grow with additional funding and support from several sources. These funding sources include financial and in-kind support from TAP, the Caring for Every Child's Mental Health Campaign, the National Evaluation Team (Macro International Inc. and Walter R. McDonald and Associates), the National Technical Assistance Center for Children's Mental Health at Georgetown University, the Federation of Families for Children's Mental Health, the Jonas Penn Fund, and the Scott Bryant-Comstock Foundation. Youth M.O.V.E.'s mission and vision are displayed in Box 10.1.

Achieving Meaningful Involvement

Building a partnership with young people requires adults to possess an understanding of their personal views of young people and a willingness to change those perceptions if necessary. Adults may view young people as objects, recipients, or partners (Innovation Center for Community and Youth Development, 1996). The Ladder of Youth Involvement (Figure 10.1) illustrates the different relationships that adults can choose to engage in with youth. As one moves closer to the

---

Box 10.1. Youth M.O.V.E.

MISSION STATEMENT

We the members of Youth M.O.V.E. will work as a diverse collective to unite the voices and causes of youth while raising awareness around youth issues. We will advocate for youth rights and voice in mental health and other systems that serve them, in the process of empowering youth to be equal partners in the process of change.

VISION STATEMENT

We the members of Youth M.O.V.E. envision a system of care in which every young person that enters any youth-serving system is successfully prepared for life. We help guide the redevelopment of the system so that no youth falls through the cracks. We advocate for youth to utilize their power to foster change in their communities and in their own lives.

Youth M.O.V.E. works toward the day when all people will recognize and accept the culture of youth, their families, and the communities that serve them in order to be truly culturally competent. We as a youth organization look forward to the day when youth are no longer treated as numbers, problems, or caseloads, but as individuals and humans. We will all stand as partners—youth, youth advocates, supporters, parents, and professionals—to see our youth become successful.

Reprinted from Matarese, M., McGinnis, L., & Mora, M. (2005). *Youth involvement in systems of care: A guide to empowerment.* Retrieved October 11, 2007, from http://www.tapartnership.org/youth/youthguide.asp.

---

top, maximum youth involvement is approached and youth–adult partnership becomes a reality. Systems of care vary in their levels of youth involvement; the primary goal is to move beyond steps 1–5 to achieve authentic youth involvement and become a youth-guided system of care. The corresponding views of youth involvement—as objects, recipients, or partners—are shown on Table 10.1.

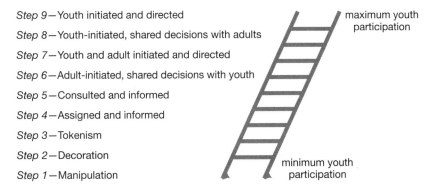

Step 9—Youth initiated and directed

Step 8—Youth-initiated, shared decisions with adults

Step 7—Youth and adult initiated and directed

Step 6—Adult-initiated, shared decisions with youth

Step 5—Consulted and informed

Step 4—Assigned and informed

Step 3—Tokenism

Step 2—Decoration

Step 1—Manipulation

maximum youth participation

minimum youth participation

Figure 10.1. Ladder of youth involvement. (*Source:* Adapted from Hart, R.A., 'Children's Participation: From tokenism to citizenship,' *Innocenti Essays No. 4,* UNICEF International Child Development Centre [now UNICEF Innocenti Research Centre], Florence, 1992. Available at: <http://www.unicef-irc.org/cgi-bin/unicef/Lunga.sql?ProductID=100>)

Table 10.1. View of youth involvement

View of youth involvement	Outcome	Steps of the ladder
Youth as objects Adults know what is best for young people.	Involves youth in adult-controlled situations at the discretion of adults; young people's contributions are insignificant and underutilized. Young people maintain a powerless position.	*Steps 1, 2, and 3* Manipulation Decoration Tokenism
Youth as recipients Adults view youth participation as an experience that will be good for them.	Creates an opportunity for young people to learn from the adult experts, which will help them when they become adult contributors	*Steps 4, 5, and 6* Assigned and informed Consulted and informed Adult-initiated, shared decisions with youth
Youth as partners Adults view youth as important contributors.	Encourages youth to become involved in all aspects of the organization, group, or project. Youth and adults share power and are equal partners in decision making. Both bring strengths, abilities, and expertise to the table. The system of care is youth guided.	*Steps 7, 8, and 9* Youth and adult initiated and directed Youth-initiated, shared decisions with adults Youth initiated and directed

Reprinted from Matarese, M., McGinnis, L., & Mora, M. (2005). *Youth involvement in systems of care: A guide to empowerment.* Retrieved October 11, 2007, from http://www.tapartnership.org/youth/youthguide.asp.

Youth and youth coordinators strive for the highest level of participation of youth-initiated and directed involvement. At this level, youth are making decisions, setting goals, and developing action strategies, with youth coordinators serving as coaches to encourage and empower them. As youth involvement is maximized, adults' roles in working with youth also evolve from being mentors to becoming partners and coaches. It is essential for adults to eliminate traditional youth–adult relationships based on power imbalances. Youth and adults must have a mutual understanding of what a partnership will entail, and roles and shared responsibilities must be clear (Drake, Ling, Fitch, & Hughes, 2000). Adults, allies, and youth coordinators must all adhere to the values of the youth movement (Table 10.2).

Shifting Gears: Youth Guided to Youth Driven

When utilized in systems of care, the term *youth guided* means that young people have the right to be empowered, educated, and given a decision-making role in the care of their own lives, as well as in the determination of policies and procedures governing care for all youth in the community, state, and nation. A youth-

Table 10.2. Values of the youth movement

Youth involvement is offered as proof that individuals with mental illness can function and be contributing members of society.

Youth have rights.

Youth are utilized as resources and part of the solutions in the development of themselves, their communities, and youth-serving systems.

Youth have an equal voice and are engaged in developing and sustaining the policies and systems that serve and support them.

Youth are active partners in creating their individual treatment and support plans.

Youth have access to information that is pertinent to their treatment and lives.

Youth are valued as experts in creating system transformation and in their own lives and needs based on their personal experiences.

Youth's strengths and interests are focused on and utilized.

Adults share power with youth.

Adults and youth respect and value youth culture and all forms of diversity.

Youth are supported in a way that is developmentally targeted to their individual needs.

Reprinted from Matarese, M., McGinnis, L., & Mora, M. (2005). *Youth involvement in systems of care: A guide to empowerment.* Retrieved October 11, 2007, from http://www.tapartnership.org/youth/youthguide.asp.

guided approach allows for a continuum of power to be given to young people based on their understanding and maturity (Youth M.O.V.E., 2006). Moving from *youth guided* to *youth driven* is an evolutionary process that occurs at the individual youth, community, and policy-making levels (Table 10.3).

DEVELOPING YOUTH PARTNERSHIPS IN SYSTEMS OF CARE

Developing youth partnerships in systems of care involves steps including hiring a youth coordinator, forming a youth group, providing training, and supporting youth involvement in multiple roles. Each of these steps is discussed below.

Role of Youth Coordinators

One of the first steps necessary for commencing a youth-based initiative for social change involves hiring a youth coordinator. In doing so, it is important to consider the voice that the youth coordinator will be representing. In many instances, communities hire youth coordinators who represent the voice of youth consumers who have been involved in the mental health system. It can be challenging to identify someone who has recently been involved in the mental health system, is sufficiently healthy to help others, and is ready to speak publicly about his or her experiences. Although challenging, many communities have identified people who fit this description. Talking with mental health organizations may help to identify young adults who may potentially fulfill this role. The youth coordinator job announcement should be disseminated to a variety of mental health organizations with a request to post it in areas that are visible to consumers. It is ideal to have young people participate on the interview team for the youth coordinator

Table 10.3. Moving from youth guided to youth driven

Youth guided

Individual	Youth are empowered in their treatment planning process from the beginning and have a voice in decision making. Youth receive training. Equal partnership is valued.
Community	Community partners and stakeholders are open and willing to partner with youth and have created safe spaces for young people.
Policy	Youth are invited to meetings, and training and support is provided. Youth can speak about their experiences. Adults value what youth have to say in an advisory capacity.

Youth directed

Individual	*The young person is:* Telling his or her story. Building relationships with supportive people and making decisions in his or her own care. Developing a deeper knowledge and understanding of the system. Not in a consistent period of crisis, and his or her basic needs are met.
Community	Youth have positions and voting power on community boards. More youth are involved and recruit other youth. Community members respect the autonomy of youth voice and spread the word of its importance.
Policy	Youth understand the policy process and have experience being involved and receiving and giving training. Youth understand policy issues and speak their opinions. Youth opinions are heard, which leads to action being taken. There is an increased presence of youth and a decrease in tokenism.

Youth driven

Individual	Youth set visions and goals for treatment with input from their teams. Youth are aware of their options and are able to utilize and apply knowledge of resources. Youth are able to stand on their own and take responsibility for their choices. Youth serve as mentors and peer advocates for other youth. Youth give presentations based on their personal experiences and knowledge. Youth make the transition into adulthood.
Community	Community partners listen to youth and make changes accordingly. Young people have a safe place to go and be heard. Multiple paid positions for youth are established in every decision making group. Youth form and facilitate youth groups in their communities. Youth provide training within their communities.
Policy	Youth call meetings and set agendas in policy making. Youth hold trainings on policy making for youth and adults. Youth inform the public about policy and have a position platform. Youth lead research to drive policy change.

Reprinted from Matarese, M., McGinnis, L., & Mora, M. (2005). *Youth involvement in systems of care: A guide to empowerment.* Retrieved October 11, 2007, from http://www.tapartnership.org/youth/youthguide.asp.

because this person will be connecting, supporting, and organizing youth. Youth coordinators must have the ability to connect with youth, as well as with adults and professionals.

The role of youth coordinator is inherently challenging. In a focus group study of youth coordinators hired within systems of care, youth coordinators reported that they (and youth) may feel disrespected, marginalized, and discounted in their work (Lampron, Poirier, & Quinn, in progress). To decrease the potential for marginalization, systems of care should create opportunities for training around youth–adult partnerships, as well as respecting and supporting one another's roles. Another challenge involves support for the youth coordinator. Youth coordinators are generally hired at a young age and may have minimal professional experience; they may require intensive support and supervision. Systems of care should identify staff members who have time and demonstrate the dedication to provide this level of support to their youth coordinators. Examples of support include providing a list of office expectations, assisting in time management, helping with communication styles, providing support in the governance structure, and providing assistance with understanding system of care language and values. Youth coordinators may have ideas or suggestions that seem unconventional to others, but it is important to focus on the creativity that younger people bring to an organization and system. One way to stay connected to the needs of youth coordinators is to have biweekly or monthly meetings between youth coordinators and system of care leaders to develop and implement strategies for the youth movement.

The youth coordinators' salaries are often directly related to their perceived value within the systems of care. When hiring a youth coordinator, system of care leaders should ask themselves important questions (e.g., How important is this position to our system and community? Is this position as vital as a director of evaluation or social marketing?) If meaningful youth involvement is critical and a key value in the system of care, the salary offered to the person who accepts this position should be reflective of this. Too often, communities have provided minimal compensation, despite the fact that youth coordinators take on tremendous job responsibilities.

The role of the youth coordinator is to be a coach for youth. Coaching involves providing encouragement, support, and guidance, as well as being energizing, empowering, and supportive. The coach is a vital part of the team, but he or she does not actually play the game. Youth coordinators should be coaches in all aspects of forming and maintaining youth groups, but they should not be directors or disciplinarians, and they should be careful not to dominate discussions or step in as experts. Instead, they should be present as a resource and a support. Youth coordinators should advocate for their youth, empowering them and enhancing their leadership skills.

Youth coordinators hired within systems of care have similar characteristics and roles (Table 10.4). As noted, youth coordinators also need support because their work as change agents can be both challenging and isolating. Administrators, supervisors, and peers all play roles in providing support. Support should

Table 10.4. Characteristics and roles of youth coordinators

Youth coordinators should:

Be flexible

Be youth focused

Understand the various child-serving systems—ideally from personal experience

Respect youth culture

Relate to young people

Have a strengths-based perspective

Be willing and able to build partnerships

Partner with youth

Focus on creating a youth-driven and youth-run process

Be willing to share or relinquish power

Understand the complexities in the lives of young people

The roles of the youth coordinator should include the following:

Raising awareness of the importance of valuing youth voice and incorporating youth voice into policy development and service delivery

Building a bridge between the youth and professional worlds

Educating adults and professionals on the importance of youth involvement

Continually advocating for increased authentic youth involvement within the system of care and the broader community

Supporting youth and advocating for their participation on governance boards and other committees

Coordinating the development of a youth-run group in the community for youth who are involved in the mental health system

Providing training to youth members to enhance their leadership skills

Attending trainings to enhance personal skill sets

Serving as a representative on relevant committees at the state and local levels

Connecting youth with community-based resources

Reconnecting youth with the community

From Matarese, M., McGinnis, L., & Mora, M. (2005). *Youth involvement in systems of care: A guide to empowerment.* Retrieved October 11, 2007, from http://www.tapartnership.org/youth/youthguide.asp.

also come in the form of opportunities for training and skill development through conferences and national activities. In addition, it must be recognized in systems of care that the youth coordinator should not be the only person advocating for youth engagement or supporting youth activities. True transformation toward the development of youth-guided care is the responsibility of all stakeholders within a system of care.

Forming a Youth Group

The development of the youth group is an important step in creating partnerships with youth because it provides the support and foundation for youth involvement in other areas within systems of care. When forming a youth group, the youth coordinator should begin by identifying youth who may be interested in participating. Although some youth coordinators get started without youth partners, it is essential to involve youth from the outset to ensure a youth-driven process. Youth can be found in family organizations and schools or through care coordinators, teachers, therapists, and child welfare workers. A youth coordinator need not worry if only one or two interested young people can be identified initially because those youth are linked to others. A small number of youth is all that is necessary to move to the next stage in developing the group.

From the beginning, it is important to explain to young people that this is an opportunity for them to reclaim their identities, to become empowered to create system change, and to improve their lives and the lives of their families and peers. Once young people are involved, the development of a mission statement, goals, objectives, and strategies that will guide the group through its work can be developed. The place where youth meet should be a place where young people feel welcome, respected, and comfortable, and where there are opportunities for youth development and positive relationships between peers and adults (Pittman & Cahill, 1992). This should be a physical space that is accessible to youth and that youth can consistently count on as their own. It is not, for example, a room next to a CEO's office or a room in the basement of a building. Giving youth their own space—a youth-friendly zone where young people feel at ease—will help to instill a sense of value and importance in the fledgling group. Box 10.2 relates the initial experience of a youth coordinator in attempting to engage youth participation in a new youth group and the lessons that were learned.

Providing Training and Skill Development

Young people need education and training in order to develop the knowledge and skills necessary to be successful in their endeavors. Systems of care can provide local training opportunities to youth by engaging speakers or consultants. In addition, national training events and conferences give youth and youth coordinators the opportunity to collaborate with individuals from other youth groups, share successes, and strategize on how to address challenges. Conferences can provide youth with direct contacts to system of care leaders at state and national levels, thus encouraging a mutually beneficial dialogue. Many conferences offer workshops to help young people develop the skills needed for effective youth participation (e.g., public speaking, knowledge of laws and regulations, leadership training). Each new activity or group endeavor may require additional training to help young people become stronger advocates and contributors.

Youth coordinators also need opportunities for growth, and training is an important support for their work. Conferences offer a vehicle for youth coordinators to connect to the national youth coordinator community for acquiring support, generating ideas, and exchanging resources. Youth coordinators have identified the need for gaining new professional skills specifically connected to their work with youth (Lampron et al., in progress).

Roles of Youth

Systems of care across the nation currently support more than 60 groups for young people. These groups have different missions and activities, but they all share the common goal of supporting youth voice and involvement within the system of care. Young people nationally have undertaken a variety of tasks:

- Organizing fundraisers and communitywide events

- Providing peer support, advocacy, and bonding activities for other youth

- Participating on governing boards and committees

- Developing social marketing campaigns

- Engaging in evaluation and research

- Developing presentations and products such as tips sheets for professionals

- Creating web sites, chat rooms, and Internet-based bulletin boards

---

Box 10.2. Reflections on the experience of a new youth coordinator in engaging youth by Myrna Carpenter, Former Youth Coordinator, STARS for Children's Mental Health, St. Cloud, Minnesota

When I was working with a local system of care, one of the counties heard that I was speaking up about youth involvement, and people came to see me as somewhat of an expert in this area. I was invited to a meeting and asked what to do about transitional services for youth. I told them in order to find out, they needed to ask youth. "Great," they said, "but we're on a small budget." I wasn't shocked that county funding was limited, but I thought we would try and get creative.

We found a local pizza place where we could get a room and they didn't charge a fee. Then came the hard part . . . the county insisted that youth coming had to be ones that had received services from them and the flyer needed to advertise this. I wondered how I could get youth to expose themselves like this to me if all I'm offering is some pizza. I worked on a flyer explaining my story and opening myself up. I let youth know it was okay to say, "I've received county services, and I've been involved in the mental health system." I made the poster fun and brightly colored, and let them know that this was their chance to make a change so that if they had a bad experience, others wouldn't have to have the same. And to top it off, I put a fun picture of myself on there to show that I am a happy "normal" person. I was proud of my work and knew there were youth that could relate, and I was hoping to touch them.

When the county saw my flyer, they said it wouldn't work. They were worried that since we were putting it in public places, it may expose me too much. Well, I didn't use my last name, and I had already had a story in the local paper telling a lot about this, so I didn't see the problem, but it wasn't my call. The end result was a bland poster with a drawing of pizza and a picture of someone drinking coke. It said, "Come have fun and talk about your experience!" I'm sure that sounded like a blast for our target audience of people 16–20! In the end, no one showed up. The social worker looked at me and asked what went wrong. I told her she was asking too much of youth and not giving enough in return. You have to realize you are asking youth to take a big risk and open up a very hard part of their lives when you are asking them to get involved. You have to make it something that they feel is going to be worthwhile, and a lot of times, when you ask them to take a big risk, you have to be willing to do the same.

Many youth groups in systems of care organize community events to create change, decrease stigma, forge partnerships, and involve other young people. In the beginning stage of organizing a group, a kick-off event may be helpful in engaging youth consumers and stakeholders. Careful planning is needed, including specifying the purpose of the activity, who will be invited, appropriate venues for advertising the event, the number of staff needed, the tasks each youth will be responsible for completing, and possible compensation. It is important for the group to seek community support for each event or project to increase its visibility within the community and to generate support.

Peer-to-peer support and mentoring are key components of a youth movement. Young people gain a sense of validation when they relate to others with similar challenges and life experiences. Participation in socialization and recreational activities often decreases loneliness and isolation and also provides an opportunity for normalization for young people who do not always feel "normal." In addition, young people can help other youth become aware of their rights and find resources within the community to address their mental health and support needs.

Young people are also taking on roles within systems of care as voting members on governing boards, advisory groups, and committees. Significant roles must be given to youth to engage them in policy and system management activities, as well as to develop their leadership skills. Youth involvement on governing and advisory bodies, however, may not be successful if adult mentors are not carefully selected, do not have time to adequately support young people, or expect that everyone will immediately know how to work together (Hoover & Weisenbach, 1999). Solutions to some of these challenges include selecting adult mentors who have time and are dedicated to providing support and encouragement to interested youth. Adults should make sure that youth have transportation to and from meetings and that meetings are held at times that do not require young people to miss school. To involve young people successfully in decision-making roles in systems of care, the following steps should be taken (Hoover & Weisenbach, 1999):

- Promote local legislation and policies to stipulate the inclusion of youth on nonprofit boards and local governing bodies

- Train youth so that they feel confident to stand up and assert themselves

- Train adults so that they better understand youth involvement, the needs of youth, and ways to partner with youth for training on positive youth development

Furthermore, the implementation of the strategies shown in Table 10.5 will enhance the success of youth involvement in policy and system management roles.

Meaningful youth participation is also essential in social marketing activities. Young people understand other young people in ways that adults never will. Social marketing is an area in which young people can tap into their experience-based knowledge and develop campaigns that will best reach their peers. Young people have had success assisting with the conceptualization of social marketing

Table 10.5.   Strategies for supporting youth involvement at the policy and system level

Identify youth and adult support

Involve more than one youth in meetings; adult supports should participate as coaches to the youth.

Ensure that youth have the appropriate skill set for their role in a particular meeting. This may vary according to meeting type (e.g., governance board, committees, presentations, workshops).

Identify requirements for youth participation (e.g., presentation experience, public speaking, advocacy, understanding of the system, personal experience within particular systems).

Facilitate introductory communication (written or verbal correspondence) once the youth is identified.

Involve youth in developing the content and, if possible, setting the time and location for the meeting.

Ensure preparatory support

Send an official invitation 30 days in advance, which will include:

- Objectives for the meeting
- Meeting agenda with youth listed on the agenda
- Logistical information

Coordinate a conference call with youth and adult support.

Identify and support cultural and linguistic needs (e.g., interpreters).

Clarify roles and responsibilities

Facilitate a conference call with youth and adult supports at a time that is convenient for everyone.

Discuss specific responsibilities and youth roles with youth and adult supports.

Review meeting objectives (e.g., specifics on topics and youth roles in those topical discussion areas).

Ensure that the adult support and youth have developed a weekly coaching schedule to prepare for the meeting or presentation.

Ensure logistical support

Identify, coordinate, and provide travel arrangements to and from the meeting.

Set protocol for stipends and honorariums for youth participation; youth should be compensated for their work.

Ensure that meals and expenses related to the meeting are covered in advance; advance the per diem if travel is involved.

Coordinate early arrival to ensure adjustment to the new environment.

Orient youth on location

Orient youth to the location prior to the meeting. This will facilitate time for questions, familiarity with the meeting space, and adjustment to the new environment. For presentations, provide time for the youth to walk on stage, use the microphone, and so forth.

Reprinted from Youth Motivating Others Through Voices of Experience (M.O.V.E.). (2006). *Youth-guided.* Retrieved October 11, 2007, from http://systemsofcare.samhsa.gov/headermenus/docsHM/youthguidedlinkBreakdown.pdf.

campaigns in systems of care, as well as with the implementation of social marketing strategies.

Another area of youth involvement is in evaluation and research efforts (Sydlo et al., 2000). Young people should be involved from the beginning stages of defining problems and then collecting information, interpreting results, making decisions, and taking action based on their findings. Involvement in these activities gives young people opportunities to learn about research and evaluation (Checkoway & Richards-Schuster, 2003). In some systems of care, young people have served as co-evaluators and directors and have organized their own research projects to study problems relevant to their lives. Developing presentations, products, and Internet-related activities and resources are also important areas of youth involvement.

Youth Involvement: Making It Last

The sustainability of youth involvement depends on both philosophical and fiscal support. Philosophical support comes from a longstanding belief in the relevance of meaningful youth consumer involvement among key stakeholders. Youth involvement should be a community value that is embedded in the work of a system of care. To this end, the youth coordinator, in partnership with young people, should work to create a systemwide attitude change among stakeholders, including system of care staff, local provider agencies, elected officials, community- and faith-based organizations, educators, civic and service clubs, and business owners. These stakeholders can support the growth and sustainability of the youth group.

In addition to creating a culture that believes in youth engagement, sustaining a youth group often comes down to the need for funding. Youth groups cannot function at their optimal potential without feasible budgets. Developing a realistic budget early in the development of the youth group is essential, followed by a focused effort to reach out to stakeholders who may be willing to provide financial support. Potential funding sources include the system of care, charitable foundations, corporate sponsors, community members, provider organizations, and government agencies (federal, state, and local). Youth should know how their group is funded and should be part of developing the budget, raising funds, and determining how funds will be used. In addition to exploring funding opportunities, youth groups may also solicit in-kind donations of meeting space, office supplies, volunteers, food, and other materials.

To respond to some funding opportunities, the youth group must be under a nonprofit 501(c)(3) organization. This is often accomplished by affiliating with a local family organization and coming under its umbrella. Well-developed youth groups can complete Form 1023, Application for Recognition of Exemption Under Section 501(c)(3) of the Internal Revenue Code.

Many systems of care are successfully sustaining youth involvement. Youth 'N Action! is one of the first youth groups developed in a system of care in King County, Washington, and has since expanded statewide.

YOUTH VOICE IN PUBLIC POLICY: YOUTH 'N ACTION!

Youth 'N Action! is a youth support and advocacy organization serving all of Washington State. It is currently supported by the Statewide Action for Family

Empowerment of Washington (SAFE WA), an umbrella group for family support and advocacy organizations. Youth 'N Action! was created to support youth who have received mental health services or services from other youth-serving systems. These youth share common concerns and feel empowered by a group sharing a "been there, done that" perspective. Although it is not a treatment intervention, participation in Youth 'N Action! can be an integral part of a youth's plan of care in that it creates opportunities for peer-to-peer relationships that are supportive of constructive, strength-based interventions.

History of Youth 'N Action!

Youth 'N Action! grew out of federal system of care grants in King and Clark Counties, both initiated in 1998, in Washington State. The King County system of care staff noted the need for youth voice in addition to family involvement and empowerment. After several exploratory meetings, a youth group called Health 'N Action! was established in 1999. As its first project, it organized a successful, well-publicized, For Youth, By Youth Teen Health Summit. Health 'N Action! became a core element of the system of care. A social work graduate student was hired as an intern, with one of her prime duties involving support to the fledgling youth organization. This intern and the mental health system's medical director became part-time youth coordinators who donated considerable time due to their passion for mobilizing youth voice. The medical director's reflections on the origins of the youth organization are shared in Box 10.3.

Early in the development of Health 'N Action!, the group was invited to participate in the Surgeon General's Conference on Children's Mental Health. Several youth leaders from Health 'N Action! were chosen to be part of a group of 10 youth from around the country who attended this meeting. Youth involvement in the Surgeon General's conference set a precedent for youth inclusion across the country.

A key factor in the development of Health 'N Action! was the opportunity provided by the federal system of care program to have youth attend and give presentations at national meetings. The chance to travel and express youth voice in a setting with respectful adults was life-changing for many youth, and they contributed greatly to the substance of these meetings. Although it was difficult to mobilize resources for youth travel, the county was committed to including youth in all system of care activities and was therefore determined to include youth in each delegation sent to national system of care meetings. System of care leaders learned that it is important to bring at least two youth to each meeting to ensure peer support because meetings can be intimidating.

As the organization evolved, many opportunities were found for Health 'N Action! youth to participate in policy-level discussions. They became part of the citizen advisory board for the state Division of Mental Health's Child and Family Section, and they were instrumental in getting that section renamed the Child, Youth, and Family Section. They accompanied King County mental health staff

---

Box 10.3. Reflections on promoting an organization to mobilize youth voice by Dr. Charles Huffine, Medical Director, Child and Adolescent Programs, King County Mental Health, Chemical Abuse and Dependency Services Division, Seattle, Washington

I had long felt that mental health leaders should embrace youth voice as a critical element of consumer voice as we work our way toward a more recovery-oriented system. I was fortunate that key leaders in our county mental health authority were strongly supportive of my point of view. It seemed unusual to many to have the prime initiative for a youth empowerment movement come from a part-time medical director. My passion and motivation for this cause came from my years as a clinician serving adolescents.

Throughout my career, I had worked with youth in impossible situations where they were misunderstood by each element of the system of care they touched, labeled as "bad kids," and shunted to programs that "managed" rather then addressed their critical mental health and developmental issues. It has always impressed me that youth see strengths and weaknesses in our system of care with amazing clarity and share their common perceptions among their peers. Finding youth willing to speak up and share such perceptions with those in charge of programs had always seemed to me a rare but special treat. Finding smart and perceptive youth willing to shed their cynicism and speak up became my passion. Folding this passion into our system of care was a phenomenal opportunity. I felt that I owed it to the youth and their families to take full advantage of the window of opportunity that was being provided.

Good intentions and good will from my county partners was not enough to create a youth program. Partnering with those who had the administrative capacity to make it happen proved critical to realizing this dream. My clinician's awareness and experience was a critical element but only one element in creating a successful youth advocacy program. I appreciate the wise administrators, youth workers, parents, and the many wonderful youth who worked to realize this dream.

---

and family members to all major stakeholder meetings as the state system reorganized. They also testified before state legislative committees. Health 'N Action! youth developed an outstanding reputation as active participants in many system of care activities, including social marketing and providing technical assistance to other youth programs. They were respected, even though they occasionally testified to the ineffectiveness of certain policies and programs. In addition, they continued their national role, including a plenary presentation provided by three Health 'N Action! members at a national system of care training conference in 2002. One of the speakers became recognized as an emerging national leader and was ultimately hired as the Youth Resource Specialist for the Technical Assistance Partnership for Child and Family Mental Health. The organization's advocacy contributed to the establishment of youth partnerships as a core element of the federal system of care program requirements.

As the system of care grants were ending in 2005, King County's Health 'N Action! and Clark County's youth program began their evolution toward becoming a statewide youth organization renamed Youth 'N Action! Affiliation with a family organization (SAFE WA) provided the infrastructure for the statewide youth group and enabled a continuation of its role in providing youth voice for mental health policy at local, state, and national levels.

Members and Youth Coordinators

Youth ages 14–22 may become members of Youth 'N Action!; some youth continue after age 22 in volunteer roles. They may join Youth 'N Action! at the suggestion of a wraparound team or through referrals from peers, families, mental health counselors, probation officers, care managers, or school system personnel. Many have histories of involvement with multiple systems, including special education for behavioral disturbances, juvenile justice, and child welfare. Many have histories of drug and alcohol difficulties, mental health hospitalizations, foster care placements, and family disruptions. Peers and youth coordinators provide an accepting and supportive environment as youth share their stories and learn to become advocates for improvements in youth-serving systems.

Some youth are not involved in mental health services when they become involved in the organization because they may not perceive mental health programs as welcoming, helpful, or culturally appropriate. Youth and their families, however, may find their way into a treatment program after they become involved in Youth 'N Action! The reflections of a Youth 'N Action! member are presented in Box 10.4.

At least two youth coordinators serve as paid staff to Youth 'N Action! and are integral to the program. Many youth share their problems with youth coordinators and receive strong support from them. The youth–youth coordinator relationship has some therapeutic aspects, but youth coordinators primarily function as natural supports. It is helpful if a youth coordinator has had direct relatable experience in the system of care.

Other adults may be involved as volunteers. It is important to ensure the safety of the youth through proper background checks, insurance certificates, and safety policies. Youth 'N Action! does not specifically exclude youth coordinators and volunteers who have had challenges as youth, including a history of legal difficulties as juveniles or young adults. Individuals who have overcome such difficulties, if properly screened and supervised, may offer a uniquely inspirational relationship to youth who are at risk.

Roles and Activities

Regional branches of Youth 'N Action! meet at least once per month. Often, other activities take place throughout the month as members take part in peer support, program development, policy, cultural, community service, and fun social activities that they are interested in doing as a group. The roles of Youth 'N Action! and its affiliates include:

des of conduct defined by youth are more strict and creative than any that might be imposed by adult authorities. Youth coordinators can assist in enforcing rules established by the youth. For example, a rule against gambling was adopted by the Health 'N Action! group at an early point in its development. Youth coordinators had no idea that this was a significant issue, but they became aware of the problem, and as directed by the youth, enforced that rule on several occasions.

The prospect of being chosen for travel continues to be a prime motivator for many youth. As the national youth movement grows, identifying with that effort has become a major source of motivation to continue efforts at the local level. Helping youth to define their own code of conduct while traveling and creating their own sanctions for infractions goes a long way toward attenuating liability concerns by those who sponsor youth travel.

Providing training, speaking, and travel opportunities for Youth 'N Action! members has been challenging without federal grant funding, but the program has attempted to continue these features. SAFE WA has been able to maintain the core value that youth should be respected for their participation by paying them stipends when they are volunteering their time in meetings for which adults are preparing and attending as part of their paid employment. Youth are also provided with a youth-friendly lunch, refreshments, and transportation (e.g., bus tokens, reimbursement to parents, driving expenses for older youth). Some youth are able to gain credit in school for their activities in Youth 'N Action!, and some are able to count their time involved in the youth group toward their community service hours owed as part of their probation. Youth 'N Action! holds fast to the three Cs of compensation—*community* service, *cash*, and school/court *credit*.

Sustaining the Dream

As the federal system of care grant ended, the King County system of care worked hard to plan for sustaining Health 'N Action! The first step in sustaining the movement was to ask the youth what they wanted. Did they want to create an organization with their own 501(c)(3) status? Did they want to partner with a family organization? Did they want to stay with King County under a government agency? Youth also had many questions. What could be a funding source? Where would the group meet? Could stipends and food at meetings be continued? Who would serve as the youth coordinator? Who would arrange transportation or provide youth with rides to the meetings? How were the youth going to sustain their role in a broad system partnership? How could they maintain their independent role in their partnerships as they became a fully operational youth organization devoted to promoting youth voice in public policy? What role would they have in determining the governing of a new statewide organization? The answers to these and other questions eventually emerged.

Initial efforts to sustain the group failed. The seed money provided by the federal system of care grant was lost. The long-time youth coordinator had to find other employment and could not commit to Youth 'N Action! in the same capacity in which she had previously served. Several of the youth leaders were aging

---

Box 10.4. Reflections of a current Youth 'N Action! member
by Kayla Paulson

As I was growing up, it became obvious that I had some big issues. My temper tantrums were especially bad. I would go on kicking and screaming for hours as a child. I was easily distracted, and I never listened to my mother. My parents started getting evaluations and trying different medications when I was 5. When I was 9, I was diagnosed with bipolar disorder. I have been diagnosed with OCD, GAD, ADHD, and ODD—basically alphabet soup with a side order of bipolar. I also struggled with an eating disorder, and I became a frequent cutter. I have been on every medication you could possibly imagine. From the time that I was 12, I was in and out of hospitals and treatment centers. As a teenager, I was sick of treatment, refused medications, and was often out of control. In these bad times, I was raped, so now I am dealing with PTSD symptoms and other problems related to a really traumatic experience.

When I was 14 and in my era of being discouraged with treatment, I met Stephanie Lane and Charley Huffine (youth coordinators for Youth 'N Action!). Stephanie came to talk at my mental health center and spoke to us about Youth 'N Action! Through this program, I began to feel empowered by speaking at conferences and meeting public officials. I was a speaker at the Orlando Georgetown Training Institutes, but my life was still out of control. I had dark periods when I had trouble respecting myself. My mom insisted that I get back on meds. I had had terrible experiences with psychiatrists. I refused to see anyone but Dr. Huffine, who I got to know well from Youth 'N Action! He had already agreed to be a natural support on my wraparound team. I just call him Charley. Charley and I talked about what it would be like for him to be my psychiatrist and my youth coordinator. We talked about it and agreed to try it.

So far, it's worked out great. He is the coolest psychiatrist that I have ever had. He was patient with me and didn't force me to go on medications, but he didn't let me rule them out either. After one more stupid mistake, it was obvious to me that I needed to be on medication. I feel like a partner in my treatment team as well as Youth 'N Action! I feel I have better control over my treatment process. I am actually taking bipolar meds, not hating it, and I can see that they help me. I now feel supported by my family and friends. Stephanie and Charley believed in me throughout my bad times with bad choices and unpleasant consequences. They keep telling me that I have a "great gift of gab" and that I need to keep talking about the system of care that I know so well. I now feel like a leader instead of a loser.

My goal as a youth leader is to improve the system for those who come after me. I will advocate for more relevant services in elements of the system that touched my life. My passion is for getting better help for girls who have been traumatized in addition to having mental health problems. I think we need more prevention programs so that teen girls know how to avoid being sexually assaulted. I want to help girls know it's not their fault and that it's okay to come forward and talk about what happened rather than feel ashamed. I think young women need to know that they are still strong, beautiful people.

Having a mental illness has really affected my life in some terrible ways, but my life is now back on track. Those like me, the ones who live life with a mental illness, know what it is like. We know what the services are really like. We know what could be improved. It empowers me when I tell my story and give youth voice to how to improve the system of care for youth.

- Supporting the role of youth consumers in guiding their own individualized services through exposure to general peer support and, when appropriate, requesting peer involvement on their wraparound team

- Supporting the role of peers in providing support to individual peers with mental health challenges, including involvement as team members for peers involved in a wraparound process

- Participation and decision making in agency-level program development to assure that services are more relevant to youth consumers

- Contributing to the development of relevant public policy with respect to youth services and legislation.

Mobilizing youth to speak at local and national meetings is a core activity for Youth 'N Action! Many youth are eager to share their stories openly with one another and in public speaking settings, whereas others are more reticent. Youth stories are personal, and young people should always be in charge of how much or how little they disclose. It is important that youth coordinators prepare them for any feelings they might have after they share their stories publicly. Sharing is not a requirement for Youth 'N Action!, but many roads to recovery have begun with one young person sharing stories with another. Bonds develop that let each person know that he or she is no longer alone.

Youth 'N Action! members have made substantial contributions to policy events. Recent examples include participation in a meeting of child and adolescent program directors from King County contract agencies held to discuss the nature of recovery from mental health difficulties in children and youth. They also allied with several other youth programs from around the state to participate in a Youth Legislative Advocacy Day with the 2007 Washington State Legislature. In addition, a youth partnership art project has been organized to combine the talents of all of the Youth 'N Action! members, which involves the making of a quilt that speaks out against stigma to be put on display around the state in different malls.

Training youth to tell their stories and offer their perspectives on systems of care is a continuous process. As new youth emerge wanting to participate, the monthly meetings are devoted in part to training new members and helping them learn how to speak in public and tell their personal stories. Youth coordinators have critical roles in facilitating this process, but it is owned by the members. Training focuses on such issues as how government works, how to fit into the culture of government meetings, which may be boring and not youth-friendly, and tolerating and coping with tokenism.

Youth have clearly expressed that a prime reason to be involved with Youth 'N Action! is to participate in local, state, and national meetings because it allows them to be involved in discussions of issues of importance to youth and to offer a clear and substantive youth voice. A plan for funding youth travel locally, statewide, and nationally is emerging. SAFE WA has contributed the perspective that parents need to know their children will be safe when participating in Youth

'N Action! activities and that funders need to ensure compliance with regulations designed for safety. The new rules can sometimes be d youth to understand, and tension over this issue remains unresolved.

Values and Principles of Youth Voice

Values and principles are important in sustaining any youth organizati to support and advocacy. The central value for such organizations is th consumers deserve respect and honor for their expertise. In Youth 'N A the intention that youth voice is respected and serves as the force tha entire process. Three key guiding principles are as follows:

- Youth shall set the agenda for the organization.

- Youth shall choose which opportunities they want to pursue.

- Youth shall determine how they want to govern themselves.

Core values of mutual respect, inclusion, and collaboration rema even though group membership changes over time and subgroups Subgroups can emerge naturally within a group, and it often falls on y nators and leaders to ensure that these subgroups integrate into the Many factors contribute to these subgroups, such as geographic origi in upbringing, ethnicity, level of maturity, social groups from school experiences (e.g., dropping out of school, homelessness, gang involve

In addition, the nature of a group such as Youth 'N Action! is th eventually leave due to natural aging out. As youth begin as gene they learn to articulate their personal stories, gain perspective on pa and come to accept that their stories may have meaning for others. ready to take on speaking engagements and internal leadership ro this process, many emerge as positive forces in their own families within their peer and community networks. A few go on to take na ship roles. Others drift away to follow developmental prerogatives su more schooling. Accepting every members' course through their tin 'N Action! is a strong group value. There is a continuous dynamic defining the group.

If the group's values and principles are clearly established and the group members and then repeatedly acknowledged, members are full partners in observing them. Meetings are opportunities fe ceive training on how to relate to one another. Teaching interpers ness is a constant learning task for participants and permeates all tions that youth coordinators, administrators, and volunteers ha and their families.

Developing youth-driven policies and procedures is critical to ing the core values and principles of Youth 'N Action! This is a co undertaken in monthly meetings. When youth set the policies, likely to feel obligated to follow them. Youth 'N Action! has foun

out. Initial attempts to affiliate with a family organization to provide an infrastructure for the group were unsuccessful. The group was faced with no money, no home base, and a great deal of fear. During this process, some youth worked to keep the dream alive, whereas others left in frustration.

The development of a statewide youth organization began at a youth retreat in the summer of 2005. The retreat was strongly supported by SAFE WA and by the state Division of Mental Health. The group included a complex mix of youth from urban King and Clark Counties, rural youth from Eastern Washington, and youth from other smaller towns. A set of governing principles were accepted and officers were elected; however, without the financial support of the federal grants, efforts to create a statewide group faltered.

Ultimately, a primary partnership was developed with SAFE WA. This family organization had a long history of being youth friendly and was the recipient of some Substance Abuse and Mental Health Service Administration (SAMHSA) funding. Benefiting from the family organization's tax exempt status, the group could engage in fund raising. With the assistance of SAFE WA, youth leaders wrote a grant proposal and were awarded $10,000 from Washington State's Mental Health Transformation Project—the first cash award Youth 'N Action! received based on its own merits. The former youth coordinator was engaged as a consultant by SAFE WA to undertake some statewide youth organizing. Based on this work, the Health 'N Action group folded into the statewide organization Youth 'N Action! In 2006, the first paid youth coordinator was hired for the new statewide organization, and a second was hired in 2007.

Support for youth voice has also developed through the state's mental health transformation initiative. Washington State was one of the first nine states to receive a federal transformation grant from SAMHSA. The state's mental health transformation initiative is committed to youth partnership and has dedicated resources to incorporating youth voice by contracting with SAFE WA. These resources have enabled the hiring of the two part-time youth coordinators—one for the eastern region of the state and one for the western region. This has further supported the growth and establishment of the statewide youth organization. Statewide status has brought new challenges, such as constraints on youth travel due to liability concerns and the need to educate new partners about the importance of youth-guided, youth-directed, and youth-driven service systems; however, the group continues to evolve, preserving the values and principles of youth inclusion in systems of care.

Evaluation

The impact of youth organizations such as Youth 'N Action! on the system of care in Washington State has been great. The impact of youth organizations on the mental health and development of its members must be carefully defined and measured to provide evidence that participation can enhance treatment and recovery from mental health problems. Avenues of funding would likely open up for well-evaluated youth support and advocacy programs that are found to be effective. Youth 'N Action! is considered a promising practice with anecdotal evidence to substantiate its impact. Although participation in youth programs such as Youth 'N Action! is not specifically a treatment element per se, youth report feeling relieved that they are included and respected for who they are and that they are not defined by the challenges they have endured. Youth 'N Action! provides a strength-based experience for youth. The experience of sharing their stories and opinions regarding the system of care, being mentors to youth still struggling, and receiving appreciation for community service helps youth to shape their emerging adult identities. Experience has demonstrated that youth often reduce or cease self-destructive behavior, renounce gang activity and violence, reduce their use of drugs, return to school, and forge partnership relationships with adults for the first time as a direct result of participation in Youth 'N Action! Membership in Youth 'N Action! plays a positive role in young people developing protective factors, diminishing risk factors, and becoming involved in growth-promoting, positive community experiences.

Little formal evaluation of youth organizations has been conducted as yet; however, in 2006, with the Youth 'N Action! minigrant from the Mental Health Transformation Project, some funds were specified for developing an evaluation process. The group will collaborate with local youth-friendly evaluators to realize the ideal of a youth-driven measurement process in which Youth 'N Action! members will participate in drafting questions; receive training on how to administer the survey; and evaluate the effectiveness of their youth voice in public policy, peer-to-peer support, community service, and other activities.

CONCLUSION

Youth voice in driving their own care, supporting peers, and determining public policy is an uplifting, spirit-enhancing experience for youth involved in systems of care. Youth often come into Youth 'N Action! with broken spirits after years without any voice in the care they had received. The author and activist Pat Deegan (1999) stated,

> The experience of spirit breaking occurs as a result of those cumulative experiences in which we are humiliated and made to feel less than human, in which our will to live is deeply shaken or broken, in which our hopes are shattered and in which giving up, apathy, and indifference become a way of surviving and protecting the last vestiges of the wounded self.

Young people joining Youth 'N Action! find developmentally supportive pathways to self-recovery, as well as opportunities to contribute to the recovery of the system. In combination with competent and recovery-oriented treatment, participation in a youth organization such as Youth 'N Action! helps youth build on their inherent strengths and realize that they can make a difference.

REFERENCES

Bernard, B. (1996). Fostering resiliency in kids: Protective factors in the family, school and community. In *Advancing youth development: A curriculum for training youth workers.*

Washington, DC: Academy for Educational Development, Center for Youth Development and Policy Research.

Burns, B., Hoagwood, K., & Mrazek, D. (1999). Effective treatment for mental disorders in children and adolescents. *Clinical Child and Family Psychology Review, 2*(4), 199–254.

Checkoway, B., & Richards-Schuster, K. (2003). Youth participation in community evaluation research. *American Journal of Evaluation 24*(1), 21–33. Retrieved October 29, 2004, from http://www.ssw.umich.edu/youthandcommunity/pubs/AJE_Paper.pdf

Deegan, P. (1999). *Advocacy I: Seize the power!* Salt Lake City, UT: Independent Living Network.

Drake, I.N., Ling, S., Fitch, E., & Hughes, D. (2000, Fall). Youth are the future of America. In *Focal Point: A National Bulletin on Family Support and Children's Mental Health, 14,* 32–34. Retrieved October 29, 2004, from http://www.rtc.pdx.edu/pgPubsScript .php?documentID=346&choice=download

Fischhoff, B., Crowell, N., & Kipke, M. (Eds.). (1999). *Adolescent decision making: Implications for prevention programs: summary of a workshop.* Washington, DC: National Academies Press.

Hart, R.A. (1992). Children's participation: From tokenism to citizenship. In *Innocenti Essay, 4,* 8. Florence, Italy: UNICEF International Child Development Centre.

Hoover, A., & Weisenbach, A. (1999). Youth leading now! Securing a place at the table. *New Designs for Youth Development, 15*(3), 29–35. Retrieved October, 29, 2004, from http://www.cydjournal.org/NewDesigns/ND_99Sum/Hoover.html

Innovation Center for Community and Youth Development. (1996). *Creating youth/adult partnerships: A training curricula for youth, adults, and youth/adult teams.* Takoma Park, MD: Author.

Institute for Mental Health Initiatives. (1999, Fall). Resilience. *Dialogue: Insights into Human Emotions for Creative Professionals, 7*(1). Retrieved October 29, 2004, from http://www.gwumc.edu/sphhs/imhi/downloads/dialogue/Resilience_Vol7_Fa99.pdf

Kirshner, B., O'Donoghue, J.L., & McLaughlin, M.W. (Eds.). (2003). *New directions for youth development: Youth participation improving institutions and communities.* San Francisco, CA: Jossey-Bass.

Lampron, S., Poirier, J.M., & Quinn, M.M. (in progress). *Systems improvement activities to enhance children's mental health services: Youth involvement report.* Washington, DC: American Institutes for Research.

Lewis, A. (Ed.). (2003). *Shaping the future of American youth: Youth policy in the 21st century.* Washington, DC: American Youth Policy Forum. Retrieved October 29, 2004, from http://www.aypf.org/publications/shaping_future_youth.pdf

Matarese, M., McGinnis, L., & Mora, M. (2005). *Youth involvement in systems of care: A guide to empowerment.* Retrieved October 11, 2007, from http://www.tapartnership.org/ youth/youthguide.asp

National Clearinghouse on Families and Youth. (1996). *Reconnecting youth and community: A youth development approach.* Silver Spring, MD: U.S. Department of Health and Human Services, Administration for Children and Families, Administration on Children, Youth and Families, Family and Youth Services Bureau. Retrieved October 29, 2004, from http://www.ncfy.com/Reconnec.htm

Pittman, K., & Cahill, M. (1992, February). *Youth and caring: The role of youth programs in the development of caring.* Paper commissioned by the Lilly Endowment Research Grants Program on Youth and Caring and presented at the Conference on Youth and Caring.

President's New Freedom Commission on Mental Health. (2003) *Achieving the promise: Transforming mental health care in America. Final report* (DHHS Pub. No. SMA-03-3832). Rockville, MD: Author.

Roach, C., Yu, H.C., & Lewis-Charp, H. (2001). Race, poverty, and youth development. *Poverty and Race, 10*(4), 3–6. Retrieved October, 29, 2004, from http://www.prrac.org/full _text.php?text_id=21&item_id=167&newsletter_id=57&header=Poverty+%2F+Welfare

Sydlo, S.J., Schensul, J.J., Owens, D.C., Brase, M.K., Wiley, K.N., Berg, M.J., et al. (2000). *Participatory action research curriculum for empowering youth.* Hartford, CT: The Institute for Community Research.

Thomlison, B. (2003). Characteristics of evidence-based maltreatment interventions. *Child Welfare, 82,* 541–569.

Youth Motivating Others Through Voices of Experience (M.O.V.E.). (2006). *Youth-guided.* Retrieved October 11, 2007, from http://systemsofcare.samhsa.gov/header menus/docsHM/youthguidedlinkBreakdown.pdf

Zeldin, S. (1995). *An introduction to youth development concepts: Questions for community collaborations.* Washington, DC: Academy for Education Development, Center for Youth Development and Policy Research.

11

Cultural and Linguistic Competence and Eliminating Disparities

MAREASA R. ISAACS, VIVIAN HOPKINS JACKSON,
REGENIA HICKS, AND ED K.S. WANG

A merica's unique contributions to the world and its most persistent challenges at home derive from the same roots—the diversity of its population. This diversity fuels strength in the arts, sports, science, technology, literature, and other areas of achievements. That same diversity, however, fuels persistent and seemingly intractable inequities in the quality of life and opportunity for many Americans, including those in rural and urban core communities; members of various faith communities; those who are gay, lesbian, bisexual, or transgender; and especially those who are people of color—Hispanics/Latinos, African Americans, Asian Americans, American Indians, Alaskan Natives, Native Hawaiians, and Other Pacific Islanders. In 2004, people of color accounted for more than 30% of the U.S. population, with Hispanics/Latinos being the largest ethnic population group at 14%, followed by African Americans at 12%; Asian Americans at 5%, and American Indians/Alaskan Natives at 1% (U.S. Census Bureau, 2002). By 2025, these groups are projected to make up 40% of the U.S. population, and by 2050, nearly one in four Americans will be of Hispanic origin.

There is growing demographic evidence that the characteristics of people of color are very different from the characteristics of the White population in the United States. These differences include the following:

- **Larger proportions of children and young adults**

Although the White population is growing older, the population growth within other ethnic groups is concentrated in children and young adults. Among Whites, 22% of the population is under the age of 18, compared with 34% of Hispanics/ Latinos, 33% of American Indians/Alaskan Natives, and 31% of African Americans.

- **Populations with larger proportions of immigrants and refugees**

A much larger proportion of populations of color are made up of immigrants and refugees than in the White population. Those in the United States who are foreign born or have at least one foreign-born parent total more than 55.9 million individuals, or approximately 20% of the total U.S. population (U.S. Census Bureau, 2002). Although they enter this country with an identity based on the traditions of their home countries, they often become *racialized* as they continue to live in this country.

- **Higher rates of poverty (socioeconomic status)**

The evidence has been consistent in demonstrating a relationship between mental health status and poverty. Differential rates of poverty are staggering between mainstream America and people of color. In 2002, the overall poverty rate in the United States was 12%, meaning that 34 million people were living in poverty. In 2002, 8% of Whites were living in poverty, as compared with 24% of African Americans, 21% of Hispanics/Latinos, and 26% of American Indians/Alaskan Natives. Across all ethnic groups, children are more likely to live in poverty than adults. This statistic is among the highest in the developed world (Annie E. Casey Foundation, 2004a), and the numbers are fueled by the high levels of poverty among children of color.

- **Place matters and exacerbates disadvantage**

A recent study by Acevedo-Garcia, McArdle, Osypuk, Lefkowitz, and Krimgold (2007) found that more than 80% of American children live in metropolitan areas. Within these metropolitan areas, however, African American and Hispanic children lived in vastly different neighborhoods than did White and Asian children. These inequalities go far beyond what can be explained by income differences, suggesting that place really does matter in a myriad of critical ways. Within rural and frontier communities, where the other 20% of American children live, children and families of color have even fewer resources compared with their urban counterparts.

ADDRESSING DISPARITIES AND QUALITY THROUGH CULTURAL AND LINGUISTIC COMPETENCE

People of color and other historically underrepresented populations have experienced disparities in mental health services. These disparities are caused by multiple factors and will require a variety of strategies to achieve resolution. The implementation of culturally and linguistically competent services offers significant opportunities to address the unique needs of racially, ethnically, and culturally diverse populations.

Disparities and Unmet Needs in Children's Mental Health

These differential demographics, in combination with differing cultural values, mores, and practices, have contributed to historical and deeply embedded inequities and disparities in mental health care for these populations. As noted by the Surgeon General's Report on Mental Health,

Ethnic and racial minorities in the United States face a social and economic environment of inequality that includes greater exposure to racism and discrimination, violence, and poverty, all of which take a toll on mental health. Living in poverty has the most measurable impact on rates of mental illness. . . .The cultures of ethnic and racial minorities alter the types of mental health services they use. (U.S. Department of Health and Human Services, 2001, p. 42)

Thus, disparities have been defined as "differences in the incidence, prevalence, mortality, and burden of diseases and other adverse health conditions that exist among specific population groups in the United States" (National Institutes of Health, 2000). In children's mental health systems, disparities exist in access to care, availability of appropriate services, quality of care, and the beneficial outcomes that should be the products of mental health treatment interventions.

The issues of racial, ethnic, and cultural disparities are further complicated in U.S. children's mental health systems simply because all children experience high levels of unmet mental health needs. Mental health and substance abuse services for children and adolescents are severely limited and underfunded, thus creating a great demand for scarce resources. When services are so limited, poor youth and families of color experience significant disadvantages in gaining access to quality treatment due to financial constraints, racial bias, culture and language barriers, fear and distrust, stigma, and different help-seeking behaviors (Cooper-Patrick et al., 1999; Pfeifer, Hu, & Vega, 2000; Pouissant & Alexander, 2000; U.S. Department of Health and Human Services, 2001; Vega et al., 1998; Zhang, Snowden, & Sue, 1998). There is growing evidence that African American and Latino children have higher rates of mental health need (i.e., 11%) than the national average of 7% (National Advisory Mental Health Council Workgroup, 2001; Sturm, Ringel, Stein, & Kapur, 2001). Kataoka, Zhang, and Wells (2002) found that 75% of youth with emotional and behavioral problems do not receive needed services in a given year, and children of color, especially Latino children, have even higher rates of unmet mental health service needs. Data also suggest that biracial children and youth have high unmet mental health and substance abuse service needs compared with White children and other youth of color (McClurg, 2004; Milan & Keiley, 2000).

There are other population groups that have higher rates of unmet mental health needs that also encounter disparities in access, availability, quality, and outcomes of mental health services. These groups include youth who reside in rural areas. Although nearly two thirds of the counties in the United States are rural, less than one fifth of the U.S. child population lives in rural America (Annie E. Casey, 2004b). Due to geographic distances and high levels of poverty (48 of the 50 poorest counties in America are rural), these youth and their families are at a distinct disadvantage when it comes to having access to scarce mental health resources.

Youth who have a different sexual orientation face social stigmatization and higher risks of abuse and traumatic experiences compared with heterosexual youth, and those youth of color face the challenges of having multiple minority status. These youth are often struggling with their own identity formation processes within a hostile social environment. In a 2003 survey of lesbian, gay, bisexual, transgender, and questioning (LGBTQ) youth in American schools, the Gay, Lesbian, Straight Education Network (GLSEN) reported that 33% of LGBTQ students stated that they had attempted suicide in the previous year, compared with 8% of their heterosexual peers. Eighty-four percent of LGBTQ students reported being verbally abused or having their safety threatened; 45% of LGBTQ youth of color experienced verbal harassment or physical assault; and many LBGTQ youth experience homelessness, having been ejected from their homes by their parents upon learning of their children's sexual orientation (Killen-Harvey & Stern-Ellis, 2006). For these youth, there is a sense of uncertainty as to which mental health providers they can trust and a lack of confidence in the likelihood that these providers will be knowledgeable about their issues and concerns.

An additional variable is the experience of youth within all of these groups who have dual diagnoses (e.g., mental health and substance abuse, mental health and intellectual disability) and find themselves without access to adequate mental health services and supports. Thus, racial, ethnic, and cultural disparities have a tremendous impact on many members of America's increasingly diverse youth population. The President's New Freedom Commission (2003) recognized those issues and included a national goal of eliminating racial, ethnic, and rural disparities in mental health.

Cultural and Linguistic Competence as a Strategy to Address Disparities

Walrath, Ybarra, and Holden (2006) conducted a study of factors associated with differential outcomes among children receiving services within systems of care. This study examined a subset of data from the national evaluation of federally funded system of care communities to investigate the characteristics and experiences of children and youth in care. Results revealed that children and youth from minority racial and ethnic backgrounds were *four times* more likely than their nonminority counterparts to deteriorate while receiving services through systems of care.

In 1989, Cross, Bazron, Dennis, and Isaacs, introduced the concept of *cultural competence* to the children's mental health field as a strategy for addressing the inherent racial and ethnic disparities that prevailed in mental health systems for children and their families. Cross and colleagues (1989) aptly noted that children of color lacked access to mental health services and often found themselves in more punitive settings (e.g., juvenile justice and child welfare systems) rather than therapeutic settings in mental health (i.e., *access disparity*). When these children were involved in mental health systems, they were more likely to be placed in restrictive settings such as residential and other out-of-home placements (i.e., *setting disparity*). Even when children of color did receive treatment, they did not often receive the same quality of care as their White counterparts (i.e., *quality of care disparity*). Cross and colleagues (1989) also noted that mental health service systems lacked diversity in their workforces (i.e., *provider disparity*). The outcomes from these disparities often meant that children of color and their families suffered tremendous burdens, disabilities, and truncated opportunities from un-treated and poorly treated mental health conditions (i.e., *outcome disparity*).

In response to these and other disparities, Cross and colleagues (1989) rec-ommended that mental health services and other systems serving children with emotional disturbances strive to become more culturally competent. They intro-duced the concept of cultural competence as a process for addressing existing dis-parities based on race, ethnicity, and culture within mental health services for children of color and their families. Cross and colleagues defined *cultural compe-tence* as follows:

> A set of behaviors, attitudes, and policies that come together in a system, agency, or among professionals that enables them to work effectively in cross-cultural situa-tions. . . .Cultural competence is the acceptance and attention to the dynamics of difference, the ongoing development of cultural knowledge, and the resources and flexibility within service models to meet the needs of minority populations. (1989, p. 1).

Cultural competence was viewed as a developmental process in which both individuals and organizations were engaged. The core elements of cultural compe-tence (i.e., valuing diversity; cultural self-assessment; understanding cross-cultural differences; institutionalization of cultural knowledge; and adaptation of policies, services, and structures based on diversity) implied the types of strategies that might be utilized to implement cultural competence. In addition, as a part of the initial conceptualization, Cross and colleagues (1989) suggested that cultural com-petence could be viewed as a continuum, ranging from cultural destructiveness to cultural proficiency (steps include cultural destructiveness, cultural incapacity, cul-tural blindness, cultural precompetence, cultural competence, and cultural profi-ciency), along which an individual or an organization could establish a baseline and measure progress. Later, *linguistic competence* was added to provide greater em-phasis on the role of language in cultural competence (Goode & Jones, 2006; Goode, Sockalingam, Brown, & Jones, 2000; Office of Minority Health, 2000).

Throughout this time, cultural and linguistic competence has been recog-nized as one of the guiding principles in the development of systems of care (Stroul & Friedman, 1986). Not only is cultural and linguistic competence an ap-proach to address disparities, but more fundamentally, it is a necessary compo-nent for quality of care.

Cultural and Linguistic Competence as a Strategy to Achieve Quality

Effective mental health services require a relationship between the service provid-ers and those who are receiving services. One cannot attain ultimate quality ser-vice without cultural and linguistic competence. Bordin (1979) asserted that ther-apeutic alliance occurs when the client and the practitioner come to an agreement on: 1) the goals of therapy, 2) the tasks needed to achieve the agreed-on goals, and 3) the development of an interpersonal bond. To be effective in any such relationship, the service provider must understand the child, youth, and family's view of the problem; the strategies the child, youth, and family have used and want to use to address the problem; and the criteria the child, youth, and family will use to evaluate success. Although these components may appear to be self-evident, the definition of the problem, the expected role of the helper, and the expected role of the client are each defined within the cultural context. The service journey includes several very important steps:

1. Identifying the need to seek help

2. Determining who to approach for help

3. Following the process and theory supporting an assessment or diagnosis

4. Following the process for creating the content of a treatment or service plan

5. Following the process of plan implementation

6. Defining successful or unsuccessful outcomes

7. Determining relationships at the conclusion of formal service delivery

The steps are all influenced by the cultural lenses of every participant in the service experience (Jackson, 1997). This includes the cultural lenses of the children, youth, families, and their communities, as well as the cultural lenses of the service providers as individuals, their disciplines, the organizations offering the services, the larger service system, and the overarching community within which the service system exists.

Cross and colleagues (1989) defined the term *culture* as "the integrated pattern of human behavior that includes thoughts, communication styles, actions, customs, beliefs, values, and institutions of a racial, ethnic, religious, or social group" (p. 13). The challenge for the providers of services and supports is to develop those services and supports in a manner that links with the thoughts, communication styles, actions, customs, values, beliefs, and institutions to ensure that the needs of the children, youth, and families are met within the context of their culturally informed world view.

In addition to attention to the values and beliefs of children, youth, and families, cultural and linguistic competence must also address issues related to social justice. This perspective acknowledges that different population groups have had different types of experiences with the dominant society in general and with service delivery provided by the dominant society in particular. The racism, ethnocentrism, stereotypes (positive and negative), discrimination, bias, and prejudice that diverse cultural groups have experienced, both historically and currently, influence the nature of emotional and behavioral distress, their understanding of the experience of emotional and behavioral distress, and the identities of the people from whom they seek assistance for relieving that distress. These parallel and intertwining processes create the cultural variables that the service system must address to be effective. These factors are relevant to both the quality of services and the elimination of racial and ethnic disparities.

IMPLEMENTING CULTURAL AND LINGUISTIC COMPETENCE IN CHILDREN'S MENTAL HEALTH

Against this backdrop, a system of care providing services must acknowledge and respond to the multiple cultures within the community and address the history of *isms* that are salient within that community. It must do so in full recognition that every person who works within the system of care as a board member, agency executive, staff person, manager, volunteer, family member, community member, child, and youth enters the system of care with their personal experiences, knowledge, skills, attitudes, biases, prejudices, and history framed from within their own cultural communities. All these factors influence their approach to diversity within the service system.

The work of creating a culturally and linguistically competent system of care is a complex task that affects every component of the system. It requires the focused and sustained attention of those in positions to make decisions and allocate resources. It requires a set of values, policies, and structures to institutionalize processes and practices that promote the creation and adaptation of services and supports that address the cultural and linguistic needs of the service population. The process of creating a culturally and linguistically competent system of care must address both the learning needs and the attitudes of all system participants in a manner that allows for effective cross-cultural interactions.

External Drivers for Change

Although some organizations, agencies, and providers have understood the need for effective cross-cultural and culture-specific practice, many have only instituted change because of external expectations. There is a growing body of legislation, guidelines, and standards that have set expectations for organizations to seriously address the unique cultures and languages reflected in the communities they serve. The legal mandate for language access was articulated in Title VI of the Civil Rights Act of 1964 (PL 88-352), as well as the subsequent Executive Order No. 13166 and guidance from the U.S. Department of Health and Human Services. Additional standards for cultural and linguistic competence include the following:

- Cultural Competence Standards in Managed Mental Health Care Services: Four Underserved/Underrepresented Racial/Ethnic Groups (Center for Mental Health Services, 2000).

- National Standards for Culturally and Linguistically Appropriate Services in Health Care (CLAS Standards) (Office of Minority Health, 2000).

- Guidelines on Multicultural Education, Training, Research, Practice, and Organizational Change for Psychologists (American Psychiatric Association, 2002)

- Indicators for the Achievement of the National Association of Social Workers (NASW) Standards for Cultural Competence in the Social Work Profession (NASW, 2001, 2007)

As levers to promote change, these standards have stimulated progress by affirming the importance of cultural and linguistic competence and offering examples and strategies to achieve it. Some practitioners and agencies have chosen to use these standards as both a guide for practice and an advocacy tool. Even so, standards alone have not transformed services and supports.

Elements of Transformative Change

Organizations that are successful in the provision of effective services for multicultural service populations operate from a value base that supports that work. The field has produced various types of technical assistance materials and guidance on what to do to facilitate this type of culture change in organizations, offering strategies to help organizations make this type of transition. A report from the Commonwealth Fund entitled *Taking Cultural Competency from Theory to Action* (Wu & Martinez, 2006) offers the following six factors as critical elements for implementation of cultural competency in the health sector:

1. Community representation and feedback is essential at all stages of implementation.

2. Cultural competency must be integrated into all existing systems of a health care organization, particularly quality improvement efforts.

3. Changes made should be manageable, measurable, and sustainable.

4. Making the business case for undertaking cultural competency initiatives is critical for long-term sustainability.

5. Commitment from leadership is a key factor to success.

6. Ongoing staff training is crucial.

Getting Started . . . and Moving On, published by the National Center on Cultural Competence at Georgetown University (Goode & Jackson, 2003), offers a similar set of 12 tasks that can help mobilize an organization toward this organizational change process:

1. Create a structure.

2. Clarify values and philosophy.

3. Develop a logic model for cultural and linguistic competence.

4. Keep abreast of community demographics.

5. Assess family and youth satisfaction.

6. Create structures for family and youth involvement.

7. Conduct a self-assessment.

8. Determine staff and volunteer development needs and interests.

9. Engage communities.

10. Create a plan for achieving cultural and linguistic competence.

11. Adopt or adapt lessons learned.

12. Create a refuge for sharing and learning.

Key themes from these and other guides on approaches to the transformation of organizations suggest the need to have an entity within the organization responsible for guiding its work in this transformational journey. Guidance suggests that leadership, staff at all levels, consumers, and the community must all be engaged in the process, and the change process must be deliberative. In addition, the organization must engage in a process to think through its values and its change theory, create a plan, and monitor the implementation of the plan. Furthermore, addressing staff needs is critical. Although training is important, service providers must also have a safe place to authentically address their feelings.

Thus, there are clear mandates that require organizations to pursue this course, growing evidence on the benefits of culturally and linguistically competent practice, and guidance to help organizations pursue the journey.

Achieving Transformation

Although system of care communities acknowledge and embrace the values and guiding principles of systems of care, many have struggled with effective implementation. Cultural and linguistic competence is one area of challenge for the majority of communities funded through the federal Comprehensive Community Mental Health Services for Children and Their Families Program. Since 1999, the Technical Assistance Partnership for Child and Family Mental Health (TA Partnership) has been responsible for providing technical assistance, training, and support for the federally funded system of care communities. During this time, the TA Partnership has been the technical assistance leader in the area of cultural and linguistic competence. The provision of technical assistance and support has been a coordinated effort involving the resources and expertise of other organizations and consultants, including the National Center for Cultural Competence at Georgetown University, the Louis de la Parte Florida Mental Health Institute at the University of South Florida, and the National Alliance of Multi-Ethnic Behavioral Health Associations.

Several critical factors, however, have limited the successful implementation of cultural and linguistic competence within systems of care. It is discouraging to note that these are some the same factors that were documented in 1991 by Isaacs and Benjamin and have been recounted by others. They include a need for:

1. A full-time position responsible for cultural and linguistic competence

2. A dedicated budget and resources for cultural and linguistic competence

3. Cultural and linguistic competence to be integrated throughout all aspects of service planning, delivery, and evaluation

4. Key policy makers and administrative authorities to support and ensure the implementation of cultural and linguistic competence within government, agencies, and organizations

5. Governing and advisory boards composed of culturally and ethnically diverse members that are representative of the community served

Similar conclusions were found in the 2003 Technical Assistance Planning Interview on Cultural Competence conducted by the National Center for Cultural Competence (Goode & Jackson, 2005). Thirty system of care communities participated in a process that involved interviews with project directors, lead family contacts, and staff or committees with responsibilities related to cultural and linguistic competence. At the time, these system of care communities identified staffing as a major barrier to serving culturally and linguistically diverse populations, as well as recruiting consultants and providers. Additional issues included the following:

- Low numbers of staff possessed the knowledge and skills necessary for serving refugee and immigrant populations.

- Staff responsible for leading organizational efforts felt overwhelmed by the magnitude of the work.

- Rural system of care communities were concerned with the increase of Latino families and their lack of knowledge and skill in providing services to this population.

The participants also reported major barriers resulting from a limited understanding of the basic framework of cultural competence and strategies for implementation, the inability to identify and create tools to monitor organizational performance, the leadership's lack of commitment to the promotion of diversity, the negative impact of racism and discrimination within the service area, a limited ability to ensure language access, an unwillingness to involve and share power with families, and the leadership's reluctance to acknowledge the extent of the problem (Goode & Jackson, 2005).

Goode and Jackson (2005) summarized the difficulties faced by system of care communities in implementing cultural and linguistic competence within four major themes:

1. *Strategies used by communities did not address the nature of the problem*—Training, expanding workforce diversity, and increasing translation and interpretation services were common interventions, but they did not have an impact on critical barriers of prejudice, discrimination, and racism.

2. *The vision for cultural and linguistic competence was not supported by planning or resources*—System of care communities articulated a desire to achieve cultural and linguistic competence, but they did not have a coordinated plan or dedicated resources for implementation.

3. *Difficulty was evident when it came to translating theory into practice in system of care communities*—Several communities were immersed in analyzing the concepts of cultural and linguistic competence, but they could not move into the action steps of creating a logic model or a change strategy for improving service delivery.

4. *The concept of culture was confused with race and ethnicity*—Some system of care communities used these terms interchangeably. This resulted in their inability to recognize and respond to cultural variables (e.g., geography, class, region, faith communities, sexual orientation) among racially homogeneous groups and to only apply cultural competence to people of color (Goode & Jackson, 2005).

The literature and direct responses from individuals working within systems of care provide overwhelming support for the role of cultural and linguistic competence and acknowledge the challenges faced in effective implementation. *The Cultural and Linguistic Competence Implementation Guide* (Martinez & Van Buren, 2008), developed by the TA Partnership at the American Institutes of Research, is a technical assistance tool designed to help communities shift their thinking and action. It identifies six key domains that organizations and communities must address to improve outcomes for diverse populations (Box 11.1).

EXAMPLES OF IMPLEMENTING CULTURAL AND LINGUISTIC COMPETENCE IN SYSTEMS OF CARE

Several system of care communities utilize the framework from the Implementation Guide to implement cultural and linguistic competence and are receiving ongoing coaching and support through regularly scheduled community of practice calls. Three of these systems of care have been identified as practice examples with strategies in place to address the various domains. These include the state of Maine; Butte County, California; and Monroe County, New York. In addition, an example of a statewide approach to implementing cultural and linguistic competence is found in Massachusetts.

Connecting Circles of Care: Butte County, California

There are approximately 55,000 children younger than 18 years old living in Butte County, California, a rural county that encompasses a small city and several

---

Box 11.1. Domains for implementation of cultural and linguistic competence in systems of care

- *Organization infrastructure*—This domain addresses the organizational resources, policy making leadership, and other oversight vehicles an organization needs to deliver or facilitate the delivery of culturally competent care.

- *Services and supports*—This domain addresses how organizations plan, deliver, and facilitate services, supports, and interventions that respond to the unique cultural and linguistic needs of the population served.

- *Planning and continuous quality improvements*—This domain includes the mechanisms and processes that an organization or agency can use to assess its level of cultural and linguistic competence. Strategies include organizational self-assessment, collection and use of cultural and linguistic information, and tracking and maintaining data.

- *Collaboration*—This domain describes specific strategies that support the development of effective working relationships between provider organizations, consumers, and the community at large to promote cultural and linguistic competence.

- *Communication*—This domain describes strategies for promoting the exchange of information and the development of collaborative relationships among system of care providers, consumers, and the community at large to develop, implement, and evaluate the effectiveness of services to diverse populations.

- *Workforce development*—This domain addresses an organization's effort to recruit and retain a culturally and linguistically representative staff to ensure that staff and other service providers have the skills and knowledge for effective services delivery.

Source: Isaacs (2005).

---

small towns, as well as isolated rural mountain areas and four rancherias. One fifth of all families with children in this county live in extreme poverty. The ethnic composition of children is 75% European American, 13.8% Latino, 7.6% Asian (primarily Hmong), 1.8% African American, and 1.75% Native American.

In 1998, Feather River Tribal Health, a Native American nonprofit tribal organization, received a 3-year Circles of Care grant from the Center for Mental Health Services of the Substance Abuse and Mental Health Services Administration to assess, plan, and design a mental health system of care for Native American children experiencing severe emotional disturbance. With the success of Circles of Care as their foundation, Feather River Tribal Health gained support from the Butte County Children's Coordinating Council and the community at large to evolve a broader system of care that would include reaching their most underserved and diverse communities. Feather River Tribal Health, Butte County Behavioral Health, and Rowell Family Empowerment of Northern California, a family organization, committed to jointly lead their county initiative entitled Connecting Circles of Care (CCOC). The service planning process was driven by data collected on youth of color from county and state tracking systems. The data were not surprising. They revealed that African American and Native American youth were six times more likely to be served in residential care than Whites. Hmong children and youth were underrepresented in services, suffering from multigenerational trauma, and becoming increasingly involved in antisocial activities, whereas Latino children and youth were found to be overrepresented in the juvenile justice system. According to Michael Clark, Co-Project Director, reviewing this information caused an "awakening of social consciousness," a call to action for the community. There were too many youth in deep-end services or rapidly heading in that direction.

Implementation efforts were guided by a governing board under the leadership of Rosilind Hussong, the second Co-Director, a Native American psychologist. She was well-known in the community for her knowledge and skills in providing culturally competent services to Native Americans and served as a catalyst or initial champion for the work. The governing board was initially chaired by two Native Americans. The majority of the board members represented the consumer perspective, with an ethnic/racial composition in alignment with the diversity of the community served.

Reaching the desired board composition required a strategic and well-coordinated outreach to the communities of color. The system of care utilized staff and other individuals familiar with the racial and ethnic groups to organize community meetings where the data could be presented. Outreach to the Latino community was done through the church, to the African American community through ministerial and social/civic organizations, and to the Hmong community through the social/cultural institution and the elders.

The community meetings became the vehicles for identifying indigenous leaders who worked with the system of care leaders to design and implement focus groups for the Latino, Hmong, and African American populations. These focus groups followed a process similar to the earlier Circles of Care planning process. The meetings focused on identifying strategies to improve child, youth, and family outcomes, and the representatives participating in these groups became cultural brokers for each population. Dr. Clark also noted that the meetings were a way of overcoming years of broken promises. The Butte County system of care hired many of the community leaders in key staff positions and recruited them to serve on the governing board. These individuals had credibility and the trust of their communities, as well as an understanding of the leverage points essential to system transformation.

Service delivery approaches were designed and staffed in accordance with the needs of the cultural groups within the county. Feather River Tribal Health hired Native American staff, and Rowell Family Empowerment hired, trained, and supported diverse family advocates. Culturally and linguistically competent wraparound teams were developed and staffed to work with each of the diverse communities. The system of care utilized the expertise and experience of many well-established nonprofit organizations in the respective communities to provide services. For example, Northern Valley Catholic Services, which had a history of working with the Latino community, was contracted to implement the wraparound approach to service delivery.

The CCOC system of care also worked with African American and Hmong community leaders to build capacity within their respective communities to implement the wraparound approach to services and increase access to care. These communities are seen as being the center of services, thus not requiring consumers to come to the mental health clinic. For the Hmong community, project directors went to the Hmong cultural center and met with elders. They were told that there *must* be a male on the team because the Hmong have a patriarchal culture. Elders were asked to identify who they wanted on the team and selected their representative. The head of the Hmong organization was recruited to work as a parent advocate; as such, he is the one who makes the first contact with the child's father, who must consent to services. This change has greatly increased the number of children and youth served. Other nontraditional helpers and practices have been integrated within the various treatment interventions (e.g., a Shaman with the Hmong animist families, drumming groups with Native Americans, faith-based organizations in the African American and Latino communities).

Thrive: Building Trauma-Informed Systems of Care in Maine

According to the 2005 census, Androscoggin County was the most ethnically diverse county in the state of Maine, with 96.2% of the population being White, 1.4% Black or African American, 0.3% Native American, 0.7% Asian, 1.4% from two or more races, and 1.2% Hispanic or Latino. Ethnic diversity decreases in the more rural communities of Oxford and Franklin, which are at least 98% White. Of particular note is that in recent years, the population identified in the census as Black or African American are predominantly refugees and immigrants from African countries such as Somalia, Sudan, Togo, and Ghana. The newly arrived immigrant population, referred to as *New Mainers*, pose interesting challenges for service delivery due to cultural, religious, and language differences. In addition, the Hispanic or Latino population is primarily composed of migrant workers who arrive from the Caribbean and Central America.

In 2005, the state of Maine was awarded a federal system of care grant to establish Thrive, a trauma-informed system of care, in the counties of Androscoggin, Franklin, and Oxford. *Trauma-informed* means that individuals working with families and youth understand the nature of trauma and the potential to retraumatize families and youth by providing services and interacting in a manner that is not sensitive to their experiences. The goal is to incorporate seven key principles within service planning and delivery:

1. Safety

2. Trustworthiness

3. Choice

4. Collaboration

5. Empowerment

6. Language access

7. Cultural competence

The Thrive approach to implementing a culturally and linguistically competent system integrates the trauma principles throughout all aspects of their work. It has been strengthened by a strong collaboration with the state's Office of Multicultural Affairs, specifically with the state coordinator, Luc Nya, who was originally from Cameroon. As the state coordinator, he played an instrumental role in writing the grant and served as a liaison with the child-serving agencies at the state level. The cultural and linguistic competence work of Project Thrive has been built on the existing Androscoggin Valley Refugee and Immigrant Mental Health Collaborative, which also includes the cities of Lewiston and Portland. The Mental Health Collaborative has a 7-year history of operation and was formed by the state cultural and linguistic competence coordinator. Its operations are guided by a public health approach that offers the opportunity to address a wide range of community concerns and provide education, prevention, and treatment strategies.

Major activities include the creation of a Public Health Division for the City of Lewiston, community-based immunization clinics for New Mainers, and two companion initiatives involving community policing and educating law enforcement about the mental health needs of the immigrant and refugee communities. This latter effort began with the collection of data from police officers to ascertain their knowledge about refugee communities and what they wanted to learn. There was also an analysis of arrest data on the populations of focus. Cultural brokers were used to conduct impromptu focus groups at shops, churches, and other natural gathering places. Through this process the planning group identified a high number of calls related to family conflict and domestic violence. It was also noted that there was a negative escalation of events in many of these police–resident situations because neither group understood the intentions of the other. To address this need, training was implemented at the police academies in Lewiston, Portland, and Auburn, the three largest cities in Maine, on the refugee/immigrant experience, trauma, and culture. Using cultural brokers, training was presented for the refugee/immigrant population on law enforcement policies and procedures, as well their legal rights as residents. Because many members of the refugee population are Muslims, special consideration was given to the gender and religious orientation of the trainers.

The governing board for Project Thrive is a subgroup of the Mental Health Collaborative and comprises service providers and community residents. Fifty percent of the board members are New Mainers. As part of the development of a trauma-informed system, special emphasis has been placed on linguistic competence. Under the direction of the governing board and in partnership with the United Way, an initiative entitled Language Access for New Americans was implemented. This major effort involved access to sign language along with translation and interpreter services. Policies and procedures have been implemented to match consumers with providers who have had special training to meet their needs. Because there are no national standards for interpretation, the work group is identifying core competencies for interpreters that are not based on having an advanced degree. This policy created new job potential for many New Mainers who were highly trained professionals in their countries of origin.

Project Thrive placed signs in all state and provider locations in the indigenous languages of the various groups. The signs informed residents of their right to services and the ways to access them. Thrive is also partnering with local stakeholders (e.g., the Lewiston Public Library, the Harward Center for Community Partnerships, the City of Lewiston's Department of Social Services). A grassroots effort in the city of Lewiston includes the local college and library and involves creating study circles, an initiative that is geared toward addressing issues facing teenagers in the community. Collaborations with universities and technical colleges have assisted in conducting cultural and linguistic needs assessments among the populations served. Diverse community members, families, and youth—including youth who are gay, lesbian, bisexual, transgendered, or questioning—are involved at all levels within the system of care from governance, to involvement on committees, to agency staffing. To supplement recruitment efforts, Thrive has developed a cultural competence training curriculum to aid in the development of cultural and linguistic competence champions.

Another significant accomplishment is the strong relationship with the various ethnic self-help organizations, which offer opportunities to consult and conduct focus groups on cultural and linguistic competence needs. Project Thrive has also used existing and new data to develop protocols for conducting culturally and linguistically appropriate assessments for diagnosing mental health needs and cognitive disabilities within the refugee and immigrant populations. Several meetings have been held with partner agencies, the state Office of Cognitive Disabilities, the Department of Health and Human Services, and the Lewiston Public Schools Office of English Language Learners and Special Education to work on cultural and linguistically appropriate tools for screening refugee and immigrant youth with severe emotional disturbances. These assessments include consideration of community norms and cultural traditions.

Monroe County Coordinated Care Services, Inc.

Monroe County's population of 750,000 includes the urban city of Rochester and the surrounding suburbs. The population is 80% White, 15% African American, 3% Asian, 6% Hispanic, and 3% other. Monroe County is an excellent example of a community that has built its approach to cultural and linguistic competence on the success of existing initiatives. In the early 1990s, predating the introduction of a system of care, the county conducted a cultural competence site review. This served as their introduction to cultural competence. This process generated a Cultural Competence Advisory Committee to carry out the resulting recommendations. While the focus was primarily on physical space issues, it helped to lay the foundation for future efforts to more comprehensively address cultural and linguistic competence.

The Cultural Competence Advisory Committee gained direction and momentum from the New York State Commissioner of Mental Health, who had a strong commitment to the work. Through the state mental health authority, each county was asked to develop a local cultural competence advisory group. One representative from each county was then selected to become part of a regional work group that provided support and advice to state efforts.

Under the leadership and guidance of a Cultural and Linguistic Competence Coordinator employed by Coordinated Services, Inc., the administrative service organization for substance abuse and mental health services in Monroe County, an organizational cultural competence assessment instrument was developed in 1999 and 2000. This tool assessed more than 200 indicators of cultural and linguistic competence. As part of the contracting process, potential providers were required to use this self-assessment and narrative tool. The assessment was mandated in agency contracts, and funds could be withheld for noncompliance. Site review reports were generated to indicate the results of the assessment. Recommendations for improvement and technical assistance were provided. The county also hired a clinical oversight coordinator to ensure the integration of cultural and linguistic competence within all services. Provider agencies began producing results, developing diverse services and staffs, and implementing ongoing cultural and linguistic competence assessments.

With the award of a system of care grant in 2005, the status of the Cultural and Linguistic Competence Advisory Committee was changed to a council, giving it a more powerful role. The Cultural and Linguistic Competence Coordinator, now the Director, continues to support the ACCESS system of care. This work is shared with the cultural broker, who works with the various ethnic communities as a relationship manager or navigator through the service delivery system. The role of the cultural broker is to connect people to appropriate care and train care coordinators and other service providers on a monthly basis. These trainings cover such topics as White privilege, racism, and the identification of cultural variables. The trainings are highly experiential in order to touch the underlying feelings and values of the participants. An additional person has been hired to spearhead advocacy, engagement, and social marketing efforts for underserved populations.

The budget for cultural and linguistic competence is smaller, but much of the early work has been institutionalized in the county's behavioral health system. The contracting process established in 2001, which required the use of a cultural and linguistic competence self-assessment, uses an abbreviated version of Siegel's Cultural and Linguistic Competence Assessment (Siegel, Haugland, & Chambers, 2004). A database has been developed to house and manage cultural and linguistic competence data collected through this process. As of 2005, this instrument has become the focus of research to establish its psychometric properties and to look at critical outcomes regarding organizational infrastructure. This has allowed Monroe County to monitor progress toward achieving cultural and linguistic competence. Unfortunately, site reviews of provider agencies have been terminated. Sharp declines in cultural and linguistic competence assessment scores have been noted since the discontinuation of the site reviews and are attributed to the lack of accountability structures in place to review, critique, and make recommendations to improve cultural and linguistic competence in provider agencies.

To address this issue, a new procedure has been implemented that incorporates a tool called Ethnicity at a Glance. This one-page document is completed by all contractors and describes the ethnic makeup of the board, staff, and the populations served. All providers are required to identify cultural and linguistic competence challenges from the prior year and any attempts made to address them. This data is collected on an annual basis and is analyzed for trends that help indicate where program improvements are needed. One significant challenge was identified in the area of linguistic competence for all providers. After examining the data, a decision was made by the Director of Cultural and Linguistic Competence that required a broad system-level intervention. Individual provider agencies could not cover the cost of recruiting and hiring the most qualified interpreters because they were all serving small numbers of Spanish-speaking populations. By blending funds and coordinating resources, staff were hired and shared by various agencies.

Another important aspect of incorporating a cultural and linguistic competence perspective into the infrastructure and service delivery components of the system of care is examining evaluation data through a cultural competence lens. The Cultural and Linguistic Competence Council has a subgroup that focuses on evaluation and serves on the system of care's evaluation team. Evaluation data is reviewed by this subgroup and is used to inform service development and delivery with respect to issues of disparities and cultural and linguistic competence.

STATE APPROACH TO ELIMINATION OF RACIAL AND ETHNIC DISPARITIES: MASSACHUSETTS

State mental health authorities are also poised to address the issues involved in serving culturally and linguistically diverse populations. They have an obligation to examine and address the disparities that may exist within their service systems. Massachusetts has undertaken a series of steps and strategies to implement cultural and linguistic competence with the goal of reducing such disparities:

1. Creation of a structure

In 1999, the state established the Office of Multicultural Affairs (OMCA) of the Massachusetts Department of Mental Health. This action served as a concrete demonstration of the role of culture and cultural competence in the mission of the department. OMCA has the focal responsibility of ensuring that the cultural and ethnic diversity of clients and staff is respected in the design and delivery of services.

2. Preparation

In preparation for its work, OMCA reviewed and built on existing knowledge and resources in the field including *Towards a Culturally Competent System of Care*

(Cross et al., 1989), *Getting Started . . . and Moving On: Planning, Implementing, and Evaluating Culturally and Linguistically Competency for Comprehensive Community Mental Health Services for Children and Families* (Goode & Jackson, 2003), *Mental Health: Culture Race and Ethnicity. A Supplement to Mental Health: A Report of the Surgeon General* (U.S. Department of Health and Human Services, 2001), *Unequal Treatment: Confronting Racial and Ethnic Disparities* (Institute of Medicine, 2002), and *Achieving the Promise: Transforming Mental Health Care in America* (President's New Freedom Commission on Mental Health, 2003).

3. Development of a logic model

OMCA sought to develop a visual operational logic model to guide its work (Hernandez & Hodges, 2003). The logic model is used to clearly articulate the theory of change and to organize and specify outcomes that can then be evaluated and tracked. In this case, the model is used to target outcomes that demonstrate that the mental health system is attentive to the needs of culturally and linguistically diverse populations. A logic model was created as the operational model for planning and evaluation and continues to be used and modified as needed. The latest version is shown in Figure 11.1.

4. Development of an annual action plan

OMCA develops an annual Cultural Competence Action Plan to put the department's mission of culturally and linguistically competent care into action. The annual plan is important in responding to the developmental process of attaining cultural and linguistic competence and resisting the temptation of some to claim an end to the process after a limited number of goals have been met. The purpose of the Cultural Competence Action Plan is to operationalize the department's mission on culturally competent care to ensure that the unified public behavioral health system is attentive to the mental health needs and effective care of culturally and linguistically diverse populations, including at-risk immigrants and refugees. An excerpt of the action plan for fiscal years 2005–2007 is shown in Table 11.1.

5. Inclusion of cultural and linguistic competence in ongoing initiatives

A key strategy has been to infuse cultural and linguistic competence into activities that were in process independently. In 2006, the Massachusetts Department of Mental Health embarked on a reform initiative referred to as the United Behavioral Health Initiative, which was designed to evaluate and reform the public mental health system. This initiative provided an opportunity for OMCA to address a major service system transformation by planning for racially, ethnically, culturally, and linguistically diverse populations as an integral part of the larger reform effort.

6. Creation of a strategic plan for the elimination of disparities

A strategic plan to eliminate disparities was developed that included: 1) a description of the level of access across racially and ethnically diverse populations at the

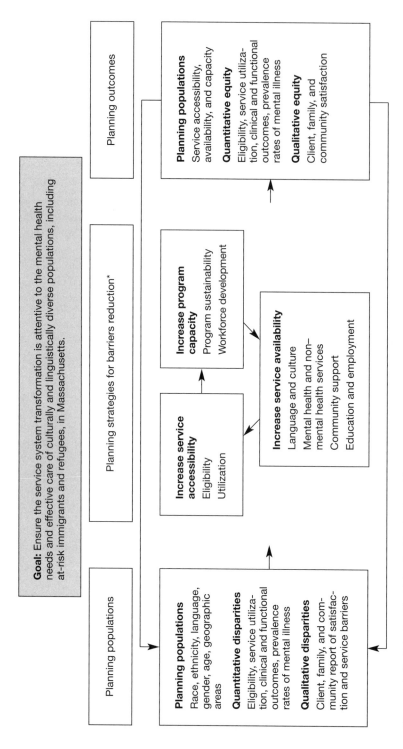

Figure 11.1. The Behavioral Health Service Planning Logic Model for Racially, Ethnically and Linguistically Diverse Populations.

system level; 2) identification of the availability of appropriate cultural and linguistic services; 3) strategies to ensure population-based, geographic-based, language, information and referral access to services for the underserved populations; 4) strategies to ensure availability of timely culturally and linguistically appropriate services; and 5) strategies to accomplish planning outcomes, document processes and progress, retool planning strategies, and measure outcomes for children, adolescents, and their families.

Strategies for Transformation of System Access

Goal: Achieve quantitative and qualitative understanding of population-based access, geographic access, language, and information and referral access among ethnically and linguistically diverse populations to provide a starting point for system planning and strategies for access improvement.

Data Analysis   The department analyzed data by comparing the differences in enrollment and utilization in mental health services among various population groups by race, ethnicity, age, gender, and primary language, and also estimated prevalence rates of mental illness of children and adolescents based on race, ethnicity, socioeconomic status, and environmental risk factors. In addition, the department solicited qualitative community knowledge from clients utilizing services and from community informants to identify needs and issues affecting access to services.

By comparing population census, service enrollment, and prevalence rates of mental illness based on race and ethnicity, and with input provided in several ethnic and linguistic consumer and family member forums, the department was able to plan and implement actions for specific populations of focus. The following are some examples of how the data were used:

- With a strong community partnership, OMCA was awarded a grant from the Blue Cross/Blue Shield Foundation of Massachusetts to implement a comprehensive needs assessment of the mental health experiences, service needs, and barriers to treatment for Latino residents in a city that has experienced a significant growth in this population. The partnership produced an assessment report that was published in a professional journal so that the assessment methodology can be replicated elsewhere. The needs assessment resulted in strategies to address identified needs. Community partners also provided ongoing training on mental health services for this population, including education and outreach for health and human service providers, consumers, and families.

- OMCA partnered with a Massachusetts grantee of the federal Office of Refugee Resettlement, the Harvard Program in Refugee Trauma at the Massachusetts General Hospital, to implement a comprehensive health and mental health care pilot program in a community health center for Cambodian

Table 11.1. Excerpt from Massachusetts Cultural Competence Action Plan

Area of focus	Goal/objective	Outcome, fiscal year 2005	Outcome, fiscal year 2006	Outcome, fiscal year 2007
Community partnerships	Goal: Partner with multicultural communities in the planning, development, and implementation of culturally and linguistically effective mental health services within a unified public behavioral health system. Objective A: Increase cultural competence[a]/diversity to reduce mental health disparities[b].	(A.1) Multicultural Advisory Committee (MAC)[c] and the Office of Multicultural Affairs (OMCA) will produce system recommendations, including promising practices on data, workforce development, bilingual/bicultural specialist team, and interpreter service, that will better serve the mental health needs of racially/ethnically/culturally diverse communities. (A.2) The Multicultural Advisory Committee will affiliate as a subgroup to the State Mental Health Planning Council (SPC) and will designate two members to join the State Mental Health Planning Council.	(A.1) The Multicultural Advisory Committee will produce at least one new performance measure for the 2006–2007 State Mental Health Plan based on the system recommendations, (e.g., data analysis on eligible clients based on race compared to population census) that address the reduction of mental health disparities. (A.2) The Multicultural Advisory Committee continues to partner with the State Mental Health Planning Council to promote the needs of identified multicultural and multilinguistic communities (e.g., adopt the Department's Cultural Competence Action Plan to address the reduction of mental health disparities of the identified communities).	(A.1) The Multicultural Advisory Committee will monitor the outcome of its proposed measure(s) and develop new measures from system recommendations (e.g., data analysis on clients' service enrollment based on race compared to population census) to reduce mental health disparities. (A.2) The Multicultural Advisory Committee continues to partner with the State Mental Health Planning Council (e.g. develop a multicultural committee of the Council) to promote and monitor progress of the Department's Cultural Competence Action Plan and develop further actions towards the reduction of mental health disparities.

Data and research	Goal: Use demographic information about Department of Mental Health (DMH) clients and applicants to inform decisions about policy development, clinical practice, research, program development, service delivery, and workforce development. Objective A: Improve accuracy of demographic information about DMH clients.	(A.1) Generate report from Mental Health Information System (MHIS) to determine current demographic collection status. (A.2) Revise DMH service applications to improve likelihood of correct and complete data entry for race, ethnicity, and preferred language. • Separate race and ethnicity • Provide drop-down lists (A.3) Provide training on collecting accurate information. • Append instructions to application for users • Develop pilot for users	(A.1) Demographic information in report is available (entered) for 100% of case managed clients and all new applicants. (A.2) Review audits on collected information biannually by local Multicultural Committees/CCAT[d] and make additional adjustments to collection procedures as needed (A.3) Provide training on collecting accurate information, as needed, to ensure complete information is collected. • Provide assessment skills instruction to all eligibility determination specialists.	(A.1) Demographic information in report is available (entered) for 100% of case managed clients and all new applicants. (A.2) Review audits on collected information biannually by local Multicultural Committees/CCAT. (A.3) Provide training on collecting accurate information, as needed, to ensure complete information is collected.

[a]"Cultural competence is the integration and transformation of knowledge, information and data about individuals and groups of people into specific clinical standards, skills, service approaches, techniques, and marketing programs that match the individual's culture and increase the quality and appropriateness of health care and outcomes" (Davis, 1997).

[b]Disparities reported in President's New Freedom Commission on Mental Health (2003), Institute of Medicine (2002), and U.S. Department of Health and Human Services (2001). Disparities conceptualized in areas of prevalence, incidence, services, treatment, rehabilitation, recovery, prevention, participation, outcomes, acceptable norms, personal choice, and racial causation (Davis, 2003).

[c]The Multicultural Advisory Committee (MAC) provides regular input and guidance for the department's cultural competence activities. Members include community-based providers, researchers, policy makers, clients and family members, gatekeepers, and stakeholders who understand the needs of the racial and ethnic diversity in communities.

[d]Cultural Competence Action Team (CCAT) consists of senior and middle management and front-line staff of the Department of Mental Health. The broad department participation enables the team to take the entire departmental operations into consideration when developing an annual Cultural Competence Action Plan.

refugees. A number of studies have indicated a particularly high prevalence rate of mental illness in this population, as well as in other refugee populations. The comprehensive care provided through this pilot program includes integrated medical and mental health care, care management, life and parenting skill development, and health promotion services for all health and behavioral health clients. The partnership also provides statewide training for primary care and mental health providers on practical skills for assessing, treating, and supporting the recovery of refugees suffering from the effects of mass violence.

- Each year, the Executive Office of Health and Human Services, MassHealth (Medicaid), the Department of Mental Health, and the Massachusetts Behavioral Health Partnership (a managed care organization) solicit recommendations from stakeholders to improve quality of care. These initiatives, known as *performance incentives*, are negotiated with MassHealth. Each performance incentive has an associated payment contingent on the completion of the project. Because of the significant increase in ethnic and linguistic diversity in Massachusetts, coupled with research results on mental health disparities, a performance incentive project is dedicated each year to the reduction of mental health disparities for the linguistically and culturally diverse individuals who are covered by MassHealth.

Resource Directory   OMCA developed a Multicultural Populations Resource Directory that contains information on health and human services providers in Massachusetts that offer culturally and linguistically specific services. The directory was originally designed as a resource tool for direct care providers working with culturally and linguistically diverse clients. It is also utilized as an ongoing resource-mapping tool to identify the availability and gaps of cultural and linguistic programs in areas with a critical mass of diverse racial and ethnic populations.

Linguistic Access   Based on the 2000 census, approximately 19% of Massachusetts residents 5 years and older speak a language other than English. Of that group, 41% speak English less than "very well." The rapidly changing demographics of Massachusetts require that individuals have access to the services and programs they need and to which they are entitled. This includes linguistic access. Language preference is collected from the clients when they enroll in a mental health program. OMCA has dedicated resources for interpreter and translation services. These resources are used to provide services to clients and staff of the Department of Mental Health who are in need of a professional interpreter to facilitate communication, as well as for translation of written materials. The Massachusetts Interpreter Services Act requires competent interpreter services in emergency rooms and acute psychiatric inpatient wards at no cost to those seeking services.

Information and Referral   OCMA organizes ongoing community education and outreach activities to increase public awareness, remove the stigma associated with mental illness, and increase awareness that treatment is effective.

Strategies for Transformation of Service Availability

Goal: Assure that mental health services are in the communities where people are, and strengthen the availability of bilingual and bicultural specialists within service delivery teams and Community Health Centers.

Workforce Enhancements   A strategy used in Massachusetts that addresses cultural and linguistic competence in the design of services and in the workforce is the creation of *bilingual bicultural specialist* positions within service delivery teams. Because ethnically and linguistically diverse licensed clinicians are frequently unavailable, bilingual and bicultural paraprofessionals are used as equal members of treatment teams. Treatment teams are composed of licensed clinicians and bilingual bicultural specialists who work in a vital, dynamic two-way process. The English-speaking clinician relies on the bilingual bicultural specialist to provide not only culturally relevant interpretation with clients, but also critical cultural information, education, and guidance to ensure that the clinical assessment, treatment plan, individual and family support, and follow-up is culturally and linguistically appropriate and effective. The bilingual bicultural specialists also do outreach through home visits and link clients to natural supports in the community. This approach is an example of the use of cultural brokers in human service systems (see Goode, Sockalingam, & Snyder, 2004, for more information). One positive unintended consequence of this program has been that some bilingual and bicultural specialists have pursued professional education to become licensed clinicians.

Strategies for Transformation of Practice

Goal: Increase acceptability and service participation by integrating client's culture and choice into practice.

Specialized Training   OMCA developed a curriculum called *Integrate Culture Into Practice.* The training is designed to examine the expression and treatment of mental illness in the context of culture through ethnographic narratives and group discussions. The curriculum explores how cultural concepts, values, beliefs, and language influence the perception and expression of mental distress, symptoms, and help-seeking behavior of individuals, their families, and their communities. Different perceptions of a diagnosis and reactions to treatment are also explored in the context of culture. A cultural assessment and formulation tool is used to illustrate these concepts. Psychiatric residency and internship programs, care management and wraparound services, child protective agencies, and advocacy organizations are the intended audience of this training. All initial trainings have been done by the Director of OMCA, and subsequent trainings designed to address specific cultural groups are being facilitated by cultural brokers and providers using examples of their work.

CONCLUSION

Although cultural and linguistic competence activities have been undertaken by many systems of care and state mental health agencies, the actual results have been disappointing thus far. The lack of definitional and population clarity, synergistic activities, uniformity in training curricula and approaches, evaluation and research, and sustained political will have hampered the recognition and adoption of cultural and linguistic competence as an essential and critical element in mental health systems (Isaacs, 2005).

The system of care and state examples described in this chapter demonstrate a range of strategies that can be used to achieve improvements in the quality of care for racial, ethnic, linguistic, and other cultural groups. These same strategies can reduce the disparities in access, quality, and outcomes of mental health services. The children's mental health field is challenged to address the multiple domains needed to achieve cultural and linguistic competence and eliminate disparities. Many resources are available, and additional tools are in development, including a cultural and linguistic competence primer created by a collaborative composed of the American Institutes for Research, the National Technical Assistance Center for Children's Mental Health at Georgetown University, the National Alliance of Multi-Ethnic Behavioral Health Associations, and the National Center for Cultural Competence; however, it is incumbent on the states and systems of care to exercise the will to use these resources effectively.

REFERENCES

Acevedo-Garcia, D., McArdle, N., Osypuk, T.L., Lefkowitz, B., & Krimgold, B.K. (2007). *Children left behind: How metropolitan areas are failing America's children.* Cambridge, MA: DiversityData.Org.

American Psychological Association. (2002). *Guidelines on multicultural education, training, research, practice, and organizational change for psychologists.* Washington, DC: Author.

Annie E. Casey Foundation. (2004a). *2004 KIDS COUNT data book: Moving youth from risk to opportunity.* Baltimore: Author.

Annie E. Casey Foundation. (2004b). *Special report 2004: City and rural KIDS COUNT data book.* Baltimore: Author.

Bordin, E.S. (1979). The generalizability of the psychoanalytic concept of the working alliance. *Psychotherapy: Theory, Research and Practice, 16*(3), 252–260.

Center for Mental Health Services. (2000). *Cultural competence standards in managed mental health care services: Four underserved/underrepresented racial/ethnic groups.* Rockville, MD: U.S. Department of Health and Human Services, Substance Abuse and Mental Health Services Administration.

Civil Rights Act of 1964, PL 88-352, 20 U.S.C. §§ 241 *et seq.*

Cooper-Patrick, L., Gallo, J., Gonzales, J., Vu, H., Powe, N., Nelson, C., et al. (1999). Race, gender, and partnership in the patient–physician relationship. *Journal of the American Medical Association, 282,* 583–589.

Cross, T., Bazron, B., Dennis, K., & Isaacs, M. (1989). *Towards a culturally competent system of care: A monograph on effective services for minority children who are severely emotionally disturbed.* Washington, DC: CASSP Technical Assistance Center, Georgetown University Child Development Center.

Goode, T., & Jackson, V. (2003). *Getting started . . . and moving on: Planning, implementing, and evaluating culturally and linguistically competency for comprehensive community mental health services for children and families.* Washington, DC: National Center for Cultural Competence, Georgetown University Center for Child and Human Development.

Goode, T., & Jackson, V. (2005). *Cultural and linguistic competency: What systems of care are telling us.* Unpublished report.

Goode, T., & Jones, W. (2006). *A definition of linguistic competence.* Washington, DC: National Cultural Competence Center at Georgetown University.

Goode, T., Sockalingam, S., Brown, M., & Jones, W. (2000). *Linguistic competence in primary health care delivery systems: Implications for policy makers.* Washington, DC: National Center for Cultural Competence, Georgetown University Child Development Center.

Goode, T., Sockalingam, S., & Snyder, L. (2004). *Bridging the cultural divide in health care settings: the essential role of cultural broker programs.* Washington, DC: National Center for Cultural Competence, Georgetown University Center for Child and Human Development.

Hernandez, M., & Hodges, S. (2003). *Crafting logic models for systems of care: Ideas into action.* Tampa: University of South Florida, Louis de la Parte Florida Mental Health Institute, Department of Child & Family Studies.

Institute of Medicine. (2002). *Unequal treatment: Confronting racial and ethnic disparities in health care.* Washington, DC: National Academies Press.

Isaacs, M. (2005). *Making cultural competence real: Practical strategies for reducing racial/ethic disparities in system of care communities.* Washington, DC: Draft paper prepared for the TA Partnership, American Institutes for Research.

Isaacs, M., & Benjamin, M. (1991). *Towards a culturally competent system of care: Vol. II. Programs which utilize culturally competent principles.* Washington, DC: Georgetown University Child Development Center, National Technical Assistance Center for Children's Mental Health.

Jackson, V. (1997, May). *How to provide culturally competent services.* Presentation at Public/Private Healthcare Summit sponsored by The Partnership for Behavioral Healthcare, Arlington, VA.

Kataoka, S.H., Zang, L., & Wells, K.B. (2002). Unmet need for mental health care among U.S. children: Variation by ethnicity and insurance status. *American Journal of Psychiatry, 159,* 1548–1555.

Killen-Harvey, A., & Stern-Ellis, H. (2006). *Effectively working with gay, lesbian, bisexual, and transgender youth.* Retrieved September 21, 2007, from http://www.nctsnet.org/nctsn_assets/pdfs/Culture_Trauma_Killen_Harvey_Stern_Ellis_3-22-07.pdf

Martinez, K., & Van Buren, E. (2008). *The cultural and linguistic competence implementation guide.* Washington, DC: Technical Assistance Partnership for Child and Family Mental Health. Available online at http://www.tapartnership.org/cc/

McClurg, L. (2004). Biracial youth and their parents: Counseling considerations for family therapists. *Family Journal, 12*(2), 170–173.

Milan, S., & Keiley, M.K. (2000). Biracial youth and families in therapy: Issues and interventions. *Journal of Marital and Family Therapy, 26*(3), 305–315.

National Advisory Mental Health Council Workgroup. (2001). *Blueprint for change: Research on child and adolescent mental health.* Rockville, MD: National Institute of Mental Health.

National Association of Social Workers. (2001). *NASW standards for cultural competence in social work practice.* Washington, DC: Author.

National Association of Social Workers. (2007). *Indicators for the achievement of the NASW standards for cultural and linguistic competence in social work practice.* Washington, DC: Author.

National Institutes of Health. (2000). *Strategic research plan to reduce and ultimately eliminate health disparities: Fiscal Years 2002–2006.* Bethesda, MD: Author.

Office of Minority Health. (2000). *National standards for culturally and linguistically appropriate services in health care (CLAS standards).* Washington, DC: U.S. Department of Health and Human Services.

Pfeifer, K., Hu, T., & Vega, W. (2000). Help seeking by persons of Mexican origin with functional impairments. *Psychiatric Services, 51,* 1293–1298.

Poussaint, A.F., & Alexander, A. (2000). *Lay my burden down: Unraveling suicide and the mental health crisis among African Americans.* Boston: Beacon Press.

President's New Freedom Commission on Mental Health. (2003). *Achieving the Promise: Transforming mental health care in America. Final report* (DHHS Pub. No. SMA-03-3832). Rockville, MD: Author.

Siegel, D., Haugland, G., & Chambers, E.D. (2004). *Cultural competence assessment scale with instructions: Outpatient service delivery agency level.* Orangeburg, NY: Nathan S. Kline Institute for Psychiatric Research, Center for the Study of Issues on Public Mental Health.

Stroul, B., & Friedman, R. (1986). *A system of care for children and youth with severe emotional disturbances.* Washington, DC: National Technical Assistance Center for Children's Mental Health, Georgetown University Child Development Center.

Sturm, R., Ringel, J.S., Stein, D., & Kapur, K. (2001). Mental health care for youth: Who gets it? How much does it cost? Who pays? Where does the money go? *Research Highlights, RAND Health,* 1–4.

U.S. Census Bureau. (2002). *Current population survey.* Washington, DC: U.S. Department of Commerce.

U.S. Department of Health and Human Services. (2001). *Mental health: Culture race and ethnicity. A supplement to mental health: A report of the Surgeon General.* Rockville, MD: Author.

Vega, W.A., Kolody, B., Aguilar-Gaxiola, S., et al. (1998). Lifetime prevalence of DSM-III-R psychiatric disorders among urban and rural Mexican Americans in California. *Archives of General Psychiatry, 55,* 771–778.

Walrath, C.M., Ybarra, M., & Holden, E.W. (2006). Understanding the pre-referral factors associated with differential 6-month outcomes among children receiving system of care services. *Psychological Services, 3*(1), 35–50.

Wu, E., & Martinez, M. (2006). *Taking cultural competency from theory to action.* New York: The Commonwealth Fund.

Zhang, A.V., Snowden, L.R., & Sue, S. (1998). Differences between Asian and White Americans' help seeking and utilization patterns in the Los Angeles area. *Journal of Community Psychology, 26,* 317–326.

12

Evaluation and Continuous Quality Improvement

Angela Sheehan, Brigitte Manteuffel,
Chris Stormann, and Teresa King

Evaluation and the use of data to inform program improvement, outcomes, and sustainability have been central to the development of systems of care. The national evaluation of the Comprehensive Community Mental Health Services for Children and Their Families Program has been an integral component of the federal system of care initiative. This evaluation has informed Congress, the Substance Abuse and Mental Health Services Administration (SAMHSA), and other stakeholders about the program's progress, needs, and achievements. The ability to describe achievements with both qualitative and quantitative evaluation data has promoted the sustainability and growth of the initiative at the federal level, which is evidenced by continued funding by Congress and the expansion of the program to additional communities. In addition to the national evaluation, local community-based evaluations of systems of care have documented positive outcomes and have contributed to the sustainability of local systems of care.

Data have also been used to guide quality improvement efforts in systems of care. For example, information has been collected on the extent to which a system of care develops according to its core values and guiding principles. Knowing whether the system of care is developing according to these principles allows communities to actively seek improvement in weaker areas. Each system of care begins its development at a different place, has different community-driven goals, and is faced with different local circumstances. Articulation of goals and development strategies—often outlined through a logic model—provides a framework for development and evaluation. Each area of the logic model must be assessed to ascertain progress and determine the areas where improvements and increased focus are necessary. When such information is gathered and reviewed, leaders and advisory groups can assess their progress and prioritize areas where improvement is needed.

Evaluation and the use of data for continuous quality improvement (CQI) can seem like an expensive and confusing undertaking. National-level data reporting has become a common requirement, but the use of these data at the local level for decision making and CQI is often much more limited. Community members and system of care staff who have limited experience performing evaluations and using data may find it difficult to identify the type of evaluation that is needed. Similarly, when information is available, it can be a struggle to prioritize attention and efforts. This chapter describes an approach to the evaluation of systems of care and the collection and use of data for CQI.

EVALUATING SYSTEMS OF CARE

The use of evaluation data at both national and community levels to inform implementation, outcomes, and ultimately, the sustainability of systems of care has been a component of the federally funded system of care initiative since its inception. The 1992 authorizing legislation for the Comprehensive Community Mental Health Services for Children and Their Families Program (i.e., the Children's Mental Health Initiative [CMHI]), which provides funding for the development of systems of care in cities, counties, states, American Indian and Alaska Native tribes and organizations, and territories, requires that program evaluation occur at various levels to provide regular information about program development, performance, and outcomes. The evaluation requirement is addressed through a commitment to the national evaluation and through the development of evaluation capacity at the local level as a component of the system of care. Specifically, federally funded systems of care are required to hire evaluation staff; participate in the national evaluation; and use evaluation data for program improvement, social marketing, and sustainability purposes. Required participation in the national evaluation has furthered the local use of data to inform stakeholders about the achievements and needs of the system of care.

The evaluation requirements of the CMHI are consistent with program performance reporting requirements established in 1993 by the Government Performance and Results Act (GPRA, PL 103-62). GPRA requires federal programs to track a limited set of outcome indicators for performance reporting. These indicators are expected to address key domains that are relevant to the program and consistent with requirements of the Office of Management and Budget's Program Accountability Rating Tool categories (Government Printing Office, 2002). For example, indicators are required to address the reach of the program through the number served, child-level outcomes, and impact on costs. Performance indicators established for the CMHI at the federal program level have evolved since 1993 and address program implementation at the infrastructure level, outcomes at the child level, and costs. The national evaluation established for the CMHI has provided reports of program performance on the program's GPRA indicators.

The national evaluation of the CMHI offers a comprehensive approach to the evaluation of systems of care and addresses core areas of the federal program through six study components:

1. Characteristics of children and families served by systems of care (Cross-Sectional Descriptive Study)

2. Child and family emotional, behavioral, and functional outcomes (Longitudinal Child and Family Outcome Study)

3. System of care implementation and development (System of Care Assessment)

4. Service experience (Service Experience Study)

5. Services and costs (Services and Costs Study)

6. System of care sustainability (Sustainability Study)

Each area is addressed using a different methodology that generates information with a periodicity appropriate to the area of assessment. Since 1993, the national evaluation protocol has evolved to refine research questions, methodology, approaches to data collection, and instrumentation in accordance with evolving program developments. These studies have been conducted since the beginning, with the exception of the sustainability study, which was added as a core component with programs funded in 1997. Table 12.1 shows the research questions for each of the core study components.

Table 12.1 Core Children's Mental Health Initiative national evaluation research questions

Study	Research questions
Cross-Sectional Descriptive Study	Who are the children and families served by the program and by the funded communities? Does the served population change over time as systems of care mature?
Longitudinal Child and Family Outcome Study	To what extent do children's clinical and functional outcomes improve over time? How are family outcomes affected? How are changes in child, family, and system outcomes associated with efforts to implement and develop systems of care?
System of Care Assessment	How do systems of care develop according to system of care principles (e.g., family driven and youth guided, culturally competent, interagency collaboration) over time? In what ways does funding accelerate system development?
Service Experience Study	To what extent are children's and families' experiences consistent with the system of care philosophy? How satisfied are children and families with the services they receive? To what extent are family members and youth involved in systems of care?
Services and Costs Study	What are the service utilization patterns (specific services, treatments, and supports) for children and families in systems of care and what are the associated costs? How cost-effective are systems of care over time?
Sustainability Study	To what extent are systems of care able to sustain themselves after federal funding has ended? What factors facilitate or impede sustainability?

Components of the National Evaluation

The following provides a brief description of each component of the national evaluation.

Cross-Sectional Descriptive Study This study collects information about demographic, descriptive, and diagnostic characteristics of all children served. The information is collected on a form completed at service intake or through a review of administrative records.

Longitudinal Child and Family Outcome Study Conducted among a sample of children and youth in each community who meet the definition of serious emotional disturbance and are eligible for system of care services, the Longitudinal Child and Family Outcome Study examines changes over time in children and families who receive services. Areas of child clinical and functional status assessed include symptomatology, diagnoses, strengths, functioning, development among young children, substance use, school attendance and performance, delinquency and juvenile justice involvement, and stability of living arrangements. Assessment of families includes family support, communications, resources, and caregiver strain. Study enrollment and initial outcome study interviews with caregivers and youth age 11 years and older are conducted within 30 days of a child or youth's entry into services. Follow-up interviews occur at 6-month intervals for up to 36 months.

System of Care Assessment The System of Care Assessment examines whether systems have been implemented in accordance with system of care theory and documents how systems develop over time to meet the needs of the children and families they serve. Of particular interest is whether services are delivered in a family-driven, individualized, youth-guided, culturally competent, and coordinated manner in community-based and least restrictive service environments, as well as whether the system of care involves multiple child-serving agencies. Interviews are conducted during three site visits to each system of care community beginning in the second year of funding and repeating at 18- to 24-month intervals during the 6-year grant period. Information is collected through a combination of semi-structured interviews with multiple stakeholders, review of randomly selected case records, document review, and follow-up telephone interviews as needed. Respondents include project directors, representatives from core child-serving agencies, representatives from family organizations, local program evaluators, care coordinators, direct service providers, youth coordinators, caregivers, and youth served by the system of care.

Service Experience Study The Service Experience Study captures information on services that were received, locations where services were delivered, agencies involved in providing services, and experiences with services, including the extent to which services met family needs, the cultural and linguistic competence of service providers, and the family's satisfaction with the services. Information is obtained during follow-up interviews for the Child and Family Outcome Study beginning at 6 months after intake into services.

Services and Costs Study　The Services and Costs Study describes the types of services used by children and families, their utilization patterns, and the associated costs. Of interest are the types of services, the combination of services, continuity or gaps in care, and the length of treatment children and their families experience. The relationships among service use, service costs, and outcomes are also explored. Information for this study is obtained from local management information systems and budgets.

Sustainability Study　Using a web-based survey, this study captures information in five areas relevant to system of care sustainability:

1. The continued availability of specific services in the system of care

2. The continued implementation of system of care principles

3. Continued success in achieving objectives related to system of care implementation

4. The impact of a variety of factors affecting sustainability (whether each factor has played a role in the development or maintenance of the system of care, and if so, the extent to which each has impacted the system of care)

5. The effectiveness of various strategies for sustaining systems of care including financing strategies

Locally hired evaluation staff collect data for the first three studies following a national protocol and assist in coordinating data collection efforts for national evaluation staff for the remaining study components. The instrumentation used to evaluate each of these components is shown on Table 12.2. Although these instruments have been selected or developed specifically for the national evaluation of the federal system of care initiative, any state or community may find them useful for evaluating their systems of care in accordance with their own specific theory of change, system of care goals and objectives, and evaluation questions.

System of Care Evaluation and Data Use

Through the five core study components, the national evaluation captures information relevant to program development, improvement, and sustainability. To inform local programs about their progress, the national evaluation provides local-level data reports from data collected for the core study components. The various reports include information about program development related to implementation of system of care principles; characteristics of children and families served; child and adolescent behavioral, emotional, and functional outcomes; family outcomes; services received; families' satisfaction with services; and sustainability.

Table 12.2.   Instrumentation for national evaluation of systems of care

Substudy	Instruments used or data source	Reference for instrument (if applicable)
Cross-sectional Descriptive Study	Enrollment and Demographic Information Form	Developed for national evaluation
Longitudinal Child and Family Outcome Study	Behavioral and Emotional Rating Scale	Epstein, M.H. (2004). *Behavioral and Emotional Rating Scale: A strength-based approach to assessment. Examiner's manual* (2nd ed.). Austin, TX: PRO-ED.
	Caregiver Strain Questionnaire	Brannan, A.M., Heflinger, C.A., & Bickman, L. (1998). The Caregiver Strain Questionnaire: Measuring the impact on the family of living with a child with serious emotional disturbance. *Journal of Emotional and Behavioral Disorders, 5,* 212–222.
	Child Behavior Checklist	Achenbach, T.M., & Rescorla, L.A. (2000). *Manual for ASEBA Preschool Forms & Profiles.* Burlington: University of Vermont, Research Center for Children, Youth, & Families.
		Achenbach, T.M., & Rescorla, L.A. (2001). *Manual for ASEBA School-Age Forms & Profiles.* Burlington: University of Vermont, Research Center for Children, Youth, & Families.
	Columbia Impairment Scale	Bird, H.R., Shaffer, D., Fisher, P., Gould, M.S., Staghezza, B., Chen, J.Y., et al. (1993). The Columbia Impairment Scale (CIS): Pilot findings on a measure of global impairment for children and adolescents. *International Journal of Methods in Psychiatric Research, 3,* 167–176.
	Delinquency Survey–Revised	Developed for national evaluation
	Education Questionnaire	Developed for national evaluation
	Family Life Scale	Developed for national evaluation
	GAIN Quick–R-Substance Problems Scale	Titus, J.C., & Dennis, M.L. (2005). *Global Appraisal of Individual Needs–Quick (GAIN–Q): Administration and scoring guide for the GAIN–Q* (version 2). Retrieved August 30, 2006, from http://www.chestnut.org/LI/gain/GAIN_Q/GAIN-Q_v2_Instructions_09-07-2005.pdf
	Living Situations Questionnaire	Developed for national evaluation
	Reynolds Adolescent Depression Scale–Second Edition	Reynolds, W.M. (1986). *Reynolds Adolescent Depression Scale* (2nd ed.; RADS2). San Antonio, TX: The Psychological Corp.

Substudy	Instruments used or data source	Reference for instrument (if applicable)
	Revised Children's Manifest Anxiety Scale	Reynolds, C.R., & Richmond, B.O. (1978). What I think and feel: A revised measure of children's manifest anxiety. *Journal of Abnormal Psychology, 6*(2), 271–280.
	Substance Use Survey–Revised	Developed for national evaluation
	Vineland Screener	Sparrow, S., Carter, A., & Cicchetti, D. (1993) *Vineland Screener: Overview, reliability, validity, administration and scoring.* New Haven, CT: Yale University Child Study Center.
System of Care Assessment (SOCA)	SOCA Interview Guides	Developed for national evaluation
Service Experience Study	Multi-sector Service Contacts Form–Revised	Developed for national evaluation
	Cultural Competence and Service Provision Questionnaire	Developed for national evaluation
	Youth Services Survey; Youth Services Survey for Families	Brunk, M., Koch, J.R., & McCall, B. (2000). *Report on parent satisfaction with services at community services boards.* Richmond: Virginia Department of Mental Health, Mental Retardation, and Substance Abuse Services.
Services and Costs Study	MIS Data Abstraction	N/A
Sustainability Study	Sustainability Survey	Developed for national evaluation

Qualitative and quantitative reports on program development and change describe the extent to which a system of care is being implemented according to required principles and identify issues encountered in system implementation. These reports include feedback about areas for improvement, as well as successes with and concerns about sustainability.

Local system of care leaders review national evaluation reports with their advisory and governing bodies. They use the reports and the input provided by community stakeholders (including agency representatives, family members, and others) to make decisions about next steps. For example, a system of care may determine from a data report that the percentage of Latino children served by their program is well below the percentage of Latino families in their jurisdiction. The staff may then develop outreach efforts by working with a local Latino cultural center to facilitate referrals, training Latino community members to be care coordinators, or outstationing staff at a cultural center.

Just as evaluation findings are reviewed at the local level, national level leadership and advisory groups use data from the national evaluation to inform decision making. Reports detailing areas in which communities have struggled (e.g., family involvement, cultural and linguistic competence, sustainability) have informed the development of guidance for program applicants for more recently funded grantees to strengthen requirements and technical assistance in these areas. Evaluation reports at the national level provide documentation of program achievements and provide information about the program to Congress, SAMHSA, the Office of Management and Budget, and the general public.

To foster the use of evaluation for CQI efforts, the federal system of care initiative has invested in the development of a progress report for local systems of care that provides performance information relative to a set of indicators in key program areas. This CQI system was designed to further the local use of data and to support a culture of data-driven decision making for systems of care. As a first step, systems of care received graphical reports of the GPRA indicators, with updates in subsequent reports showing change as data were accumulated. GPRA reports provided a program-level snapshot of performance in required areas. Building on the GPRA reports, the CQI Progress Report was developed to include multiple indicators in key program areas with ratings of performance. These reports drew on national evaluation data and assessed performance relative to system of care goals and objectives as outlined in the program logic model. The following section reviews the fundamentals of the CQI process and outlines a practical approach for implementing this CQI process in systems of care.

IMPLEMENTING CONTINUOUS QUALITY IMPROVEMENT IN SYSTEMS OF CARE

CQI as a concept has been used in the business world for decades (LeVitt, 1997; Walton, 1986). Since then, principles of total quality management and CQI have received increasing attention in the health and mental health care fields (Berwick, 1989; Blumenthal & Kilo, 1998; Hermann & Provost, 2003; Lichiello, Skariba, & Thompson, 2000). CQI involves planning and organizational improvement efforts that are grounded in "empirical data; careful consideration of customer preferences; ongoing monitoring of processes and outcomes to continuously improve quality; strong support by leadership; and involvement of employees in cross-functional teams" (Berwick, 1989). Using evaluation data to support quality improvement has long been encouraged in the health and mental healthcare fields, and more recently, at multiple levels of government (Berwick, 1989; Epstein, Coates, Wray, & Swain, 2006; Fountain et al., 2003).

Although the use of evaluation data for performance measurement and CQI efforts is becoming increasingly common, there are still significant challenges for systems of care in their efforts to develop effective data-driven CQI processes.

These challenges include the development of consensus on indicators and associated benchmarks of care, the lack of reliable data across systems, variations in resources to support service provision, and the lack of consistent definitions of measures (Dougherty Management Associates, 2004; Hermann et al., 2004). Using evaluation data as part of a CQI approach, however, is critical for system of care communities to ensure high-quality service systems and service delivery mechanisms for children and families.

The concept of CQI offers a simple framework for systems of care to identify intended system-level and service delivery-level outcomes and to support efforts designed to achieve them. Accordingly, a CQI Progress Report and Benchmarking Initiative was implemented in 2004 for the CMHI by the Child, Adolescent, and Family Branch of the federal Center for Mental Health Services (CMHS). The purpose of the CQI Progress Report and Benchmarking Initiative was to support system of care communities in their CQI efforts, to better target technical assistance efforts, and to support the continuous improvement of services and service systems for children and their families.

The CQI Progress Report and Benchmarking Initiative offers a practical approach designed to help systems of care utilize evaluation data for CQI purposes. It provides a data-driven tool to better understand performance related to system of care goals and objectives, identify technical assistance needs, allocate system of care resources, and monitor progress. Implementing the CQI approach outlined by this initiative involves specific strategies to be implemented by each system of care. These strategies have been identified as key components of CQI in the literature and are integral to the CQI Progress Report and Benchmarking Initiative for the CMHI. These strategies include the following:

1. Establishing community partnerships that include families and youth

2. Setting organizational goals, objectives, and desired outcomes for system change

3. Utilizing evaluation data to develop process and outcome measures to monitor performance

4. Reviewing and analyzing evaluation data to support continuous quality improvement

5. Developing an infrastructure to support continuous quality improvement

Establishing Community Partnerships that Include Families and Youth: Implementing a Team Approach to Continuous Quality Improvement

Consistent throughout the organizational improvement literature is the need to involve internal and external stakeholders in CQI efforts (Lichiello et al., 2000; Scholtes, Joiner, & Streibel, 2003). CQI efforts in system of care communities must involve those who have a stake in ensuring the quality of service systems and service delivery mechanisms. These stakeholders include families, youth, policy makers, system of care administrators, service providers, evaluators, technical assistance providers, community members, and representatives of other child-serving agencies. CQI teams must include members who represent various roles and responsibilities, all of whom bring value to the CQI process. It is important to have participants in the CQI process who understand system-level issues (e.g., administrators knowledgeable about budget, personnel, policy, and grant management), practice-level issues (e.g., family members, youth, providers, supervisors), and support issues (e.g., evaluators, contractors, program coordinators, technical assistance providers).

Those who participate in the CQI process should be an extension of those who participated in the system of care's logic modeling process. As outlined by Hernandez and Hodges (2003), multiple perspectives are required to establish an effective theory of change displayed graphically in the form of a logic model. Because the theory of change provides the framework for CQI efforts, these same perspectives are critical to implementing an effective CQI process. Although it may seem natural for an evaluator to be solely responsible for identifying process and outcome measures, it is crucial for administrators and consumers (i.e., youth and family members) to be involved in the selection of indicators for assessing the quality and outcomes of services that are intended to help them. Building a bridge between evaluation staff, system of care staff, and consumers and families is essential in the CQI process. Various stakeholder groups must be engaged in the CQI process because they represent the perspectives needed to understand the performance of the system of care and to develop strategies to improve its quality. A team approach is needed at every stage of the CQI process, including identifying outcomes of interest, performance measures, goals for performance (e.g., benchmarks), and appropriate strategies to improve performance.

Setting Organizational Goals, Objectives, and Desired Outcomes for System Change: Crafting a Logic Model

Once community partnerships are developed and a team is established to implement and monitor CQI efforts, the CQI cycle begins. Figure 12.1 illustrates the CQI Process for Monroe County, NY, which was adapted from the Deming CQI model (Walton, 1986), and provides an excellent and replicable example for how CQI processes can be structured in system of care communities. In Monroe County, the CQI process starts with the development of the logic model for the system of care. Among the commonly cited recommended practices in data-driven CQI is the alignment of performance measures with the organization's strategic direction (Lichiello et al., 2000; National Performance Review, 1997). In the system of care context, this translates into alignment of performance measures with the program's intent as defined in a logic model that expresses program components and activities in a logical flow, including a program's goals, guiding principles, and desired outcomes (Hernandez & Hodges, 2003).

The logic model identifies the goals and objectives of the program, as well as the inputs and outputs of the program that are intended to lead to the achieve-

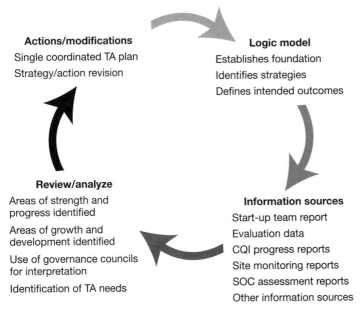

Actions/modifications
Single coordinated TA plan
Strategy/action revision

Logic model
Establishes foundation
Identifies strategies
Defines intended outcomes

Review/analyze
Areas of strength and
progress identified

Areas of growth and
development identified

Use of governance councils
for interpretation

Identification of TA needs

Information sources
Start-up team report
Evaluation data
CQI progress reports
Site monitoring reports
SOC assessment reports
Other information sources

Figure 12.1. Continuous quality improvement cycle. (From Levison-Johnson, J. [2007, March]. Monroe County logic model process. In A.K. Sheehan [Chair], *Theories of change from a continuous quality improvement [CQI] perspective: Logic modeling, measuring performance and benchmarking.* Symposium conducted at the 20th Annual Research Conference, A System of Care for Children's Mental Health: Expanding the Research Base, Tampa, FL; reprinted by permission.) (*Key:* CQI, continuous quality improvement; SOC, systems of care; TA, technical assistance.)

ment of those goals and objectives. A well-crafted logic model simply and clearly defines the desired outcomes for a program and the necessary steps to reach the desired outcomes. These outcomes provide the basis for developing performance measures and benchmarks. For example, the CMHI Logic Model (Figure 12.2) includes *child and family satisfaction with services is improved* as an outcome. Accordingly, indicators on the CQI Progress Report (Macro International Inc., 2006) include measures of child and family satisfaction. Furthermore, if the CQI process determines that child and family satisfaction is an area that requires improvement, the implementation of activities postulated as contributing to this outcome are also specified on the logic model. In this way, the logic model provides the framework for identifying implementation and technical assistance strategies to address areas that require improvement.

Utilizing Evaluation Data as Information Sources: Developing Process and Outcome Measures to Monitor Performance

The logic model identifies desired outcomes for a system of care, but for many communities, identifying measures for the desired outcomes is a challenging task. Evaluation data comprise a rich source of information to measure the desired outcomes included in the logic model, along with contextual information, historical

>> Adaptation >>

Logic Model

The mission of the Comprehensive Community Mental Health Services for Children and Their Families Program is to encourage the development of intensive community-based services for children with serious emotional disturbance and their families based on a multi-agency, multi-disciplinary approach involving both the public and private sectors.

>> Quality Improvement >>

Population

Practice Context

Practices have traditionally promoted the use of restrictive placements and services

Service providers need to meet multiple needs of children and families that cross agency boundaries

Need coordination among service providers

Child & Family Context

Children under 22 years of age and their families

Diagnosis of emotional, behavioral, or mental disorder

Level of functioning in family, school, and/or community environments is limited

Two or more community agencies invoved

Disability must be present at least one year

System Context

Federal Center for Mental Health Services funds and supports systems of care with: Leadership, Technical assistance, Consultation, Evaluation

Local matching funds and resources

Need for comprehensive array of community-based, culturally competent and family-focused services

Need for family advocacy

Guiding principles

Family-focused: Services and supports should consider the needs and strengths of the entire family.

Individualized: Services and supports should be tailored to the needs and strengths of each child and family.

Culturally competent: Services and supports should be sensitive and responsive to the cultural characteristics of children and their families.

Least restrictive: Service planning should balance a child and family's need to interact in school and community settings with the most appropriate service and supports.

Core Values are Family-driven and Culture-based

Community-based: Services and supports should be provided in the child and family's community.

Accessible: Access to services and supports should not be limited by location, scheduling or cost.

Interagency: Core agencies providing services and supports should include mental health, child welfare, juvenile justice, and education.

Coordination/collaboration: Partner agencies, providers and organizations should provide a seamless system of services and supports for children and families.

<< Internal Evaluation <<

Figure 12.2. Program logic model. (Used with permission by Hernandez, M., & Hodges, S., [2003]. [Making children's mental health services successful series, 216-1]. *Crafting logic models for systems of care: Ideas in to action.* Tampa: University of South Florida, The Louise de la Parte Florida Mental Health Institute. Available online at http://www.usf.edu/institute/pubs/pdf/cfs/CMHseries/IdeasintoAction/IdeasintoActionprint.pdf)

Services for Children & Their Families

System of Care Strategy

Local Service Delivery Process

System entry, service planning, service provision, and review/monitoring of the care of individual children and families

Individualized & flexible services/supports

Family & child partners

Community member partners

State & federal agency partners

Local agency & organizaton partners

Community ownership and planning

Local Infrastructure Development

Governance, management, quality monitoring, and array of services/supports

Outcomes

Practice Outcomes

Service providers integrate system of care principle and values into practice

Children and families receive coordinated and useful services and supports in the community

Child and Family Outcomes

Children's distressing symptoms are reduced

Children have an improved ability to function at home, in school, and in their community

Improved family functioning and reduced caregiver strain

System Outcomes

Families are full partners in policy and implementation

Agency partnerships are broadened and deepened

Comprehensive, coordinated, efficient, and accountable service array is developed

Resources are appropriately allocated and utilized locally

System of care is sustained with stable, long-term funding

Child and family satisfaction with services is improved

Evaluation and Feedback to Suport Improved Service Delivery

experiences, and practical knowledge from stakeholders. Utilizing evaluation data for CQI efforts requires the development of appropriate performance measures and the achievement of consensus on these measures among members of the CQI team. Developing good performance measures is critical to the CQI process because these measures are used for a variety of purposes, including identifying areas of performance that require improvement, monitoring progress, and providing comparative information so that administrators can make better decisions and consumers and families can make better choices (Sorian, 2006).

There are three commonly accepted types of performance measures:

1. Workload and capacity measures

2. Process measures

3. Outcome measures

These three types of measures are defined on Table 12.3.

A comprehensive approach to CQI includes workload, process, and outcome measures that are both qualitative and quantitative and that accurately measure progress toward meeting system of care goals and objectives. When planning a CQI effort, it is important to balance use of existing sources of data with investing resources in new data collection efforts. Multiple data sources should be explored to identify performance measures for a system of care. Existing data sources should be used to the extent possible and should involve administrative data, including management information system (MIS) data and secondary data such as existing survey data, school data, and other types of existing data. The viability of using existing data sources should be assessed prior to deciding that new data collection efforts are required. The descriptive and outcome studies of the CMHI national evaluation provide an available source of data for the CQI Progress Report. Communities receiving these reports are encouraged to supplement information included in these reports with other information obtained from local data sources to provide additional measures of performance.

Table 12.3. Types of continuous quality improvement measures

Workload measures

Assess the level of work (inputs and outputs) and efficiency. Examples include timeliness of services, number of clients served, percent of inquiries responded to, and so forth.

Process measures

Assess what an organization does as part of the delivery of services. Process measures are used as a proxy for a desired outcome, assuming that improving the process will improve outcomes. The majority of measures in the mental health field are process measures.

Outcome measures

Assess a change or lack of change due to participation in the system, both functional (improved functioning in community) and clinical (psychological changes). Difficulties in using outcome measures include ways to define a positive change and the variation in interpretation of measures depending on the audience.

When developing the CQI Progress Report for the CMHI, performance indicators were identified that were actionable and measurable. *Actionable* refers to an indicator that can be influenced by actions or strategies put in place at the local level. As part of a CQI approach, indicators as measures of performance that will be able to show change must be selected or developed according to their ability to show the results when specific actions are taken. *Measurable* refers to the ability to measure performance relative to a specific program goal using the indicator. Table 12.4 provides an example of a performance measure—*timeliness of services*—and the assessment of the appropriateness of an indicator (*length of time between intake assessment and first service*) to gauge performance based on its measurability and actionability.

Once data sources and performance measures (e.g., *timeliness of services*) are identified, potential indicators (e.g., *number of days between intake and first service*) should be generated and discussed by the CQI team to ensure that the data represent what was intended. It is difficult for evaluators to develop measures that are functional (i.e., directly related to objectives), credible, and understandable to stakeholder groups without input from those who are involved in program administration, service delivery, and service receipt (Lichiello, 2000). For example, developing appropriate measures of family-driven and youth-guided care requires input from both youth and family members. Once appropriate performance measures are identified, tools must be developed and used to review and analyze performance.

Issues to consider when testing indicators include the reporting period, quality of data, frequency of data collection, and consumer perspectives. As part of the development of the CQI Progress Report and Benchmarking Initiative, several listening sessions were held over a period of 3–4 months to obtain feedback on the proposed indicators and the frequency of data reporting. Evaluators, family members, project directors, youth, and representatives from the Council for Collaboration and Coordination (the group guiding the federal CMHI), the Technical Assistance Partnership for Child and Family Mental Health, the Federation of Families for Children's Mental Health, Macro International Inc., and four systems

Table 12.4. Assessing the appropriateness of an indicator to measure the timeliness of services. *Indicator:* The average number of days between date of intake assessment and date of first service.

	Measurable	Actionable
Appropriate	This indicator is appropriate if it is possible to measure the time between an intake assessment and service receipt.	This indicator is appropriate if it is possible for program stakeholders to implement strategies that impact the number of days between intake and service receipt.
Inappropriate	This indicator is inappropriate if there is no mechanism to track the date of service intake and the date of first service receipt.	This indicator is inappropriate if there is no ability by program staff to influence the date of service receipt (e.g., due to short-term budget or personnel issues).

of care initially funded by the CMHI in 2002 and 2003 contributed to the development of the CQI Progress Report. Cuyahoga Tapestry System of Care; Bridgeport, Connecticut; Fort Worth, Texas; and Guam all participated as pilot sites for the development of a process to guide systems of care in their use of the report for technical assistance planning.

Reviewing and Analyzing Performance: Developing and Using Tools to Monitor Progress

The CQI Progress Report for the CMHI was developed using the previously outlined process, a team approach using the program logic model as a framework, and developing performance measures and accompanying indicators and benchmarks for assessing performance. The CQI Progress Report is a tool designed to review and analyze performance in five key areas for systems of care:

1. System-level outcomes

2. Child and family outcomes

3. Satisfaction with services

4. Family and youth involvement

5. Cultural and linguistic competency

The CQI Progress Report is a tool available to support system of care communities in their CQI efforts, but it also provides a practical example of how communities can engage in developing their own local CQI tools. The CQI Progress Report utilizes administrative data and longitudinal caregiver and youth-reported data to measure performance on indicators within the five domains. Raw scores are provided for each indicator, as well as benchmarks for performance and a scoring index to measure the extent to which benchmarks are achieved. The scoring index was designed to provide a construct for identifying areas of strength that can be replicated as recommended practices and areas of opportunity that can be targeted with technical assistance.

Each key area of performance includes specific indicators that generate a measure of performance related to that area, as well as performance on the specific indicator. There are 35 indicators across the key areas of performance assessed with the CQI Progress Report. Raw scores for each indicator are generated using data collected as part of the national evaluation. Each federally funded system of care community receives a community-level CQI Progress Report three times per year. In addition, a national-level CQI Progress Report, generated to assess program performance as a whole, is released on the same schedule in April, July, and December.

Figure 12.3 presents a sample section of the CQI Progress Report for an individual community. Each of the lettered circles identifies a feature of the report. To achieve the fundamental goal of continually improving the quality of systems of care, the CQI Progress Report includes benchmarks. Establishing performance goals through benchmarks provides clear and documented expectations for performance, as well as a means for communities and national program partners to measure progress in achieving those expectations or goals. The scoring index measures the ability to achieve benchmarks on specific indicators and allows communities and technical assistance providers to identify areas of strength and opportunity so that technical assistance resources can be appropriately targeted.

The benchmarks for each indicator included in the CQI Progress Report were established using a comparative approach. Indicators reported across communities were ranked, and the raw score that fell at the 75th percentile was established as the benchmark. This is a common benchmarking approach when trying to consider variations across sites and when clear performance criteria are not established. When more extensive historical data are available related to the indicators included on the CQI Progress Report, a criteria-based approach (i.e., setting benchmarks based on a widely expected level of performance) may be used to establish new benchmarks.

Identifying and Implementing Improvement Strategies: Developing an Infrastructure to Support Continuous Quality Improvement

Critical to CQI efforts is the development of an infrastructure to identify and implement improvement strategies based on system performance information derived from the review and analysis of data. Once tools are developed to monitor and analyze performance, a process for identifying and implementing strategies to improve performance closes the CQI loop. The communication feedback process that was developed as part of the CQI Progress Report and Benchmarking Initiative offers a practical example that can be replicated in systems of care. The CQI communication feedback process is designed to facilitate dialogue at the community level around CQI and between community representatives and technical assistance providers. This process uses the CQI Progress Report as a tool to identify areas that can be targeted for improvement and to develop technical assistance plans. Community-level representatives and federal program partners (e.g., the Technical Assistance Partnership for Child and Family Mental Health, the National Indian Child Welfare Association) use the CQI Progress Report to discuss the performance of their systems of care and whether that performance is meeting local and national benchmarks. Areas of strength are highlighted, opportunities for improvement are identified, and strategies to improve performance are developed. Individuals at the local level are responsible for providing the context for their performance and for identifying strengths and challenges that contributed to their performance. Federal program partners are responsible for assisting communities by helping to identify strategies to improve performance and by providing technical assistance to communities in carrying out those strategies. Specific discussion items mentioned in the communication feedback process include areas in which performance exceeded expectations, areas in which the community improved from the previous reporting period, areas in need of improvement, strategies and action steps to improve those areas, and expectations for the next reporting period.

COMPREHENSIVE COMMUNITY MENTAL HEALTH SERVICES FOR CHILDREN AND THEIR FAMILIES PROGRAM
CONTINUOUS QUALITY IMPROVEMENT (CQI) PROGRESS REPORT
COMMUNITY A, JULY 2006

	Date Service Started:	Oct-03
	Number Enrolled in the Descriptive Study:	355
	Number Enrolled in the Outcome Study:	345

	ACTUALS		CHANGE		INDEX		
	Performance Mark	Raw Score	Previous Raw Score	Change From Previous Report	Benchmark	Max Points	Actual Points
TOTAL SITE SCORE						100.00	78.50
System Level Outcomes							
Service Accessibility							
1. Number of children served (with descriptive data)	?	325	254	↑	n/a		
2. Linguistic Competency Rate	?	75.0%	88.0%	↓	98.9%	2.06	1.56
3. Agency Involvement Rate—Service Provision	? +	88.7%	96.5%	↓	92.9%	3.50	3.34
4. Caregiver Satisfaction Rate—Access to Services	? ++	4.63	4.54	↑	4.42	3.46	3.46
5. Timeliness of Services (average days)	? ++	2.00	2.07	↓	10.18	3.24	3.24
Service Quality							
6. Agency Involvement Rate—Treatment Planning	—	5.6%	9.5%	↓	64.1%	3.16	0.28
7. Informal Supports Rate	—	20.9%	25.6%	↓	51.4%	3.07	1.25
8. Caregiver Satisfaction Rate—Quality of Services	? ++	4.24	4.45	↓	4.13	3.30	3.30
9. Youth Satisfaction Rate—Quality of Services	? ++	4.22	4.21	↑	4.02	2.94	2.94
10. Caregiver Satisfaction Rate—Outcomes	? +	3.89	3.75	↑	3.61	2.72	2.72
11. Youth Satisfaction Rate—Outcomes	? ++	4.06	4.10	↓	3.92	3.41	3.41
System Level Outcomes Subtotal	?					37.00	29.53

Callout labels: a, b, c, d, e, f, g, h, i, j, k, l

Figure 12.3. Sample section of the CQI Progress Report. (Reprinted from Macro International Inc. [2006]. *Continuous Quality Improvement [CQI] Progress Report user's guide: Understanding the Center for Mental Health Services' (CMHS) Comprehensive Community Mental Health Services for Children and Their Families Program CQI Progress Report.* Available online at http://www.systemsofcare.samhsa.gov/hottopics/cqi.aspx)

a. **CQI Progress Report title**—Provides the name of the community represented on the report and the date the report was issued. The National Aggregate Report represents data across all communities with available data. The indicators in the report will represent data collected through the previous quarter (July 2006 report represents data collected through May 2006).

b. **Descriptive information**—The date services started and the number of families enrolled in the descriptive and outcome studies are provided for contextual information. The date services started reflects the first services provided as part of the funded system of care. The number enrolled in the descriptive study reflects the number of Enrollment and Descriptive Information Forms (EDIFs) submitted to the Interactive Collaborative Network (ICN) as of the data download date (e.g., July 2006 report reflects EDIFs submitted through May 2006). The number enrolled in the outcome study reflects the number of baseline outcome study cases that have been submitted to the ICN as of the data download date (e.g., July 2006 report reflects data submitted through May 2006). The baseline instrument with the largest number of cases is used as the number enrolled in the outcome study.

c. **Key areas of performance**—The CQI Progress Report is organized according to six keys areas of performance, including 1) system level outcomes, 2) child and family level outcomes, 3) satisfaction with services, 4) cultural and linguistic competency, 5) family and youth involvement, and 6) evidence-based practices.

d. **Subdomain of key area of performance**—Where appropriate, the key area of performance is grouped by subdomain to represent separate categories within the key area of performance.

e. **Performance indicators**—Within each key area of performance is a set of indicators that represent performance in that key area. For some key areas of performance, indicators are grouped by subdomain to further group indicators.

f. **Raw score**—The raw score represents the raw calculation for the specific performance indicator based on available data during the reporting period.

g. **Performance mark**—This column represents how well the community is performing relative to other communities in the cohort. The symbols represent the quartile at which the raw score falls; √++ represents the top quartile (75%-100%), √+ represents the quartile just below the top (50%-75%), √ represents the quartile just under the halfway mark (25%-50%), and – represents the lowest quartile (0%-25%).

h. **Previous raw score and change from previous report**—The previous raw score column represents the raw score from the previous report for each indicator. This allows for comparison across reporting periods. The change from previous report column indicates whether performance improved or declined from the previous report. An up arrow represents a positive change, and a down arrow represents a decline in performance.

i. **Benchmark**—For each indicator, a benchmark was established that represents the 75th percentile across sites on the April 2006 CQI Progress Report. Benchmarks are the established raw score that communities should attempt to achieve.

j. **Index**—The index represents a score calculated based on the proportion of the established benchmark achieved by the raw score. Max points represent the total number of points available for the indicator. Actual points represent the number of points assigned to the indicator based on the raw score. The proportion of the established benchmark achieved by the raw score is assigned to the max points to calculate the actual points.

k. **Subtotal**—The subtotal represents performance at the domain level. Subtotals will be provided for max points and actual points. The subtotal represents performance relative to benchmarks across all indicators in the domain. This allows for assessment of performance in the key areas that parallel the goals and objectives of the program. A performance mark will also be provided for each domain to represent how performance compares with other communities in the cohort.

l. **Total site score**—The total site score represents the sum or points across all indicators included on the report. A total site score will be provided for max points and actual points. The total site score represents performance relative to benchmarks across all indicators and domains. This allows for an assessment of overall performance.

Continous Quality Improvement
Progress Report Tool and User's Guide

As noted, the CQI Progress Report organizes performance measurement information into five critical areas for assessing systems of care:

1. *System-level outcomes*—includes indicators for service accessibility, service quality, and service appropriateness

2. *Child and family outcomes*—includes indicators at the child and family levels as reported by a caregiver and indicators reported by youth

3. *Satisfaction with services*—includes indicators for caregiver and youth satisfaction

4. *Family and youth involvement*—includes indicators for caregiver and youth satisfaction with their participation in service delivery, as well as caregiver and youth involvement in the service plan

5. *Cultural and linguistic competency*—includes indicators for family and youth satisfaction regarding cultural and linguistic competency

A sixth area assessing performance relative to the use of evidence-based practices is under development. Currently, 35 indicators within these areas are included in the CQI Progress Report. Table 12.5 displays the indicators within each of these areas and details how each indicator is defined and measured.

The *Continuous Quality Improvement (CQI) Progress Report User's Guide* (CQI User's Guide; Macro International Inc., 2006) was developed to provide instructions and guidance to systems of care and others seeking to use the CQI Progress Report. The *CQI User's Guide* can be found on the system of care web site at http://www.systemsofcare.samhsa.gov and can serve as a resource to states and communities interested in implementing a CQI process for their systems of care, regardless of whether they have received a federal grant for this purpose.

IMPLEMENTING THE CONTINUOUS QUALITY IMPROVEMENT PROGRESS REPORT IN CUYAHOGA TAPESTRY SYSTEM OF CARE (CLEVELAND, OHIO)

Cuyahoga Tapestry System of Care (Tapestry) was funded in 2003 with a grant from the CMHI, with the goal of improving outcomes and the integration of child-serving systems for youth with serious emotional disturbances. The level of need for services to this population and the backdrop of poverty in and around Cleveland are staggering. A needs assessment study conducted by the Federation for Community Planning (Johnsen, Marountas, Biegel, & Peters, 2003) estimated that 26,002 Cuyahoga County youth younger than age 21 suffered from a serious emotional disturbance. In 2005, Cleveland, the county's largest city, had the highest poverty rate among America's big cities (U.S. Census Bureau, 2006). Approximately 80% of the families enrolled in Tapestry live at or below the pov-

Table 12.5. Performance measurement areas and indicators in the CQI Progress Report

	Indicator definition

System-level outcomes

Service accessibility

1. Number of children served — Total number of children who received system of care services since the start of grant funded program

2. Linguistic competency rate — % of caregivers who indicated the provider spoke the same language or that interpreters were available to assist them always (5) or most of the time (4) during the first 6 months of services, excluding children/youth where English is the primary language spoken in the home

3. Agency involvement rate: Service provision — % of caregivers who identified more than one agency involved in providing services to their child and family during the first 6 months of services

4. Caregiver satisfaction rate: Access to services — Mean score across all children/youth on a scale of 1 (strongly disagree) to 5 (strongly agree) measuring agreement with access to service statements at 6 months after service intake

5. Timeliness of services: Average days — Average number of days between the assessment date and the first date of service

Service quality

6. Agency involvement rate: Treatment planning — % of children/youth with staff other than mental health involved in the development of the child's service plan

7. Informal supports rate — % of caregivers who reported receiving informal supports during the first 6 months of services

8. Caregiver satisfaction rate: Quality of services — Mean score across all children/youth on a scale of 1 (strongly disagree) to 5 (strongly agree) measuring caregiver agreement with quality of service statements at 6 months after service intake

9. Youth satisfaction rate: Quality of services — Mean score across all youth on a scale of 1 (strongly disagree) to 5 (strongly agree) measuring youth agreement with quality of service statements at 6 months after service intake

10. Caregiver satisfaction rate: Outcomes — Mean score across all children/youth on a scale of 1 (strongly disagree) to 5 (strongly agree) measuring caregiver agreement at 6 months after service intake with statements concerning the outcomes resulting from the services their child or family received

11. Youth satisfaction rate: Outcomes — Mean score across all youth on a scale of 1 (strongly disagree) to 5 (strongly agree) measuring youth agreement at 6 months after service intake with statements concerning the outcomes resulting from the services their child or family received

Service appropriateness

12. Increase in individualized education plan (IEP) development — % increase in the number of children/youth that had an IEP at intake to the total number of children/youth that had an IEP at 6 months after intake

13. Substance use treatment rate — % of caregivers who reported that their child had a problem with substance abuse and reported that the child received at least one service during the first 6 months of services that was related to the child's substance abuse problem

(continued)

Table 12.5. *(continued)*

	Indicator definition

Child and family outcomes

Caregiver Report child level

14. School enrollment rate
% of caregivers who reported that their child attended school at any time during the first 6 months after service intake, excluding caregivers who reported that the youth graduated from high school or obtained a GED

15. School attendance rate
% of caregivers who report that their child attended school at least 80% of the time in the first 6 months after service intake

16. School performance improvement rate
% of children/youth where the child/youth's grades improved during the first 6 months of services

17. Stability in living situation rate
% of children/youth where the child/youth lived in one living situation during the first 6 months of services

18. Inpatient hospitalization days per youth
Average number of days per child/youth spent in inpatient hospitalization during the first 6 months of services

19. Suicide attempt reduction rate: Caregiver report
% change from intake to 6 months in the percent of caregivers who reported a suicide attempt for their child in the previous 6 months. A negative raw score indicates a positive outcome (i.e., fewer suicide attempts).

20. Emotional and behavioral problem improvement rate
% of children/youth demonstrating improvement from intake to 6 months in emotional and behavioral total problem scores on the Child Behavior Checklist according to the reliable change index (RCI; Jacobson & Truax, 1991)

Family level

21. Average reduction in employment days lost
Difference from intake to 6 months in the average number of days missed work due to child's problem for children/youth. A negative raw score indicates a positive outcome (i.e., fewer average days lost).

22. Family functioning improvement rate
% change from intake to 6 months in mean score on the family functioning scale for children/youth with complete data at intake and 6 months.

23. Caregiver strain improvement rate
% of children/youth demonstrating improvement from intake to 6 months in caregiver strain on the Caregiver Strain Questionnaire, according to the reliable change index (RCI).

Youth report

24. Youth no arrest rate
% change from intake to 6 months in the percent of youth who reported no arrests in the previous 6 months.

25. Suicide attempt reduction rate: Youth report
% change from intake to 6 months in the percent of youth who reported a suicide attempt in the previous 6 months for cases. A negative raw score indicates a positive outcome (i.e., fewer suicide attempts).

26. Anxiety improvement rate
% of children/youth demonstrating improvement from intake to 6 months in total scores on the Revised Children's Manifest Anxiety Scales (RCMAS) according to the reliable change index (RCI).

27. Depression improvement rate
% of children/youth demonstrating improvement from intake to 6 months in total scores on the Reynold's Adolescent Depression Scale (RADS) according to the reliable change index (RCI).

Indicator definition

Satisfaction with services

28. Caregiver overall satisfaction

Score for caregiver overall satisfaction is the mean score across all satisfaction items on the Youth Services Survey–Family (YSS–F), on a scale of 1 (strongly disagree) to 5 (strongly agree). This indicator represents a compilation of all questions on the YSS–F.

29. Youth overall satisfaction

Score for youth overall satisfaction is the mean score across all satisfaction items on the Youth Services Survey (YSS) on a scale of 1 (strongly disagree) to 5 (strongly agree). This indicator represents a compilation of all questions on the YSS.

Family and youth involvement

30. Caregiver satisfaction rate: Participation

Mean score across all children/youth on a scale of 1 (strongly disagree) to 5 (strongly agree) measuring agreement at 6 months after service intake with statements related to caregiver participation in treatment, services and setting treatment goals.

31. Youth satisfaction rate: Participation

Mean score across all children/youth on a scale of 1 (strongly disagree) to 5 (strongly agree) measuring agreement at 6 months after service intake with statements related to youth participation in treatment, services and setting treatment goals.

32. Family/caregiver involvement rate: Treatment planning

% of children/youth with caregiver or other family members involved in the development of the child's service plan.

33. Youth involvement rate: Treatment planning

% of children/youth with a child age 11 or older, where the child was involved in the development of the child's service plan.

Cultural and linguistic competency

34. Caregiver satisfaction rate: Cultural competency

Mean score across all children/youth on a scale of 1 (strongly disagree) to 5 (strongly agree) measuring caregiver agreement at 6 months after service intake with statements related to the cultural competency of staff.

35. Youth satisfaction rate: Cultural competency

Mean score across all children/youth on a scale of 1 (strongly disagree) to 5 (strongly agree) measuring youth agreement at 6 months after service intake with statements related to the cultural competency of staff.

Reprinted from Macro International Inc. (2006). *Continuous Quality Improvement (CQI) Progress Report user's guide: Understanding the Center for Mental Health Services' (CMHS) Comprehensive Community Mental Health Services for Child and Their Families Program CQI Progress Report.* Available online at http://www.systemsofcare.samsha.gov/hottopics/cqi.aspx

erty level. In sum, Tapestry is serving the most economically challenged families in the most economically depressed city in the country.

In what is proving to be a unique strategy, Tapestry is integrating system of care implementation efforts with those of the Annie E. Casey–funded Neighborhood Collaboratives that are being implemented through the county Department of Children and Family Services. This partnership is proving beneficial for families because family and youth voice and choice are implemented on the ground in the very communities in which they live. Within this partnership, Tapestry uses a wraparound team process to blend formal Medicaid billable mental health services, coordinated by care managers, with informal family supports facilitated by parent advocates who are themselves caregivers of children with serious emotional disturbances. Care managers are colocated in the neighborhood collaboratives with parent advocates and supported administratively by the Positive Education Program (PEP) agency. PEP, which has been recognized nationally by the U.S. Department of Education as a model program for serving troubled youth, provides a strong foundation for CQI initiatives.

Continuous Quality Improvement Initiative

Tapestry was selected as a pilot site and development partner for the CQI Progress Report and Benchmarking Initiative that is part of the national evaluation. At the core of the local CQI initiative is a strong partnership between the evaluator and the system of care project director. It is important for the project director and evaluator to understand the data being collected in relation to the service delivery process so that a CQI team can be created with individuals that possess the knowledge and experience required to effect change. Trust is also critical for the CQI team because a high level of openness is necessary to accurately assess the circumstances and context surrounding the CQI data. The CQI team for the Tapestry system of care includes:

- Two family members with children in the system of care

- Two Parent Advisory Council members

- The Tapestry project director

- A Family and Children First Council representative

- Three evaluation team members from Kent State University

- A parent lead for Tapestry

- A juvenile court program officer

- The clinical director for Tapestry

- A Community Mental Health Board representative

- A school-based mental health programming representative

- A therapist from a leading private provider in the county

Much has been learned from the CQI pilot, and Tapestry continues to discover benefits and challenges resulting from the infusion of data into normal operations and decision making for the system of care. Challenges with the CQI process have been principally associated with the diffuse nature of service delivery in a system of care, meaning that treatment is a collaborative effort across multiple people and agencies working in teams and providing multiple services. This makes it difficult to understand the mechanisms that drive a particular outcome or to determine a cause and effect relationship that can be connected to new interventions or unique components of an intervention. Understanding why and how change occurs in the CQI Progress Report data is difficult, but without such data, stakeholders would not necessarily know the questions that should be asked to improve in important areas.

Communicating the Big Picture   With literally millions of data points coming and going in a system of care, it can be deceptively difficult and complex to take stock and answer such questions as "How are we doing?" The CQI total site score found at the top of the CQI Progress Report helps the Tapestry system of care regularly assess its overall achievement, progress over time, and success when compared with other system of care communities at a similar developmental stage.

Understanding Strengths   The domains, subdomains, and individual indicators included in the CQI Progress Report represent different facets of the principles important to a system of care. Each indicator tells a story, and understanding the service delivery mechanisms hypothesized to be causing or moving those scores informs the system of care about a strength in a particularly area. For example, Tapestry regularly sees success in the education domain on its CQI Progress Report. This strength is attributed to the strong relationships that PEP, Tapestry's care coordination provider, has developed with local schools and its commitment to ensuring that youth are attending and performing well in school as part of their individualized wraparound plans. The CQI data has helped to identify this as a strategy that works, which has led to the application of this strategy of collaboration with other system partners (e.g., probation officers, the juvenile court) to achieve a similarly positive impact.

Prioritizing Areas for Improvement   Those people reviewing the data presented in the CQI Progress Report have a tendency to go directly to the negative indicators. Based on Tapestry's experience, it is recommended that communities first establish priorities and then use the CQI tool as an aid to address, benchmark, and improve these priorities over time. It is important to look intuitively for answers when prioritizing the CQI indicators and developing plans of action to improve them. For Tapestry, the *timeliness of services* indicator represented the first level of engagement for families, and it made sense to focus on this CQI indicator because treatment, clinical outcomes, and satisfaction all follow from timely engagement and the quick provision of assistance to families seeking services.

Using the Continuous Quality Improvement Progress Report to Improve Service Delivery

The CQI process is invaluable in helping systems of care identify areas that need improvement and providing the impetus for implementing corrective strategies.

Data from the CQI Progress Report on the indicator *timeliness of services* demonstrates how CQI data are used to improve the system of care and its services. Timeliness of services is defined in the *CQI User's Guide* as "the average number of days between assessment date and date of first service" (Macro International Inc., 2006). The CQI tool uses data collected from the enrollment and demographic information form that is part of the national evaluation to calculate the mean value and benchmark for this indicator. Based on Tapestry's first CQI Progress Report, it was clear that too many families were waiting several weeks or more to begin services following the diagnostic assessment. To address this, the system of care took concrete steps. These included creating a *floater* position to make up for time lost due to staff turnover and leaves of absence, introducing an intake specialist, and relying more heavily on welcome meetings to quickly engage families. Despite these interventions, the mean number of days between assessment and the initiation of services remained relatively unchanged, and a meeting was convened to further address *timeliness of services*.

The next step was to review the raw data to analyze the distribution of the days making up the mean value seen in the CQI Progress Report. It was discovered that a large group of families received their first service incidents within 30 days, and a smaller group received their first services in 60 days or more. It appeared, therefore, that families were either being seen fairly promptly, or had to wait a significantly longer time for service delivery to begin, thus inflating the mean number of days from assessment to first service. This analysis suggested that other factors (e.g., engagement in services) could be playing a role for some families, and these needed to be addressed with different strategies.

Recognizing the importance of the 30-day threshold in initiating services, the CQI team created a new measure called *percent of families seen within 30 days*. PEP provides data to the CQI team on a weekly basis to monitor progress on this indicator. The percent of families seen within 30 days is a new local CQI measure that is reset each month to show the number of enrollments from the previous month and the percent of those who were seen within 30 days. This indicator has benefits because it does not reflect the impact of outliers in the time it takes to receive a first service after assessment. After sharing data with PEP managers and supervisors on the *percent seen within 30 days* indicator, a commitment was made to closely monitor this indicator and place those families that pass the 30-day mark for a first service after assessment into a special category of observation and follow-up. Results from this meeting and from instituting the local CQI indicator into a feedback loop have been dramatic. In the 2-month period of April and May 2007, the percentage of Tapestry families seen within the first month of enrollment has more than doubled (Figure 12.4).

Thus, CQI is a powerful tool that helps communities begin asking questions about the quality of their services and methods that might foster improvement. The first time a report is generated and a CQI team asks the questions "What is this number telling us?" and "What can we do about this?" the quality improvement journey is underway. By empowering people with the necessary data and creating feedback loops, remarkable outcomes are possible. Although there are en-

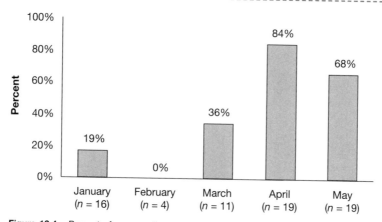

Figure 12.4. Percent of new enrollments each month seen with a face-to-face service within 30 days after intake/assessment. (*Note:* Data from Tapestry System of Care service enrollment counts; used by permission.)

gagement factors beyond the control of the system of care that are likely to affect the ability to serve every family within 30 days of assessment, this example makes a powerful case that demonstrates how families can be better served when the right data reach the right people.

CONCLUSION

The CQI process for systems of care described in this chapter builds on a history of evaluation and the use of evaluation data to provide information about system characteristics and outcomes at the local and national levels. This process clearly links goals to outcomes, thereby facilitating the use of evaluation information for the ongoing improvement of systems of care. Knowing what needs to change and how a system of care is progressing toward the desired change allows efforts to be directed to the specific target areas that require attention.

The CQI Progress Report and Benchmarking Initiative marks a significant advance toward the focused use of evaluation data for the improvement of systems of care. Buy-in to this CQI process was achieved across critical constituents involved with systems of care by fully involving funded communities, advisory groups, and other key stakeholders in the developmental process. It offers a tool that can be used by all parties—system of care communities, technical assistance providers, and federal CMHI leadership—as a template for assessing progress in system of care development. By developing a reporting tool and establishing benchmarks, the CQI Progress Report and the approach for rating indicators has the greatest potential for utility and buy-in at all levels.

Ultimately, CQI is not about *having* information regarding performance, but about *acting* on that information. The challenge for systems of care is in determining which areas require action, and if they do require action, what action is needed and in what priority order or relationship to one another various areas should be addressed. A performance rating on a specific indicator cannot determine the type of improvement effort to employ. The *why* behind performance is not answered by an indicator score or by comparison of that score to an established benchmark for performance. Further evaluation and contextual information are often needed to address questions about why a program is or is not achieving desired outcomes, as well as to inform next steps in the development of an approach to address program needs. Thus, a challenge for CQI processes is to determine not just where a challenge exists in a system of care but also why the challenge exists and what strategies will best address that challenge.

Although the CQI Progress Report was developed for communities funded by the federal system of care initiative and utilizes evaluation generated by the national evaluation, the method is applicable to nonfunded communities developing systems of care for youth with emotional disorders and their families. It is becoming more common for mental health boards at the county level—either by mandate or necessity due to increasing fiscal constraints—to implement comprehensive outcomes instrumentation in combination with structured billing and reporting techniques to better understand the effectiveness of treatment services being covered by Medicaid, state, and local dollars. The CQI Progress Report's use of benchmarking at the 75th percentile, along with its use of indicators over time that represent important system of care principles, is a model that can be used by all communities to assist in the allocation of finite resources aligned with local priorities to monitor improvements and provide data-driven technical assistance across an array of service providers.

REFERENCES

Achenbach, T.M., & Rescorla, L.A. (2000). *Manual for ASEBA Preschool Forms & Profiles.* Burlington: University of Vermont, Research Center for Children, Youth, & Families.

Achenbach, T.M., & Rescorla, L.A. (2001). *Manual for ASEBA School-Age Forms & Profiles.* Burlington: University of Vermont, Research Center for Children, Youth, & Families.

Berwick, D. (1989). Continuous improvement as an ideal in health care. *New England Journal of Medicine, 320,* 53–56.

Bird, H.R., Shaffer, D., Fisher, P., Gould, M.S., Staghezza, B., Chen, J.Y., et al. (1993). The Columbia Impairment Scale (CIS): Pilot findings on a measure of global impairment for children and adolescents. *International Journal of Methods in Psychiatric Research, 3,* 167–176.

Blumenthal, D., & Kilo, C.M. (1998). A report card on continuous quality improvement. *Milbank Quarterly, 76*(4), 625–648.

Brannan, A.M., Heflinger, C.A., & Bickman, L. (1998). The Caregiver Strain Questionnaire: Measuring the impact on the family of living with a child with serious emotional disturbance. *Journal of Emotional and Behavioral Disorders, 5,* 212–222.

Brunk, M., Koch, J.R., & McCall, B. (2000). *Report on parent satisfaction with services at community services boards.* Richmond: Virginia Department of Mental Health, Mental Retardation, and Substance Abuse Services.

Dougherty Management Associates, Inc. (2004). *Children's mental health benchmarking project: Fourth year report.* Lexington, MA: Author.

Epstein, M.H. (2004). *Behavioral and Emotional Rating Scale: A strength-based approach to assessment. Examiner's manual* (2nd ed.). Austin, TX: PRO-ED.

Epstein, P., Coates, P.M., Wray, L.D., & Swain, D. (2006). *Results that matter: Improving communities by engaging citizens, measuring performance, and getting things done.* San Francisco: Josey-Bass.

Fountain, J., Campbell, W., Patton, T., Epstein, T., Cohn, M., Abrahams, M., et al. (2003). *Reporting performance information: Suggested criteria for effective communication.* Norwalk, CT: Government Accounting Standards Board.

Government Performance and Results Act of 1993, PL 103-62, 107 Stat. 285.

Government Printing Office. (2002). *Rating the performance of federal programs.* Retrieved December 2007 from http://www.gpoaccess.gov/usbudget/fy04/pdf/budget/performance .pdf.

Hermann, R.C., Palmer, H., Leff, S., Shwartz, M., Provost, S. Chan, J., et al. (2004). Achieving consensus across diverse stakeholders on quality measures for mental health care. *Medical Care, 42*(12), 1246–1253.

Hermann, R.C., & Provost, S. (2003). Interpreting measurement data for quality improvement: Standards, means, norms, and benchmarks. *Psychiatric Services, 54*(5), 655–657.

Hernandez, M., & Hodges, S. (2003). Building upon theory of change for systems of care. *Journal of Emotional and Behavioral Disorders, 11*(1), 19–26.

Hernandez, M., & Hodges, S., (2005). *Making children's mental health services successful series: Vol. 1. Crafting logic models for systems of care: Ideas in to action* (Rev. ed.). Tampa: University of South Florida, The Louise de la Parte Florida Mental Health Institute

Jacobson, N.S., & Truax, P. (1991). Clinical significance: A statistical approach to defining meaningful change in psychotherapy research. *Journal of Consulting and Clinical Psychology, 59,* 12–19.

Johnsen, J., Marountas, L., Biegel, D., & Peters, J. (2003). *Cuyahoga County Community Mental Health Board Assessment.* Cleveland, OH: Federation for Community Planning.

Levison-Johnson, J. (2007, March). Monroe County logic model process. In A.K. Sheehan (Chair), *Theories of change from a continuous quality improvement (CQI) perspective: Logic modeling, measuring performance and benchmarking.* Symposium conducted at the 20th annual research conference, A System of Care for Children's Mental Health: Expanding the Research Base, Tampa, FL.

LeVitt, R. (1997). Quality 1 on 1. *Center for Quality of Management Journal, 6*(2), 29–40.

Lichiello, P. (2000). *Turning point guidebook for performance measurement.* Seattle: University of Washington, School of Public Health and Community Medicine, Health Policy Analysis Program.

Lichiello, P., Skariba, K., & Thompson, J. (2000). *Performance measurement in mental health final literature review.* Joint Legislative Audit and Review Committee, 2000 Mental Health System Performance Audit, Washington State.

Macro International Inc. (2006). *Continuous Quality Improvement (CQI) Progress Report User's Guide: Understanding the Center for Mental Health Services' (CMHS) Comprehensive Community Mental Health Services for Children and Their Families Program CQI Progress Report.* Available online at http://www.systemsofcare.samhsa.gov/hottopics/ cqi.aspx

National Performance Review (renamed National Partnership for Reinventing Government). (1997). *Serving the American public: Best practices in performance measurement, Benchmarking study report.* Available online at http://govinfo.library.unt.edu/npr/ library/papers/benchmrk/nprbook.html

Reynolds, C.R., & Richmond, B.O. (1978). What I think and feel: A revised measure of children's manifest anxiety. *Journal of Abnormal Psychology, 6*(2), 271–280.

Reynolds, W.M. (1986). *Reynolds Adolescent Depression Scale* (2nd ed.; RADS2). San Antonio, TX: The Psychological Corp.

Scholtes, P.R., Joiner, B., & Streibel, B.. (2003). *The team handbook: How to use teams to improve quality* (3rd ed.). Madison, WI: Oriel.

Sorian, R. (2006). *Measuring, reporting, and rewarding performance in health care.* New York: The Commonwealth Fund.

Sparrow, S., Carter, A., & Cicchetti, D. (1993) *Vineland Screener: Overview, reliability, validity, administration and scoring.* New Haven, CT: Yale University Child Study Center.

Titus, J.C., & Dennis, M.L. (2005). *Global Appraisal of Individual Needs–Quick (GAIN–Q): Administration and scoring guide for the GAIN–Q* (version 2). Retrieved August 30, 2006, from http://www.chestnut.org/LI/gain/GAIN_Q/GAIN-Q_v2_Instructions_09-07-2005.pdf

U.S. Census Bureau. (2006). *American fact finder.* Available online at http://factfinder.census.gov

Walton, M. (1986). *The Deming management method.* New York: Putnam Publishing Group.

13

Monitoring Fidelity to System of Care Principles in Service Delivery

MARIO HERNANDEZ, KEREN S. VERGON, AND JOHN MAYO

The system of care approach has been described as an explicit organizational philosophy emphasizing services and supports that are family focused, individualized, provided in the least restrictive environment, coordinated among multiple agencies, and culturally competent (Hernandez & Hodges, 2003). This conceptualization views systems of care as mutable strategies for improving interorganizational relationships and partnerships with youth and families so that access to a combination of seamless services and supports can be created in the context of system of care values and principles. The complexity associated with this conceptualization is far reaching and challenges system of care stakeholders with the need to ensure that the system's practices reflect its values and principles across all organizational levels. This important challenge, which is necessary at all levels of the system, is most needed at the point where children and their families receive services from the system of care.

Although system of care values and principles may be evident within organizational or management structures and processes, they may not be evident within service delivery practices. To address this challenge, methods are needed that assess the extent to which system of care values and principles are actualized within a system's direct service provision or in conjunction with fidelity to the system of care philosophy. Furthermore, it is important to continually monitor the extent of system of care implementation at the level of practice to ensure that the philosophy associated with systems of care is evident in practice, regardless of which services or supports are being provided to a child and family.

To effectively determine the depth of implementation of the values and principles at the direct service level, it is necessary to have a tool that supports the assessment of adherence to the system of care philosophy and to use this tool for ongoing fidelity monitoring and quality improvement purposes. The System of Care Practice Review (SOCPR) is such a tool, and its use enhances the ability of a system of care to achieve congruence between what its stakeholders, including policy makers and funders, have written and verbally expressed regarding their service delivery intentions and how the system's direct service practitioners actually implement services. The SOCPR uses a ratings-based intensive case study methodology that relies on multiple data sources to determine how existing services and supports address the needs of individual children and their families. This chapter describes the SOCPR and how it can be implemented and used to assess fidelity to system of care principles and to identify areas in need of improvement. An example of the use of the SOCPR for these purposes in a system of care in Hillsborough County, Florida (THINK) is also provided. THINK (Tampa-Hillsborough Integrated Network for Kids) was a community-based initiative intended to integrate mental health, juvenile justice, education, social, and other services for children with serious emotional disturbances (SEDs) and their families in Hillsborough County, Florida. It was funded through a federal system of care grant from 1998 to 2004.

THE SYSTEM OF CARE PRACTICE REVIEW

The SOCPR collects and analyzes information about the process of service delivery to document the service experiences of children and their families and then provides feedback and recommendations for improvement to the system. The process yields thorough, in-depth descriptions that reveal and explain the complex service environment experienced by children and their families. Feedback is provided through specific recommendations that can be incorporated into staff training, supervision, and coaching and may also be aggregated across cases at the system level to identify strengths and areas in need of improvement within the system of care. In this manner, the SOCPR provides a measure of how well the overall system is meeting the needs of children and their families relative to system of care values and principles.

The reliability of the SOCPR has been evaluated, and high interrater reliability has been reported in its use (Hernandez et al., 2001). The validity of the protocol is supported through triangulating information obtained from various informants and from document reviews. The SOCPR was found to distinguish between a system of care site and a traditional services site. Moreover, Hernandez et al. (2001) found in their study that the SOCPR identified system of care sites as being more child centered and family focused, community based, and culturally competent than services in a matched comparison site offering traditional mental health services. System of care sites were more likely than traditional service systems to consider the social strengths of both children and families and to include informal sources of support such as extended family and friends in the planning and delivery of services. In addition, Stephens, Holden, and Hernandez (2004) found that SOCPR ratings were associated with child-level outcome measures. In their comparison study, Stephens and colleagues discovered that children who received services in systems that functioned in a manner consistent with system of care values and principles compared with traditional services had significant reductions in symptomatology and impairment 1 year after entry into services, whereas children in organizations that did not use system of care values demonstrated less positive change. The study also found that as system of care–based practice increased, children's impairments decreased.

Method

The SOCPR relies on data gathered from face-to-face interviews with multiple informants, as well as through case files and record reviews. Document reviews precede face-to-face interviews and provide an understanding of the family's service history, including the presence and variety of services from sectors outside of mental health. These reviews also provide the chronological context of service delivery and help to orient the reviewer with the child and family's strengths, needs, and participation with services.

The face-to-face interviews are based on a set of questions intended to obtain the child and family's perceptions of the services they have received. Questions related to accessibility, convenience, relevance, satisfaction, cultural competence, and perceived effectiveness are asked. These questions are open-ended and designed to elicit both descriptive and explanatory information that might not be found through the document review. The questions provide the reviewer with the opportunity to obtain information about the everyday service experiences of the family and therefore gain a glimpse of what life is like for a child and family in the context of the services they have received.

The SOCPR uses a case study methodology informed by caregivers, youth, formal providers, and informal supports. The unit of analysis is the *family case*, with each case representing a test of the extent to which the system of care is implementing its services in accordance with system of care principles. The family case consists of the child involved in the system of care, the primary caregiver (e.g., biological parent, foster parent, relative), the primary formal service provider (e.g., lead case manager, mental health counselor, social workers), and if present, a primary informal helper (e.g., extended family member, neighbor, friend).

Domains

The SOCPR assesses four domains relevant to systems of care—Child Centered and Family Focused, Community Based, Culturally Competent, and Impact. The Child Centered and Family Focused domain is defined as having the needs of the child and family dictate the type and combination of services provided by the system of care. It is a commitment to adapt services to children and families, as opposed to expecting children and families to conform to preexisting service configurations. This domain has three subdomains: 1) Individualization, 3) Full Participation, and 3) Case Management.

The Community Based domain is defined as having services provided within or close to the child's home community in the least restrictive and most appropriate setting possible, and coordinated and delivered through linkages between a variety of providers and service sectors. This domain is composed of four subdomains: 1) Early Intervention, 2) Access to Services, 3) Restrictiveness, and 4) Integration and Coordination.

The Cultural Competence domain is defined by the capacity of agencies, programs, services, and individuals within the system of care to be responsive to the cultural, racial, and ethnic differences of the population they serve. This domain has four subdomains: 1) Awareness, 2) Sensitivity and Responsiveness, 3) Informal Supports, and 4) Agency Culture.

The Impact domain examines the extent to which families believe that services are appropriate and are meeting their needs and the needs of their children. This domain also examines whether services are seen by the family to produce positive outcomes. This domain has two subdomains: 1) Improvement and 2) Appropriateness.

Taken individually, these measures allow for assessment of the presence, absence, or degree of implementation of each of the domains and subdomains. Taken in combination, they speak to how close a system's services adhere to the values and principles of a system of care. The findings can also highlight which aspects of system of care–based services are in need of improvement. Ultimately, results provide the basis for feedback that allows a system's stakeholders to maintain fidelity to system of care values and principles.

Organization of the SOCPR

The SOCPR is organized into four major sections, as shown on Table 13.1:

- *Section 1*—Includes demographic information and a snapshot of the child's current array of services

- *Section 2*—Organizes the case records review and comprises the Case History Summary and the Current Service/Treatment Plan. The Case History Summary requires the reviewer to provide a brief case history based on a review of the file. It also provides information about all of the service systems with

Table 13.1. Components of the System of Care Practice Review

Section 1: Demographic Profile	Includes a brief overview of the current service array
Section 2: Document Review	Organizes and summarizes the case history and current service/treatment plan
Section 3: Interviews Primary caregiver Child/youth Case manager/provider Informal helper	Interview questions for the four informant types across domains
Section 4: Summative Questions	Reviewer ratings and discussion of the extent to which system of care values and principals are actualized

which the child and family are involved (e.g., special education, mental health, juvenile justice, child welfare). It summarizes major life events, people involved in the child's history and current life, outcomes of interventions, and the child's present status. Review of the service and treatment plan provides information about the types and intensity of the services received, integration and coordination, strengths identification, and family participation. The Document Review is completed prior to any interview so that the information gathered through the documents can inform and strengthen the interviews. Table 13.2 displays sample items from Sections 1 and 2 of the SOCPR.

- *Section 3*—Consists of the interview questions organized by the type of informant (primary caregiver, youth, formal service provider, informal helper). The interviews are designed to gather information about each of the four identified domains (Child Centered and Family Focused, Community Based, Cultural Competence, and Impact). Questions for each of the four domains are divided into subdomains that define the domain in further detail and represent the intention of the corresponding system of care core value. Questions in each of the subdomains are designed to indicate the extent to which core system of care values guide practice. Data are gathered through a combination of closed-ended questions (i.e., quantitative) that produce ratings and explanatory responses from participants through more open-ended questions and narrative responses (i.e., qualitative). The open-ended questioning provides an opportunity for the reviewer to probe issues related to specific questions so that answers are as complete as possible. In addition, direct quotes from respondents are recorded whenever appropriate and possible. Sample questions exploring each of the four domains with each type of informant are shown on Table 13.3.

- *Section 4*—Includes summative questions for each domain and subdomain. Sample summative questions are displayed in Table 13.4.

Table 13.2.   Sample items in sections 1 and 2

Section 1: Demographic Profile	Child's age, race, date of birth, gender, grade, language
	Service systems utilized
	Treatments and interventions
	Diagnosis
Section 2: Document Review	*Education*—Labels/conditions, type of school, resources
	Mental health—Diagnoses, interventions, and outcomes
	Summary—Summary of goals, services, and supports, as well as the extent to which they uphold system of care values/principals

Table 13.3. Section 3: Sample interview questions by domain and respondent type

	Primary caregiver	Child/youth	Formal provider	Informal provider
Child Centered and Family Focused	Do the people who are providing your child and family with services know about the strengths, concerns, and needs that you have just described? Do you think the current combination of services and supports is too intense, not intense enough, or just right for your child and family? How are your child and family involved in service planning? Is this person (case manager) helpful in coordinating the various services that your child and family receive?	Do you have any worries or concerns about your family? Is there someone in your life who you feel close to and go to for help when you need it? Do you and your family have a say in the final plan and the goals that are set? Does (primary coordinator) ask for your opinion about what kind of help you need?	What are the strengths of this child and family? How well do these types of services and supports (in plan) fit with the combination of needs and strengths you described for this child and family? Do the child and family directly influence the final plan that is developed and the goals that are set? How do you maintain communication with all of the child and family's service providers and informal supports?	What are the child and family's current needs? Do you participate in any of these services (provided) with child and his/her family? Do you feel like these services and supports are appropriate types for child and his/her family to be participating in at this time? Does (case manager) create a sense of teamwork among the various service providers, friends, and family who are helping the family?
Community Based	Once the providers clarified your needs, how long did it take before your child and family started getting help?	Is it easy for you to get to the places where you meet with (formal service providers)?	Do you think the child and family would be better off if they had received help sooner from systems and providers in the community?	Do the child and his/her family seem comfortable spending time in the places where they get help?

	Are the locations of the meetings and services convenient for your child and family? Does it seem like there is a smooth and seamless process to link your child and family with additional services as needs arise?		Do the child and family need any support to increase their access to services? To what extent are the services for this child and family provided in the least restrictive while also most appropriate environment(s) possible?	
Culturally Competent	Do the people working with your child and family seem to understand your culture, as you just described it?	Is the written information from (providers) in your language? Do the people who are helping your family understand what things are like in your neighborhood?	What is the cultural identity of this child and family as reflected in their values, beliefs and lifestyle? How do the child and family's culture impact their lives and relate to their concerns? Does the family understand how your agency works and how the agencies of other service providers work?	What is this family's culture? Do the service providers seem to recognize how their own culture influences their work? Do child and his/her family seem to understand how the different agencies and organizations work? Are you involved in the service planning process?
Impact (rating and explanation)	My family has made progress toward meeting its goals. Services have improved my child's overall situation	How much have services helped you?	The primary care giver is better able to deal with his/her child's problems. Services have improved this family's overall situation. What do you think has been most helpful about the services and supports provided to this child and family?	The child has made progress toward meeting his/her goals. Services have improved the child's overall situation

Table 13.4. Section 4: Sample summative questions by domain and subdomain

Child Centered and Family Focused	The strengths of the child have been identified.
	There is a primary service plan that is integrated across providers.
	The child and family influence the service planning process.
	The child and family actively participate in services.
	Service plans are responsive to the emerging and changing needs of the child and family.
Community Based	As soon as the child and family entered the service system, the service system responded by offering the appropriate combination of services and supports
	Services are provided within or close to the child and family's home community.
	Services are provided in the least restrictive and most appropriate environment(s).
	There is ongoing two-way communication among and between all team members, including formal service providers, informal helpers, and family members including the child.
Culturally Competent	Service providers recognize that the child and family must be viewed within the context of their own cultural group, and their neighborhood and community.
	Service providers know about the family's concepts of health and family.
	Service providers are aware of their own culture (values, beliefs, and lifestyle) and how it influences the way they interact with the child and family.
	Service providers translate their awareness of the family's culture into action.
	Service providers assist the child and family in understanding/navigating the agencies they represent.
Impact (rating and explanation)	The services/supports provided to the child have improved his/her situation.
	The services/supports provided to the family have appropriately met their needs.

Selecting Cases and Informants

Implementing the SOCPR involves the selection of cases for review and the selection of the key informants for interviews. The number and type of cases to be examined is determined by the agency or system of care using the SOCPR and should be tailored to meet the specific needs and interests of that agency or system. Cases are selected based on characteristics such as the child's age, gender, and the service sector with which the child is involved. For example, an agency or system may be interested in assessing its service delivery for young children who are not yet in school or for youth involved within the juvenile justice sector. A system may only include families with children who have certain challenges or youth who have been involved for short or long periods of time with services. Other criteria that could help guide case selection may be to select cases from a particular provider or a particular service modality such as case management. A system of care should be purposeful in its approach to sampling to ensure the usefulness of the results. If a few cases are drawn from too large a pool of services and programs, then it will be difficult to understand the results and to later know how and to whom to provide feedback. Determining the number of cases to be examined and the system's reason for implementing the SOCPR is critical to the usefulness of the results. For example, THINK focused its reviews only on child and families receiving care management services.

The SOCPR produces findings including mean ratings that reveal to what extent the services or system under review adhere to the system of care philosophy, that is, to what extent services are child centered and family focused, community based, and culturally competent. A mean rating is also completed that assesses the impact of services on children and their families. The ratings are supported and explained by reviewers' detailed notes and direct quotes from respondents in order to provide feedback that is objective, yet evocative and indepth. The findings are used to document the specific components of service delivery that are effective or that need to be further developed and improved to increase fidelity to the system of care approach.

Data Analysis and Reporting

The results of the SOCPR are organized and presented on the basis of the four domains: Child Centered and Family Focused, Community Based, Cultural Competence, and Impact. Each summative question is rated on a scale of –3 (disagree very much) to +3 (agree very much). These scores are then transformed, as shown in Figure 13.1, on a scale from 1 (disagree very much) to 7 (agree very much) to eliminate the – and + signs. Thus, –3 is transformed to 1; –2 to is transformed to 2; –1 is transformed to 3, and so forth.

Thus, a rating ranging from 1–7 is derived for each of the domains and their embedded measurements. Scores from 1 to 3 represent lower implementation of a system of care principle, and scores from 5 to 7 represent enhanced implementation of a system of care principle. A score of 4 indicates a neutral rating, meaning a lack of support for or against implementation.

The analysis of the SOCPR follows a sequential process in which data are coded, sorted, rated, and examined. Data are integrated, and ratings are determined for each question, embedded within a subdomain of one of the four main domains, with higher scores indicating that a family's experiences are more consistent with system of care principles. All of the interview questions in the SOCPR are organized into a predetermined coding scheme. This allows for questions to be sorted by interview (e.g., primary caregiver, child, formal provider) and by domain. Once all of the required data for the protocol have been collected, the information is integrated to rate the summative questions, each relating to a specific domain. The ratings specified for each subdomain are averaged to provide a global rating for that domain. In addition, the summative questions for each domain are clustered, with their average rating representing a

-3	-2	-1	0	1	2	3
1	2	3	4	5	6	7
Disagree very much	Disagree moderately	Disagree slightly	Neither agree nor disagree	Agree slightly	Agree moderately	Agree very much

Figure 13.1. Summative question rating scale.

measurement of the individual components in each domain. Finally, reviewers support their final ratings with a brief explanation and direct quotes from the interviews.

The report is structured so that each domain and its subsections are individually reviewed to complement the overall summary score data table. Each section is defined, and then the average ratings found in the summary score data table are reviewed with a translation to implementation level. An analysis of the overall scores and qualitative findings is then given, followed by illustrative quotes from actual respondents. This format was chosen to allow for examination of individual sections in isolation without having to continuously reference other parts of the report. Box 13.1 provides a sample summary report for the SOCPR, including sample sections from the qualitative analysis.

Training of the Interview Team

Before data collection begins, the team administering the SOCPR process must be identified and trained. The teams are composed of a team leader and reviewers. Case reviews may be conducted using single reviewers or paired review teams. The use of single reviewers allows for more cases to be reviewed at a lower cost. Pairing reviewers provides the advantage of being able to validate and discuss what is being learned through the review process. The use of paired reviewers is obviously more costly and may not always be feasible; however, when individual reviewers are conducting the SOCPR, it is recommended that reliability checks be conducted with another reviewer.

Training sessions should be provided to the reviewers to enhance interrater reliability and the validity of ratings for the SOCPR, as well as to familiarize reviewers with the SOCPR's structure. To achieve these goals, training sessions include a review of the values and principles of systems of care, an orientation regarding the purpose and objectives of the SOCPR, and practice sessions for interviewing and rating the summative questions within the SOCPR. Because much of the useful information about a family is collected through interviews, it is important to train reviewers in the proper methods for conducting interviews and documenting in-

Box 13.1. Sample section qualitative analysis

The overall mean score (see Figure 13.2) at the case level falls on Agree Slightly (M = 5.16, SD = 0.97). This indicates that, overall, the system of care's services operate at a slightly enhanced level of implementation of system of care (SOC) principles. Mean scores show that the SOC performed best in the Community Based domain, followed by the Culturally Competent domain. The Child Centered and Family Focused and Impact domains follow; however, the ratings were in the neutral range overall. The standard deviations of 0.86–1.46 show that three of the domains experienced variability in implementation, with some cases showing higher levels of implementation, while others evidenced more room for improvement. The SOC scored highest in subdomains related to access to services and restrictiveness level.

SAMPLE SECTION FROM THE CHILD CENTERED AND FAMILY FOCUSED DOMAIN: CASE MANAGEMENT

Case management is intended to ensure that youth and families receive the services they need in a coordinated manner, that the types and intensity of services are appropriate, and that services are driven by the youth and families' changing needs over time. The protocol assumes that for case management to take place, the presence of someone with the title of *case manager* is not required as long as someone is assigned the responsibility of service coordination or case management.

The average rating for this subdomain fell in the neutral SOC implementation range. The large standard deviation shows that while some cases did evidence strong case management, other cases would have benefited from a single person who successfully coordinated the planning and delivery of services and supports. In fact, about half of the cases rated the question about a single person coordinating the service planning and delivery as low. The existence of multiple plans from multiple providers and, in some cases, multiple formal providers acting as case managers, made identification of a single point of coordination difficult to achieve. In addition, there was one case in which there were multiple plans and two people who were managing the plans, yet the family felt the arrangement worked well for them.

Some caregivers voiced strong frustration. One caregiver said, "[Case manager] does not help me get services. She only comes to do paperwork." Another caregiver made several statements about her case management service: "I've been on my own." "She'll say she'll do something, but it rarely happens." "I had to take care of most of the problems . . . " However, when case management and coordination are successful, families are happy: "[Provider] really connected with them (service) and got us the fit." Thus, efforts to place a single person in charge of service planning and delivery can have a large positive impact on families' service receipt experiences.

SAMPLE SECTION FROM THE COMMUNITY BASED DOMAIN: INTEGRATION AND COORDINATION

For a system to be truly community based, integration and coordination between components of the system of care and between service providers should be evident. This assists in communication between child and family team members and contributes to a smooth and seamless process for linkages to new and needed services.

(continued)

Box 13.1. (continued)

The average rating for this subdomain was in the neutral implementation range; however, the size of the standard deviation for this rating indicates that some cases within the system of care do show integration and coordination.

One caregiver said, "I think they try to direct [care in a coordinated way], but I don't know if they communicate." Another caregiver reported, "There's no team—everybody's doing their own thing." Still another caregiver said, "They talk to us to coordinate what we need and then get us help." These very different experiences—confusion, difficulty, and ease—show that sometimes integration and coordination are very apparent, yet at times seem to be lacking.

---

formation from the responses that emerge during the review. Without this part of the training, reviewers may not probe adequately, or they may overlook information that helps with both the summative ratings and with the feedback that is later provided to the system of care. In addition, interview training is important so that the reviews are respectful, effective at ensuring that all questions are answered, and able to create a comfortable experience for informants.

During the training of reviewers, it is recommended that each trainee be shadowed by the trainer or another person with experience using the SOCPR protocol. This hands-on training includes the shadowing of a trainee by an experienced reviewer who participates in all aspects of the case review. The trainee conducts the interviews and leads the case review, and the shadow is available to provide support, clarify procedures, answer questions, and complete a separate set of ratings for comparison. Once a training case is completed, the trainee and shadow debrief about the case. It is essential that the debriefing include a discussion of why the ratings were given and how the notes resulting from the review will be used to give feedback to system stakeholders. Trainees, shadows, and the primary trainer typically meet together for group debriefing. The process of shadowing and debriefing continues until each trainee attains acceptable levels of agreement with their experienced shadow based on Spearman-Brown reliability coefficients (Hernandez et al., 2001).

The shadowing of two cases per trainee allows for an examination of the trainee's ability to conduct the SOCPR in an appropriate and reliable manner. The reliability of a trainee can be examined through the calculation of three different measures: 1) the percentage of summative question ratings that were exact matches between the trainee and the shadow, 2) the percentage of summative question ratings that were scored in the same direction (positive or negative scores) by the trainee and the shadow, and 3) the discrepancy value between the trainee and shadow scores displayed as a percentage. Figure 13.3 provides an example of reliability scoring.

Overall Score—all cases: 5.16 (0.97)		
	Areas X (SD)	Subdomain X (SD)
Domain I: Child Centered and Family Focused: 5.03 (1.01)		
Individualized		4.84 (1.09)
Assessment/inventory	6.02 (0.75)	
Service planning	4.37 (1.29)	
Types of services/supports	4.26 (2.05)	
Intensity of services/supports	3.79 (2.44)	
Full participation		5.63 (1.15)
Case management		4.39 (2.03)
Domain II: Community Based Domain Score: 5.58 (0.86)		
Early intervention		4.42 (1.88)
Access to services		6.36 (0.59)
Convenient times	6.16 (1.57)	
Convenient locations	6.11 (1.40)	
Appropriate language	6.84 (0.41)	
Minimal restrictiveness		6.21 (1.22)
Integration and coordination		4.42 (1.53)
Domain III: Culturally Competent Domain Score: 5.13 (1.46)		
Awareness		5.48 (1.63)
Awareness of child/family's culture	5.56 (1.64)	
Awareness of providers' culture	5.16 (2.09)	
Awareness of cultural dynamics	5.58 (1.84)	
Sensitivity and responsiveness		4.53 (2.17)
Agency culture		5.42 (1.82)
Informal supports		3.95 (1.99)
Domain IV: Impact Domain Score: 4.68 (1.40)		
Improvement		5.03 (1.33)
Appropriateness		4.34 (1.68)

Figure 13.2. Sample section qualitative analyses.

Reviewee/shadow	Case	Metric	Case total	Child Centered and Family Focused total	Community Based total	Cultural Competence total	Impact total
Reviewee 1	1	% Same Score	19.0	11.8	45.5	10.0	0.0
		% Same Direction	70.7	76.5	70.0	60.0	75.0
Shadow 1		% Total Scoring Distance	25.0	24.5	15.0	36.7	29.2
Reviewee 1	2	% Same Score	78.6	88.2	63.6	70.0	100.0
		% Same Direction	97.6	94.1	100.0	100.0	100.0
Shadow 2		% Total Scoring Distance	4.0	3.9	5.0	5.0	0.0

Figure 13.3.   Sample reliability scoring.

The first score, *% Same Score,* represents the percentage of times the reviewer and the shadow scored the summative question with the exact same rating. Thus, if both people scored a summative question as +2, then this summative question would be counted as positive for this percentage score. There are a total of 42 summative questions, so the number of same responses divided by this total number of summative questions yields the *% Same Score.* A high percentage in this score is desirable.

The second score, *% Same Direction,* represents the percentage of times the reviewer and the shadow scores the summative question in the same direction, either positive or negative. As previously explained, the –3 to +3 scale is used to rate summative questions. Each time the reviewer and the shadow both score the summative question with either a positive or a negative number, the summative question is counted as positive for this percentage score. Because a score of 0 does not indicate directionality (0 = Neither Agree or Disagree), a score of 0, by default, cannot count as a match in directionality. A high percentage in this score is desirable.

The third score, *% Total Scoring Distance,* represents the percentage of total possible distance that is reported between all of the reviewer's ratings and the shadow's ratings. This score can be used to determine if the reviewer is moving in the right direction in terms of his or her ratings. Because the –3 to +3 scale is transformed to a scale of 1–7, a total distance of 6 is possible for each summative question. Thus, if the reviewer and the shadow were the maximum rating apart on every summative question, a total of 252 units of difference could be recorded. The actual distance between all of the reviewer's rating and the shadow's ratings is converted into a percentage score. A low percentage in this score is desirable. Desirable ratings are indicated by achieving a total scoring distance of less than 10%, indicating a high degree of consistency between the reviewers being trained and the experienced shadows.

EXAMPLE OF SYSTEM OF CARE PRACTICE REVIEW USE: FROM APPREHENSION TO PARTICIPATION

The SOCPR was implemented during the first 2 years of the development of a system of care in west central Florida known as the THINK. As mentioned previously, THINK was a community-based initiative intended to integrate mental health, juvenile justice, education, social, and other services for children with SEDs and their families in Hillsborough County, Florida. The THINK system of care was one of more than 100 sites around the United States funded by a grant from the Center for Mental Health Services in the federal Substance Abuse and Mental Health Services Administration. THINK served children in Hillsborough County who were referred by either the school system or a mental health practitioner (Davis, Dollard, & Vergon, 2003). Five area case management agencies were involved in the THINK project, including THINKids, a case management pilot program funded by the THINK system of care grant.

Initial Implementation

At the time of SOCPR implementation, THINKids was serving 25 children and their families. The service delivery team consisted of three traditionally trained system navigators/case managers and a program director. The four-person team had extensive years of mental health experience—two were licensed mental health counselors, one was a license-eligible marriage and a family therapist completing her internship, and one was the parent of a child with special needs. THINKids' program director, one of the four providers, was a licensed clinical social worker responsible for liaison work between the community and the school's SED programs. At the time of the SOCPR's introduction to THINKids, the service delivery team was beginning its orientation and training in wraparound techniques. The THINK project's evaluators from the University of South Florida conducted the SOCPR implementation.

After the initial review using the SOCPR was completed, THINKids' program director was asked to provide feedback on the experience of using the SOCPR to assess service delivery. The director reported that the team perceived the review process to be substantially different from their past experiences with quality assurance and quality improvement processes within mental health organizations. The team was initially apprehensive about the level of exposure and review their practices would receive, but they were made comfortable with the nonjudgmental and strengths-based manner in which the review was conducted. Team members, however, also reported that the instrument was very lengthy and required more time to complete than they had anticipated. Families who participated in the review gave overwhelmingly positive reports, with none expressing discomfort with either the interview protocol or the reviewers.

Feedback to the System of Care

The director also reported on the feedback process, which was provided during a meeting with the entire case management team and the staff that had conducted the review. The feedback was perceived to be provided in a timely manner, and the meeting was reported to have been conducted in a comfortable and casual style. The case managers reacted positively to the practical nature of the feedback process and described it as strength based, nonjudgmental, and clear about which practices needed improvement.

The feedback that resulted from the reviews was reported to be interesting, and in some cases, surprising to the team. One important suggestion based on the SOCPR chart reviews was that there was no documentation of family voice and choice in service planning and delivery. Although the team believed that their practice was anchored in family voice and choice, there was no documentation that this had occurred in the process of service planning and delivery. This is a direct example of feedback that quickly resulted in a change to the team's approach to documentation. It was later reported by the team that it was important to redesign forms to document family input and choice of services and supports, but it was even more important to have this emphasized in the documentation as a prompt to case managers to remind them of the importance of the family role. Box 13.2 provides an example of feedback from the SOCPR based on the service experience of one family served by the system of care.

Another benefit of the initial SOCPR feedback was the provision of information that reinforced what they were doing well and pointed out ways to improve their practice in implementing strengths-based and culturally competent care. For example, the team received high ratings for giving families information about resources available in the community and incorporating community resources into the service plans. The team was also assessed positively for finding and creating individualized solutions that included nontraditional services, explaining agency cultures to families, considering culture when planning services, and being aware of neighborhood characteristics that might affect a family's par-

---

Box 13.2.   Vignette based on the System of Care Practice Review
feedback for one family

The "Diez" family was referred to the THINK program in August 2002 and discharged in April 2005. The immediate family consisted of the mother, her two sons, and two nephews she was caring for. The father had died while serving a prison sentence. Extended family included the maternal grandfather, who was a pastor of a local church, and others who resided out of town. The family identified themselves as Hispanic and reported that they were fully Americanized. The mother was bilingual. The children spoke English, but they also understood some Spanish. Both sons had severe mental health and substance abuse issues. The youngest son was attending the SED Center at the time of his admission to THINK.

The family team varied a great deal during the Diez family's involvement with the program, ranging from 4 to 12 members. During this time, the sons had several crisis center admissions; the oldest was committed to a Department of Juvenile Justice facility, and the youngest was placed in a substance abuse facility. At the time the family was discharged from THINK, the youngest son was living at home, the oldest son (now an adult) was living on his own, and the nephews had been reunited with their mother. At discharge, the mother reported much greater stability, but she was concerned about the potential for future substance use by both sons. The natural supports available at discharge included the extended family, the church, and the mother's supervisor at work. Formal providers continuing services at discharge included Job Corp, substance use outpatient treatment, and the Department of Juvenile Justice.

The results of the System of Care Practice Review included high ratings in the areas of cultural competency, community-based services, and child-centered and family-focused service delivery. The review process also revealed areas needing improvement in practice at the program and system levels. Program issues included the need to focus support plans on long-term stability of the family rather than on responding to crises and the need to develop strategies for educating families to become advocates for the services they needed. It was also suggested that staff could decrease the time it takes to get families into services after a need has been identified. The main systemic issue that was identified was the need to offer smooth and timely transitions between child-serving systems—particularly between mental health and substance abuse treatment services—and exceptional student education and juvenile justice facilities.

---

ticipation in services and quality of life. High ratings were also received for conducting team meetings in nontraditional locations that were more convenient and comfortable for families. The main area assessed as needing improvement was the inclusion of more informal supports in the service planning and delivery process. Figure 13.4 provides an example of feedback given to providers from the SOCPR in the Cultural Competence domain.

The review was also helpful in delineation between program and system traits. It was discovered that the service delivery system in the county was rela-

System of Care Practice Review Findings

Cultural Competence Domain

1–7 point scale 1 = Disagree very much 7 = Agree very much	Mean
1. Service providers are aware of the dynamics inherent when working with families whose cultural values, beliefs, and life style may be different from their own.	7
2. Service providers know about the family's concepts of health and family.	6
3. Service providers recognize that the child and family must be viewed with the context of their own cultural group, neighborhood, and community.	7
4. Service providers recognize that the family's values, beliefs, and lifestyle influence the family's decision-making process.	7
5. Service providers are responsive to the family's values, beliefs, and lifestyle.	6
6. Service providers include informal/natural sources of support for the child and family in service delivery.	5

Comments:

In many ways, System Navigators are culturally competent. They are responsive to the family's native language and seem to be aware of cultural dynamics when working with families. They are intentional about explaining agency cultures to the family. They are respectful of the families' cultures and consider cultural variables when planning services. They are aware of family relationships and community or neighborhood characteristics and often exhibit respect for them. However, one ongoing challenge is including extended family and informal supports in team meetings or, to a lesser extent, Family Support Plans. There are, however, notable examples in which extended family members are present both in the team meeting and in the FSP. The main challenge to including informal support seems to be reluctance on the part of the family. This should be a long-term goal for the family—to build a personal support network. Incorporating church youth groups or the YMCA in the service array are nice examples of success in including informal supports. THINKids' forms include a cultural competence checklist, which helps System Navigators maintain an awareness of the family's culture.

Figure 13.4. Sample feedback to providers.

tively devoid of strengths-based procedures and opportunities for family voice and choice. Across mental health, child welfare, juvenile justice, and education, the practice of a deficit-based approach was common among workers. It was helpful for the team members to be able to distinguish between their use of strengths-based planning, for which they were personally responsible, and the systemwide deficiencies in this area, which required a community effort to influence practice across different sectors. Another example of a system issue identified through the SOCPR process was in the linkages between THINK and county agencies. This was seen in the lack of a coordinated process for obtaining services outside of THINK's typical partners and was also specifically noted in the inconsistent attendance of these partners at child and family team service planning meetings.

At the conclusion of the first round of SOCPR reviews, overall recommendations for the THINK team were provided. The suggestions were as follows:

- Include more informal supports in meetings

- Use strengths in a more relevant manner that better relates identified strengths to family goals or needs

- Set goals that are more measurable, behaviorally specific, and have clear steps for implementation such as time frames for review

- Write the entire support plan *with* the family rather than *for* the family

- Update plans more frequently to include subsequent goals

- Engage youth to a greater degree in service planning

- Practice better meeting management skills (e.g., draw up and follow agendas, summarize the meeting at its conclusion)

    The review also identified team strengths. These included the following:

- Developing good relationships with families

- Demonstrating the ability to move families beyond initial crises

- Engaging other providers in the planning

- Engaging families in planning

- Acknowledging culture in the planning and delivery process

- Addressing multiple life domains in a holistic plan

- Conducting meetings in nontraditional locations that are convenient for the family

- Creating individualized solutions that include nontraditional services to meet a family's needs.

CONCLUSION

The SOCPR is useful in providing feedback to service providers as they attempt to make quality improvements to their systems of care. Results from the SOCPR can highlight successes and challenges at the level of the individual service worker, team, program, and the system of care as a whole. The SOCPR seeks to accomplish this quality improvement task by documenting the experiences of children and their families enrolled in systems of care, documenting adherence to the system of care philosophy by direct service providers, and generating recommendations for improvement. In this manner, information learned through the SOCPR can be used as part of a system's continuous quality improvement strategy. At the service provider level, the SOCPR is helpful in identifying staff training, supervision, and coaching needs. The SOCPR can identify service delivery practices such as the failure to complete child and family assessments, a lack of prioritization of the needs and strengths of a child and family by life domains, or a lack of involvement of families in the creation of service plans. Because these lapses in the practice of the system of care are believed to affect child and family outcomes, it is important that they be identified and addressed in a system's quality improvement efforts.

By aggregating results at the system level, the SOCPR can also identify gaps in service access that prevent families from obtaining the help they need. This may be due to the lack of services offered in or near their communities, as well as issues of interagency coordination and implementation of services that impair a system's ability to provide seamless services. Aggregate findings may also indicate systemwide needs such as improved cultural competence throughout the service system. Because it is also possible to use the SOCPR to assess the needs of a community prior to the development of a system of care, emerging systems can determine what specific areas need to be addressed at both the practice and system levels.

Overall, the SOCPR is a promising tool for assessing the degree of implementation and fidelity to system of care values and principles at the level of practice (Hernandez et al., 2001). Rosenblatt (1998) asserted that regardless of the intentions of a system of care, it is the direct service strategies that will most likely achieve the positive results that system of care stakeholders seek for children and families within their communities.

REFERENCES

Davis, C.S., Dollard, N., & Vergon, T. (2003, April). *The reconstruction of meaning in creating a system of care in community mental health care.* Paper presented at Top Papers in Health Communication, Eastern Communication Association Conference. Washington, DC.

Hernandez, M., Gomez, A., Lipien, L., Greenbaum, P. E., Armstrong, K., & Gonzalez, P. (2001). Use of the system of care practice review in the national evaluation: Evaluating the fidelity of practice to system of care principles. *Journal of Emotional and Behavioral Disorders, 9,* 43–52.

Hernandez, M., & Hodges, S. (2003). Building upon theory of change for systems of care. *Journal of Emotional and Behavioral Disorders, 19,* 19–26.

Rosenblatt, A. (1998). Assessing the child and family outcomes of systems of care for youth with severe emotional disturbance. In M.H. Epstein, K. Kutash, & A. Duchnowski (Eds.), *Outcomes for children and youth with emotional and behavioral disorders and their families: Programs and evaluation best practice* (pp. 329–362). Austin, TX: PRO-ED.

Stephens, R.L, Holden, E.W., & Hernandez, M. (2004). System-of-care practice review scores as predictors of behavioral symptomatology and functional impairment. *Journal of Child and Family Studies, 13*, 179–191.

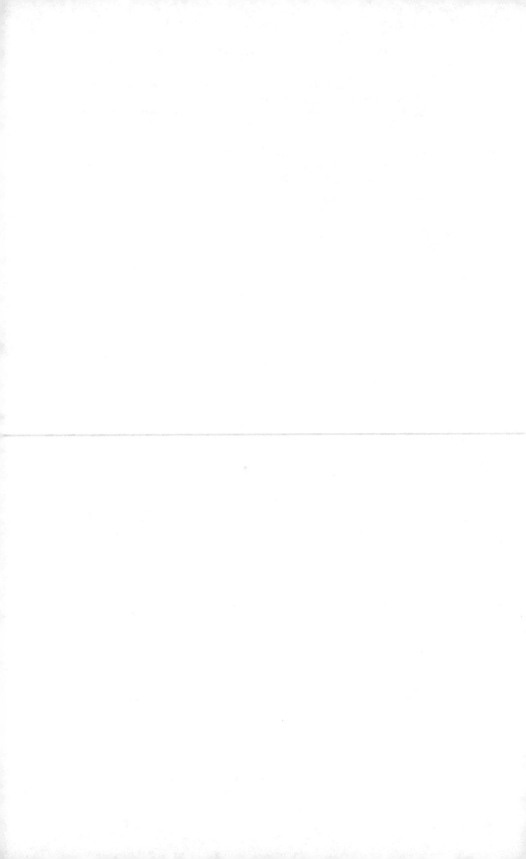

14

Social Marketing

MARIA J. RODRIGUEZ, LISA RUBENSTEIN, AND BARBARA HUFF

It is hard to imagine what the world would be like if there were no social change campaigns. Over the years, people have been encouraged to quit smoking, say no to drugs, not drink and drive, buckle their seatbelts, and do a myriad of other things to improve themselves and the world around them. Many of the most successful campaigns use social marketing, which essentially is the application of commercial marketing practices to promote ideas or causes. Instead of persuading people to buy a certain brand of soap or see a hit movie, these social marketing strategies are designed to encourage people to take actions that will lead to better health or some other social good.

As early as 1951, experts were exploring the use of commercial marketing practices to sell social causes and behavior change. In his visionary article, Gerhardt Wiebe (1951) asked if brotherhood could be sold like soap and implied that the more a social cause campaign mimicked the marketing of commodities, the more likely it was to be successful. Twenty years later, Philip Kotler and Gerald Zaltman answered Wiebe's question with a resounding "yes," and in doing so, they forever changed the marketing industry. Together, they coined the term *social marketing*, which was then defined as "the design, implementation and control of programs calculated to influence the acceptability of social ideas and involving considerations of product planning, pricing, communication, distribution and marketing research" (Kotler & Zaltman, 1971, p. 5). The rest is history.

By the mid 1990s, social marketing techniques had proven their worth. Americans were smoking less, designating drivers, and preventing forest fires. Youth were saying no to drugs, women were getting mammograms, whales were being saved, and recycling had become law in some parts of the country.

Despite the explosive growth in the use of social marketing and its obvious effectiveness, its application by the mental health community was cautious. The tremendous stigma associated with mental health challenges prevented people from talking openly about mental health issues. Many blamed the media for perpetuating the stigma by depicting violent and negative portrayals of people with mental health problems. More often than not, mental health professionals distrusted the media and avoided it altogether. They were also reticent to pursue or accept other opportunities to speak publicly about mental health service delivery and treatment. The notion of proactively seeking media and public attention for mental health programs was rarely given serious consideration.

Given the success of social marketing in other areas, the U.S. Congress recognized the important role it could play in overcoming stigma when it mandated investment in the design of systems of care for children, youth, and their families. In 1992, when federal funding became available to develop systems of care across the country and in tribal nations, the government included a social marketing component—the Caring for Every Child's Mental Health Campaign. Since then, the campaign has undertaken national social marketing efforts and provided technical assistance in social marketing to federally funded system of care communities. Specifically, the campaign has helped system of care communities design and implement social marketing initiatives that have led to increased access to care by all children and youth with serious mental health needs and their families. In addition, the campaign has produced public information materials that systems of care use to educate children, youth, families, and their system partners on children's mental health issues.

The first federally funded system of care communities reluctantly embraced social marketing. Many decision makers in these communities believed that they had bigger issues on which to focus (e.g., sustaining their systems beyond federal funding, building partnerships among local agencies and organizations, hiring and training staff, building service capacity, overcoming stigma). They felt that they had to dedicate their resources to these issues and failed to understand how social marketing could support those priorities. Social marketing was viewed by many in the field as sales or marketing of existing services.

These decision makers, however, did understand that they needed to change the attitudes and behaviors of many players to establish and sustain this new way of serving children and youth with mental health needs. Whether support was needed from families, community leaders, local service providers, or all of these groups, many professionals recognized that social marketing techniques could, in fact, help system of care communities garner the support necessary to forge strong partnerships. As the use of social marketing exploded among system of care communities, more professionals in the mental health care field saw the practical—and essential—application of this tool to their work. The federal program also noticed its impact, and for the first time, required new system of care communities to hire social marketing staff as part of their funding agreements. The combination of early successes and in-house expertise led to better integration of social marketing into the day-to-day affairs of system of care communities.

WHAT IS SOCIAL MARKETING?

To determine how a system of care can best implement social marketing techniques to achieve its goals, it is important to understand what communicators mean when they use the term *social marketing*. According to the National Cancer Institute's "Pink Book" (U.S. Department of Health and Human Services, n.d.), a leading manual on health communications, *social marketing* is:

The application and adaptation of commercial marketing concepts to the planning, development, implementation, and evaluation of programs that are designed to bring about behavior change to improve the welfare of individuals or their society. Social marketing emphasizes thorough market research to identify and understand the intended audience and what is preventing them from adopting a certain health behavior, and to then develop, monitor, and constantly adjust a program to stimulate appropriate behavior change. Social marketing programs can address any or all of the traditional marketing mix variables—product, price, place, or promotion. (n.d., p. 251).

The inclusion and accounting for the Four *P*s of Marketing—product, price, place, and promotion—are what separates social marketing from simple mass media campaigns (Social Marketing National Excellence Collaborative, n.d.). In social marketing, the *product* is what is being offered to the intended audience and its benefits. This can be an item, idea, practice, or a combination of all three. Examples could include human immunodeficiency virus (HIV) prevention through the use of new hypodermic needles (i.e., item), personal freedom through equal rights (i.e., idea), and personal wellness through healthy eating habits (i.e., practice).

The *price* can be an actual monetary cost, but it may also be another type of sacrifice such as time and effort. For example, a campaign promoting solar power might ask people to pay monetary costs for purchasing and installing solar panels, as well as the time and effort costs for installation—especially if the marketer is asking people to do it themselves.

Place involves the way in which the product reaches the intended audience. Place includes distribution systems and points of purchase. Depending on the actual nature of the product, the place can include anything from the Internet and direct mail to classrooms and health clinics. For instance, community health clinics often place transit ads on buses and subways (i.e., place) to promote the importance of seeking early prenatal care (i.e., product) in addition to handing out flyers at health fairs and other community gatherings (i.e., place).

Promotion may overlap with place, but the key difference is that promotion is the way in which knowledge of the product's existence is communicated. Promotion can be done through a wide range of channels (e.g., radio, television, print media, the Internet, interpersonal contact). A good way to tell the difference between place and promotion is to look at the content. If a campaign promotes a web site through banner advertising, the web site is the place because it contains the product (i.e., the message), and the banner ads are considered promotion because they are the means by which the web site is promoted.

The Center for Substance Abuse and Prevention of the Substance Abuse and Mental Health Services Administration (SAMHSA) has been successful in promoting awareness of issues involving mental health and substance abuse by using a six-stage social marketing process that integrates the Four *P*s (Center for Substance Abuse Prevention, n.d.). This process is particularly relevant to systems of care because they often market themselves as a solution to the problem of meeting the mental, emotional, and behavioral needs of children, youth, and families,

Table 14.1. Social marketing process

Stage 1: Plan your approach

Research the scope of the problem.

Review the research literature.

Define your audience.

Develop your concept.

Set goals and objectives.

Stage 2: Define your messages and channels

Identify the message(s) you want to send.

Choose appropriate and effective channels of communications.

Stage 3: Develop and pretest your materials

Develop message statements and concepts.

Test materials with target audience(s) and important community gatekeepers; determine whether the target audience responds to the product(s) and ensure that the message is clear; revise the product(s) based on pretests.

Stage 4: Implement the program

Promote and distribute through all channels chosen.

Review activities and track audience reactions.

Review as necessary.

Stage 5: Evaluate the program

Determine what has worked well based on the goals and objectives established at the beginning of your program.

Assess how the program has affected the beliefs, attitudes, and behaviors of the target population.

Stage 6: Use feedback to refine the program

Revise the community's prevention program to maximize its effectiveness.

Receive feedback.

Source: Center for Substance Abuse Prevention, http://preventiontraining.samhsa.gov/THEORY/communications.htm

with serious attention and consideration given to substance abuse needs when these needs are present. A summary of this process is shown on Table 14.1.

MARKETING MENTAL HEALTH AT THE NATIONAL LEVEL

A social marketing approach is used in SAMHSA's National Anti-Stigma Campaign, which was launched in 2006. The campaign is an outgrowth of the Elimination of Barriers Initiative (EBI), an extensive research effort conducted across eight states over 3 years to identify effective approaches in addressing the stigma and discrimination associated with mental illnesses.

SAMHSA started the initiative with a two-part situational analysis that assessed the state of stigma both nationally and within the participating states. SAMHSA also convened key public and private sector representatives, mental health consumers, and state-level representatives to provide advice and guidance on the strategic planning, implementation, and evaluation of the EBI. In addition, a series of town hall–style meetings were held in each of the eight states to give interested constituents, consumers, and advocacy groups an opportunity to learn about the program and provide input to its planning, as well as its message and materials development.

Based on all of this research, SAMHSA identified audiences, messages, channels, and milestones that have guided the development of a social marketing plan. Because participating states had varying levels of expertise in communications and social marketing, the plan also accounted for the provision of social marketing and communications training, as well as technical assistance for state representatives.

With a social marketing plan and a technical assistance program in place, SAMHSA began refining messages and developing materials that included broadcast and print public service announcements, a web site, and an informational brochure—all of which were created in English and Spanish. In addition, a variety of other products and programs were developed—posters, fact sheets, drop-in articles, training curricula, and a national recognition program—that were used to reach out to schools, workplaces, and the greater media community. Ongoing evaluation helped SAMHSA identify which components were most and least successful, making it possible for SAMHSA to make corrections before launching the national campaign and making materials available beyond the eight pilot states (Center for Mental Health Services, 2006b).

SAMHSA's Caring for Every Child's Mental Health Campaign has also focused its national social marketing efforts on reducing the stigma associated with mental health, specifically for children, youth, and their families. For more than 50 years, the mental health community has conducted wide-ranging public awareness activities related to mental health during the month of May, which has been designated Mental Health Month. Since the late 1990s, the Federation of Families for Children's Mental Health, a national advocacy group, has placed special emphasis on children and youth during Children's Mental Health Week, which also occurs in May.

In collaboration with system of care communities, the national Caring for Every Child's Mental Health Campaign sought to create an opportunity during the month of May to demonstrate the effectiveness of systems of care among important stakeholders (e.g., primary health providers, educators, juvenile justice professionals, policymakers). On May 8, 2006, SAMHSA joined with the Federation of Families for Children's Mental Health and a host of other national partners, including Mental Health America, the National Alliance on Mental Illness, and the National Association of Social Workers, to launch National Children's Mental Health Awareness Day. This annual observance is designed to promote resilience, recovery, and the transformation of mental health services delivery for children and youth with mental health needs. Awareness Day provides an opportunity for the national public and private sectors to join with local and tribal communities to show how children and youth with mental health needs can thrive at home, in school, at work, and in their communities. As of 2006, hundreds of communities have utilized social marketing strategies to engage their current and potential partners in staging audience-specific events and activities. Whether holding communitywide events such as health fairs, carnivals, art contests, and walk-a-thons or engaging specific audiences with events in schools, mayors' offices, and courthouses, Awareness Day has become a rallying point for advancing effective programs to meet the mental health needs of children and youth.

The national stage for Awareness Day features a briefing on Capitol Hill in Washington, D.C., with testimonials from national mental health advocates, youth, families, business leaders, and policymakers. In 2007, national attention for Awareness Day was amplified through the participation of well-known celebrity Howie Mandel, whose long career includes serving as host of NBC's top-rated game show *Deal or No Deal* and other well-known television and stage roles. Mandel has lived with obsessive-compulsive disorder since childhood and has spoken openly about his struggles and the need for services and supports for all young people on popular television and radio programs, including *The Oprah Winfrey Show, Larry King Live, The Tonight Show with Jay Leno,* and *The Martha Stewart Show.*

WHY DO SYSTEM OF CARE COMMUNITIES NEED SOCIAL MARKETING?

As noted, the notion that social marketing can further the overall goals of systems of care has not always been a widely held belief among system of care communities. System of care decision makers are challenged with many competing priorities. Traditionally, staff for social marketing is usually the last resource allocation made, if such resources are designated at all. In 1999, the Caring for Every Child's Mental Health Campaign conducted research that included interviews with members of federally funded system of care communities throughout the country. In interviews conducted for this study, system of care staff reported that social marketing was not being implemented in their sites because "it would be taking away dollars which could be used for services for families" (Center for Mental Health Services, 1999, p. 38).

By 2005, this prevailing negative attitude toward social marketing among system of care leaders changed considerably. In a follow-up research study, several interviewees said that social marketing should be seen as integral to every aspect of the system of care. Each interviewee agreed that the goals of the Caring for Every Child's Mental Health Campaign were congruent with the goals of their systems of care (Table 14.2). In fact, many decision makers said that they regretted not beginning social marketing activities during the first year of federal funding instead of waiting until the second or third years (Center for Mental Health Services, 2005).

This dramatic change in attitude occurred in part because system of care communities became more familiar with social marketing and realized that it was compatible with their core values (family driven and youth guided, community based, culturally and linguistically competent). Because social marketing demands the implementation of research-based strategies that are tailored to the target audience, its application in system of care communities easily lends itself to being family driven, youth guided, community based, and culturally and linguistically competent.

In addition to seeing social marketing as an important part of their work, interviews conducted for the follow-up study revealed that system of care staff also

Table 14.2. Social marketing goals for systems of care

Reduce stigma associated with mental illness and promote mental health.

Use social marketing strategies to help increase the likelihood that children and youth with serious emotional and behavioral disturbances and their families are appropriately served and treated.

Increase awareness of mental health needs and services for children and youth among mental health providers, system of care communities, intermediary groups and organizations, and the public.

Demonstrate to communities that the mental health needs of children and youth with serious emotional and behavioral disturbances and their families are best met through utilization of systems of care.

Use social marketing strategies to help build capacity within system of care communities to sustain services and support to children and youth with serious emotional and behavioral disturbances and their families.

Source: Substance Abuse and Mental Health Services Administration, http://systemsofcare .samhsa.gov/ResourceDir/Caring.aspx

saw social marketing as an essential component to their sustainability after the conclusion of the initial federal support. One system of care leader stated, "Social marketing strategies, based on evaluation data, are used to raise awareness of systems of care and demonstrate the effectiveness to key decision makers such as state legislatures, county boards of supervisors, interagency meetings, and the community at large" (Center for Mental Health Services, 2005, p. 10).

How did such a major change in opinion occur over the span of 6 years? A recent study offers some insight (Stroul, 2006; Stroul & Manteuffel, 2007). In this study, the researchers assessed the ability of systems of care to sustain themselves after the conclusion of federal funding. The study involved examining the extent to which specific components of a system of care are maintained during the period in which federal funds are phased out and during the postfunding period. Through this research, 11 strategies for sustaining systems of care were identified. Of those 11, the 5 that received the highest effectiveness ratings can all benefit from social marketing, with the top 2 almost exclusively depending on social marketing for success:

1. Cultivating strong interagency relationships

2. Involving stakeholders

3. Establishing a strong family organization

4. Using evaluation results

5. Creating an ongoing focal point for managing the system of care

The importance of social marketing to sustainability is well-illustrated in St. Charles County, Missouri. When facing the challenge of sustainability, the St. Charles County Partnership with Families, a federally funded system of care, turned to its local community for help. After working on a focused advocacy effort with its partners, local voters supported a one eighth cent sales tax to fund all of the county's services for children and families, including the system of care.

Getting people to agree to a new tax was difficult and required the efforts of numerous community members and organizations. The St. Charles Partnership with Families joined part of a grass roots organization called the Putting Kids First Coalition, which was made up of citizen activists; nonprofit, religious, and business leaders; and staff from social service agencies, as well as others who wished to be involved. After the state legislature passed various measures to allow such a tax to be approved directly by voters—no easy feat—the team from the St. Charles County Partnership with Families helped launch the Putting Kids First Campaign, an all-out effort to win voter approval.

The entire campaign was grounded in audience research. The coalition held voter focus groups with participants from across the county and augmented them with a professional telephone survey. The survey randomly asked potential voters what they knew about children's services and children's mental health needs in their community. Through the focus groups and survey, they learned that child abuse prevention, treatment of youth with drug addictions, and helping runaways were major concerns. The focus groups and survey also helped them learn that people would respond best to messages about cost savings in long-term social services expenditures. In addition, the coalition learned that a significant challenge would be to convince families in the largely upper middle class areas that these types of problems existed in their own community.

Informed by these findings, the campaign took a multifaceted approach. First, the campaign needed to educate voters about problems in their communities, as well as how these problems were and were not being addressed. They then faced the daunting task of convincing voters that the solution to these problems ultimately involved taxing themselves. To do this, the campaign identified three core messages:

1. There are substance abuse, suicide, and other problems in this community.

2. The families suffering in these situations are just like the families you know and may even be the families you know. They are your neighbors and friends; they are here in our community.

3. These problems can be addressed, and tragedies don't need to happen—and it takes money to take care of children.

The campaign also realized that their resources would not allow them to reach out to all people of voting age in the community. As a result, they focused their efforts on those most likely to turn out at the polls. Relying on conventional wisdom that voters tend to read newspapers and that people with college educations are most likely to vote, the campaign worked to obtain positive coverage in the news media about the importance of children's services.

Believing that any single newspaper article or opinion column was unlikely to convey information potential voters needed to make an informed choice, the campaign explored additional ways to convey its core messages through this channel. As chance would have it, a community mental health center board member was the publisher of three weekly newspapers that reached virtually every resident in St. Charles County with a college education or higher. At the publisher's suggestion, the team ran a full-color newspaper insert that was delivered to everyone who received any of the three newspapers. To control costs to the campaign, the publisher agreed that for every page of paid advertising the campaign could secure, it would provide one full page to the campaign's insert. After finding partners to advertise, the agencies constituting the system of care provided articles that told the real stories of families in the community that emphasized and illustrated the campaign's core messages. Visuals for the insert were also carefully selected for cultural competence.

After the insert was published, the St. Charles County Children and Family Service Authority received numerous telephone calls requesting information. In addition, campaign volunteers noticed a significant increase in name recognition for the Putting Kids First Campaign among those they contacted in the community, and the businesses that agreed to purchase advertising were also satisfied with their investment. Although the sales tax effort failed by a slim margin its first time on the ballot, the social marketing effort forged the way for legislative approval of the tax in 2006. The sales tax not only secures sustainability for the system of care, but it also secures services for children and families in the county for the foreseeable future (Center for Mental Health Services, in press).

TIPS FOR SOCIAL MARKETING SUCCESS

How does a system of care community achieve results like the St. Charles County Partnership with Families? This section includes some tips based on the social marketing experience of more than 100 diverse system of care communities from across the United States, its territories, and its tribal nations.

Dedicate Staff and Resources to Social Marketing Activities

A system of care's social marketing or communications coordinator should be at least a half-time position. This position may be filled by a staff person within the system of care, an outside hire, or through a contract with a social marketing firm. Each approach to filling this position has its benefits and limitations. Internal candidates are likely to be most familiar with the system of care's values and audiences, but may not have a comprehensive understanding of social marketing across disciplines. Outside hires may bring a greater understanding of marketing theory and how it relates across disciplines, but they may not fully grasp the unique needs of the system's community. Contracted firms may be able to bring a range of individuals with varying subspecialty expertise (e.g., media outreach, materials development, partnership outreach, special events) but at an initially greater cost than that of an internal hire. No matter which option the system chooses, all candidates should have specialized experience in developing and implementing marketing campaigns designed to promote specific behavior change among their intended audiences. In addition, it is important for candidates to understand the role that marketing and communications can play in sustaining change among the audiences. Once a hiring decision has been made, the coordinator should be integrated into all system of care activities and be trained in system of care vision and values.

In addition to dedicating a permanent social marketing position within the system of care, system members should create a social marketing committee to guide all marketing efforts. In support of system of care core values, this committee should include a combination of families, youth, system partners, community organizations, system of care evaluation staff, and other system of care stakeholders. Families, youth, and others volunteering personal time should be reimbursed for their participation. Some systems of care make the social marketing committee a subcommittee of the greater governance council that facilitates final decision making and resource allocations. Also, some systems of care contract with family organizations to conduct significant portions of their social marketing efforts. Family participation enriches social marketing programs by bringing a strong voice of firsthand experience to the planning and implementation of specific strategies. Furthermore, family organizations already engage in robust advocacy outreach with diverse audiences, which can be used to leverage a system of care community's overall outreach efforts (Box 14.1).

Finally, when budgeting for social marketing, a system of care must look beyond the mere costs of materials production such as printing. Funds should be included for planning; stipends for family, youth, and child participants; research; materials development and testing; materials dissemination; events; and, finally, the evaluation of social marketing activities.

Develop a Social Marketing Plan

A good social marketing plan will serve as a roadmap to achieving a system of care's goals and objectives. It should be informed by the overarching goals of the system of care, and it should include an evaluation component. The plan should be developed in collaboration with families, youth, and system of care evaluators. Engaging as many system of care partners as possible in the planning stages yields tremendous benefits to the success of the social marketing efforts and has the added benefit of keeping partners engaged in the overall system of care's programs.

At a minimum, the social marketing plan should identify the expected outcome of the effort (i.e., goal), individual milestones necessary to achieve that goal (i.e., objectives), clearly defined audiences, culturally and linguistically competent messages and tactics, and a method for measuring the success of the work completed (i.e., evaluation). It also is important to know that a good social marketing plan is a living document that must be modified throughout the life of the system of care to reflect its current goals and priorities. Whenever possible, the system of care's governance body should approve the plan to encourage a sense of ownership and support throughout the system of care.

Understand the Audience and Community's Perceptions

The best way to understand a system of care's audience and community's perceptions is to conduct a variety of formal and informal research activities to gain an understanding of the messages and tactics that resonate best. The information gained from these queries helps identify cultural and linguistic needs and informs

Box 14.1. Family voices as power players

Project I Famagu'on-ta, the system of care in Guam, presented its social marketer with a lofty goal: to obtain political and financial support from the community to sustain its children's mental health services. In a relatively small community like Guam, drive-time radio is a natural channel for reaching a broad range of the public, including political leaders and other influential people. However, a fleeting public service announcement or on-air appearance would not be enough to achieve the goal. Instead, the social marketer conceived of producing an entire radio program featuring local families whose children were successfully served by Project I Famagu'on-ta.

One of the island's largest stations signed on to air the program on National Children's Mental Health Awareness Day in May. The station was particularly eager to highlight the real stories of Guam's families. That turned out to be the easy part. The hard part came when the social marketer met with serious resistance from families who were either nervous about appearing on the radio or felt that their stories were too personal to share with strangers. Fortunately, the program staff had developed trusting relationships with many families in the system of care, so they worked together with the social marketer to address the specific needs articulated by the families.

To ensure a comfortable environment, the project convinced the radio station to broadcast from the conference room at the system of care, a setting that was familiar to the participating families. The social marketer also accompanied program staff to meet with each family individually. They talked about how many other families struggling with mental health challenges would benefit from hearing these stories directly from families just like them. They also talked about how much more powerful it would be for political and business leaders to hear directly from families. Finally, the system of care provided each family with training on how to tell their story, including practicing a mock radio program. On the day the 4-hour program aired, a few political leaders dropped into the live remote after tuning in to the show on their way to work. They were especially interested in meeting the families who were on the program. By working in true partnership, the families and system of care succeeded in engaging influential people in the local community.

Successful systems of care have learned that even a brochure can be a powerful tool if it is developed in partnership with the intended audience. In the case of the Cuyahoga Tapestry System of Care in Cleveland, Ohio, a simple, unbound, 8″ by 6″ booklet printed on white paper paved the way for families to obtain services and develop strong partnerships with the system of care. Families in the Cleveland area had sought help for their children before, and the system had failed them. Consequently, families didn't trust that the Tapestry program was anything new or different.

To present the system of care philosophy and illustrate that systems of care are not "business as usual," the Tapestry team enlisted the help of their social marketing committee, which was made up of family members and marketing professionals. The committee decided to develop the simple booklet and recruited additional families to help them write, design, and produce it. Thanks to so much family involvement, the text was easy to understand, free of jargon, and depicted youth and families of African American, Hispanic, Asian, and Caucasian cultures, which were the main cultural populations served by the project. Even though families were involved at every step of the way in the booklet's development, the Tapestry project followed a key principle of social marketing and tested the copy and design with many other families in the community. The booklet has proven to be so popular that the project has already had to update and reprint it.

Adapted from Center for Mental Health Services, Substance Abuse and Mental Health Services Administration, U.S. Department of Health and Human Services. (in press). *Reaching out: Using communications and social marketing to support children's mental health*. Washington, DC: Author.

the process used to test draft communication materials. Most importantly, these research activities work toward assuring that the system's social marketing efforts are truly family driven, youth guided, community based, and culturally and linguistically competent.

Feedback can be gathered through formal focus groups, in-depth interviews, surveys, or other tools. If resources are limited, system of care staff can look to partners, especially youth and family organizations, to help organize less expensive, informal discussion groups or one-on-one interviews. Surveys are another effective strategy for obtaining information about knowledge and attitudes of community members. Whenever possible, social marketing staff should partner with evaluation staff, families, and youth to conduct research (Box 14.2).

Box 14.2.   The audience is king/queen

The importance of understanding and tailoring social marketing and communications approaches to the intended audiences' specific needs cannot be overemphasized. The Proyecto Iniciativa system of care in Puerto Rico embraced this basic tenet of social marketing when it was looking for ways to reduce the stigma associated with serious mental health needs among its youth. They knew that an easy way to reach youth would be through the classroom, but they also learned that teachers are busy meeting curriculum requirements and do not have time to add extra programs to their class schedules. To develop a tailored approach that would address the needs of both of their audiences—youth and classroom teachers— Proyecto Iniciativa involved them in the development of their outreach strategy. The outcome, a 4-month theater workshop about mental health for youth, turned out to be a win–win strategy for everyone. Youth enjoyed writing about their mental health attitudes and experiences in their own words and then acting them out on stage. Teachers were able to use the playwriting and performance process as a way to teach their students critical thinking, creative writing, editing, and public speaking skills.

   When Community Solutions, a system of care in Forth Worth, Texas, faced a similar challenge, they, too, turned to youth and teachers in their community to develop an outreach strategy that would meet their needs. Local school district officials had discouraged Community Solutions from developing curricula because teachers could not fit more material into their state-mandated curricula; however, the system of care learned that the textbooks chosen to teach some of the newly mandated topics were not yet available. They seized this opportunity and offered to develop a curriculum that would incorporate mental health education with another mandate, specifically with instruction in the development of electronic slide presentations. To develop a product that would engage both audiences, Community Solutions recruited the participation of health education teachers and middle and high school students. The effort resulted in the production of a slide presentation on mental health, including a teacher's guide with talking points and a list of additional student activities that complemented the slide presentation.

Adapted from Center for Mental Health Services, Substance Abuse and Mental Health Services Administration, U.S. Department of Health and Human Services. (in press). *Reaching out: Using communications and social marketing to support children's mental health*. Washington, DC: Author.

Make Sure Everyone is a Social Marketer

Despite having a dedicated social marketer on staff and an established social marketing committee, other individuals affiliated with the system of care should acknowledge the important roles they play in social marketing. As ambassadors of the system of care, it is important that they are on message when communicating system of care core values and benefits to external and internal audiences. This, in turn, facilitates the development of meaningful partnerships, especially with groups that have something to gain from an alliance with the system of care and have the ability to enhance its work.

When serving as ambassadors to external audiences, system of care staff should look beyond money as the only form of support that a partner can provide. They should also consider the following:

- *The system of care's needs*—Identify what is needed and desired from a partnership.

- *The total scope of possible partners in the community (e.g., families and youth within the system of care, as well as those unaffiliated with the program)*—Think outside the box to brainstorm potential partners that can help the system reach its goals.

- *The most likely partnership candidates*—Concentrate initial efforts on those most likely to say yes.

- *The strongest allies*—Identify those affiliated with the system of care who might be willing to introduce the system of care to the potential partner's decision makers. Often, families are the strongest allies in these efforts. Their voices are given great credence because they speak from personal experience.

- *A potential partner's track record*—Look for organizations and agencies that have been involved with children's or mental health issues in the past. These organizations and agencies may be easier to partner with than those that have not shown prior interest. Also, consider who the potential partner is capable of reaching. Partnering with an organization that can reach the system of care's intended audiences—although for reasons that complement but may not match the system's goals—is also an effective partnership outreach strategy.

- *The management structure of the potential partner*—Locally owned companies with local customers such as a small business or a franchise are probably more promising than satellite offices of multinational corporations that are more interested in meeting global needs than local ones. When reaching out to nonprofit organizations, it is important to remember that local chapters or affiliates of national organizations tend to be fairly autonomous and do not necessarily take orders directly from a central office.

- *Reciprocity between the system of care and the potential partner*—Determine how the potential partner can benefit from working with the system of care.

- *The system of care's contacts*—Nurture and build relationships with people who introduce the system of care to key decision makers within a possible partnering organization. Be sure to find out who calls the shots; learn as much as possible about the organization.

- *The pitch*—Be specific about what is expected from partners as part of their collaboration with the system of care. Once a clear pitch has been developed, think about who may be the best person to receive it, when may be the best time to deliver it, and where and in what manner it should be delivered. Careful consideration to the who, what, when, where, and how of the pitching process will improve your chances of success (Box 14.3).

Just as it is important for system of care representatives to be good ambassadors to external audiences, it is equally important that they are good ambassadors to internal audiences. Everyone within the system of care should share the same vision and use similar language to express that vision. If people within a system of care cannot communicate consistently with one another, it is unreasonable to expect them to be consistent when communicating with external audiences. To punctuate this point, one system of care partner interviewed for the Caring for Every Child's Mental Health Campaign's 2005 research study noted this major social marketing challenge for his system of care: "Better communication— understanding each other's roles—among multidisciplinary agencies . . . each system has its own vision for system integration. Definitions of system of care are jargon. We have to be able to explain it in words that are meaningful to the audience we're talking with" (Center for Mental Health Services, 2005).

To address this need, the campaign engaged in a robust message development process to craft an easily understood definition of *systems of care*. Representatives of the campaign's target audiences, namely local system of care staff, family and youth leaders, national partners, and SAMHSA, worked together to achieve the following common language for describing a system of care:

> A system of care is a network of community-based services and supports that is organized to meet the challenges of children and youth with serious mental health needs and their families. Families and youth work in partnership with public and private organizations so services and supports are effective, build on the strengths of individuals, and address each person's cultural and linguistic needs. A system of care helps children, youth, and families function better at home, in school, in the community and throughout life. (Center for Mental Health Services, 2006a, p. 1)

This common definition appears in all written materials about systems of care developed by the campaign. Local communities can use this definition, but they are encouraged to engage their key audiences on the local level to adapt it for cultural and linguistic competence.

Good internal communications goes beyond having a common vision and using common language. As a general rule, staff should understand the role of each internal partner so communications with that partner are relevant and the credibility of the system of care is maintained. Staff should know the communica-

Box 14.3. Playing to the strength of a community's culture

Program staff at Anishnabek Community and Family Services in Sault Sainte Marie, Michigan were frustrated with the lack of community interest in their mental health materials. Time and time again, they brought their friendliest smiles to tribal community events and set up an exhibit table brimming with stacks of fact sheets, flyers, and brochures. Event-goers routinely passed up their table but flocked to the tables that provided fun and games. To help draw attention to their display table, the system of care, which serves the Sault Sainte Marie tribe of Chippewa Indians, decided to create a fun game of their own. They created the Animal Friends Fun Wheel, a spinning wheel that provided everyone who spun it with a prize. They also added a bonus of educational information on the Chippewa people and on mental health. Players would win a major prize such as a small toy or an animal card. Each animal card featured a picture of an animal and its name in English and in Ojibwe on one side, and information about the animal on the other.

As people stood in line to take a turn at spinning the wheel, system of care staff took the opportunity to talk with them about the services and values of the system of care and offer them a flier or brochure on the program. The Animal Friends Fun Wheel became a crowd pleaser, with children and even adults collecting the animal cards like baseball cards. More importantly, the local community began learning more about their culture and about where they can turn for help if they find themselves or someone in their family in need of mental health services.

Understanding an institutional or professional culture is as important as understanding a racial or ethnic community's cultural and linguistic needs. The One Community Partnership in Broward County, Florida, found this to be true when they attempted to educate primary health providers about children's mental health. Primary care providers see children and families on a regular basis, and they are trained to recognize symptoms requiring intervention. This positioned them as ideal partners to help identify a family's mental health needs early and refer them to appropriate services. Unfortunately, the One Community Partnership learned that the primary care providers in their county did not consider mental health to be part of their practice area, and most had not received mental health training in medical school.

To develop a strategy that would resonate with the culture of primary care providers, the One Community Partnership turned to the medical school at Nova Southeastern University, the largest independent university in the state of Florida, for help. Together, they decided to host a seminar on Raising Healthy Children. Health care providers were accustomed to receiving professional information in a conference or seminar setting, and the university would be received as a trusted source for information on children's health.

Cultural considerations didn't end there, though. The university and One Community Partnership also spoke directly with medical professionals to learn more about their information resources. Based on these discussions, the seminar was promoted in the local pediatric association's magazine and the university's publications, as well as in newspapers, on the radio, and in other local media. In addition, promotional information was distributed through professional networks via e-mail and direct mail. Attendance at the seminar by physicians, social workers, nurses, clinic administrators, and others from the primary care arena exceeded expectations, and even more were reached through a DVD, print publication, and web postings of the proceedings.

———————————

Adapted from Center for Mental Health Services, Substance Abuse and Mental Health Services Administration, U.S. Department of Health and Human Services. (in press). *Reaching out: Using communications and social marketing to support children's mental health*. Washington, DC: Author.

tion preferences of internal partners to optimize how messages are delivered. For instance, if a system of care partner spends a substantial amount of time in the car, sending messages via fax or postal mail is probably not the best communication strategy. In addition, systems of care should periodically train and refresh staff on the best ways to communicate with internal partners. Doing this provides internal partners with a high level of continuity, which also helps maintain credibility. Finally, systems of care should ask for, and be open to, feedback from internal partners.

Evaluate Efforts and Make Midcourse Changes as Necessary

All social marketing efforts for systems of care should be evaluated, and planning for the evaluation of social marketing efforts should begin as early as possible. Social marketing staff should partner with evaluation staff, families, and youth to design an evaluation that is robust, realistic, supportive of system of care values, and within a system of care community's means. If it is not possible to partner with evaluation staff, another option is to partner with a local university to conduct research. Universities are a great resource; they bring a public health perspective to the work, and they are always on the lookout for new areas of research investigation.

If an evaluation partnership is not possible, it does not mean that the system of care cannot evaluate the success of its work. Almost any evaluation information is better than none at all, and thus most social marketers plan to acquire a minimal amount of evaluation research, even if they have to go it alone. A system of care in this position must look for qualitative and quantitative data. Qualitative data help tell the story in compelling ways such as through a series of individual heartfelt stories. When these stories are coupled with quantitative information such as compelling statistics, they can leave a long-lasting impression.

It also is important for a system of care to strive for cultural and linguistic competence in its evaluation activities. To be most effective, evaluation tools and methodologies should be designed with consideration of cultural practices and traditions. One way to do this is to involve members of the intended audience in the evaluation process. Systems of care should partner with organizations, especially youth and family organizations, representing the culture of the intended audience.

In 2003, SAMHSA conducted an expert panel of social marketing evaluation experts who identified several factors as important when evaluating social marketing for systems of care. When designing evaluation activities, a system of care should consider the following (Center for Mental Health Services, 2003):

- The number of partnerships
- The types of partnerships
- Distribution of materials
- Audience participation

- Web hits and links

- Media coverage

- A focus on outcomes

- A logic model that identifies each desired change in knowledge, attitudes, and behavior

Celebrate Success

Celebrating success can be a huge motivation and a good way to build teamwork. Social marketing efforts should have clear goals and milestones that will help stakeholders in the system of care know they have been successful. The system of care should be positive and declare victory when reaching the goal. Also, the contributions of all partners, including families, youth, children, community members, and system of care staff, should be recognized.

CONCLUSION

In many ways, today's system of care communities are writing a new chapter in the history of social marketing as they adapt this practice for their unique needs. Just as Kotler and Zaltman could have never anticipated social marketing's profound impact, it is impossible to say how far-reaching the benefits of social marketing will be for children and youth with mental health needs and their families. If the present is any indication, the future for systems of care and social marketing is extremely promising. System of care decision makers often cite three reasons for the importance of social marketing:

1. To reduce stigma

2. To increase access to services and supports

3. To ensure long-term sustainability for family-driven, youth-guided, community-based, and culturally and linguistically competent systems of care

Social marketing has already proven to be an important tool for system of care communities to meet the mental health needs of thousands of children, youth, and families who would not have had any access to services and supports only 20 years ago. Perhaps within the next 20 years, social marketing efforts will have decreased stigma to such an extent that the mental health needs of *all* children, youth, and families will be met.

REFERENCES

Center for Mental Health Services, Substance Abuse and Mental Health Services Administration, U.S. Department of Health and Human Services. (1999). *Findings of the needs assessment/situational analysis final report: Caring for Every Child's Mental Health Campaign.* Unpublished report.

Center for Mental Health Services, Substance Abuse and Mental Health Services Administration, U.S. Department of Health and Human Services. (2003). *Caring for Every Child's Mental Health Campaign: Expert panel meeting report.* Unpublished report.

Center for Mental Health Services, Substance Abuse and Mental Health Services Administration, U.S. Department of Health and Human Services. (2005). *The state of social marketing in 21 selected system of care communities: A situational analysis: Caring for Every Child's Mental Health Campaign.* Unpublished report.

Center for Mental Health Services, Substance Abuse and Mental Health Services Administration, U.S. Department of Health and Human Services. (2006a). *Children's mental health facts. Helping children and youth with serious mental health needs: Systems of care.* Washington, DC: Author.

Center for Mental Health Services, Substance Abuse and Mental Health Services Administration, U.S. Department of Health and Human Services. (2006b). *Developing a stigma reduction initiative.* Washington, DC: Author.

Center for Mental Health Services, Substance Abuse and Mental Health Services Administration, U.S. Department of Health and Human Services. (in press). *Reaching out: Using communications and social marketing to support children's mental health.* Washington, DC: Author.

Center for Substance Abuse Prevention, Substance Abuse and Mental Health Services Administration, U.S. Department of Health and Human Services. (n.d.). *Social marketing and health communications.* Retrieved May 15, 2007, from http://preventiontraining.samhsa.gov/THEORY/communications.htm

Kotler, P., & Zaltman, G. (1971). Social marketing: An approach to planned social change. *Journal of Marketing, 35,* 3–12.

Social Marketing National Excellence Collaborative. (n.d.). *The basics of social marketing: How to use marketing to change behavior.* Retrieved May 15, 2007, from http://turningpointprogram.org/Pages/pdfs/social_market/smc_basics.pdf

Stroul, B. (2006). *The sustainability of systems of care: Lessons learned: A report on the special study on the sustainability of systems of care.* Atlanta, GA: ORC Macro.

Stroul, B., & Manteuffel, B. (2007). The sustainability of systems of care for children's mental health: Lessons learned. *Journal of Behavioral Health Services and Research, 34*(3), 237–259.

U.S. Department of Health and Human Services. (n.d.). *Making health communication programs work: A planner's guide.* Washington, DC: U.S. Government Printing Office.

Wiebe, G.D. (1951). Merchandising commodities and citizenship on television. *Public Opinion Quarterly, 15,* 679–691.

IV

Recommended Practice Examples

The Service Delivery Level

15

Strengths-Based, Individualized Services in Systems of Care

KNUTE ROTTO, JANET S. MCINTYRE, AND CELIA SERKIN

This chapter considers the individualized service delivery process used in systems of care operated by Choices, Inc., a nonprofit care management organization that coordinates services for individuals and families involved in one or more governmental systems. Choices uses the system of care philosophy and approach with wraparound values and blends them with managed care technologies to provide a wide range of services and supports to high-risk populations with multiple and complex service needs. Choices programs serve both children and adults, with services that are family centered, community based, culturally competent, outcome driven, and fiscally accountable.

Choices was created in 1997 by four Marion County, Indiana, community mental health centers to coordinate the Dawn Project, a collaborative effort among child welfare, education, juvenile justice, and mental health agencies to serve youth with serious emotional disturbances and their families. Launched in May 1997, the Dawn Project served 82 youth during its first year. In 1999, a 5-year federal grant from the Comprehensive Community Mental Health Services for Children and Their Families Program was awarded to the Dawn Project, enabling an increase in the number of children and families that could be served. This included an expansion in the target population to serve children at risk for out-of-home care, as well as support for the development of Families Reaching for Rainbows, a family support and advocacy organization, and evaluation activities.

Choices was conceived as a separate and independent entity to manage the Dawn Project system of care. In its role as a care management organization, Choices provides the necessary administrative, financial, clinical, and technical structure to support service delivery and manages the contracts with the provider network that serves youth and their families. Choices' responsibilities include providing financial and clinical structure; providing training; organizing and maintaining a comprehensive provider network; providing system accountability to the interagency consortium; managing community resources; creating community collaboration and partnerships; and collecting data on service utilization, outcomes, and costs. Choices operates several programs that serve youth with serious emotional disorders—the Dawn Project in Marion County, Indiana; Hamilton Choices in Hamilton County, Ohio; and Maryland Choices in Montgomery County, Baltimore City, and St. Mary's County, Maryland.

The goal of Choices' programs for youth and families is to improve services for youth with serious emotional disorders and to enable them to remain in their homes and communities by providing a system of care comprised of a network of individualized, coordinated, community-based services and supports using managed care technologies. Dawn and Hamilton Choices in Ohio are funded by case rates provided by the participating child-serving systems. The programs in Maryland are not yet risk based.

In addition to its direct services, Choices has become a resource for technical assistance in Indiana. The Indiana Divisions of Mental Health and Family and Children began providing start-up resources in 2000 for the development of systems of care based on Dawn's experience in other areas of the state. Choices has been a key technical assistance resource for these sites, and in 2002, it was officially funded by the state as a technical assistance center (Choices TA Center) to provide assistance in developing similar community-based systems of care throughout Indiana.

While state and local structures, laws, and political and fiscal environments vary considerably among sites, Choices has helped local leaders implement systems of care using a common set of values and principles, as well as management and fiscal tools:

• *Wraparound process*—The systems of care are based on the wraparound process and philosophy. Service delivery is organized according to the four phases of wraparound as articulated by the National Wraparound Initiative—*engagement, planning, implementation,* and *transition.* In addition, the systems of care are guided by the 10 principles of wraparound: 1) family voice and choice, 2) team based, 3) natural supports, 4) collaboration, 5) community based, 6) culturally competent, 7) individualized, 8) strengths based, 9) persistence, and 10) outcome based (Miles, Bruns, Osher, Walker, & National Wraparound Initiative Advisory Group, 2006). At the center of the wraparound process are child and family teams and care coordinators who play the pivotal dual roles of team facilitator and coordinator of services and supports. Coordinators are responsible for assuring that all team members are heard and for helping the team gain consensus around an individualized service plan that utilizes the child's and family's strengths to address areas of concern. Fidelity to the wraparound process is monitored by clinical directors, as well as by supervisors who meet with care coordinators at least weekly and advise them on individual cases as often as necessary. The culture of Choices encourages all employees and subcontractors to model wraparound principles in their interactions with one another and with the families they serve. Fidelity to the wraparound process is also gauged by administration of the Wraparound Fidelity Index (Bruns, Suter, Force, Sather, & Leverentz-Brady, 2006).

- *Braided funding*—Across sites, Choices utilizes braided or blended funding, paid through a case rate structure in Indiana and Ohio. Once funds reach Choices, they lose their identity and can be used for any legitimate need identified and approved by the team. In addition, Choices makes flexible funding available to care coordinators quickly to meet specific needs of children and families. Despite a strict process of authorization and claims adjudication, funds are usually made available to care coordinators and families in less than an hour. In all five communities, Choices provides high-quality services and achieves strong outcomes without receiving new funds. Rather, the services and supports are provided with resources that have been redirected, allowing Choices' system of care sites to contain public spending.

- *Broad provider network*—Another hallmark of Choices' approach to care is the development of a vibrant provider network. Each site has a community resource manager whose job is to identify and enter into contracts with a large number of local providers to meet the service needs identified by child and family teams. Providers are paid on a fee-for-service basis, but Choices has incorporated flexible funding arrangements to allow small and nontraditional providers to gain a foothold and become part of the provider network. Furthermore, the role of the community resource manager includes locating providers and resources for a specific child and family, including faith-based and culturally matched providers.

- *Quality improvement and outcome measurement*—Choices employs a doctoral-level director of outcomes and evaluation and a quality manager. This team works closely with outcomes teams in each state. Quality improvement at Choices includes training staff in measurement tools, closely and routinely scrutinizing client outcome data, providing annual outcome reports for community partners, reporting other data as requested, and carefully monitoring costs. The outcomes and evaluation team has developed a cost modeling process that allows the Choices' senior management team to quickly spot trends in referral patterns, service utilization, and spending.

- *Community partnerships and trust*—Wherever Choices operates, staff members endeavor to be dependable and valued partners with local community leaders. Trust is earned over time, and being a catalyst for a change in the way children and families are served creates stress in even the strongest relationships. Choices management team members understand their responsibility for being capable, collaborative, and attentive partners and for modeling this behavior for all staff.

In addition to these common systemic features, Choices' service delivery process reflects a strength-based, individualized philosophy and approach. The approach to services centers around the role of the care coordinator, the role of the child and family team, and the role of providers. Each of these roles is described in detail, with illustrations from the experience of a boy referred to Choices by the child welfare system. In addition, an effective strategy for training and supervising care coordinators is offered to support their critical role as facilitators of the planning and delivery of individualized care.

ROLE OF THE CARE COORDINATOR

The care coordinator is a bachelor's- or master's-level clinician who is skilled at engaging family members, system representatives, and community stakeholders in an individualized wraparound process focusing on child needs and family strengths. A master's-level clinician supervises all care coordinators. Care coordinators must be skilled in identifying resources and facilitating the team process to assist families and youth by locating, developing, coordinating, and monitoring care in the community. They ensure that families and youth have a voice in identifying their needs while helping child and family teams to develop and implement individualized wraparound plans to achieve permanency, safety, and well-being. The role of the care coordinator is detailed within each phase of the wraparound process.

Engagement and Team Preparation Phase

This initial wraparound phase is characterized by the care coordinator getting to know the child and family by hearing their story, addressing any immediate and urgent needs, creating a list of child and family strengths, and identifying potential team members, as well as choosing a date and location for the first team meeting (Miles et al., 2006).

Strengths Discovery   During this phase of wraparound, the care coordinator facilitates an initial strengths discovery process that assists in identifying child and family strengths, strategies that have been helpful in the past, and practices that are important to family members from their cultural perspective (see Figure 15.1). Strengths are qualities that contribute to the family's life in a functional way and are descriptors that reveal the family's distinctive attributes. All family members and children have unique strengths. Strengths discovery helps to balance the picture when so much emphasis has been placed in the past on what has not been working for the child and family. This helps to reframe the family's situation by acknowledging positive attributes and by transforming challenges into strengths. It also allows the care coordinator and other team members to understand and appreciate the family's culture. By building on strengths, the wraparound process supports the family's journey toward self-advocacy and self-efficacy.

Strengths and Needs-Based Assessment

Client name: _____ Date: _____

Mental health

Briefly discuss any significant psychological/psychiatric child and family history; current behavioral, emotional, and psychological state; mental status and functioning; access to needed care; and crisis management.

General summary/significant events: _____

_____

_____

Strengths/resources: _____

_____

_____

Concerns: _____

_____

_____

Needs: _____

_____

_____

Family/relationships

Briefly describe the family constellation, relationships among family members, extended family resources, and support network. Discuss family involvement in plans for child, service coordination abilities, and empowerment.

General summary/significant events: _____

_____

_____

Strengths/resources: _____

_____

_____

Concerns: _____

_____

_____

(continued)

Figure 15.1. Strengths and needs-based assessment.

Figure 15.1.   *(continued)*

Needs: _____

_____

_____

Financial

Briefly describe child/family's access to shelter, safety, food, transportation, and other basic needs. Describe the source of financial resources and money management skills.

General summary/significant events: _____

_____

_____

Strengths/resources: _____

_____

_____

Concerns: _____

_____

_____

Needs: _____

_____

_____

Home/place to live

Briefly describe the living situation (space, privacy, safety, comfort, and availability of respite), status of placement, and changes planned in the long-term arrangement.

General summary/significant events: _____

_____

_____

Strengths/resources: _____

_____

_____

Concerns: _____

_____

_____

Needs: _____

_____

_____

Safety/crisis

Describe the current situation in terms of safety of the child and ability to handle crisis and emergency situations. Attach crisis plan to summary.

General summary/significant events: _____

_____

_____

Strengths/resources: _____

_____

_____

Concerns: _____

_____

_____

Needs: _____

_____

_____

Social/recreational

Describe social interactive skills and current/past relationships for the child and family. Also include access to other community resources, both current and desired, and feelings of belonging in or contribution to the community.

General summary/significant events: _____

_____

_____

Strengths/resources: _____

_____

_____

Concerns: _____

_____

_____

(continued)

Figure 15.1. *(continued)*

Needs: _____

_____

_____

Vocational/educational

Describe educational status, including grade level, type of educational placement, attendance, and behavior. If applicable, describe work experience, preemployment skills and goals/interests, and independent living skills.

General summary/significant events: _____

_____

_____

Strengths/resources: _____

_____

_____

Concerns: _____

_____

_____

Needs: _____

_____

_____

Cultural/spiritual

Describe any ethnic or national traditions important to the child/family, as well as their ability to acess these traditions. Also, describe religious or spiritual beliefs, practices, and support.

General summary/significant events: _____

_____

_____

Strengths/resources: _____

_____

_____

Concerns: _____

_____

_____

Needs: _____

_____

_____

Legal

Describe history of involvement with police and courts and current status, including any identified community safety and accountability concerns.

General summary/significant events: _____

_____

_____

Strengths/resources: _____

_____

_____

Concerns: _____

_____

_____

Needs: _____

_____

_____

Health/medical

Briefly describe physical and dental history and current status, including medications and special physical health needs, as well as access to medical care.

General summary/significant events: _____

_____

_____

Strengths/resources: _____

_____

_____

Concerns: _____

_____

_____

(continued)

Figure 15.1.   *(continued)*

Needs: _____

_____

_____

Summary

_____

_____

_____

_____

_____

Preliminary plan: ☐ Completed and signed off

Care coordinator: _____ Date: _____

Care coordinator supervisor: _____ Date: _____

Supervising M.D.: _____ Date: _____

Features of the strengths discovery include attitudes and values, skills and abilities, attributes and history, and preferences. Family members identify their assets, dreams, and expectations, and share good news about what they have experienced in the past. The care coordinator understands that this process is an unusual experience for families in the system. Using a conversational format, the care coordinator asks the family and the youth what they are good at, what they enjoy doing, what hobbies they have, what their customs and traditions are, and what they do as individuals and as a family to have fun. The family and the youth discuss their positive characteristics and what motivates them; they also explain where they go for support and comfort.

Strengths-based discovery is an advanced skill that care coordinators must possess in order to assist the family and team in using all available resources and talents to meet the needs of the family and youth. Strengths are initially identified across 10 life domains:

1.   Mental health

2.   Family/relationships

3.   Financial

4. Home/place to live

5. Safety/crisis

6. Social/recreational

7. Vocational/education

8. Cultural/spiritual

9. Legal

10. Health/medical

The care coordinator shares the initial strengths discovery with team members, and the team updates the strengths list regularly with the family. The team members use strengths to select interventions to address needs. During team meetings, the care coordinator also facilitates a discussion about the strengths of the team members. The strengths discovery process helps to identify potential team members, including natural supports. William's story illustrates how the individualized service process begins with the strengths discovery process.

William was referred to the Dawn Project at the age of 11 by his child welfare case manager, Scott. William had spent more than 4 years in institutions—in a state hospital and then in a residential treatment center. Scott hoped that the Dawn Project could help William make the transition back to the community and into the care of his aunt or possibly his mother. William's diagnoses included major depressive disorder, oppositional defiant disorder, and attention-deficit/hyperactivity disorder. He also suffered from asthma. He was considered an *unbonded* child and had been diagnosed as a baby with failure-to-thrive. He had increasingly negative acting-out behavior, problems in school, and a conflicted relationship with his mother. William had never known his father, and his mother told him he was the product of rape.

Immediately upon referral to the Dawn Project, William was assigned Barbara as his care coordinator. She was an experienced coordinator who worked well with child welfare. Despite his difficulties, William was able to identify strengths across several life domains after being referred to Dawn. He was actively involved in a spiritual group (i.e., cultural/spiritual); he practiced excellent personal hygiene (i.e., health/medical); he attended school regularly and was good at spelling and art projects (i.e., vocational/education); members of his family felt responsible to one another (i.e., family/relationships); he could identify his personal strengths and talents (i.e., mental health); and he knew how to obtain support in a crisis situation (i.e., safety/crisis).

Building Trust   The care coordinator works to build trust with family members during the engagement phase. The coordinator is respectful and caring, does not judge or devalue the family members, and shares power and authority with them. The coordinator understands that families define themselves and their own culture and recognizes that a child's family is the group of individuals who support that child emotionally, physically, and financially. Family members can include individuals of different ages and backgrounds, and they may be biologically related, related by marriage, or not related at all.

William's family consisted of his mother and a maternal aunt. Upon referral, William's mother wanted William to be placed with her sister. This aunt, however, could not control William's behavior. Although she continued to participate on William's team, she did not want him to live with her.

Upon leaving the residential center, William was placed with a therapeutic foster family. These caregivers also became part of William's family, and they worked with William, his mother, and a specialist in bonding therapy. After many months of difficult therapy, William's mother decided that she could not provide enough stability for him and therefore chose to relinquish her parental rights. After this event, William again demonstrated his feelings of rejection, anger, and grief by acting out his negative feelings in the therapeutic foster home, which resulted in the foster family requesting his removal. After several periods of intense instability and several placements, Barbara finally found a "forever family" for William, and he was eventually adopted.

Team Member Identification   The care coordinator helps the family members to identify possible members for their child and family team. The role and responsibilities of team members and the value of having natural supports and formal supports on the child and family team are explained and discussed with the family. The care coordinator and the family members discuss recruiting and orienting team members. The family members may want the care coordinator to invite potential team members to the child and family team meeting, or they may choose to approach potential team members about joining the team on their own. The participation of a peer support person on the team is a key to the success of many families, and this practice is encouraged by Choices at all sites. In Maryland, the family support partner is an integral part of the process and is included on the child and family team. In Indiana, a staff member of the family support group may serve as a family mentor and participate on the team.

During the 4 years that William was in the Dawn Project, more than 20 different people participated on his child and family team. At any given time, the team was comprised of William, his mother until her rights were terminated, his aunt, his care coordinator Barbara, his child welfare case manager Scott, his foster family members, his teachers and school counselors, an educational mentor or tutor, the guardian ad litem appointed by the court, respite providers, therapists, and David, William's friend who was a pastor of a local church.

Initial Crisis Plan   Working in partnership with the family, the care coordinator quickly develops an initial crisis plan to address the most immediate crisis and safety concerns and to stabilize the family (see Figure 15.2). This initial effort is not a substitute for the development of the more comprehensive crisis plan that is created with team members during the implementation phase of the wraparound process, but rather addresses immediate needs. The crisis plan is created by asking family members and the youth about recent and current crises, safety concerns, and crises that could occur in the very near future. Care coordinators discuss with youth and families strategies that have worked in the past in the home, school, and community and then jointly identify triggers that may lead to crises. The care coordinator explores with the youth and family any life threatening situation or immediate crises, including those resulting from a lack of basic needs, such as the family not having food, shelter, or heat. The care coordinator also asks the referring sources, agency representatives, potential team members, and other knowledgeable people about crisis and safety concerns and the actions that have been taken in the past in response. Efforts are then made to provide immediate relief to the family.

Over the years, William had harmed peers and physically assaulted staff members in various placement settings. At school, William was disruptive, talkative, easily distracted, and attention seeking. More than once, he was expelled from school for threatening to bring a gun to school, requiring him to be schooled at home. Each time there was a major disruption in William's life, his behavior at home and school deteriorated significantly. William's crisis plan recommended that he be provided with specific expectations of what was going to occur if he did not follow requests. William did not respond productively to nagging or arguing. The plan suggested that allowing William time and space to make the appropriate decision would be the best strategy for redirecting him. He had to understand the consequences of his actions and be held accountable if he

Crisis/Safety Plan

Name: _____ Date of birth: _____ Age: _____

Parent name: _____

Current placement: _____ Phone: _____

Medications: _____ Doctors: _____

Respite home: Back-up home:

Name: _____ Name: _____

Phone: _____ Phone: _____

Dangerous potential: ☐ Low   ☐ Medium   ☐ High   ☐ None

Background information:

_____

_____

Anticipated problems (home, school, and community):

_____

_____

What approaches are most useful (home, school, and community):

_____

_____

Recommended interventions (home, school, and community):

_____

_____

Hospital procedure (who will hospitalize, access for hospitalization):

_____

_____

Care coordinator: _____ Date: _____

Parent(s): _____ Date: _____

Team member: _____ Date: _____

Team member: _____ Date: _____

Figure 15.2.   Crisis/safety plan.

made inappropriate choices. His crisis plan named the hospital that would be used for acute care for William if necessary and included five other names and telephone numbers of people, including a respite provider, who could be called in the event of a crisis.

Initial Plan Development Phase

A major role for the care coordinator is facilitating the child and family team by helping the newly formed group become a cohesive team unit and by developing supportive relationships with all members. Choices provides ongoing training and coaching to ensure that coordinators have the support they need to perform this pivotal role. One of the most critical and difficult duties of the coordinator is keeping the team focused on the client's and team's strengths and helping them develop a plan that incorporates those strengths.

After the strengths of the family and client are identified in each domain, the team identifies concerns they may have. Concerns are typically broad and can encompass all domains. Needs are then identified from the concerns and are prioritized by the team and family. The care coordinator may need to remind the team that "needs are not services," a mantra used by Choices to emphasize that there are often a number of ways to meet needs and that a categorical service may or may not be the best way for doing so. The top three to five needs become the outcomes that will be addressed during the initial 30 days of service delivery (see Figure 15.3 and Box 15.1). Outcomes must be measurable, and there must be a person assigned to each outcome who will report back to the team about progress at the next team meeting.

Interventions are the specific services or resources necessary to address the outcomes. The interventions included in the plan of care are the authorized services and supports that Choices manages. Each month, the care coordinator submits authorizations for the services and supports decided by the team for the following month. Supervisors, along with Choices' finance department, review the authorizations that are used to verify and pay provider invoices.

From the first meeting, the care coordinator is responsible for keeping team members informed about all activities and decisions. Written team notes, as well as reports for schools or the court where appropriate, provide accountability to referring agencies. As differences of opinion arise during team meetings, the coordinator is responsible for mediating conflicts so that members are satisfied that everyone has been heard and treated fairly.

William's initial team included his care coordinator Barbara, his child welfare worker Scott, his aunt, and the teacher and therapist from the residential cen-

---

Individualized Care Plan

Client: _____ ICP number: _____ Dates covered: _____

Life domain: _____

Vision: _____

Concerns of all: _____

Needs: _____

Strengths: _____

1. **Outcome** _____

    Source: _____ Baseline: _____ Goal: _____ Current:_____

    Intervention: _____

    Date: _____ Current: _____ Met: Yes/No

    Intervention: _____

    Date: _____ Current: _____ Met: Yes/No

    Intervention: _____

    Date: _____ Current: _____ Met: Yes/No

2. **Outcome** _____

    Source: _____ Baseline: _____ Goal: _____ Current:_____

    Intervention: _____

    Date: _____ Current: _____ Met: Yes/No

    Intervention: _____

    Date: _____ Current: _____ Met: Yes/No

    Intervention: _____

    Date: _____ Current: _____ Met: Yes/No

Figure 15.3. Individualized care plan.

3. **Outcome:** _____

  Source: _____ Baseline: _____ Goal: _____ Current:_____

  Intervention: _____

  Date: _____ Current: _____ Met: Yes/No

  Intervention: _____

  Date: _____ Current: _____ Met: Yes/No

  Intervention: _____

  Date: _____ Current: _____ Met: Yes/No

Individualized care plan summary

Summary statement:

Summarize the team goals and the outcomes you are looking to achieve in the next 60 days.

_____

_____

_____

_____

_____

Program completion criteria:

1. Stable psychiatric symptomatology
2. Stable system involvement
3. Mutual agreement of client/guardian and community team that project services and resources are no longer needed.

Signatures:

Parent/guardian: _____ Date: _____

Care coordinator: _____ Date: _____

Team member: _____ Date: _____

Team member: _____ Date: _____

Care coordinator supervisor: _____ Date: _____

Supervising M.D.: _____ Date: _____

Box 15.1.   Individualized care plan instructions

1. *Life domain*—An overall look at a person's life; the long-term goals and outcomes will focus on a life domain. This is the framework for asking about needs and strengths: mental health, social/recreational, family/relationships, vocational/education, financial, cultural/spiritual, home/place to live, legal, safety/crisis, and health/medical.

2. *Vision*—Defined by the individual or family regarding the way they want their future to look. Ask, "What do you want to be different? What will your life look like when the plan is completed?"

3. *Concerns of all*—This is where the team members have stated their concerns regarding the specific domain to be addressed. The concerns are taken from the team meetings and discussions with parents and providers and are addressed through the needs.

4. *Needs*—Needs are ways to address the concerns presented by the team. The needs should relate to the life domain and the reason for the long-term goal. This sets the baseline in which progress will be measured.

5. *Strengths*—The strengths are taken from the strength-based assessment and incorporated to show how the needs can be addressed through the strength of the client. These strengths should be functional and useful.

6. *Outcomes*—This area describes the desired outcomes for the life domain. Outcomes are the behaviors and areas targeted for change. They should be descriptive and measurable. Outcomes will be the focus of the team and measure progress toward completion of the long-term goal. The desired outcome is one behavior or area that when combined with several other accomplished desired outcomes will create the successful completion of the long-term goal. Ask, "How will you know the long-term goal has been achieved?" or "What is the child or family member expected to accomplish within a specified period of time?"

7. *Source*—This is *who* will be measuring the progress and *how* the information will be collected (e.g., self-report, parent report, teacher checklist).

8. *Baseline*—Using a scale 1–7, define where the client starts and how future progress will be measured.

9. *Goal*—This is where the client is at the time of the review. Justification for this level is summarized in the progress section, case record notes, and team meeting summaries.

10. *Current*—This is where the current level of the behaviors being measured is stated using a 1–7 scale. This will be compared against the baseline level. Use the same measurement tool used to create the baseline score.

11. *Interventions*—This area describes the interventions used to meet the outcomes in the life domain. These strategies can be both formal and informal resources and services.

12. *Met*—Progress is evaluated as to whether the goal has been met. Circle yes or no at each review.

ter where he was placed. Initially, his mother did not participate as she was in-carcerated for a brief time; however, the original plan for William was reunifica-tion with his mother after they had completed bonding therapy and she demonstrated sobriety for a certain amount of time; the initial plan of care was developed in accordance with the goal of reunification.

Needs were identified for William by domain:

- William needs help identifying the right educational program so that he can be successful in school (i.e., vocational/education).

- William and his caregiver need adequate medical care and skills to manage mental health needs (i.e., health/medical).

- William needs to live in a family setting after release from the residential center (i.e., home/place to live).

- William needs a comprehensive plan of care (i.e., mental health).

- William and his family need to be safe from violence (i.e., safety/crisis).

- William and his mother need to be drug and alcohol free (i.e., health/medical).

The highest priorities were set for finding a stable home for William and an ed-ucational setting that worked for him. The initial plan listed several outcomes:

- William and his mother will have their basic material needs met.

- William will succeed in school as evidenced by attending school for the full day, receiving average grades, and not engaging in behavior that will lead to suspensions throughout his time in the Dawn Project.

- William and his family will demonstrate the understanding, skills, and abil-ity to access resources to manage his medical care.

- William will live successfully in a family setting until his final court review prior to his Dawn graduation.

- William will have a comprehensive plan of care to address his psychiatric needs throughout his enrollment in Dawn.

- William and his family will live in a safe environment as evidenced by fewer crisis calls to service providers or the police, and will have fewer emer-gency room visits throughout his enrollment in Dawn.

- William's mother will remain in recovery and not relapse into alcohol abuse.

The initial plan called for a number of interventions:

- Barbara and Scott will facilitate HUD Section 8 certificate.

- Pastor David will help the family provide for basic needs.

- An educational consultant will advise the school on appropriate classroom interventions for William.

- William will receive individual support in the classroom provided by an educational mentor.

- William will attend public school for as many hours as possible, supplemented by home-bound instruction if necessary.

- William will receive skill development assistance in interpersonal and communication skills from a Dawn Project case manager.

- William's mother will arrange for annual physical, dental, and eye exams.

- William and his mother will attend intensive bonding and attachment therapy sessions two times per week with a local therapist who specializes in this field.

- Monthly child and family team meetings will be facilitated by Barbara.

- William will receive 10 hours of clinical mentoring per week.

- Barbara will assist family members in effectively communicating their needs and thoughts to fellow team members and professionals.

- William and his family will receive home-based therapy and care management from a local mental health center.

- The child and family team will monitor William's mother's sobriety at each contact.

Implementation and Refinement Phase

After the initial plan is developed, the team meets to review the plan of care every 30–45 days. The care coordinator asks each team member to report on progress related to the specific outcome they have been assigned. This allows the team to monitor progress and make decisions about changes in services and supports based on the status of each outcome. Crisis plans also are periodically reviewed, particularly in the aftermath of a crisis that required activation of the plan, to assess its success or the need for revisions.

During the implementation phase of wraparound, the care coordinator is responsible for keeping the team proactive, rather than reactive. Both verbal and written communication with members and referring entities is crucial, and care coordinators have cell phones, voice mail, and e-mail that allow them to communicate easily with team members and supervisors. During this time, the coordinator and team closely monitor the provision of formal services and community supports, and the coordinator ensures that high-quality services are delivered as planned. The care plan may need only fine tuning, or it may need to be completely overhauled if the desired results are not forthcoming. Outcomes that are attained are celebrated, and families or youth may begin to take over some of the care coordinator's responsibilities such as facilitating some team meetings.

During William's rather lengthy stay in the Dawn Project, interventions and service provision changed a number of times in response to or in anticipation of events. It became apparent that William's mother was not in a position to care for him when he left residential treatment, so William was initially placed in a therapeutic foster home associated with the bonding specialist. After William's mother decided to relinquish her parental rights, the permanency plan for William was changed to adoption, and thus preadoptive homes were sought. William experienced two more therapeutic foster families and removals from these families after incidents when his mother reappeared in his life. He also spent brief periods of time in the hospital for stabilization. Each time he was removed or rejected by a family, his positive behavior deteriorated into disruptive and threatening rages both at home and school.

After William was in the Dawn Project for about 3 years, Barbara was at last successful in finding a preadoptive therapeutic foster home with Paul, who had known William for several years as a case manager in an agency that had provided services to William. Paul was thrilled to be adopting William, and William readily settled into family life with him. William bonded with Paul, which has had a profound effect on his feeling safe and secure. William was given a chance to experience life, as he said, "like a normal kid." A combination of mentors, mental health providers, and intense care coordination finally convinced William that many people cared about him and were willing to stay by him no matter what. He learned that he was safe and loved.

Transition Phase

Transitions occur during all phases of wraparound. Throughout all phases, the care coordinator and other team members support family members as they strive toward attaining their vision. Beginning with the first child and family team meeting, members consider what needs to be accomplished to help family members sustain themselves after wraparound ceases. The care coordinator and the services and supports provided during wraparound help family members to gain the skills, knowledge, and support network that will enable them to address future needs and crises.

The final transition to complete wraparound is the team's decision. The team recognizes that outcomes are being realized, and family members have acquired the skills and knowledge needed to obtain services and supports in the future. Family members are comfortable expressing what they want and need. All necessary help and supports are in place. Family members may have chosen to become part of the family movement and may be connected to a peer support network. They possess the skills and knowledge to address future needs. At this important crossroad, the team develops a transition plan, a postwraparound crisis plan, and a transition schedule. The final steps needed before wraparound ends typically include the following:

- A family member or the youth regularly facilitates team meetings.

- The care coordinator engages the team in a conversation about plans for follow-up care.

- The team ensures that the transition plan is sustainable and that the family can manage resources and knows how to obtain services that may be needed in the future.

- The team discusses how to celebrate success in a culturally appropriate manner.

- If the family agrees, the team members may conduct or participate in a commencement ceremony that recognizes the work, accomplishments, and successes of the family, the youth, and the team.

- The care coordinator completes a formal discharge report that outlines these accomplishments and successes, and then documents those interventions that were beneficial.

- The care coordinator works with the team to establish a procedure for checking in with the family and the youth after the completion of wraparound.

If family members need assistance in the future, they can choose to hold a team meeting or they can ask the care coordinator or individual team members for help to obtain needed services.

As the time approached for William's adoption by Paul to be finalized, most services and supports for William were tapered off. His remarkable success in school—both social and academic—continued after he enrolled as a freshman in high school. William came to really enjoy school. Paul reported to Barbara that William planned to attend his homecoming dance with a date in October. This was a child who could not look another person in the eye until his work with the bonding therapist. William was finally capable of making decisions about goals for his life and interacting with others in a responsive and pleasant manner. He recently told a close group of caring adults, including Paul, that he loved them. William and Paul planned to continue with home-based individual and family therapy through a local mental health center after William's graduation from Dawn. This would ensure that William had ample opportunity to continue dealing with his issues of abandonment, anger, and grief regarding his mother, as well as any problems that might arise as the result of his adoption. William's team quietly celebrated his graduation with a special cake and ice cream requested by Paul and William.

ROLE OF THE CHILD AND FAMILY TEAM

The child and family team is the cornerstone in developing a strengths-based, individualized care plan. The team is the eyes and ears for child and family needs, the purchaser of services within the provider network, the resource creator and developer, and the accountability monitor. The child and family team is composed of the people who know the youth best, including a representative of the referring agency, the care coordinator, the youth, his or her family or other caregivers, parent advocates, providers, informal family and community supports, and anybody else who knows the child and family well and can offer resources and support. The child and family team includes representatives of the public human service systems involved with the child, including probation, schools, child welfare, mental health, and corrections. Each representative is responsible for presenting his or her system's critical issues to the team so that the team can incorporate them into a single individualized care plan. Maximum coordination of care is assured when the appropriate agencies are involved and active in the team process. Court orders, individualized education programs, probation rules, and parole orders are critical elements that must be recognized by the care coordinator and integrated into the plan of care.

Clinical and Fiscal Control

In Choices' systems of care, the child and family team is able to manage service delivery because it has responsibility for designing the care plan, authorizing payment for the services and supports included in the plan, monitoring progress made toward desired outcomes, and modifying the plan in a real-time manner. The dynamic of controlling the payment for and modifying services creates the locus of control at the team level, encouraging child and family team members to be engaged and actively involved in the care process. Teams do not have to wait for approval as services and supports included in the plan are considered to be authorized. If the team decides on a course of action, then it is the team's job to carry it out. Care coordinators, who facilitate the teams, are trained in their responsibility for guiding financing decisions and understand the consequences of high-cost plans that can cause financial challenges for the entire system. Team members learn that plans are closely monitored to provide assurance that scarce resources are being used wisely. To monitor progress, Choices utilizes a robust information management system, The Clinical Manager, which captures clinical and fiscal outcome data for the care coordinator to share with the team and also provides data for teams and supervisors to monitor child and family progress. Thus, a culture of accountability is created for teams, along with discipline for the child and family team process.

Developing and Implementing the Plan of Care

Using a high-quality team process (Walker, Koroloff, & Schutte, 2003), the child and family team develops a plan of care that is family driven, youth guided, and reflective of wraparound values. As noted, when a youth and family are enrolled in the system of care, the care coordinator meets with them within 5 days to identify strengths, devise a preliminary list of team members, create an initial plan of care and a crisis/safety plan, and authorize initial services. When referral information is incomplete, the care coordinator is responsible for gathering the relevant information. The first team meeting occurs within 30 days of enrollment. The care coordinator prepares an agenda for the meeting, which he or she uses to keep the meeting on task and to move from the brainstorming of ideas to a completed plan of care. After each meeting, the care coordinator distributes meeting notes to all team members and copies them into the electronic clinical record. These notes serve as a record of decisions made and tasks to accomplish before the next meeting.

The agenda for the first team meeting includes results of the Child and Adolescent Needs and Strengths (CANS) assessment (Lyons, 2004), which is completed with the family. The CANS is used at all Choices locations as a clinical needs and strengths assessment, a service planning instrument, and a quality assurance and outcomes measurement tool. The CANS is administered at intake and at 60- to 90-day intervals thereafter.

The family and the team create a plan of care based on needs identified by the referral source, as well as those cited by the family and youth. To facilitate full team participation, all barriers that prevent family involvement at team meetings are addressed, including transportation, time of day, child care, and conflicts with work. No team meeting occurs without the family's involvement unless a parent has designated a spokesperson other than the care coordinator to attend on his or her behalf.

The development of the plan does not begin with a conversation about which services are needed. The starting points for plan development are determining the family's vision and identifying strengths and needs. The plan groups the family's strengths and needs by life domain and then addresses the family's specific needs and desired outcomes in each.

After strengths and needs are identified and outcomes are selected, the family and team members design creative and practical interventions to address the issues. When the team is looking for resources to meet the needs of the family, the first question asked is whether the need can be met through the use of a family, nonprofessional, or community resource. Choices believes that the intensive wraparound intervention is a brief time in the family's life and that the resources employed should be ones that the family can use and sustain after the formal child and family team is no longer available. The use of existing, no-cost, or low-cost resources supports the goal of creating self-sufficiency for families over the long term. The plan specifies informal supports in addition to more formal treatment and interventions needed by youth and their families.

The family codevelops and commits to the plan, which integrates the multiple perspectives of the different team members. The plan is practical, action oriented, and individualized, and it includes measurable goals. It documents the family's experience from a strengths-based and culturally competent perspective as it incorporates the family's vision for the future. It blends different existing plans that the family may have, thereby combining different viewpoints and mandates into a single more manageable plan. The plan specifies which team members are responsible for accomplishing designated interventions. It is a dynamic and living document that is revisited and regularly updated during each team meeting. The written plan of care helps to hold all team members accountable for their contributions to the ultimate success of the youth and family.

In Montgomery County, Maryland, during the engagement phase of the wraparound process, a family support partner from the family organization administers a Family Support Needs Assessment Survey to determine the family's needs in terms of family-to-family support. During meetings, the team members discuss how to integrate family support goals and efforts into the care plan. The family support partner and the family also use the survey to recognize successes, monitor and track results, and identify barriers and gaps, thereby helping family members recognize the point they have reached in their journey toward self-advocacy and self-efficacy.

Importance of Many Points of View

With multiple perspectives from 5–8 team members, the care plan created is rich with diverse points of view and ideas. Choices believes a variety of points of view have the ability to generate creative options for the team to consider. As Walker et al. (2003) stated, "Discipline in generating multiple options also has great potential to increase the extent to which the plan will be family driven and culturally competent" (p. 30).

Child and family team meetings occur every 30–45 days to ensure that the team remains focused on the plan, addresses the outcomes, makes changes to service packages, and adds new team members when necessary. Team meetings last from 30 to 90 minutes depending on the needs of the team and the information being discussed. On average, team meetings last 60 minutes. The care coordinator, the convener of the child and family team, is respectful of each member's time and ensures that the agenda is both focused and flexible.

Building on the Family's Vision

As noted, the care coordinator from Choices meets with the youth and family during the engagement phase of wraparound to explore individual and family strengths, needs, culture, and vision. The care coordinator listens to the family members as they tell their stories, share their hopes and dreams, and explain their immediate needs. In their own words, members express their vision for the future, which helps to shape the care plan and to determine which needs are addressed. With help from the care coordinator, the family and the youth create a clear and focused statement of where they want to be in 6 months to a year. The family members share their vision with the team members during the first child and family team meeting; it may be displayed visually or included on the agenda at each subsequent meeting to remind team members of the family's vision. If the family agrees, team members can add to the vision statement, and the family's vision may change over time. The team builds on the family's vision throughout the wraparound process.

Celebrating Successes

The child and family team celebrates successes throughout the wraparound process. Acknowledging these successes, no matter how small, is important because it helps to empower the family and the youth. Team members celebrate efforts that the youth and family have made, try to find the positives in every situation, and recognize the family's movement toward independence. During the transition phase, the family may want to have a celebration with team members, other family members, and friends. If the family agrees, the team can have a ceremony to honor the work done by the family, the youth, and team members. The team celebrates in a way that is meaningful to family members and their culture. Celebrations often include sharing a meal or having a pizza party.

ROLE OF PROVIDERS

Each Choices' system of care community has a network of providers, both formal and informal. The provider networks are purposefully created and managed so that there are many options available for teams to build individualized, coordinated care plans.

Community Resource Manager

Choices uses a community resource manager in each site to develop and manage the provider network. The community resource manager recruits providers for the network (e.g., agencies, individual providers), administers contracts with providers, and sets rates and service expectations for network providers. In addition, as needs are identified by teams, the community resource manager is contacted, and a search begins for a specified service or individual to fit the needs of a specific youth and family. For example, locating respite providers who are interested in working with clients and becoming members of teams as active participants in the treatment process is a task frequently completed by the community resource manager. Family members, kin, and family-designated caregivers who are willing to care for the client if they can be paid for their services may be contacted by the community resource manager to become providers for a family.

At each Choices location, the community resource manager is the main point of contact with agencies and individual providers. The manager assists with complaints and grievances, acts as a liaison for providers, and interfaces with teams and families when they are unhappy with services. Issues about payment for services, quality of care, and a lack of referrals are all managed through the resource manager. The manager also works with providers to develop standards of practice for specific services. The community resource manager meets with providers at least quarterly to discuss the global needs of clients, provide training, and encourage program development for community-based alternatives to out-of-home placements.

Provider Network

Each Choices system of care is responsible for developing a communitywide provider network made up of the traditional human service providers who may already have contracts with local child-serving systems and new providers. Agencies and individual providers are part of the network, which includes providers who offer nontraditional, community-based support for specific youth. Nontraditional providers may include faith-based organizations, Boys and Girls Clubs, and community centers located in the neighborhoods served by the system of care. Providers are paid by Choices on a fee-for-service basis.

Because the needs of the youth and family dictate the combination of services provided, providers who are willing and able to think flexibly and creatively about their services receive priority when Choices seeks treatment centers, group homes, and other services and supports that serve youth and families. For example, Choices may offer a financial incentive in a contract for a residential provider to move children home more quickly than usual and to provide smooth transitions, or it may encourage a residential center to maintain 24-hour crisis respite capacity to be used as needed for crisis stabilization. In each community, Choices' goal is to create the capacity to provide a broad array of services and supports that gives families options when choosing their providers. The family, youth, and team members determine which providers can offer the types of interventions that will be most helpful in addressing the family's needs; family voice, choice, and culture are critical in this determination. Furthermore, natural supports are potential providers seen as essential for helping the family sustain its success after wraparound ceases. Table 15.1 shows the broad array of services available to youth and families through the provider network.

Quality Control and Improvement

One of the challenges in building and operating a community provider network is finding enough providers that are aligned with the core values of a system of care. Choices assumes that values of new providers may not be in concert with system of care and wraparound values, so specific strategies are required to create values alignment. Working with community providers to incorporate the principles of

Table 15.1. Choices service array

Behavioral health	Psychiatric	Mentor	Placement
Behavior management	Assessment	Community case management/ case aide	Acute psychiatric hospitalization
Crisis intervention	Medication follow-up, psychiatric review	Clinical mentor	Nontherapeutic foster care
Day treatment	Nursing services	Educational mentor	Therapeutic foster care
Evaluation		Life coach/ independent living skills mentor	Group home care
Family assessment			Relative placement
Family preservation		Parent and family mentor	Residential treatment
Family therapy		Recreational/ social mentor	Shelter care
Group therapy		Supported work environment	Crisis residential
Individual therapy		Tutor	Supported independent living
Parenting/family skills training		Community supervision	
Substance abuse therapy (individual and group)		Intensive supervision	
Special therapy			

Respite	Service coordination	Discretionary	Other
Crisis respite (daily or hourly)	Case management	Activities	Camp
Planned respite (daily or hourly)	Service coordination	Automobile repair	Team meeting
Residential respite	Intensive case management	Child care/ supervision	Consultation with other professionals
		Clothing	Guardian ad litem
		Educational expenses	Transportation
		Furnishings/ appliances	Interpretive services
		Housing (rent, security deposits)	
		Medical	
		Monitoring equipment	
		Paid roommate	
		Supplies/groceries	
		Utilities	
		Incentive money	

systems of care into their practice is a challenge that Choices addresses on an on-going basis. One of the primary responsibilities of the community resource manager is to ensure not only that providers are credentialed and highly qualified in their fields but that they are also committed to the system of care and wraparound philosophy and approach. Ongoing training opportunities, as well as interaction with the community resource manager and child and family teams, offer vehicles for ensuring increasing alignment of providers in the network with this philosophy and approach to service delivery. Furthermore, teams are responsible for assessing the performance of the providers they choose and replacing them or withholding payment if the articulated goals of the care plan are not met or the services are not performed to the team's satisfaction. Linking provider performance, payments, and outcomes helps to achieve high-quality and family-responsive performance. If the family and youth have a good experience, and the provider assists the family in achieving good outcomes, the provider will become a valued member of the network and will be used more often.

TRAINING AND SUPERVISION OF CARE COORDINATORS

Training and supervision are essential to support care coordinators as team facilitators and managers of service delivery and to retain skilled staff. Extensive initial orientation and training are supplemented by weekly staff training meetings at each Choices site and also by weekly individual and group supervision. Topics covered at staff meeting trainings are suggested by management and supervisory staff. They are also selected in response to local needs and requirements. In addition, special on-site training sessions for individuals or small groups are offered as needed by the Indianapolis and Cincinnati training managers.

Care Coordinator Training Modules

The Dawn Project training manager has grouped care coordinator training into specific topic modules that can be accessed electronically by anyone at any Choices site. These modules contain PowerPoint presentations, interactive training exercises, and written materials. Training modules include the following:

- *Assessment tools and electronic records*—Care coordinators at all three sites receive training in the CANS assessment, which is utilized as a treatment planning and outcome measurement tool by Choices. Slightly different versions of the CANS are used in the three sites, but testing for reliability is required, and as of 2007, annual recertification is required in Indiana. In addition, all care coordinators must become proficient in the use of The Clinical Manager, the software used to track both clinical and authorization data, as well as costs for every Choices client. Additional assessment and evaluation instruments are completed in Ohio and Maryland per local contracts, and Choices assures that coordinators are well-trained in their use.

- *Provider network*—It is critical for facilitators of wraparound child and family teams to be knowledgeable about local providers available to supply the services and supports determined by the teams. Although all services are individualized for each youth and family, a large number of providers have existing contracts with Choices. Care coordinators learn about the provider network and how to initiate the process of recruiting new providers, if necessary, to meet a need identified by the team.

- *Practice components*—This training module contains the meat of the care coordinator's work. It includes wraparound values and system of care principles, strengths-based practice, crisis and safety planning, the four phases of the wraparound process, successful teams, and fiscal requirements unique to each community that Choices serves.

- *Technology*—Care coordinators are trained to use the technology that allows them to work efficiently and effectively away from the office. Technology includes laptop computers for coordinators to use at home and at team meetings, as well as desktop computers, cell phones, voice mail systems, e-mail accounts, and Choices' office telephone systems.

- *Boundaries and ethics*—A training module, along with ongoing supervision, is devoted to helping care coordinators understand the critical importance of highly ethical conduct and the ways to navigate the sometimes murky waters of boundary issues in the wraparound process.

- *Other modules*—Other training modules covered with care coordinators include orientation to the local and national system of care movement, diagnosis and medication, outcomes and evaluation, the Health Insurance Portability and Accountability Act (HIPAA) of 1996 (PL 104-191) and client rights, safety in the workplace, and the Wraparound Fidelity Index.

Strength-Based Supervision

Some experts have posited that the real cost to a company from the turnover of a single employee is the equivalent of 1 year of pay (Goleman, 1998). The ongoing stress associated with social service work makes care coordinators at high risk for early burnout if they are not carefully nurtured through strength-based supervision. High turnover results not only in the loss of revenue and hard-won experience and knowledge but also the loss of continuity with clients. Choices has developed an approach to provide strength-based supervision for care coordinators. Successful supervision begins with careful screening and hiring. Once employees are hired, the following components are required:

- *Orientation and welcome*—Most organizations have orientation programs designed to acquaint employees with regulations and paperwork requirements for HIPAA and Medicaid, as well as employee benefits. All new employees, including supervisors, must also gain familiarity with the core values and guiding principles for a system of care, as well as the historical context for systems of care at local, state, and national levels.

- *Initial training*—Specific training for new hires comprises all of the material, including training regarding the previously described modules. Such training is provided to care coordinators and to those who supervise them. Studies have shown, however, that only 10% of skills taught in training are actually used in practice (Walker et al., 2003) and that true learning requires ongoing coaching and supervision. Knowledge transfer is dramatically increased when these elements are added, especially when supervision follows a structured process that sets and monitors specific goals.

- *Ongoing training and professional development*—To create and maintain a learning environment, each Choices site holds a weekly staff meeting to provide ongoing training, employee recognition, support, and networking opportunities for care coordinators. Supervisors provide consistent recognition and use unique ways to honor employees for their hard work in the belief that employees need opportunities for personal as well as professional growth in order to give their best performance.

- *One-on-one coaching and feedback*—Choices believes that individualized coaching is critical for employees to internalize the training they receive. Fixsen, Naoom, Blase, Friedman, and Wallace (2005) stated, "Training by itself seems to be an ineffective approach to implementation" (p. 43), while "coaching makes clear contributions to the preparation of practitioners, both in the experimental and other research literature" (p. 47). Although this vital aspect of supervision may be overlooked, individualized coaching can provide much needed opportunities to celebrate and reinforce successes, as well as chances to correct mistakes and encourage growth. An important role for all coaches is to provide feedback to coordinators. Feedback given in a positive way at the appropriate time provides an opportunity for personal and professional growth. It can also result in an employee and coach jointly deciding that the employee's current role is not appropriate for his or her talents.

- *Regular group clinical support*—Peer-to-peer support, brainstorming, networking, and problem solving are valuable supervisory tools. Any staff member can play the role of teacher in group supervision. The supervisor's role is to facilitate the group process.

- *Modeling strength-based behavior*—It is crucial for employees to see strength-based practices in action. Although agencies often take care to be strength based with clients, they sometimes forget to model the same approach with their own staff members. Walker and colleagues (2003) reported, "Employees were adamant that facilitators could truly learn to be strengths based within agencies that treated them in a strength-based way" (p. 39). Assessing employee strengths and needs is an important part of the supervision process. This assessment process must include an awareness of the employee's cultural background and how this affects his or her behavior in the workplace. A way to model strength-based behavior is to encourage trust by having fun together. Successful supervisors may plan out-of-office retreats to celebrate successes, encourage employees to get to know one another on a personal level, and provide opportunities for personal growth (Lencioni, 2002).

- *Performance planning and employee evaluation*—Choices' supervisors collaborate with employees to create a performance plan. These plans include agency must-do items such as meeting productivity standards or performing daily duties inherent in the operations of the unit. Performance plans also include individualized professional development goals jointly identified by the employee and supervisor. The plans may address strengths and plans for improvement, as well as plans for the future. Just like families, employees have strengths and needs that can be used to create positive solutions for concerns. Brainstorming solutions that utilize strengths can help to build trust between the supervisor and the employee. When real trust exists between the employee and the supervisor, difficulties can be resolved through conversation and planning rather than through supervisory orders (Buckingham & Coffman, 1999).

• *Policy/system level support*—Supervisors and their employees face an uphill battle without both organizational and system-level support for their work. Walker and colleagues (2003) defined this support in terms of strong leadership by system champions who share the philosophy, vision, and commitment to providing the necessary resources and policy back-up to support the innovation. In their literature review, Fixsen and colleagues (2005) described system interventions as core components for implementation of effective models of care.

CONCLUSION

For more than a decade, Choices has provided care for youth with multiple and complex challenges and their families. From its inception, Choices has striven to "walk the talk" of strengths-based, family-driven, individualized, community-based care. Guided by wraparound values and system of care principles, day-to-day operations are supported by a structure that employs people who truly believe that children and their families can successfully reach the goals they set for themselves. Whether employed in accounting, information technology, communications, human resources, or as frontline staff that work directly with clients, all staff members understand that Choices only exists because of the people who are served.

This chapter outlined the structures and processes necessary for successful service provision. Critical for individualized services is a strong and well-managed provider network whose members are encouraged to think creatively as they participate on child and family teams and provide individualized services. Consistent ongoing training and coaching to support care coordinators in their ever-expanding understanding of the meaning of strengths-based care, as well as support and guidance for supervisors when tough challenges arise, are critical components of the system of care. Open communication with community partners coupled with an understanding of their legal mandates and needs for public financial accountability must also guide the system. A strengths-based appreciation of the challenges partners face goes a long way toward gaining support for the values of systems of care.

Many details go into the day-to-day clinical operations of a strong system of care based on wraparound values. Care coordinators must be accountable for strict adherence to agreed-on timelines that move children and families through the phases of wraparound. A well-structured crisis/safety plan must be crafted with a family at the very first point of contact and revised whenever necessary to ensure that everyone involved knows what to do if or when something goes wrong. Intrateam communication is key. Care coordinators complete and distribute child and family team minutes and timely court reports as needed. Families and individual team members are consulted between meetings whenever the need arises. Families are always at the center of decision making, and the family and youth are coached to take leadership roles on their team, including the facilitation of meetings when they are ready.

A system of care is organic—an almost living, breathing, changing life form that must be nurtured to survive. All participants in the system from managers to care coordinators and their supervisors, as well as other service providers, should be committed to excellence and be willing to change and grow to keep the system vital. Quality improvement dictates that procedures and policies be strategically reexamined on a regular basis to ensure that the values and beliefs of systems of care are known and followed by all.

It would be simplistic to assert that adherence to beliefs alone can account for the successes of the youth and families served, however, one cannot underestimate the power of care that is guided by strong philosophical underpinnings. Choices' care coordinators' workspaces are surrounded with banners that remind them of the 20 wraparound values and urge them to remember, "If your service decision meets this test, go ahead." These values, shown on Figure 15.4, are covered in orientation, discussed at staff meetings, and used in continuing super-

---

Wraparound Values

Family centered	Community based
Strength based	Responsive
Individualized	Unconditional
Normalized	Outcome driven
Culturally relevant	Cost effective
Collaborative	Promote independence
Flexible	Team based
Comprehensive	Consumer driven
Needs driven	Integrative
Innovative	Least restrictive

If your service decision meets this test, go ahead.

Figure 15.4. Wraparound values.

Table 15.2.   Phrases That Pay

LISTEN, LISTEN, AND THEN LISTEN!
What are the strengths, the strengths, and the strengths?
Needs aren't services.
Make the decision value driven.
With every decision who do we empower/disempower?
Families don't fail—plans do.
A crisis is when the adults don't know what to do.
Find the positive intent and reframe.
Be part of the solution, not the problem.
Incremental, not instantaneous.
You can't fail without trying.
See with the magic eye. Listen with the third ear.
How we voice our concern is as important as the concern being voiced.
You tell us!
If your service decision meets the Wraparound Values test, go ahead!
You can't burn out if you've never been lit!
No parents, no solutions. Know parents, know solutions.
Change agents change first.

From Matthews, B. (2004). Phrases that pay: A celebration of their roots! *Collaborative Adventures: A Quarterly Newsletter of Choices Technical Assistance Center, II*(IV), 4. Available online at http://www.ChoicesTeam.org. Reprinted by permission.

vision. The meaning of these values and an understanding of how each value is put into practice are topics for conversations throughout Choices.

Finally, the care that Choices provides for youth and families is also guided by statements called Phrases That Pay (Matthews, 2004). While the origin of many of these cannot be attributed to a particular person, together they represent the thoughts and words of many early wraparound pioneers. These phrases, displayed on Table 15.2, are embedded in the culture of Choices, provided to employees and trainees on laminated cards, and used as prompts for coaching individuals. From the first phrase that states, "LISTEN, LISTEN, AND THEN LISTEN!" to the last which observes "Change agents change first," they form a compelling reminder of the huge role that values play in the ongoing work of a system of care.

WEB RESOURCES

- *CANS information*—http://www.buddinpraed.org/cans/

- *National Implementation Research Network*—http://nirn.usf.edu

- *National Wraparound Initiative*—http://www.rtc.pdx.edu/nwi

REFERENCES

Bruns, E.J. (October, 2004). *Wraparound fidelity report for Dawn*. Seattle: University of Washington, Department of Psychiatry.

Bruns, E., Suter, J., Force, M., Sather, A., & Leverentz-Brady, K. (2006). *Wraparound Fidelity Index 4.0: Manual for training, administration, and scoring of the 4.0 (for use in WFI 4.0 pilot sites only)*. Seattle: University of Washington, Wraparound Evaluation and Research Team.

Buckingham, M., & Coffman, C. (1999). *First, break all the rules: What the world's greatest managers do differently*. New York: Simon & Schuster.

Fixsen, D.L., Naoom, S.F., Blase, K.A., Friedman, R.M., & Wallace, F. (2005). *Implementation research: A synthesis of the literature* (FMHI Publication No. 231). Tampa: University of South Florida, Louis de la Parte Florida Mental Health Institute, The National Implementation Research Network.

Health Insurance Portability and Accountability Act (HIPAA) of 1996, PL 104-191, 42 U.S.C. §§ 201 *et seq.*

Goleman, D. (1998). *Working with emotional intelligence*. New York: Bantam Books.

Lencioni, P. (2002). *The five dysfunctions of a team*. San Francisco: Jossey-Bass.

Lyons, J.S. (2004). *Redressing the emperor: Improving our children's public mental health system*. Westport, CT: Praeger Publishers.

Matthews, B. (2004). Phrases That Pay: A celebration of their roots! *Collaborative Adventures: A Quarterly Newsletter of Choices Technical Assistance Center, II*(IV), 4. Available online at http://www.ChoicesTeam.org

Miles, P., Bruns, E.J., Osher, T.W., Walker, J.S., & National Wraparound Initiative Advisory Group (2006). *The wraparound process user's guide: A handbook for families*. Portland, OR: Portland State University, Research and Training Center on Family Support and Children's Mental Health, National Wraparound Initiative.

Walker, J.S., Koroloff, N., & Schutte, K. (2003). *Implementing high quality collaborative individualized service/support planning: Necessary conditions*. Portland, OR: Portland State University, Research and Training Center on Family Support and Children's Mental Health.

16

Improving Services Through Evidence-Based Practice Elements

JASON SCHIFFMAN AND CHRISTINA M. DONKERVOET

The children's mental health system in the state of Hawaii is administered by the Child and Adolescent Mental Health Division (CAMHD) of the Hawaii Department of Health. CAMHD's mission is to provide timely and effective mental health services to children and youth with emotional and behavioral challenges and their families within a framework that integrates system of care principles, evidence-based services (EBS), and continuous monitoring. Major system emphases include ensuring that all services and supports are individualized, youth guided, and family driven, as well as locally available, community based, and least restrictive.

The origins of Hawaii's child and adolescent mental health system are unique. First, Hawaii's geographic isolation with rich cultural and economic diversity creates an environment that is simultaneously—and proudly—independent and interdependent. There is an acute awareness of the need to adapt ideas and practices to make them effective in this system because there is a sense that what may work in other places will not necessarily work in Hawaii. This isolation and diversity creates a strong sense of independence and autonomy that simultaneously strengthens local partnerships, collaboration, and a sense of community.

Another unique contributor to the development of Hawaii's system of care is the federal court involvement in two lawsuits settled during the 1990s that motivated the state to strengthen children's mental health practice. The first case involved a settlement agreement with the Department of Justice regarding the violation of the civil rights of people residing in mental health care institutions. Because the children's system moved institutional services from a state hospital to acute care hospitals and residential treatment programs, there was a need to strengthen clinical practice in these settings. The second lawsuit related to a violation of the state's compliance with the Individuals with Disabilities Education Act (IDEA) of 1990 (PL 101-476) as it pertained to students with disabilities who also had mental health needs. The state entered into the Felix Consent Decree,

437

agreeing to implement a statewide integrated system of care consistent with the system of care philosophy (Stroul & Friedman, 1986).

As the state implemented activities to come into compliance with all aspects of the Department of Justice settlement agreement and the Felix Consent Decree, the significantly increased funding for children's mental health services resulted in a magnification of the need for accountability and the demonstration of improved outcomes. Both funding sources and advocates expected assurances that not only would the state meet the expectations of the lawsuits, but also that the mental health of local youth would improve on the receipt of the mandated services. Despite the initial investment of resources in response to the lawsuits, as well as the substantial cost of services, outcomes were poor. A high percentage of youth were served in high-cost residential treatment settings on the mainland and in Hawaii, and youth continued to have law violations and problems in school.

In an effort to meet the treatment needs of youth and provide accountability, CAMHD leadership collaborated with a diverse group of stakeholders to create a comprehensive, community-driven plan to improve children's mental health services in the state of Hawaii. This group of families, private providers, and public partner organizations took on the challenges of identifying new strategies that would offer a means of improvement and accountability for children with mental health needs. The group adopted a philosophy of evidenced-based services and decision making, providing a core foundation for the system of care. The result of these efforts was the statewide adoption of the system of care approach, an integrating and individualized approach to services with evidence-based practices (EBPs).

CREATING AN EVIDENCE-BASED CULTURE

An important first step in creating an evidence-based culture was the creation of the Evidence-Based Services Committee (EBS Committee). Established in 1999, the ultimate charge of the committee is to evaluate and distill the mental health treatment literature in a way that makes sense for local communities and service providers. In a collaborative approach, the committee is comprised of family representatives, advocacy groups, university partners, providers of various disciplines, and representatives from all child-serving agencies (Chorpita & Donkervoet, 2005). An important key to sustaining a broad, systemwide commitment to EBS was the initial engagement of local partners with diverse viewpoints.

Defining and Reviewing the Evidence Base

This group's earliest goal was to achieve a consensus on a definition of the term *evidence-based* for Hawaii, recognizing that the term does not conform to a single, universal definition. Similar to national debates at the time, the committee wrestled with complex questions:

• Who defines the evidence base?

• What is the evidence for?

- What constitutes evidence?

- How much evidence is required?

Other early factors considered included understanding what the evidence relays, deciding whether studies considered to be contributing to the evidence base provide information on long-term follow-up or just short-term posttreatment effects, determining which outcome variables are of interest and must be included, and ascertaining a definition for the term *improvement* (e.g., improvement in functioning vs. a reduction of target symptoms vs. no longer meeting diagnostic criteria). Although these questions are not unique to Hawaii, providing stakeholders with the opportunity to deliberate and resolve these issues at a local level established an early context for the engagement of local- and state-level participants in the process.

Early EBS Committee meetings established guidelines for reviewing the literature, partially adopting the Chambless and Hollon (1998) model of defining evidence-based protocols. This model originated from the American Psychological Association and its task forces, which examined empirically supported interventions. National guidelines, however, were not forced on the system, but rather the committee was provided guidance from national sources to use in conjunction with their own autonomy to make decisions. Based on the developed guidelines, the EBS Committee reviews and codes posttreatment outcomes cited in studies and links these outcomes to problem areas within diagnostic categories. One important decision agreed on by the committee was that there were various levels of evidence, with some studies providing more compelling evidence than others. Therefore, the committee established a system of levels, indicating varying degrees of evidence-based support (Child and Adolescent Mental Health Division, 2004; Chorpita et al., 2002).

After establishing definitions for the term *evidence*, the EBS Committee took on the task of reading and coding the literature. Psychosocial treatment articles were divided into those problem areas that were most common in the children's mental health system:

- Anxious or avoidant behavior problems

- Depression or withdrawn behavior problems

- Disruptive behavior and willful misconduct problems

- Substance use

- Attention and hyperactivity behavior problems

- Bipolar disorder

- Schizophrenia

- Autism

- Eating disorders

- Juvenile sex offenders

Prioritization of the committee's review of articles is driven by the needs of the system. The initial focus included those populations that the system was having the greatest difficulty managing effectively (e.g., youth with problems related to misconduct). Over time, the committee has been able to review literature related to all major populations served by the public mental health system. As of 2007, more than 35,000 articles have been screened, with more than 300 read and coded in detail. The EBS Committee created two major written documents known as the Blue Menu and the Biennial Report (Child and Adolescent Mental Health Division, 2004).

Developing the Blue Menu

The Blue Menu, so named because it is a menu of intervention choices printed on blue paper, summarizes the committee's coding in a concise and accessible double-sided sheet of paper. One side of the Blue Menu displays evidenced-based psychosocial interventions for youth (Figure 16.1). The first column lists the problem areas, and the next five columns contain interventions with varying levels of support for the various problem areas. Levels include *best support* at Level 1, *good support* at Level 2, *moderate support* at Level 3, *minimal support* at Level 4, and *no support* at Level 5. For instance, a best support (Level 1) intervention for anxious and avoidant behaviors is Cognitive-Behavioral Therapy whereas an intervention with no support (Level 5) for this same problem area is relationship counseling.

The other side of the Blue Menu contains information on psychopharmacological interventions for youth. Like the psychosocial side, the first column is the problem area. Problem areas on the psychopharmacology menu are slightly different from those on the psychosocial menu:

- Anxiety disorders

- Obsessive-compulsive disorder

- Attention-deficit/hyperactivity disorder (ADHD)

- Aggression in autism

- Aggressive conduct

- Bipolar disorder

- Depression

- Schizophrenia (psychotic disorders)

- Tourette's syndrome

The second column lists medication classes that have been tested for the problem areas. Columns 3–6 include evaluations or *grades* of the various medications by problem areas based on *short-term efficacy* (column 3), *long-term efficacy* (column

4), *short-term safety* (column 5), and *long-term safety* (column 6). An *A* indicates adequate data to inform prescribing practices, a *C* indicates no controlled evidence, and a *B* indicates the existence of some available data. The most updated versions of the Blue Menus for psychopharmacology and psychosocial interventions and other resources for EBS can be found at http://hawaii.gov/health/ mental-health/camhd/library/webs/ebs/ebs-index.html.

Both the psychosocial and psychopharmacology sides of the menu are designed to be user friendly with basic information regarding treatment options available at a glance. The menu is updated on a quarterly basis to provide the most up-to-date information garnered from the EBS Committee coding. Over time, the Blue Menu has become a staple in the culture of mental health professionals. It is not uncommon to see the Blue Menu posted on the walls in the offices of school counselors, private providers, and Department of Health staff throughout the state. In addition, it is routinely used by service planning teams as they develop individualized service plans for each youth and family. The Blue Menu is also used by families and youth as they become more informed and confident advocates for their services. Routine Blue Menu training is provided by Hawaii Families as Allies, the state's family organization, to increase understanding of treatment options and to encourage families to expect EBS in their service plans.

Producing Biennial Reports

The Biennial Report is a comprehensive document that includes, among other details, the methodology of the committee and details about specific studies (Child and Adolescent Mental Health Division, 2007). The 2007 report included information regarding the context of the treatments reviewed (e.g., setting, gender, age, ethnicity, type of therapist, frequency of intervention, format, cost, effect size relative to a control treatment). The report also provides a thorough summary of the literature, allowing for an in-depth understanding of a variety of treatments. Although it is more comprehensive than the Blue Menu, the report is still sufficiently concise and clear to be accessible to a wide audience. Both the Blue Menu and the Biennial Report influence CAMHD policy and strategy. Many of the CAMHD resources and innovations refer to the Blue Menu and Biennial Report for guidance and decision making.

Consideration of Ethnicity in Defining the Evidence Base

Hawaii is rich in cultural and ethnic diversity, and unlike most states, it lacks a single ethnic majority. The Hawaii Vital Statistics 2001 Report stated that 21.6% of residents identified themselves as Japanese, 21.5% as other or mixed ethnicity, 21.3% as Hawaiian, 19.8% as White, and 15.7% as Filipino (Hawaii Department of Health, 2002). Factors relating to ethnicity are baseline considerations in the Hawaii system of care. For example, the EBS Committee codes the ethnic breakdown of every study and protocol represented in the Biennial Report. This information is then presented in the Biennial Report and made available for con-

"Blue Menu"—Evidence-Based Child and Adolescent Psychosocial Interventions

This tool has been developed to guide teams (inclusive of youth, family, educators, and mental health practitioners) in developing appropriate plans using psycho-social interventions. Teams should use this information to prioritize promising options. For specific details about these interventions and their applications (e.g., age, setting, gender) see the most recent Evidence Based Services Committee Biennial Report (http://www.hawaii.gov/health/mental-health/camhd/library/webs/ebs/ebs-index.html).

Notice: The Blue Menu is being substantially updated based on hundreds of additional studies. Some problem areas that are now omitted will reappear in updated form on future editions.

Problem area	Level 1 Best support	Level 2 Good support	Level 3 Moderate support	Level 4 Minimal support	Level 5 No support
Anxious or Avoidant Behaviors	Cognitive-Behavioral Therapy, Education, Exposure, Modeling	Assertiveness Training, Cognitive-Behavioral Therapy with Parents, Hypnosis, Relaxation	None	Biofeedback, Play Therapy, Psycho-dynamic Therapy, Rational Emotive Therapy	Client-Centered Therapy, EMDR, Relationship Counseling, Teacher Psycho-education
Attention and Hyperactivity Behaviors	Behavior Therapy and Medication, Self-Verbalization	Biofeedback, Contingency Management, Parent Management Training and Problem Solving, Physical Exercise, Social Skills and Medication	None	Parent Management Training and Social Skills, Relaxation, Social Skills	Client-Centered Therapy, Parent Management Training and Self-Verbalization, Self-Control Training, Self-Verbalization and Medication, Skill Development
Autistic Spectrum Disorders	Intensive Behavior Therapy, Intensive Communication Training	None	None	None	Auditory Integration Training

Problem Area					
Delinquency and Disruptive Behavior	Assertiveness Training, Cognitive-Behavioral Therapy and Medication	Anger Control, Client-Centered Therapy, Communication Skills, Functional Family Therapy, Multisystemic Therapy, Parent Management Training and Problem Solving, Problem Solving, Rational Emotive Therapy, Relaxation, Transactional Analysis	Outreach Counseling, Peer Pairing, Self-Control Training	Physical Exercise, Stress Innoculation	Catharsis, Collaboratve Problem Solving, Education, Exposure, Family Empowerment, Family Systems Therapy, Group Therapy (!!), Life Skills, Peer Pairing, Project CARE (!!), Psychodynamic Therapy, Self-Verbalization, Skill Development
Depressive or Withdrawn Behavior	Cognitive-Behavioral Therapy, Cognitive-Behavioral Therapy and Medication	Client-Centered Therapy, Cognitive-Behavioral Therapy with Parents, Interpersonal Therapy, Family Therapy, Relaxation	None	Self-Control Training, Self-Modeling	Attention, Counselors Care, Counselors Care and Anger Management, Life Skills, Problem Solving, Social Skills
Eating Disorders	None	Family Therapy (anorexia only)	None	None	None
Substance Use	None	Cognitive-Behavioral Therapy, Contingency Management, Purdue Brief Family Therapy, Family Therapy, Family Systems Therapy	None	None	Client-Centered Therapy, Education Group Therapy (!!), Project CARE, Twelve-Step Program
Traumatic Stress	Cognitive-Behavioral Therapy	Cognitive-Behavioral Therapy with Parents	None	Play Therapy, Psychodrama	Client-Centered Therapy, Cognitive-Behavioral Therapy with Parents Only, EMDR

Figure 16.1. Blue Menu, psychosocial treatments. (Reprinted from Hawaii Department of Health. [2007]. *Blue menu—Evidence based child and adolescent psychosocial interventions.* Available online at http://www.hawaii.gov/health/mental-health/camhd/library/pdf/ebs/ebs022.pdf. Published by PracticeWise, LLC.) (*Note:* Level 5 refers to treatments that were tested and found ineffective. Risk of harm is noted by the symbol (!!), which indicates that at least one study found negative effects on the main outcome measure. The risk of using such treatments should be weighed against potential benefits.) (*Key:* EMDR, Eye Movement Desensitization and Reprocessing.)

sideration in treatment planning when deciding which protocol might be most appropriate for a particular youth.

Assessing Evidence-Based Service Coverage for Youth Registered in the Child and Adolescent Mental Health Division

A question of interest to CAMHD with respect to the EBS Committee's work is the extent to which the diagnoses of the youth in the system match EBS as defined by the EBS Committee's Blue Menu. Accordingly, CAMHD initiated a study to assess the match between Blue Menu evidence-based treatments and the diagnoses found among youth in the CAMHD system (Schiffman, Becker, & Daleiden, 2006). Diagnostic profiles of all CAMHD registered youth were analyzed to determine whether a relevant EBS treatment had been identified for their diagnoses.

Based on the CAMHD system in 2004, 2,197 youth had available diagnostic information for this analysis. As noted, the EBS Committee established guidelines for what was considered evidence based for Hawaii's system of care. According to the Blue Menu, the diagnostic categories with evidence-based coverage identified in the literature to the *best, good,* or *moderate* level were:

- Anxiety and avoidant

- Attention and hyperactivity

- Autism spectrum disorder

- Bipolar disorder

- Depressed and withdrawn

- Disruptive or oppositional

- Eating disorders

- Delinquency and willful misconduct

- Psychotic disorders or schizophrenia

- Substance related disorders

According to the Blue Menu, EBS could not be identified in the literature for:

- Adjustment disorders with mixed disturbances

- Reactive attachment disorder

- Learning communication and academic disorders

- Intermittent explosive or impulse control disorders

- Cognitive disorder nonspecific

- Neglect

- Physical and sexual abuse of the child

To determine the fit between Blue Menu coverage and diagnoses within CAMHD, the diagnostic profile for each youth was examined. Of all youth in the CAMHD system in 2004 with diagnostic information, the vast majority (89%) had a primary diagnosis—regardless of secondary diagnoses—for which an evidence-based service was identified, and 94% had at least one diagnosis (primary or additional) for which an evidence-based service was identified. Overall, EBS could be identified for the primary diagnosis for 9 out of 10 youth. This suggests that despite the presence of comorbid diagnoses and multiple treatment targets, EBS have been identified in the literature for the principle concerns of many youth served by the CAMHD system of care. Although most youth have problems for which at least one evidence-based service is identified, many youth served have additional problems for which EBS have not yet been identified. Furthermore, although an evidence-based service may be identified in the literature, it may not necessarily be available in the community.

IDENTIFYING AND APPLYING PRACTICE ELEMENTS

The analyses undertaken by CAMHD and its EBS Committee determined the degree to which diagnoses of youth in the system of care are amenable to EBS identified in the literature. This approach, however, had limitations in terms of identifying which methods a therapist might employ in practice for an individual youth and family. Given that there are typically numerous evidence-based interventions for particular diagnoses and problems, CAMHD first attempted to answer the question, "Which manual do we use?" In many instances, pinning providers down to a single manual-covered intervention was met with resistance, leading providers to ask, "Of all the evidence-based protocols for a particular disorder, what are the common clinical practice elements?" A *practice elements* approach was then established to break these evidence-based interventions down into their component ingredients, weigh these components based on their frequency in existing successful intervention packages, keep them connected to the evidence base, and make them flexible enough to appeal to clinicians.

Generation of Practice Elements

To generate practice elements (i.e., clinical techniques within a manual) EBS Committee members coded all identified evidence-based interventions (i.e., protocols) in the *best* and *good* range for each disorder, identifying the presence of 55 possible clinical techniques in the manuals. Figure 16.2 shows the coding sheet used to code each *best* or *good* supported intervention. Some of the practice elements coded included techniques such as *relaxation, marital therapy, mindfulness, hypnosis, supportive listening, play therapy,* and *activity scheduling.* The committee used the coding to report the proportion of all evidence-based treatments that used each of the identified practice elements. For example, there are 36 evidence-based protocols for anxiety, and the practice of *exposure* is in 35 (97%) of these (Chorpita, Daleiden, & Weisz, 2005a, 2005b; Daleiden, Lee, & Tolman, 2004).

**Evidence-Based Services Committee
Intervention Strategies Code Sheet**

Instructions: Please read the manual or intervention description to determine which of the following list of intervention strategies is present. For definitions of intervention strategies, please use the latest codebook for the CAMHD Provider Monthly Summary (available on the web at http://www.state.hi.us/doh/camhd/ index.html). It is suggested that raters code in both directions; that is, read each strategy in the codebook to determine whether it is in the intervention *and* read the intervention or manual to code what strategies are apparent in the text. Code for the presence of a strategy by placing a checkmark in the box to the left of the name of the item. Also, please write comments below if difficulties arise, and these will be discussed in our next commitee meeting. Mahalo!

Intervention name (name of manual or program): _____

Author(s): _____

Year: _____

Name of rater: _____

Intervention strategies (check all that apply)

Activity scheduling	Eye movement, tapping	Marital therapy	Play therapy	Stimulus or antecedent control
Assertiveness training	Family engagement	Medication/pharmacotherapy	Problem solving	Supportive listening
Biofeedback, neurofeedback	Family therapy	Mentoring	Psychoeducation, child	Tangible rewards
Catharsis	Free association	Milieu therapy	Psychoeducation, parent	Therapist praise/rewards
Cognitive/ coping	Functional analysis	Mindfulness	Relationship or rapport building	Thought field therapy
Commands/ limit setting	Guided imagery	Modeling	Relaxation	Time out
Communication skills	Hypnosis	Motivational Interviewing	Response cost	Twelve-step programming
Crisis management	Ignoring or DRO	Natural and logical consequences	Response prevention	Other:
Directed play	Insight building	Parent coping	Self-monitoring	Other:
Educational support	Interpretation	Parent-monitoring	Self-reward/ self-praise	Other:
Emotional processing	Line of sight supervision	Parent praise	Skill building	
Exposure	Maintenance or relapse prevention	Peer modeling or pairing	Social skills training	

Figure 16.2. Coding sheet for practice elements. (Reprinted from Hawaii Department of Health. [2003]. *Coding form for intervention strategies.* Available online at http://www.hawaii.gov/health/ mental-health/camhd/library/pdf/ebs/ebs004.pdf) (*Key:* CAMHD, Child and Adolescent Mental Health Division; DRO, differential reinforcement of other behavior.)

Practice Elements for Diagnostic Categories

At the time of the 2004 EBS Biennial Report, 12 evidence-based protocols for attention and hyperactivity problems were coded for practice elements. Similarly, the committee had coded 36 evidence-based studies in the *anxious avoidant behaviors* category, 14 studies in the *depressive or withdrawn* category, and 37 studies in the *disruptive or oppositional* category. Figure 16.3 illustrates the coding process and the means by which the information from the coding is distilled for attention and hyperactivity problems. The vertical axis lists the practice elements such as *tangible rewards, parent praise,* and *response cost,* and the horizontal axis lists percentages. The bars within the graph indicate the percentage of evidence-based protocols that contain the particular practice elements. For instance, the most common practice element reported in the 12 *best* or *good* evidence-based intervention studies for attention and hyperactivity problems was *tangible rewards.* The committee defined *tangible rewards* as "the training of parents or others involved in the social ecology of the child in the administration of tangible rewards to promote desired behaviors. This can involve tokens, charts, or record keeping, in addition to first-order reinforcers" (Child and Adolescent Mental Health Division, 2003). As shown, 92% of *best* or *good* empirically supported treatment protocols for attention and hyperactivity contain *tangible rewards,* 83% contain *parent praise,* and 58% contain *response cost.*

For anxiety or avoidance problems, exposure is the key ingredient, with a large number of protocols also including *modeling, cognitive work,* and *relaxation.* Protocols for *depressed or withdrawn* most frequently involve the elements of *psychoeducation, cognitive work, problem solving,* and *activity scheduling,* all of which were found in more than half of the 14 coded EBPs for depression. For *disruptive behaviors,* the ingredients of *tangible rewards, commands/limit setting, time out, parent praise,* and *problem solving* were all found in more than half of the protocols.

Advantages of the Practice Elements Approach

The practice elements approach has been well-received by mental health providers, individualized service planning teams, and families in that it allows for increased flexibility rather than strict adherence to manual-covered treatments, yet it still (it is assumed) maintains the key ingredients of successful evidence-based protocols. Choosing which elements to employ, the length of time to persist with a particular element, and the order of the elements are all factors that are fixed in manuals for specific interventions. The practice elements approach frees these factors, leading to flexibility in planning and delivering individualized services, increased freedom for therapists, and greater opportunity for therapists to match the current condition of the youth with a personally tailored treatment strategy. The greater flexibility may also lead to greater portability, providing a general evidence-based framework for providers (e.g., in rural settings with few resources). Preliminary evidence suggests that the practice elements approach leads to improved satisfaction from providers relative to traditional models (Francis & Chorpita, 2003).

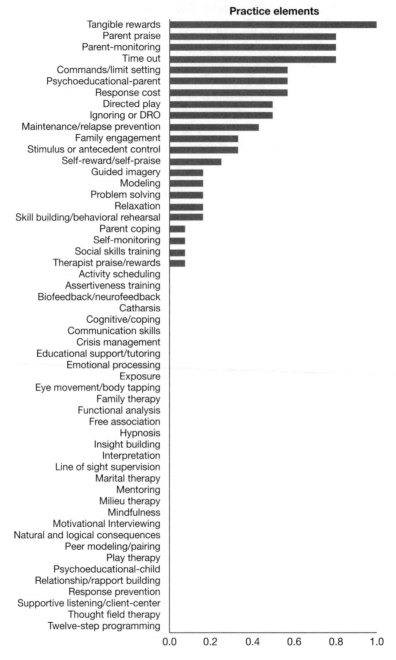

Hawaii Evidence-Based Services Practice Profile (as of 10/26/2004)

EBS Level 1 Best Support   Problem(s): 100% Attention and Hyperactivity

Figure 16.3. Distillation of practice elements from evidence-based service protocols for attention and hyperactivity. (Reprinted from Hawaii Department of Health, Evidence Based Services Committee. [2004]. *2004 biennial report* [p. 10]. Available online at http://www.hawaii .gov/health/mental-health/camhd/library/pdf/ebs/ebs011.pdf) (*Key:* DRO, differential reinforcement of other behavior.)

Combining Monthly Treatment Progress Summaries and Evidence-Based Service Practice Elements

The use of this approach is intended to arm clinicians with knowledge of particular elements that are likely to be useful for specific diagnostic categories and to increase the likelihood that providers will use these EBP elements. Initially, there was no mechanism in place to monitor the practice strategies used by providers for individual clients. To obtain feedback regarding actual services provided, as well as to assess if providers are using the practice elements commonly found in EBS, CAMHD created the Monthly Treatment Progress Summary (MTPS, see Figure 16.4), a three-page clinician report checklist completed for each client on a monthly basis.

The MTPS measures service format and setting, treatment targets, clinical progress, and intervention practice elements. The measure allows clinicians to report up to 55 predefined practice elements, as well as 3 additional write-in (i.e., *other*) intervention practice elements per month. In addition, the MTPS measures the foci of treatment, referred to as *treatment targets*. Clinicians are asked to indicate up to 10 treatment targets or concerns that were the focus of treatment during the reporting month, as well as the amount of progress made on treating those targets.

The MTPS's idiographic clinical progress ratings seem to capture valid, sensitive, and nonredundant client-specific treatment outcome information that somewhat overlaps with both the Child and Adolescent Functional Assessment Scale (CAFAS; Hodges, Wong & Latessa, 1998) and Child and Adolescent Level of Care Utilization System (CALOCUS; American Academy of Child and Adolescent Psychiatry, 1999; Nakamura, Daleiden, & Mueller, 2007). Statewide training was provided for CAMHD clinicians and providers on the completion of this form and the various practice element definitions. The MTPS and its structured codebook defining intervention practice elements are also available on the CAMHD website (http://www.hawaii.gov/health/mental-health/camhd/provider/prov-agency/index.html).

The EBS coding of practice elements provides a summary of the most common practices within evidence-based protocols for various diagnostic categories, and the MTPS tool provides a unique opportunity to examine actual practices reported by clinicians for youth served. Combining these two sets of information, CAMHD was able to assess the degree to which actual care matches guidelines derived from the literature (Daleiden, Lee, & Tolman, 2004). Figure 16.5 summarizes the findings from this analysis for the diagnostic category *attention and hyperactivity*. The figure suggests that although many practice elements found in the evidence base are employed for this diagnostic category, many other practice elements used are not found in the evidence base. For instance, 92% of the protocols coded for attentional disorders included some sort of *tangible rewards*, but only 43% of clinicians treating youth with a primary diagnosis relating to attentional problems indicated using *tangible rewards*. Although all 23 practice elements identified in the literature for attentional problems were reportedly used by

Service Provider Monthly Treatment and Progress Summary
Child and Adolescent Mental Health Division (CAMHD)

Instructions: Please complete and electronically submit this form to CAMHD by the 5th working day of each month (summarizing the time period of 1st to the last day of the previous month). The information will be used in service review, monitoring, planning, and coordination in accordance with CAMHD policies and standards. Mahalo!

Client name: _____ CR #: _____ DOB: _____

Month/year of services: _____ Primary diagnosis: _____ Eligibility status: _____

Level of care (one per form): _____

Service format (circle all that apply):

Individual   Group   Parent   Family   Teacher   Other:

Service setting (circle all that apply):

Home   School   Community   Out of home   Clinic/office   Other:

Service dates: [ ][ ][ ][ ][ ][ ][ ][ ][ ][ ][ ][ ][ ][ ][ ][ ]

Targets addressed this month (number up to 10):

Activity involvement	Contentment, enjoyment, happiness	Learning disorder, under-achievement	Phobia/fears	Sleep disturbance
Academic achievement	Depressed mood	Low self-esteem	Positive thinking/attitude	Social skills
Aggression	Eating, feeding problems	Mania	Psychosis	Speech and language problems
Anger	Empathy	Medical regimen adherence	Runaway	Substance use
Anxiety	Enuresis, encopresis	Oppositional/noncompliant behavior	School involvement	Suicidality
Assertiveness	Fire setting	Peer involvement	School refusal/truancy	Traumatic stress
Attention problems	Gender identity problems	Peer/sibling conflict	Self-control	Treatment engagement
Avoidance	Grief	Personal hygeine	Self-injurious behavior	Willful misconduct, delinquency
Cognitive-intellectual functioning	Health management	Positive family functioning	Sexual misconduct	Other:
Community involvement	Hyperactivity	Positive peer interaction	Shyness	Other:

Progress ratings this month (check appropriate rating for any target numbers endorsed above):

#	Deterioration < 0%	No significant changes 0%–10%	Minimal improvement 11%–30%	Some improvement 31%–50%	Moderate improvement 51%–70%	Significant improvement 71%–90%	Complete improvement 91%–100%	Date (if complete)
1								
2								
3								
4								
5								
6								
7								
8								
9								
10								

Figure 16.4. Monthly treatment and progress summary. (Reprinted from Hawaii Department of Health. [2005]. *Service provider monthly treatment and progress summary.* Available online at http://hawaii.gov/health/mental-health/camhd/library/pdf/paf/paf-002.pdf) (*Key:* CAFAS, Child and Adolescent Functional Assessment Scale; CALOCUS, Child and Adolescent Level of Care Utilization System; CASII, Child and Adolescent Service Intensity Instrument; CBCL, Child Behavior Checklist; CR #, central registration number; DOB, date of birth; DRO, differential reinforcement of other behavior; ID #, identification number; TRF, Teacher's Report Form; YSR, Youth Self-Report.)

CR #: _____ (please repeat the number here)

Intervention strategies used this month (check all that apply):

Activity scheduling	Eye movement, tapping	Marital therapy	Play therapy	Stimulus or antecedent control
Assertiveness training	Family engagement	Medication/ pharmacotherapy	Problem solving	Supportve listening
Biofeedback, neurofeedback	Family therapy	Mentoring	Psycho-education, child	Tangible rewards
Catharsis	Free association	Milieu therapy	Psycho-education, parent	Therapist praise/rewards
Cognitive/ coping	Functional analysis	Mindfulness	Relationship or rapport building	Thought field therapy
Commands/ limit setting	Guided imagery	Modeling	Relaxation	Time out
Communication skills	Hypnosis	Motivational Interviewing	Response cost	Twelve-step programming
Crisis management	Ignoring or DRO	Natural and logical consequences	Response prevention	Other:
Directed play	Insight building	Parent coping	Self-monitoring	Other:
Emotional support	Interpretation	Parent-monitoring	Self-reward/ self-praise	Other:
Emotional processing	Line of sight supervision	Parent praise	Skill building	
Exposure	Maintenance or relapse prevention	Peer modeling or pairing	Social skills training	

Psychiatric medications (List all)	Total daily dose	Dose schedule	Check if change	Description of change
_____	_____	_____	☐	_____
_____	_____	_____	☐	_____
_____	_____	_____	☐	_____
_____	_____	_____	☐	_____
_____	_____	_____	☐	_____

Projected discharge date: _____   ☐ Check if discharged during current month

If youth was dischaged this month, please complete items A & B.

A. Discharge living situation (check one)

☐ Home   ☐ Foster home   ☐ Group care   ☐ Residential treatment
☐ Institution/hospital   ☐ Jail/corrections facility ☐ Homeless/shelter ☐ Other:

B. Reason(s) for discharge (check all that apply)

☐ Success/goals met ☐ Insufficient progress   ☐ Family relocation
☐ Runaway/elopement ☐ Refuse/withdraw   ☐ Eligibility change ☐ Other:

_____

(continued)

Figure 16.4. *(continued)*

CR #: _____ (please repeat the number here)

Outcome measures: Optional. If you have any of the following data, please report the most recent scores:

	Date:
CAFAS (8 Scales): (1-School:) (2-Home:) (3-Community:) (4-Behavior Toward Others:) (5-Moods/Emotions:) (6-Self-Harm:) (7-Substance:) (8-Thinking:) (Total:)	Date:
CASII/CALOCUS (Total): CASII/CALOCUS (Level of care):	Date:
CBCL (Total problems T): CBCL (Internalizing T): CBCL (Externalizing T):	Date:
YSR (Total problems T): YSR (Internalizing T): YSR (Externalizing T):	Date:
TRF (Total problems T): TRF (Internalizing T): TRF (Externalizing T):	Date:
Arrested during month? (Y/N): School attendance (% of days):	

Comments/suggestions (attach additional sheets if necessary):

Provider agency and island: _____ Clinician name and ID #: _____

Provider supervisor signature: _____ Clinician signature: _____

Submitted to CAMHD (date): _____ Care coordinator: _____

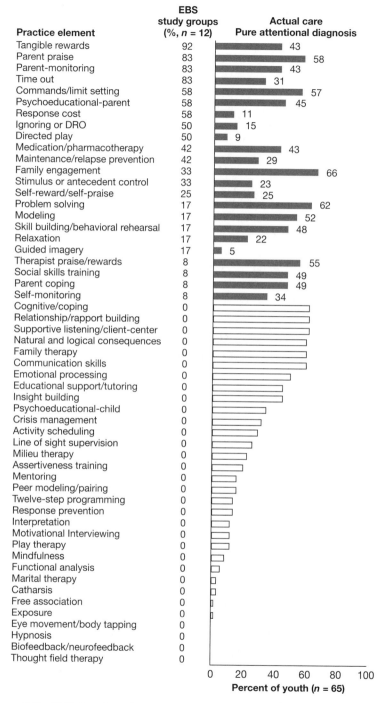

Figure 16.5. Distillation of practice elements from evidence-based service protocols and actual care reported from Monthly Treatment Progress Summary within the Child and Adolescent Mental Health Division for youth with attention and hyperactivity. (Reprinted from Daleiden, E., Lee, J., & Tolman, R. [2004]. *Annual evaluation report: Fiscal year 2004.* Honolulu: Hawaii Department of Health Child and Adolescent Mental Health Division.) (*Key:* DRO, differential reinforcement of other behavior.)

at least a portion of clinicians, the clinicians also reported using 30 practice elements not identified in the literature for youth with attentional concerns. Approximately 60% reported employing *communication skills* in treatment, an element not described in any of the 12 evidence-based protocols coded for attention problems. These conclusions were similar for the other diagnostic categories. Thus, findings revealed that practice elements commonly identified in the literature tended not to be used by clinicians as often as might be expected given their appearance in multiple evidence-based protocols, and many practice elements not identified in the literature were employed by clinicians.

In addition to assessing the alignment of practice elements used by clinicians for particular disorders with the EBS Committee's distillation of the evidence base, the MTPS also can be used to investigate whether such alignment translates into improved clinical progress. Specifically, the MTPS may shed light on the question as to whether youth who have providers using EBP elements improve faster or more dramatically than youth who have providers using non-EBP elements or elements with only partial empirical support. This would test the core assumption that use of the EBP elements will yield improved treatment outcomes.

INTEGRATING EVIDENCE-BASED PRACTICE ELEMENTS INTO INDIVIDUALIZED CARE

A major emphasis in Hawaii's system of care is placed on assuring that all services and supports are individualized. Child and family teams are organized as the cornerstone of the individualized care or wraparound process. In addition to the youth, family, and care coordinator, involved staff from other agencies and treatment providers are included on the team to develop, implement, and coordinate an individualized service plan that brings together all of the services and supports for an individual child and family. Mental health care coordinators play a pivotal role in this process by convening the team, coordinating ongoing service delivery, monitoring progress, and revising services as indicated.

The individualized approach to care provides a context for incorporating EBP elements into services, based on the unique needs of each youth. Information and resources are provided to help teams and mental health providers make appropriate decisions. The most straightforward resource comes directly from the EBS Committee's coding of practice elements for each diagnostic category, illustrating the most common elements within evidence-based protocols for that diagnosis. Although this information is simply a frequency count, it provides some indication of the relative importance of a particular element for the diagnostic category. Individualized planning teams can also use their collective judgment to match family-generated treatment goals with relevant practice elements.

Planning Documents for Individualized Care

Three documents—mental health assessments, coordinated services plans, and mental health treatment plans—are used to guide the individualized care process.

In mental health assessments, mental health professionals assess an individual youth, apply their knowledge of the research literature, and make recommendations regarding the focus of treatment and therapeutic practices. This information is then used in the individualized planning process to develop comprehensive coordinated services plans (CSPs). These overarching, strengths-based plans are family-driven, youth-guided documents identifying youth and family strengths, goals, and preferences and specifying the services and supports to be provided. From the CSP, individual mental health providers construct individualized mental health treatment plans for each youth. Family and youth are integrally involved in creating these documents and providing input on every level about their goals and priorities. There are opportunities in each of these documents to identify and include EBP elements. These documents, along with the monthly monitoring of treatment targets and practice elements included in the MTPS, guide the service delivery process.

In an ongoing effort to assess quality, CAMHD recently evaluated the consistency over time of these documents that guide and inform the delivery of individualized services. Specifically, the study examined rates of congruence between treatment targets and practice elements recommended in one stage of treatment planning with targets and practice elements at subsequent stages. Results suggested a lack of congruence between the assessment, coordinated service plan, and mental health treatment plan documents in that some recommendations offered in one stage of planning tended to get lost in subsequent stages. This pattern was especially found for more severe treatment targets such as psychosis, runaway incidents, safe environment, self-injurious behaviors, sexual misconduct, and suicidal tendencies (Young, Daleiden, Chorpita, Schiffman, & Mueller, in press). In response, CAMHD is considering steps such as attaching an MTPS form to each mental health assessment, coordinated service plan, and mental health treatment plan based on the premise that this might help the team remain focused on relevant treatment targets and practice elements for each youth. A study is being designed to test the effectiveness of this strategy. Another area of study will compare the content of recommendations made at each stage of planning with content from what is known from the evidence base. Coordination of the process of planning individualized care with the work of the EBS Committee will further the infusion of evidence-based strategies into direct care.

Clinical Dashboards

Clinical progress is another important source of information factored into individualization of care. In an effort to provide relevant information regarding clinical progress, every child in the system has a viewable clinical dashboard containing information about the child's progress over time. These dashboards provide general information such as age, sex, and diagnoses, as well as information on service history, school attendance, sentinel events such as runaway incidents and arrests, functioning (via the CAFAS), and clinical progress (via the Achenbach System of Empirically Based Assessment [ASEBA] scales). This information gives providers an indication as to whether the current services and supports are affecting the child's life and whether current treatment strategies (i.e., targets and practice elements) are appropriate. Care coordinators receive dashboards for all of the youth they serve and use this information to continually evaluate needs and progress.

Figure 16.6 shows an example of a clinical dashboard of a youth with available information between September 2003 and March 2004. Starting from the upper left of the dashboard, the ASEBA Total Problems *T*-Score figure displays the youth's composite problem score on the three Achenbach scales (Child Behavior Checklist [CBCL], Youth Self-Report [YSR], and Teacher's Report Form [TRF]) across time. In this example, a September 2003 assessment yielded a CBCL *T*-score of approximately 65, suggesting, based on parent report, that this youth is struggling with general emotional and behavioral problems at a level greater than 94% of other youth in a similar age range. This score was discrepant with the youth's own report on a YSR administration at that same time that yielded a *T*-score of slightly under 50. The youth's self-report of problems was in the average range compared with his or her peers. Several months later in February 2004, a TRF *T*-score of around 50 on the Problems scale was recorded, suggesting that per the teacher's report, the youth's general emotional and behavioral functioning were in the average range compared with his or her peers.

The ASEBA Total Competence *T*-Score figure shows the youth's composite strengths score on the Achenbach scales across time. In this example, the youth's initial assessment yielded a YSR scale score of approximately 30, indicating that approximately 98% of youth in the same age range indicated more competencies than this particular youth. Several months later, in an assessment in February 2004, a TRF score from this scale suggested that the youth was in the average range compared with his or her peers.

The CAFAS 8-Scale Total Score figure displays the total CAFAS scores over time, with the CAFAS Role Performance figure showing three subscales within the CAFAS (Home, School/work, and Community). In this case, overall CAFAS scores are improving, with a decrease from a score of 150 in September 2003, to a score of 90 in March 2004. Drilling down further on the CAFAS shows that school functioning has improved dramatically, changing from a 30 in December 2003 to a 0 in March 2004, while Community functioning worsened during that same time.

The next two figures represent information from the CALOCUS across time. Overall, at each time point, the CALOCUS Total Scores suggest that this youth's functioning is at a level where outpatient or intensive outpatient services would be appropriate. The CALOCUS Level of Care figure illustrates that at first assessment, this youth was being served at Level 5, likely a group home with 24-hour services and psychological monitoring. As treatment progressed, the level of care decreased over time to Level 3, intensive outpatient therapy. The Diagnostic History graph displays diagnoses assigned to the youth at different time points. The youth in this example received diagnoses in the Disruptive, Substance Use/Abuse, and Miscellaneous categories in September 2003. The Level of Care figure

Overall Summary for Individual Youth

CR number: Example 1
Initial registration date:

Date of birth:
Report date: 5/10/2004

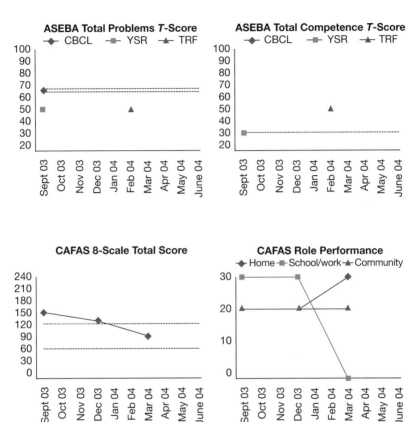

(continued)

Figure 16.6. Example of a clinical dashboard from the clinical report module of the Child and Adolescent Mental Health Management Information System. (Reprinted from Child and Adolescent Psychiatric Clinics of North America, Vol. 14, D.L. Daleiden & B.F. Chorpita, From data to wisdom: Quality improvement strategies supporting large-scale implementation of evidence-based services, pp. 329–349, Copyright © 2005, with permission from Elsevier.) *(Key:* ADAD, Alcohol and Drug Abuse Division; ASEBA, Achenbach System of Empirically Based Assessment; CAFAS, Child and Adolescent Functional Assessment Scale; CALOCUS, Child and Adolescent Level of Care Utilization System; CBCL, Child Behavior Checklist; CBR, community-based residential; CHR, community high risk; CR, central registration; CS, crisis stability; DC, discharge; Dev. Dis., developmental disabilities; DOH, Department of Health; DHS, Department of Human Services; DT, detoxification; Early Int., early intervention; FLX, flexible spending; HBR, hospital-based residential; HH, hospital home; IDS, intensive day stabilization; LI, less intensive; MH, mental health; MR, mental retardation; MST, Multisystemic Therapy; OOS, out of state; PDD, pervasive developmental disorder; PH, partial hospitalization; RH, respite home; RSP, respite; TFH, therapeutic foster home; TGH, therapeutic group home; TRF, Teacher's Report Form; YSR, Youth Self-Report.)

Figure 16.6. *(continued)*

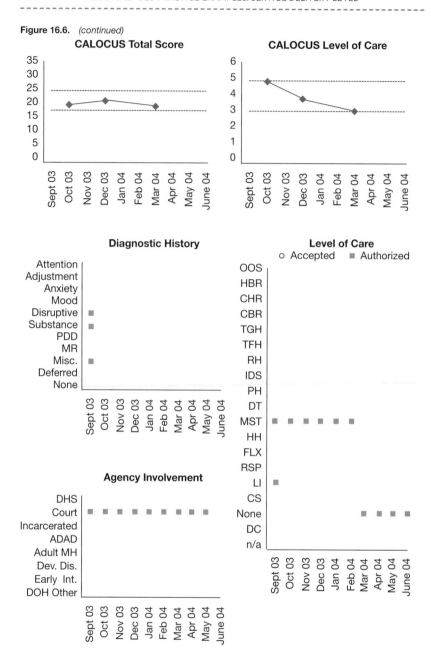

illustrates services provided to the youth. This youth began with a course of Multisystemic Therapy (MST) that lasted 6 months. The family also received less intensive services in September 2003. At the conclusion of MST, the child did not receive any services other than active case management. The Agency Involvement figure indicates other service agencies within the system of care interacting with the youth.

Collectively, this information gives relevant stakeholders a comprehensive snapshot of information such as the youth's functioning from a variety of sources, the youth's diagnostic history, as well as services provided. The information can be used in countless ways to guide treatment. For example, a quick glance at the Diagnostic History and the Level of Care figures could show a team if the treatments provided seemed relevant for the family of diagnoses the youth carried. In addition, pairing Level of Care figure with CAFAS scores, for instance, might provide some clues as to whether the employed intervention strategies are proving effective in improving functioning. In this example the youth's functioning improved over time along with the implementation of MST, suggesting the effectiveness of the service in this case.

Clinical Supervision

CAMHD utilizes clinical supervision as a means of promoting the use of evidence-based approaches in service delivery for individual youth. The model incorporates a variety of information to provide recommendations about strategies and practice elements throughout the different steps of treatment. For example, as a new youth and family enter the system, a child and family team is convened for a coordinated service planning meeting. During this meeting, the team will consult the Blue Menu to identify evidence-based strategies appropriate to the youth that might be incorporated into the service plan. If significant concerns arise (e.g., a suicide attempt, a runaway incident, an arrest) or if there is lack of progress, teams are encouraged to consult with a state-employed or contracted practice specialist for recommendations. Teams monitor clinical progress through a variety of measures, including the CAFAS, the ASEBA scales, the MTPS, and the reporting of critical incidents. Routine progress is easily monitored through reports displayed on the clinical dashboard. If the treatment selection appears to be a mismatch with the youth's challenges and goals, the team is again encouraged to consult the Blue Menu or to seek consultation. If, however, treatment appears appropriate and gains are not recognized, options such as assuring fidelity to the treatment model, evaluating service intensity, increasing community supports, or adding or changing interventions are suggested by the supervision process as depicted on a flow chart. Thus, the CAMHD clinical supervision flow chart provides a roadmap guiding the individualized care process and the incorporation of evidence-based treatment approaches.

Proprietary Evidence-Based Services

In addition to endorsing the practice elements approach to intervention, the CAMHD system of care provides an array of proprietary EBS, as determined by the Blue Menu, for youth who may be good candidates for the particular programs. For instance, as of 1999, CAMHD has offered MST, a comprehensive psychosocial approach for youth with a variety of behavioral problems. This is an evidence-based program that CAMHD adopted directly from the treatment creators. CAMHD procures all aspects of MST (e.g., measuring fidelity and outcomes, hiring MST trainers to oversee the services). CAMHD has also introduced Multidimensional Treatment Foster Care (MTFC) and Functional Family Therapy (FFT). MTFC is an evidence-based approach to foster care involving more training and support for foster families than is offered in traditional foster care; FFT is an evidence-based program with special emphasis on family engagement and motivation. Similar to its role with MST, CAMHD contracts for training, fidelity monitoring, outcome measurement, and other supports associated with implementation of these interventions.

ENGAGEMENT OF SYSTEM PARTNERS

To increase the likelihood of the adoption of evidence-based approaches, CAMHD has engaged in efforts to spread a culture of EBS among providers, families, and partner agencies.

Provider Engagement

Although mental health providers have always been openly invited to be part of the EBS Committee's work, early attempts to shift practice toward EBS initially resulted in resistance among some professionals. Many had been working in the community for years without specific guidelines and expectations as to the process and outcome of their work; the term *evidence-based* was simply not part of the local mental health vocabulary. Imposing increased structure to care was a dramatic shift for some practitioners, requiring both support and time. CAMHD addressed providers' early reluctance to implementing EBS in a variety of ways. The first method involved extensive training, which consisted of a host of ongoing CAMHD-sponsored workshops and conferences to increase working knowledge of evidence-based approaches among individual therapists and supervisors. Trainings included detailed descriptions of the principles, benefits, and techniques of EBS. Trainings were often interactive, including role plays requiring therapists to practice as they were being observed. Other learning opportunities came in the form of expert speakers hosting day-long symposiums. These trainings were offered free of charge to providers. To supplement trainings, the CAMHD Clinical Services Office is available to provide consultation, supervision, and additional literature about EBS.

In addition to continued didactic trainings for providers, CAMHD offers a wealth of information about EBS on the CAMHD web site. The Blue Menu, the Biennial Report, and other locally generated materials and research reports are all freely and readily available. An additional novelty on the CAMHD web site is the *EBS Tip of the Week*, which offers ideas, research, and general guidelines about

EBS. These practical tips impart insight into EBS and contribute to the culture of EBS within Hawaii's system of care.

The connection between data from providers regarding the youth they serve and EBS is another method used to help create an EBS culture for CAMHD providers. Information provided by clinicians is regularly transformed into easy-to-read technical reports, an annual evaluation, and other publications and presentations. These reports and presentations tangibly demonstrate positive clinical outcomes for CAMHD-registered youth. They also serve as a source of pride for providers, showing that their work is effective in improving people's lives and that the data they gather is put to good use.

Family Engagement

A core value of the Hawaii system of care is that services, programs, and policies are youth guided and family driven. As such, the system requires input from family members and youth in decision making at all levels of the system. With respect to EBS, family voices within the EBS Committee have shaped the way in which studies are coded and information is disseminated. A code for the date a study was published was added to the EBS Committee code sheet after a parent expressed concern that a potential evidence-based study from three decades ago may or may not be currently valid. In addition, parents on the EBS Committee actively share their knowledge with other families, spreading enthusiasm for EBS among families and youth.

The belief in EBS from families is a major contributor to the EBS culture within the system of care. Many parents use their knowledge of EBS, as well as the information available to them through CAMHD, to demand appropriate EBS from their providers. Informed consumers empower the evidence-based movement in a way that administrative planning and leadership cannot. In addition, parent partners are active educators when it comes to teaching the importance of EBS to students training to become mental health providers in the system. Several times throughout the year, parents present guest lectures in classes for the various university programs affiliated with CAMHD (i.e., psychology, social work, nursing, psychiatry). This infusion of parent input into the curriculum of mental health trainees serves a variety of goals, including educating students of the family perspective, reemphasizing the core values of youth-guided and family-driven care, and highlighting the importance of EBS to families.

University Engagement

CAMHD has made tremendous investments in the training of future mental health care providers in the provision of EBS. Through unique relationships with the University of Hawaii, CAMHD provides funding to students working on advanced degrees in psychology, social work, nursing, and psychiatry. In return, these students provide direct services to CAMHD-registered youth, or in some cases, perform research that informs the entire system. Through practicum experiences working directly with youth and families, as well as through class work, CAMHD-funded students learn about the system of care philosophy and approach; family-driven, youth-guided care; the vision and mission of CAMHD; and EBS. In addition, students attend EBS Committee meetings and are given opportunities to interact across disciplines to encourage interdisciplinary teamwork. The result of this investment is both knowledge and acceptance of the system of care approach and EBS among future community service providers and leaders. Although this investment in workforce development is in its relatively early stages, many students have continued contributing to the public children's mental health system following their practicum placements, and several have returned to the system after graduating to assume leadership positions.

Child-Serving Agency Engagement

Providing holistic care that coordinates services across multiple domains and agencies has required successful partnerships with education, child welfare, and juvenile justice systems. Examples of interagency collaboration include the creation of the Interagency Performance Standards and Practices Guidelines, a comprehensive, evidence-based, and interagency-driven guide for services. In addition, both the child welfare and juvenile justice systems have worked closely with the EBS Committee in an attempt to disseminate accurate and useful information about interventions for attachment disorders, trauma, and runaway and/or suicidal tendencies. CAMHD has also offered specific trainings on these topics for partner agencies.

SYSTEM INFRASTRUCTURE

The Hawaii system of care offers resources and guidelines to help support families and providers in the provision of individualized care that incorporates evidence-based treatment strategies. These supports include the Clinical Services Office (CSO) and the Interagency Standards and Practices Guidelines manual.

Clinical Services Office

CAMHD's CSO is a specialty office focusing on the development of effective practices and clinical innovations. This division performs a number of tasks that help build expertise in systems of care and evidence-based approaches. CSO regularly sponsors large-scale conferences, creates informational reading material, provides clinical trainings, facilitates clinical networking groups, and creates guiding policy and procedure documents to build an informed provider network. In addition, the CSO personnel, including CAMHD's medical director, chief psychologist, and clinical specialists, are available to serve as consulting specialists to assist clinicians and other service providers with their most challenging cases. They bring their knowledge of individualized care and EBS to assist providers as they work to solve problems in the field.

Interagency Standards and Practices Guidelines

Alongside state agency system partners (e.g., the Department of Education), CAMHD's CSO developed the Interagency Performance Standards and Practices Guidelines manual. Available for free online, this comprehensive manual contains detailed information about accessing services, treatment guidelines and strategies, levels of care available for youth, and system of care principles. The Interagency Performance Standards and Practices Guidelines are highly influenced by the EBS Committee as seen in their emphasis on EBS. They are also appropriately flexible, allowing for the individualization of services and treatments to fit the needs of individual youth and their families.

REAL LIFE APPLICATION: THE CASE OF JENNIFER

The application of the evidence-based philosophy within Hawaii's system of care is brought to life through a description of an individual youth's experiences receiving mental health services. Jennifer was a 14-year-old girl referred for mental health assessment and treatment after a suicide attempt, which resulted in her hospitalization. In conjunction with Jennifer's mother, the hospital initiated the referral to CAMHD, at which time Jennifer was assigned a CAMHD care coordinator. The care coordinator facilitated a coordinated service planning process, which decided that Cognitive-Behavioral Therapy (CBT) was an appropriate service for her mood and anxiety challenges. The care coordinator contacted the Center for Cognitive Behavior Therapy, a CAMHD-supported mental health training clinic operated by the Department of Psychology at the University of Hawaii, to provide services.

Diagnoses, Targets, and Strengths

After a thorough mental health assessment using a semi-structured interview and incorporating information from multiple informants, the assessor was able to identify diagnoses, treatment targets, and strengths for Jennifer. Jennifer met *Diagnostic and Statistical Manual of Mental Disorders, Fourth Edition* (American Psychiatric Association, 1994) criteria for major depression and generalized anxiety disorder. The targets of treatment viewed as the highest priorities by the treatment team—emphasizing the opinions of Jennifer and her mother—included suicidal tendencies, depressed mood, self-injurious behavior, and school refusal and avoidance. Jennifer also possessed personal strengths. She was an intelligent adolescent who had earned high marks in school throughout her life. She was also artistic and showed pride in several of her arts and crafts. She also enjoyed walking along the beach and playing with her 2-year-old brother. Jennifer's mother was a loving person, and she worked hard for the family, holding two jobs and dedicating every resource she could afford to her three children.

Coordination of Care

Upon seeing the Blue Menu at Jennifer's school counselor's office, Jennifer's mother requested that CBT be used for Jennifer, as she noted that it fell in the *best support* category for depression. Jennifer's newly assigned therapist had detailed information about Jennifer from her mental health assessment, including knowledge of the specific problems associated with her depression and anxiety. Based on this information, she was eager to begin CBT, but reluctant to jump into a direct treatment for depression or anxiety such as Coping Cat (Kendall, 1992) or Primary and Secondary Control Enhancement Training (Weisz, Southam-Gerow, Gordis, & Connor-Smith, 2003) because she felt that a more individualized and flexible approach might better serve Jennifer. At the first team meeting, which included Jennifer, her mother, a representative from her school, her care coordinator, and a psychiatrist from the hospital, the therapist discussed the Blue Menu and practice elements within CBT, as well as ways to individualize treatment. This conversation helped to engage Jennifer and her mother in the treatment process and also facilitated the coordination of care for other providers. The psychiatrist used this opportunity to discuss psychopharmacological interventions for Jennifer, noting his recommendations' standings on the Blue Menu.

The therapist used team input from the meeting, along with information from the mental health assessment, to develop a mental health treatment plan consisting of strategies and goals for the psychosocial aspects of therapy. In addition, a coordinated service plan was created at the meeting to delineate responsibilities of care and ensure continuity across settings for Jennifer. Among other interventions, the coordinated service plan documented the psychiatrist's role in the monitoring of medication and the school's commitment to providing a one-to-one aide for Jennifer when she attended school.

Psychosocial Treatment Approach

Jennifer's therapist spent a great deal of time determining which practice elements would be most helpful for Jennifer. The therapist started with practice elements for depression, given the fact that depression is generally the most troubling factor for Jennifer. The decision of which particular elements to employ was informed not only by the percentage of evidence-based packages containing each element, but also by the specific goals and needs of the family. The most important target for Jennifer and her family was her suicidal tendencies. Other major areas of concern included Jennifer's depressed mood, self-injurious cutting behavior, and refusal to attend school due to anxiety.

The therapist was mindful of the concerns that she believed particular practice elements would best address and how certain practice elements might match Jennifer's needs and strengths. For instance, *psychoeducation*, included in 86% of all EBS for depression, was selected as a point of departure for treatment. The therapist felt that *psychoeducation* was a relevant practice element for all of Jennifer's targets, and it seemed particularly relevant given Jennifer's intelligence in that it provided her with the opportunity to learn about depression.

Problem solving was the next practice element employed by the therapist. Problem solving is cited in 71% of all EBS for depression, and it is believed to be clinically useful for treating suicidal tendencies, self-injurious behavior, and depressed mood. Jennifer's mother was particularly involved in the early sessions introducing problem solving. Her familiarity with the techniques and the proper times to apply them allowed her to provide Jennifer with important reminders when she struggled with problems at home.

After a week of introducing *problem solving* and assigning homework, *relaxation*, which is included in 50% of EBS for depression, was added. *Relaxation* is not the next most common practice element among EBS protocols for depression, however, Jennifer's therapist believed it to be a relevant fit for Jennifer's particular concerns and her anxiety. This skill was introduced alongside *problem solving* based on the opinion that Jennifer could handle both simultaneously. The decision to employ two strategies at once is generally discouraged in strict manual adherence, but it can be appropriate from the practice elements approach.

Several weeks into therapy, the therapist consulted with Jennifer's care coordinator to discuss her progress. An issue raised by the therapist at this meeting was Jennifer's mother's workload and the resulting fatigue she experienced at the end of a long workday. The care coordinator obtained approval to offer respite care one night per week for Jennifer's mother to provide her a helping hand with her smaller children. This service ultimately led to her having more energy and an increased ability to interact even more lovingly with all of her children.

In terms of Jennifer's progress, the care coordinator accessed Jennifer's clinical dashboard to obtain a variety of data points assessing progress over time. Using information from the therapist-submitted MTPS form, the care coordinator was also able to see what specific targets and strategies the therapist was using. Jennifer's dashboard suggested treatment gains across the board, with progress beginning to level out over the last several weeks of *problem solving* and *relaxation*. After the consultation with the care coordinator and consideration of Jennifer's progress, the therapist introduced *skill building*, a strategy that focuses on increasing talents and is included in 64% of EBS for depression. In this case, Jennifer's enjoyment of the beach and her arts and crafts were blended together, and she was encouraged to make shell necklaces and sand art. This strategy built Jennifer's sense of self-efficacy and provided valuable behavior activation.

Once Jennifer's depressed mood began to lift, the therapist gradually introduced practice elements related to anxiety to address truancy. Unfortunately, Jennifer responded so negatively to early exposure attempts—the first element employed to increase school attendance—that she ran away from home for a day. Because Jennifer's brief runaway was very distressful for everyone and her school attendance was not increasing, Jennifer's therapist consulted with the Clinical Services Office's lead psychologist to discuss Jennifer's current situation in treatment. After review and direct supervision, the CAMHD specialist suggested that Jennifer's exposure be more gradual. In addition, recognizing the consistent emotional support provided by Jennifer's mother, it was recommended that exposure be scheduled in such a way as to increase her mother's ability to participate. Easing Jennifer more slowly into school with more support from her mother was a successful strategy that led to regular school attendance within several months.

Ultimately Jennifer's treatment was successful. She remained in treatment, however, for more than 1 year, a duration that exceeds the finite number of sessions in some strict manual-designated approaches. Her progress, however, made it clear that this time frame was required for Jennifer's treatment. Contrary to manuals, extending the duration and dose of treatment are acceptable strategies within a practice elements framework. By the end of therapy, Jennifer successfully overcame all of her treatment targets and no longer met the criteria for depression or anxiety.

Although Jennifer improved consistently during the months she received services, her therapist and other CAMHD staff were certainly not the only members of the team involved in helping her work toward her goals. Her success was due in large part to her own perseverance, her mother's involvement and love, and their collective investment in her mental health.

CONCLUSION

Data regarding the functioning of youth over time suggest that the previously described system of care is effective in improving lives, as measured by the Child and Adolescent Functioning Scale, the ASEBA scales, and the CALOCUS. In addition, youth are getting better faster than in years past, spending less time in the system and doing so at a decreased cost (Daleiden, Chorpita, Donkervoet, Arensdorf, & Brogan, 2006). These improvements have escalated over the years, coinciding with many of the previously described strategies and innovations such as providing individualized care and incorporating EBPs.

REFERENCES

American Academy of Child and Adolescent Psychiatry Work Group on Systems of Care & American Association of Community Psychiatrists. (1999). *Child and Adolescent Level of Care Utilization System (CALOCUS) user's manual, Version 1.1.* Washington, DC: Authors.

American Psychiatric Association. (1994). *Diagnostic and statistical manual of mental disorders* (4th ed.). Washington, DC: Author.

Chambless, D.L., & Hollon, S.D. (1998). Defining empirically supported therapies. *Journal of Consulting and Clinical Psychology, 66,* 7–18.

Child and Adolescent Mental Health Division. (2003). *Evidence-based Services Committee: Codes for intervention strategies.* Honolulu: Hawaii Department of Health.

Child and Adolescent Mental Health Division. (2007). *Evidence-based Services Committee: biennial report.* Honolulu: Hawaii Department of Health.

Chorpita, B.F., Daleiden, E., & Weisz, J.R. (2005a). Identifying and selecting the common elements of evidence-based interventions: A distillation and matching model. *Mental Health Services Research, 7,* 5–20.

Chorpita, B.F., Daleiden, E., & Weisz, J.R. (2005b). Modularity in the design and application of therapeutic interventions. *Applied and Preventive Psychology, 11,* 141–156.

Chorpita, B.F., & Donkervoet, C.M. (2005). Implementation of the Felix Consent Decree in Hawaii: The impact of policy and practice development efforts on service delivery. In R.G. Steele & M.C. Roberts (Eds.), *Handbook of mental health services for children, adolescents, and families* (pp. 317–332). New York: Kluwer.

Chorpita, B.F., Yim, L.M., Donkervoet, J.C., et al. (2002). Toward large-scale implementation of empirically supported treatments for children: A review and observations by the Hawaii Empirical Basis to Services Task Force. *Clinical Psychology: Science and Practice, 9*, 165–190.

Daleiden, D.L., & Chorpita, B.F. (2005). From data to wisdom: Quality improvement strategies supporting large-scale implementation of evidence-based services. *Child and Adolescent Psychiatric Clinics of North America, 14*, 329–349.

Daleiden, E., Chorpita, B.F., Donkervoet, C., Arensdorf, A.M., & Brogan, M. (2006). Getting better at getting them better: Health outcomes and evidence-based practice within a system of care. *Journal of the American Academy of Child and Adolescent Psychiatry, 45*(6), 749–756.

Daleiden, E., Lee, J., & Tolman, R. (2004). *Annual evaluation report: Fiscal year 2004*. Honolulu: Hawaii Department of Health, Child and Adolescent Mental Health Division.

Francis, S.E., & Chorpita, B.F. (2003, November). *An examination of clinical decision making strategies: Preliminary findings*. Paper presented at the annual meeting of the Child and Adolescent Anxiety Special Interest Group, Association for Advancement of Behavior Therapy, Boston.

Hawaii Department of Health. (2002). *Hawaii Health Survey 2001*. Honolulu: Hawaii Department of Health, Office of Health Status Monitoring.

Hawaii Department of Health. (2003). *Coding form for intervention strategies*. Available online at http://www.hawaii.gov/health/mental-health/camhd/library/pdf/ebs/ebs004.pdf

Hawaii Department of Health, Evidence Based Services Committee. (2004). *2004 biennial report*. Available online at http://www.hawaii.gov/health/mental-health/camhd/library/pdf/ebs/ebs011.pdf

Hawaii Department of Health. (2005). *Service provider monthly treatment and progress summary*. Available online at http://hawaii.gov/health/mental-health/camhd/library/pdf/paf/paf-002.pdf

Hawaii Department of Health. (2007). *Blue Menu—Evidence based child and adolescent psychosocial interventions*. Available online at http://www.hawaii.gov/health/mental-health/camhd/library/pdf/ebs/ebs022.pdf

Hodges, K., Wong, M.M., & Latessa, M. (1998). Use of the Child and Adolescent Functional Assessment Scale (CAFAS) as an outcome measure in clinical settings. *Journal of Behavioral Health Services and Research, 25*(3), 325–336.

Individuals with Disabilities Education Act (IDEA) of 1990, PL 101-476, 20 U.S.C. §§ 1400 *et seq.*

Kendall, P.C. (1992). *Coping Cat workbook*. Ardmore, PA: Workbook Publishing.

Nakamura, B., Daleiden, E., & Mueller, C. (2007). Validity of treatment target progress ratings as indicators of youth improvement. *Journal of Child and Family Studies, 16*(5), 729–741.

Schiffman, J., Becker, K., & Daleiden, E. (2006). Evidence-based services in a statewide mental health system: Do the treatments fit the problem? *Journal of Clinical Child and Adolescent Psychology, 35*(1), 13–19.

Stroul, B.A., & Friedman, R.M. (1986). *A system of care for children and youth with severe emotional disturbances* (Rev. ed.). Washington, DC: Georgetown University Child Development Center, CASSP Technical Assistance Center.

Weisz, J.R., Southam-Gerow, M.A., Gordis, E.B., & Connor-Smith, J. (2003). Primary and secondary control enhancement training for youth depression: Applying the deployment-focused model of treatment development and testing. In A.E. Kazdin & J.R. Weisz (Eds.), *Evidence-based psychotherapies for children and adolescents* (pp. 165–186). New York: Guildford Press.

Young, J., Daleiden, E.L., Chorpita, B.F., Schiffman, J., & Mueller, C. W. (in press). Assessing stability between treatment planning documents in a system of care. *Administration and Policy in Mental Health and Mental Health Services Research*.

17

Services for
High-Risk Populations
in Systems of Care

BRUCE KAMRADT, STEPHEN A. GILBERTSON, AND MARGARET JEFFERSON

W raparound Milwaukee is a system of care for children with serious emotional and mental health needs and their families serving Milwaukee County, Wisconsin. Since its inception, Wraparound Milwaukee has focused on serving youth from the juvenile justice, child welfare, and mental health systems who are at the highest risk for placement in residential treatment centers, state correctional facilities, or long-term psychiatric hospitals. The population served by the system of care includes juveniles adjudicated as sex offenders and fire setters, as well as youth who have committed serious batteries, assaults, and other offenses.

The widespread misconception about these youth and their families is that they cannot be effectively served in their homes and communities. The experience of Wraparound Milwaukee, however, demonstrates that high-risk youth and their families can, in fact, be served safely and effectively in community-based systems of care using individualized care approaches that address their specific needs. This individualized approach to services for youth with the most serious and complex mental health, emotional, and behavioral issues drew the attention of the President's New Freedom Commission on Mental Health (2003), which cited Wraparound Milwaukee as an exemplary program in its report. This chapter describes how Wraparound Milwaukee has evolved into a system of care that effectively works with high-risk youth and their families, the organization and financing of the system of care, the key service components necessary for working with high-risk youth, and the system of care enhancements needed for working with subgroups of high-risk youth, in particular, youth affected by juvenile sexual violence and their families.

DESCRIPTION AND
BACKGROUND OF WRAPAROUND MILWAUKEE

Wraparound Milwaukee is a unique system of care operated as a type of managed care system. The system of care pools funding from Medicaid, as well as mental health, child welfare, and juvenile justice. It utilizes a single care coordinator coupled with the support of family advocates to offer comprehensive, coordinated, and family-focused care to children with serious emotional disorders and their families. From a pilot program serving 10 children initiated in 1995, it has grown to a $37 million system that annually serves more than 1,000 children and their families.

History of Wraparound Milwaukee

The impetus in Milwaukee for serving a target group of high-risk youth, and for the Wraparound Milwaukee program, was the overutilization of institutional settings for treatment and the poor outcomes achieved for youth served in those settings. In the early and mid-1990s, the child welfare and juvenile justice systems operated by the Milwaukee County Human Services Department were placing an increasing number of youth in residential treatment and correctional settings. In 1995, the average number of youth placed in residential treatment centers reached 375 youth per day, with the resulting costs of such placements increasing steadily to more than $18.5 million at that time. The increased placement costs were funded with county tax levy funds because federal reimbursement was insufficient to keep up with placement costs. State juvenile correctional placements from Milwaukee County also grew steadily to more than 375 youth, and the increased placements were outstripping available state funding, resulting in an added county tax levy contribution for every delinquent youth committed to these locked state facilities.

In addition, the Wisconsin State Medicaid program was concerned about increasing Medicaid costs for these youth, many of whom had spent considerable time in inpatient psychiatric hospitals prior to going to residential treatment centers or correctional facilities. Often, these facilities subsequently found the children to have emotional disturbances too severe for their settings, and many were transferred back to inpatient psychiatric hospitals. Frequent hospitalizations and longer lengths of stay were driving up Medicaid costs.

For families with children with a serious emotional disturbance, the excessive use of institutional placements in this community was very frustrating and discouraging. When children with serious mental health needs got into trouble at home, at school, or in the community, they were labeled "bad" children, and the parents often were blamed for their children's mental health problems. Parents were frequently told that the only alternative for their children was residential treatment or correctional placement. In many instances, parents were not given any choice because the child welfare or juvenile justice systems had obtained a court order for the institutional placement. Typically, placements were ordered for at least 1 year and, in many cases, for multiple years. In fact, the first youth enrolled in Wraparound Milwaukee had been in a residential treatment center for 10 consecutive years. As a result of these institutional placements—many of which occurred in facilities far removed from Milwaukee—parents were separated from their children and had little opportunity to see them on a regular basis. Families were not regularly included in treatment decisions, leaving them with little hope, no sense of empowerment, and little choice or voice in determining what was best for their children.

In 1994, the Planning Council of Milwaukee, an independent evaluation and research firm, conducted a study for the Milwaukee County Human Service Department and found that the outcomes for youth served in residential treatment centers were very poor. The council noted high AWOL and recidivism rates, even for children deemed to be successful discharges (Planning Council of Milwaukee, 1994). Milwaukee's experience with residential care was consistent with findings from national studies and reports. As noted by the U.S. Surgeon General, there were few, if any, studies that demonstrated the long-term effectiveness of inpatient psychiatric care or residential treatment for children with serious emotional and mental health needs (U.S. Department of Health and Human Services, 1999).

Also in 1994, the Milwaukee County Mental Health Division's Children's Program collaborated with the Wisconsin Bureau of Children's Mental Health to apply for a grant under the Comprehensive Community Mental Health Services for Children and Their Families Program implemented by the Center for Mental Health Services of the Substance Abuse and Mental Health Services Administration. Funding from the grant, which was awarded to Milwaukee County in the fall of 1994, was used to create a system of care in Milwaukee to target these high-risk youth and their families.

The system of care was called Wraparound Milwaukee, and it incorporated components that included a wraparound philosophy of care, care coordination, mobile crisis services, a provider network of community services, and a strong family advocacy program. It was tested with child welfare and juvenile justice system partners in 1995 and 1996 through a pilot project called the 25 Kid Project. This pilot was designed to determine if youth who committed serious delinquent acts and youth in the child welfare system with the most complex mental health needs who were placed in residential treatment centers could be successfully returned to their communities. The 25 Kid Project targeted 25 youth selected by the child welfare agency or county juvenile justice program who had resided in residential treatment centers for 6 months or longer with no immediate discharge plan. No youth were to be rejected or ejected from the pilot. The goals were as follows:

- Returning the youth to their communities and homes
- Keeping the youth and communities safe by minimizing recidivism of delinquent behaviors
- Keeping the cost of the community placement equal to or less than the cost of the residential treatment placement

With the support of the juvenile court judges, and despite the initial skepticism of some other system partners, 17 of the 25 youth referred to the pilot were returned to their communities, and in most cases, home to their families within 90–120 days. Eventually, over a 10-month period, 24 of the 25 youth were successfully placed back in the Milwaukee community. Recidivism was kept low, and the program costs for the pilot were approximately 60% of the costs of the institutional placements (Kamradt, 1999).

As a result of the success of the 25 Kid Project, Wraparound Milwaukee was in the position to submit an innovative proposal to the Bureau of Milwaukee

Child Welfare and Milwaukee County Delinquency and Court Services to provide services to youth in or at high risk for institutional placement. The proposal and plan also involved Medicaid to address concerns about uncontrolled and unmanaged inpatient psychiatric care for many of these children.

Characteristics of Youth Served

From the inception of the 25 Kid Project, Wraparound Milwaukee has focused on children with the most serious and complex emotional needs. Of the youth served by the system of care, 63% are adjudicated delinquent, and 30% are abused, neglected, or have special needs and are referred by the child welfare system. The average age of youth served is 13.9 years, with 74% of the youth being male. Wraparound Milwaukee's population includes 68% African American families, 23% Caucasian families, 7% Hispanic families, and 2% Native American families. Fifty percent of the families served have incomes at or below the federal poverty level. Based on agreements with the child welfare and juvenile justice systems, all youth referred to Wraparound Milwaukee must be determined to be at immediate risk of residential treatment, correctional placement, or long-term hospitalization.

Based on diagnoses from the *Diagnostic and Statistical Manual of Mental Disorders, Fourth Edition* (American Psychiatric Association, 1994) nearly two thirds (63%) of the youth served by Wraparound Milwaukee have a primary diagnosis of conduct disorder or oppositional defiant disorder. In addition, approximately 40% of these youth are diagnosed with depression, 41% with attention-deficit/hyperactivity disorder, 40% with alcohol and drug abuse issues, and 25% with learning disorders. From a list of presenting issues at intake, 83% of the youth served are characterized as having serious school and community behavioral issues, 60% display severe aggressiveness, 50% have chronic runaway behavior, 45% have substance abuse issues, 35% have histories of psychiatric hospitalization, and 27% have been suicidal or had significant suicidal ideation (Seybold, 2006).

The youth coming into Wraparound Milwaukee all have a history of juvenile court involvement, and in fact, all are court ordered into the Wraparound Milwaukee program. Under Wisconsin statutes, placement in a residential treatment center or correctional facility can only be made under a juvenile court order. The youth enrolled in Wraparound Milwaukee come with a flexible court order that allows the system of care to make any out-of-home placement deemed necessary without further court review and to identify alternatives for the child in the community and with his or her family.

Organization and Funding of the System of Care

Following the success of the 25 Kid Project, Wraparound Milwaukee devised a financing strategy and organizational design to provide care to the 350 youth remaining in residential treatment and to any newly identified youth at risk for residential placement. Both the child welfare department and the county's delinquency and court services program were essential partners based on their roles in placing and funding services for high-risk children. A partnership with Medicaid was also critical to address the mental health and substance abuse treatment needs of this population. A flexible and sustainable funding model was crucial to meet the complex needs of this high-risk population of children with serious emotional disorders and their families. The answer was to create a unique, publicly operated managed care entity under a 1915(a) Medicaid waiver that could blend funding across child welfare and juvenile justice systems with Medicaid; create a unique type of benefit plan with a broad, flexible array of services; and accept risk for the cost of care it provided.

Figure 17.1 shows how the various funds are brought together using a combination of case rates, capitation, fee-for-service, and fixed funding strategies.

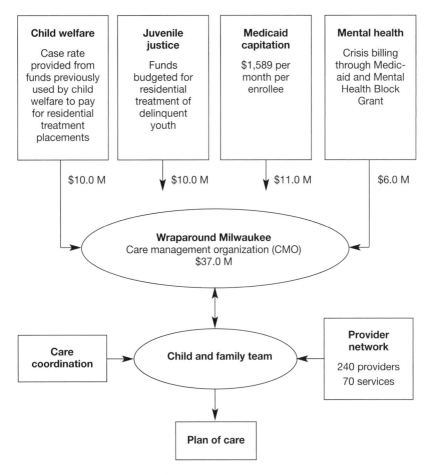

Figure 17.1. Wraparound Milwaukee pooled funds.

Wraparound Milwaukee negotiated with its system partners to develop mutually beneficial financing agreements. For youth in the child welfare system and their families, a case rate was negotiated that was substantially less than what the child welfare system paid on a monthly basis for a child's placement in a residential treatment center. Today, the case rate paid by the child welfare system is about $3,900 per month per child, significantly lower than the average cost of a residential treatment placement, which is currently $7,600 per month. For the average of 220–225 youth served, the cost to the child welfare system is approximately $10.0 million per year for Wraparound Milwaukee to provide all necessary community and institutional services. Wraparound Milwaukee assists the child welfare system to make claims under Title IV-E through a fiscal intermediary (i.e., a company contracted by the state for federal Title IV-E claiming) for eligible children. The federal funds collected by the state-contracted fiscal intermediary are returned to the state and incorporated into Wraparound Milwaukee's case rate.

For Delinquency and Court Services, two types of funding arrangements were created. For delinquent youth with serious emotional disorders who would otherwise be placed in a residential treatment center paid by that agency, Wraparound Milwaukee receives a fixed annual budget of $8.2 million and provides all necessary services to these youth; approximately 400 youth per month are served through this arrangement. For youth who would otherwise have been committed to the Wisconsin Department of Corrections for placement in a locked juvenile correctional facility, Wraparound Milwaukee receives a case rate of $3,500 per month, which is significantly less than the $6,800 average monthly cost charged to Milwaukee County when a youth is sent to the state correctional system. This case rate is paid for approximately 50 youth per month, with a total of $1.8 million in funding given to Wraparound Milwaukee.

Through written agreements with the child welfare and juvenile justice agencies, Wraparound Milwaukee agrees to provide and pay for any and all services needed by youth, including residential treatment, group home services, treatment foster care, and regular foster care, if needed, as well as all treatment and support services in the community. Youth are specifically court ordered into Wraparound Milwaukee by children's court judges. Wraparound Milwaukee receives a flexible order, allowing the system of care to determine the level and type of services required for each youth, including any type of out-of-home placement, unless a judge requires a specific initial out-of-home placement.

Wraparound Milwaukee's management team also approached the state Medicaid agency to consider the possibility of carving out the behavioral health treatment costs of these high-risk, high-cost youth. The Medicaid agency performed an actuarial analysis of claims data for the youth from the child welfare and juvenile justice systems that Wraparound Milwaukee proposed to serve and found that, based on Medicaid claims, they were the most costly youth. The youth in this group averaged approximately 2.5 inpatient episodes per year, and they received many other Medicaid-funded mental health and substance abuse services as well. After a 6-month negotiation, Medicaid contracted with Milwaukee County, designating Wraparound Milwaukee as a special managed care entity and carving out this population with an established maximum of 630 enrollees. The agreement established a monthly capitation payment to Wraparound Milwaukee for every child eligible for Medicaid coverage, which was 95% of the actuarially determined monthly cost for these youth. In 1995, the state Medicaid agency received approval for a 1915(a) waiver from Centers for Medicare & Medicaid Services (CMS) to create this blended funding model. Wraparound Milwaukee agreed to provide any and all mental health and substance abuse services deemed medically necessary ("Contract for Services Between the Wisconsin Department of Health and Family Services and Milwaukee County," 2007). In 2007, the capitation rate was $1,589.00 per month, and in 2006, the Medicaid capitation payments received by Wraparound Milwaukee totaled approximately $11 million.

In 2000, Wraparound Milwaukee was also designated by Medicaid to provide all crisis intervention services for Milwaukee County youth, including all youth and their families enrolled in the carve out. From billing on a fee-for-service basis for such things as mobile crisis teams, crisis foster and group homes, crisis one-on-one in-home stabilizers, and other eligible services, Wraparound Milwaukee has been able to capture another $6.0 million in revenue to add to its pool of blended funds. Health management organizations and private insurance carriers are billed for covered services, although the insurance plans typically offer limited coverage. In addition, federal mental health block grant funds—approximately $150,000—are provided to Wraparound Milwaukee by the state. The total available pooled funding for 2007 is $37 million.

All of the pooled funds are managed by Wraparound Milwaukee, which serves as the administrative service organization. Funds are available to the family through a child and family team process facilitated by a care coordinator, who helps the family determine needed services and supports for their child. The determination of services by the child and family team constitutes meeting medical necessity under the Medicaid contract for purposes of service authorization. Costs related to the provision of any and all mental health, substance abuse, social, and support services are billed by vendors to Wraparound Milwaukee, which then makes payment to vendors once each claim is adjudicated based on units of service authorized by the care coordinator. Wraparound Milwaukee's fiscal office utilizes managed care strategies and a sophisticated Internet-based information system called *Synthesis* to track enrollment; authorize services to vendors; adjudicate, process, and pay claims; develop care plans; enter progress notes; perform utilization review; write reports; and monitor costs.

COMPONENTS OF CARE FOR YOUTH AT HIGH RISK AND THEIR FAMILIES

Values that Underlie Work with Youth at High Risk and Their Families

Regardless of whether youth enter the Wraparound Milwaukee system of care through the child welfare or juvenile justice systems, a set of fundamental core values underlie all of the work with youth and their families. These values recognize that:

1. All youth and families have strengths that can be identified and incorporated into the strategies to meet the emotional, behavioral, and mental health needs of each child and his or her family.

2. All youth should have one care plan across child-serving systems, and that plan should be coordinated by a single care manager.

3. Children can be best cared for and usually attain the best treatment outcomes when they are cared for in community settings rather than institutions, especially when they are with their families.

4. Families usually know what is best for their children and should always be involved in making decisions about what their children and family members need. Access, voice, and ownership of the planning process are critical.

5. Care must be unconditional. Children do not fail. Plans fail, and they must be modified when they are not getting the desired results set by the child and family team.

Child and Family Teams

At the core of the Wraparound Milwaukee system of care are child and family teams. These teams consist of those individuals identified by the family that are most significant in supporting them and their children. Such teams typically include the parent(s), care coordinator, youth (if he or she wants to be part of the team), close friends and relatives, the child welfare or probation worker, an individual or family therapist, a teacher or school counselor, and a crisis one-to-one aide or mentor. The team is the planning vehicle, coordinating planning across multiple child-serving systems regardless of where the child resides. The child and family team process is used to identify needs, match them with individual and family strengths, and design strategies to meet the goals set by the youth and his or her family for themselves. Wraparound Milwaukee's child and family teams are family friendly and listen to what youth and parents say about their needs, strengths, and preferences. The child and family teams develop and implement the individualized plan of care, monitor progress, and modify services and supports as necessary. As noted, a unique part of the Wraparound Milwaukee child and family team process is that, under the program's contract with the State Medicaid Agency, all services determined necessary by the team are considered to be medically necessary by Medicaid and do not require a specific physician's order for the service to be covered.

All child and family teams follow a process of individualized, needs-driven planning and service delivery based on the values and principles of the wraparound approach. A series of steps are followed to formulate a care plan:

1. Identifying the individual strengths of the child and family to determine a *Strength-Based Inventory*

2. Developing the crisis/safety plan to anticipate emergencies

3. Developing the *family plan*, which involves having family members talk about their vision for themselves and their child, and the *family narrative* (the family's story), which reflects what has led the family to seek help

4. Identifying needs as steps in the process of reaching the family vision, including identifying needs in the life domains of safety/crisis, family, mental health, medical, educational/vocational, cultural/spiritual, living situation, and social/recreational

5. Creating a needs statement describing what the family needs help with, identifying strengths that can be used to assist the family to meet their needs, and incorporating family supports, natural supports, and community supports

6. Identifying strategies that will be used to achieve the needs, which include formal paid services (e.g., therapists, mentors, in-home aides), as well as informal supports

Care plans typically address no more than three to five active needs at any time. All child and family team members must sign off on the care plan to demonstrate their commitment to it.

Care Coordination

Critical to an effective service delivery system working with youth with serious mental health needs, particularly those youth at high risk for institutional care, are the care coordinators. Care coordinators facilitate the child and family teams that develop, implement, and monitor the care plans for the youth and their families. Care coordinators help families identify their strengths, assemble the participants on the child and family team, facilitate team meetings, identify child and family needs with families across life domains (i.e., mental health, living situation, educational, recreational, safety, medical, spiritual, vocational), develop strategies toward meeting those needs, identify and obtain formal and informal services to be incorporated into the strategies, and monitor and evaluate plans. The care coordinator also ensures the adherence to the wraparound philosophy and approach.

Wraparound Milwaukee's care coordinators are unique in that they serve as the care managers across all the child-serving systems. Staff from other system partners (e.g., child welfare workers, probation workers) join child and family teams, but the Wraparound Milwaukee care coordinator organizes the planning process, and one inclusive service plan is developed for each family. Thus, Wraparound Milwaukee implements "one plan for one family." Because the funding is pooled across systems, the care coordinator also has greater access to funds and greater flexibility in how the funds are used to obtain services for families than in more traditional service systems.

Because the youth served by Wraparound Milwaukee require high levels of daily management and support, the caseloads of care coordinators are kept small—one care coordinator per nine families. The role of care coordinators in Wraparound Milwaukee includes other unique features that that are critical to the success of this approach:

1. The care coordinator obtains a single release of information for the exchange of information across systems.

2. The care coordinator is included in the court process, preparing court letters and testifying in front of the judge.

3. The judicial order made is flexible, allowing the care coordinator to add and eliminate services and even move the child to different placements (e.g., from a residential treatment center to a group home or foster home) without having to go back to court to get the order revised.

4. Because medical necessity is determined by the child and family team, the care coordinator does not need further authorization to put services in place.

5. For disagreements with other system partners, there is a written conflict resolution protocol used across the child-serving systems, including probation and child welfare.

Provider Network Services

A key to Wraparound Milwaukee's ability to work effectively with high-risk children and their families has been its ability to individualize services based on need. The best way to achieve this has been to develop and offer a broad array of services and supports through a network of community providers who are paid on a fee-for-service basis. Wraparound Milwaukee has moved away from silo funding or a categorical approach to developing and funding services. Using a large network of providers offering multiple services, families are able to choose services and providers that best fit their needs. As needs change, funding follows the needs, and new services are developed to meet those changing needs.

Wraparound Milwaukee establishes uniform rates for all services; credentials and trains providers on working within a family-driven, strengths-based, wraparound model; and monitors and evaluates provider performance. With more than 230 agency providers, 850 individual providers, and approximately 70 different services, high-risk children receive the services determined through the child and family team process. The provider network model has increased diversity in the types and ethnicity of providers, and competition has led to the greater availability, dependability, and quality of service providers. The services provided through the provider network are shown on Table 17.1.

Table 17.1.   Services available through Wraparound Milwaukee

Care coordination	Transportation
Individual and family therapy	After school care and activities
Substance abuse counseling	Job coaches
Group therapy	Independent living
Crisis one-to-one stabilization	Housing
Mentors	Child care
Tutors	Household management
Intensive in-home therapy	Specialized educational services
Psychiatric inpatient treatment	Behavioral aides
Residential treatment	Supervised apartments
Group home	Intensive in-home monitoring for court
Foster care	Discretionary funds
Therapeutic foster care	Parent aides
Professional foster care	Interpretation
Medical day treatment	Kinship care
Crisis/respite group home	Rent/food assistance
Specialized sexual offender services	Employment training/placement
FOCUS: Alternatives to correctional care	Transitional care
Medication management	

Crisis Safety Planning and Mobile Crisis Services

The ability to anticipate, plan for, and ameliorate crises is critical when working with youth at high risk and their families. Thus, crisis safety planning is incorporated into the services provided by Wraparound Milwaukee. To accomplish this, a plan that identifies the needs, strengths, and resources of each child; describes past situations that have caused crises for the child; discerns strategies and techniques that have been effective in the past; and identifies people who may be contacted to support the child in a crisis is developed with the family. The specific questions addressed on the crisis plan are shown on Figure 17.2.

In addition, Wraparound Milwaukee developed a Mobile Urgent Treatment Team (MUTT) to support families, care coordinators, and youth. The 24-hour crisis teams include psychologists, social workers, and a nurse, all of whom are trained in assessing, interviewing, supporting, and treating youth in crisis and their families. Families who were previously reluctant to call for help have learned to trust MUTT to help de-escalate their children's presenting behaviors in the home, school, or other community settings. Typically, a child in crisis can be treated in the community. MUTT can make one-to-one crisis mentors available for the family to monitor and support the youth. If children must be temporarily removed from their homes, the crisis teams have crisis/respite homes, group homes, and foster homes available for short-term crisis stabilization. For children needing more intensive supervision, Wraparound Milwaukee purchases crisis beds from several residential treatment centers. Placements are kept to less than 14 days;

Crisis Plan

Effective date: _____

If a crisis happens, these are the steps we need to take:

- How do we define a crisis?

  Our definition of a crisis is... _____

- What strengths can we use to help us meet this crisis?

  Interests and strengths we can tap into are... _____

- Are there special risks we should be aware of?

  Risk factors should speak specifically to risk and safety concerns that the team and court may be concerned about or triggers that lead to a crisis.

  _____

- Which family and community supports can we contact?

  List the names and contact information of people and agencies in the community that the family can use when in a crisis.

  _____

- How can we help the caregiver?

  Speak to what techniques help the caregiver for the child.

  _____

- What specific steps should we use?

  _____

Figure 17.2.   Crisis plan questions.

most crisis placements are only for 24–48 hours. The availability of crisis teams has allowed Wraparound Milwaukee to drastically reduce its use of inpatient psychiatric care. Fewer than 150 inpatient psychiatric days were utilized in both 2005 and 2006 (Wraparound Milwaukee, 2006).

Family Advocacy Services

Since its inception, Wraparound Milwaukee has recognized the vital role played by families in the lives of their children. It became apparent that families of children with serious emotional disorders could benefit from support and assistance from other families who have had similar experiences and challenges. In addition, families needed advocacy help as they interacted with other child-serving systems that did not necessarily embrace wraparound values. Many of these systems blame families for their children's issues rather than seeing their strengths, and many do not effectively engage the families in the process of serving their children. Often, families relate best to other families who have had similar experiences. They are more willing to trust the advice of their peers and seek their help when necessary.

Given these observations, Families United of Milwaukee was created in 1996 as a family advocacy and support organization for families enrolled in Wrap-around Milwaukee. Families United operates from the premise that families must be empowered to best address their needs and advocate for their children. The goal of Families United is to become connected to families receiving care in an effort to assist them in obtaining needed services, as well as to provide support and advocacy that will help to preserve family units by keeping youth from being placed outside the home or by facilitating their return to their families as soon as possible. The services provided by Families United include:

- Educational advocacy to ensure that youth have an appropriate school placement and an individualized education program because success in school is critical to being successful in the community

- Skill-building training for leadership development to teach parents how to work in conjunction with professionals and system of care partners

- Crisis support for families facing financial emergencies, homelessness, domestic violence, loss of employment, or mental health crises

- Providing information and connecting families to community resources (e.g., child care, clothing, housing, health care, transportation)

- Holding family events (e.g., cookouts, holiday parties, breakfasts), so peer families can get together and have fun

Families United of Milwaukee strives to help parents develop their power, voice, and strength to enable them to make choices that will help their children and themselves to live productively and safely in their communities.

SERVING YOUTH AT HIGH RISK IN WRAPAROUND MILWAUKEE

Although all youth enrolled in Wraparound Milwaukee are considered to have complex emotional and behavioral concerns and are at risk for out-of-home care, a significant subgroup of enrolled youth has been specifically designated high risk. The purpose of the high risk designation is to bring a specialized focus to those youth whose behavioral histories have put either themselves or others at risk. The goal is to improve access to empirically derived and recommended practice strategies for assessment, treatment, and community-based risk management of youth and families with specialized risks and needs.

Youth behaviors and ecological factors considered to contribute to risk are carefully reviewed during the pre-enrollment screening process. Youth for whom highly specialized interventions are required are placed on the high risk list. Specialized clinical review is provided to assist the court and the eventual child and family team in determining needs and developing strategies for minimizing and managing risk.

This high-risk designation is often applied to youth with histories of sexual misconduct (adjudicated or nonadjudicated), fire setting, homicide or aggravated assault, self-injurious or suicidal behaviors, and psychiatric hospitalization, as well as youth who have been victims of sexual assault.

System of Care Enhancements for Youth and Families Affected by Juvenile Sexual Violence

An example of how a system of care can be enhanced to effectively serve youth designated as particularly high risk is provided by Wraparound Milwaukee's services for youth and families affected by juvenile sexual violence. Milwaukee County Children's Court adjudicates approximately 125 youth per year for sexual assault. The average age of these youth who are adjudicated is 13.6; more than half of the victims of juvenile-perpetrated sexual assault are younger relatives of a youth who has been adjudicated.

Prior to the implementation of Wraparound Milwaukee, there were limited community-based resources for risk assessment, treatment, and supervision of youth adjudicated of sexual offenses. There were no providers of empirically derived sexual offense-specific risk assessment in the Milwaukee area. There were no probation intake workers trained in managing the complexity and risk of sexual assault, which often is intrafamilial. The District Attorney's Office at Children's Court had only two prosecuting attorneys with specialized training in sensitive crimes, and there were no specialized probation staff to provide community-based supervision of juveniles adjudicated of sexual offenses. There were no providers of treatment foster care, group homes, or crisis intervention supervision and observation with specialization or training in working with youth with sexual behavior problems. Only one nonprofit agency in the Milwaukee area provided outpatient group therapy and brief individual therapy to these youth under contract with the juvenile probation department.

The lack of community-based treatment options, coupled with uncertainty about the safety and effectiveness of community management of sexual offenders, led the courts to rely heavily on residential treatment centers or correctional placements for treatment and containment of this population. Three residential treatment centers in the state offered specialized treatment to sex offenders, but two of the three were geographically distant from metropolitan Milwaukee. The state Department of Juvenile Corrections offered specialized treatment within two locked facilities outside of the Milwaukee metropolitan area. Few, if any, services were provided to the parents, families, or victims of youth adjudicated of sexual offenses by these residential treatment centers or correctional facilities.

Following a review of the professional literature and technical assistance provided by the Center for Sex Offender Management (CSOM), Wraparound Milwaukee proposed a system of care approach to serving juvenile sex offenders (see http://www.csom.org). This approach was based on the premise that by strengthening the array of specialized community-based risk assessment, treatment programming, and service coordination, Milwaukee County could reduce the number of juvenile sex offenders unnecessarily placed in residential care or within correctional placements, shorten residential lengths of stay for those who did require placement, and improve the postresidential transitioning of youth back into the community.

In 1998, Wraparound Milwaukee began to implement enhancements to its system of care to serve juvenile sex offenders. Technical assistance and financial support were obtained in 1999 through a federal grant from the U.S. Department of Justice, Corrections Program Office. A policy team was formed to guide and facilitate collaborative program development, including representatives from local legal, mental health, and social service systems involved in juvenile sex offender management.

Key research findings and recommendations from various national task forces guided the development and implementation of enhanced community-based services for youth and families affected by juvenile-perpetrated sexual assault in Milwaukee County (Hunter, 2002; National Task Force on Juvenile Sexual Offending, 1993; Righthand & Welch, 2001):

- Juvenile sexual offenders are a heterogeneous group, reflecting various types and levels of psychosexual and psychiatric disturbance and risk of reoffending (Hunter, Figueredo, Malamuth, & Becker, 2003).

- Ongoing collection of local data is needed to allow for examination of specific behavioral subtypes of juvenile-perpetrated sexual violence.

- There is a need for ongoing examination of local juvenile sexual assault recidivism data in relation to subtypes of offending, other behavioral and family history, mental health, and legal intervention (Driessen, 2002).

- Critical to the viability of community-based programming is early determination of which youth can be most effectively and safely treated in a community environment (Hunter, Gilbertson, Vedros, & Morton, 2004). Recommended practice and empirically derived offense-specific risk assessment should be available to assist decision making (Prentky, Harris, Frizzell, & Righthand, 2000; Righthand & Welch, 2001).

- There is a need for viable, credible, and comprehensive community-based alternatives to institutional care for those youth who are appropriate for community approaches to treatment (Dishion, McCord, & Poulin, 1999; Hunter, Gilbertson, Vedros, & Morton, 2004).

- There is a need to broaden the therapeutic focus, taking into consideration victim and family needs and the developmental status of juvenile offenders (Chaffin & Bonner, 1996; Gilbertson, Storm, & Fischer, 2001).

- Social-ecological models offer promise of improved clinical and costs outcomes for youth with delinquent and aggressive tendencies (Borduin & Schaeffer, 2001; Henggeler, Schoenwald, & Pickrel, 1995; Malysiak, 1997; Miller & Prinz, 1990; Zigler, Taussig, & Black, 1992). Social-ecological models are defined by their emphasis on understanding delinquent behavior as a product of multiple and oftentimes interactive individual, familial, social, and cultural determinants (Bronfenbrenner, 1979).

The enhancements to Wraparound Milwaukee's system of care for youth and families affected by juvenile sexual violence included:

- Implementation of comprehensive data collection and program evaluation processes regarding all youth referred for a sexual offense (Hunter et al., 2004)

- Utilization of empirically derived predispositional, sexual offense-specific risk and needs assessment of youth and their families (Gilbertson, Storm, & Fischer, 2001; Hunter, 2002)

- Training of specialized (sensitive crimes) probation intake workers, ongoing probation officers, public defenders, judges, and district attorneys (Hunter, 2002)

- Predisposition offering of voluntary sexual offense–specific clinical intervention with families affected by juvenile-perpetrated incest (Hunter et al., 2004)

- Cross-system training and ongoing consultation to care coordinators, probation officers, judges, clinicians, and parents regarding recommended practices in juvenile sex offender assessment, treatment, and risk management

- Ongoing evaluation and policy team review of legal and mental health responses and outcomes

- Enhancement of community-based services to families affected by juvenile-perpetrated sexual abuse, including the development of specialized home and community-based crisis, safety, and treatment services; treatment foster care; more culturally diverse outpatient providers; and group homes willing and able to provide services to adjudicated juvenile sex offenders

- Development of community-based resources to support parents, including crisis one-to-one and supervision/observation workers available through the Wraparound Milwaukee provider network to supply supervision and structure for youth, parent assistants, and multifamily education and support groups specialized to address the complexities of intrafamily abuse

Integral to the system of care enhancements has been the development of a cadre of clinicians with the skills needed to work with youth with sexual behavior problems, victims, and their families. Wraparound Milwaukee provided the leadership in this effort, along with the support of a cross-system policy team, including children's court judges, prosecuting and defense attorneys, youth probation, the Milwaukee Bureau of Child Welfare, victim advocates, and the Milwaukee Police Department. Training events were provided to highlight recommended practices in the assessment and treatment of youth and families affected by juvenile sexual violence. More than 350 clinicians and other youth-serving personnel attended these training events, which were held over the 2-year period from 1999 to

2001. Follow-up contacts were made with clinicians who expressed interest in expanding their practices to include work with this special population, and networking events were held to connect clinicians experienced in working with sexual aggression and abuse with those interested in expanding their practices. Service codes with higher reimbursement rates were established within the Wraparound Milwaukee billing system to acknowledge and compensate clinicians with documented and verified expertise in working with this high-risk population.

With a growing cadre of skilled clinicians, Wraparound Milwaukee could incorporate a broader range of specialized crisis, safety, and treatment services into its system of care. One added agency provides offense-specific individual, family, and group education and therapy for youth with sexual behavior problems. Several agencies became providers of in-home and outpatient Cognitive-Behavioral Therapy and ecologically oriented family intervention aimed at the prevention of sexual abuse and other delinquency.

Wraparound Milwaukee, in collaboration with grant-funded, community-based agencies and the Wisconsin Crime Victim Compensation program, also provides specialized services to victims of sexual abuse. Clinicians in the community with expertise in the provision of services to victims and their families were actively recruited to join the provider network. Networking and training events, along with competitive rates of reimbursement and provider-friendly billing procedures, have served as incentives for highly qualified clinicians, many with years of private practice experience, to join the Wraparound Milwaukee provider network. Recommended practices in services to child victims and family reunification processes are disseminated through the regularly scheduled high risk reviews. Wraparound Milwaukee has collaborated with others to promote broad-based sexual abuse prevention programming and the establishment of STOP IT NOW! Wisconsin (http://stopitnow.wi.gov).

Status of Services for Youth and Families Affected by Juvenile Sexual Violence

Since 1998, all Milwaukee County youth deemed at risk for residential treatment due to complex emotional or behavioral needs have been enrolled in Wraparound Milwaukee. At that time, only 9% of youth enrolled in Wraparound Milwaukee were adjudicated of sexual offenses. By 2005, 20% of youth enrolled in Wraparound Milwaukee were juvenile sex offenders. Wraparound Milwaukee serves an average of 100–130 youth adjudicated of sexual assault at any given time. On average, 80% of youth enrolled in Wraparound Milwaukee with sexual offenses reside in their communities, outside of residential treatment centers.

Decisions regarding treatment and level of supervision for sexually aggressive youth rely on an initial (predispositional) assessment and ongoing holistic assessment of youth and family strengths, needs, and risks (Gilbertson, Storm, & Fischer, 2001). High risk reviews are held weekly, during which care coordinators review newly enrolled youth on the high risk list with a high risk consulting psychologist. In addition, the consulting psychologist visits each of the care coordination agencies on a monthly basis to review all youth on the high risk list. Reviews consist of an examination of the services provided, youth and family response to the services, and any instances of risky or concerning behavior. Strategies for managing risk and for preventing harm are discussed, and safety plans are reviewed. The consultant is also available to attend child and family team meetings as requested and has access in real time to all progress notes, plans of care, critical incident reports, and service authorizations through the Internet-based management information system. All requests for out-of-home care and preauthorization for residential treatment and group homes are reviewed by the consultant. The consultant also meets regularly with district attorneys, probation officers, and specialized treatment providers to promote collaboration and to share empirically derived recommended practices and local outcomes in the care of the high-risk youth and families served.

Population Served, Service Utilization, and Outcomes

Between 1998 and 2005, Wraparound Milwaukee served 528 youth who were adjudicated delinquent on sexual assault charges and were deemed at risk for residential treatment. The average age of these youth was 13 years, 7 months; 68% were in sixth through eighth grade; and 54% were identified as special education students. Seventy percent of the youth were African American, 22% Caucasian, 6% Latino, and 1% Native American. The majority (60%) were residing in single-parent (maternal) homes at enrollment; only 16% were residing with both biological parents. Annual gross family income was below $15,000 for 47% and below $25,000 for an additional 26%. For Wraparound Milwaukee–enrolled youth, touching the victim's genitalia (34%) and rubbing together of bare genitalia (24%) were the most common sexual behaviors resulting in adjudication. This is in contrast to those Milwaukee County youth receiving correctional placements since 2000, for whom fellatio by the victim (47%) and penile–vaginal penetration (32%) were the most common behaviors resulting in adjudication. Twelve percent of the youth receiving a correctional placement threatened their victims with weapons during the commission of their crimes.

The average age of sexual assault victims of enrolled in Wraparound Milwaukee is 8 years, 5 months. Seventy percent are female; 30% are male. Approximately 50% are a relative of the offender, 20% are child neighbors, 21% are peers, and only 3% are strangers. Sixty-eight percent of the offenses occurred in either the perpetrator or the victim's home. In 60% of the cases, the victim was more than 4 years younger than the perpetrator. In 47% of cases, physical force was evident; however, weapon threats were evident in only 1% of the cases.

Access to a more comprehensive and data-based understanding of Milwaukee's sexually aggressive youth, their victims, and their families, along with the development of community-based services, has led to a shift toward utilization of services that seem to better match youth and family needs. This shift in utilization has resulted in a significant reallocation of monies spent to serve adjudicated juvenile sex offenders and their families in Milwaukee. More than 80% of all Milwaukee County youth adjudicated of sexual offenses in 2005 were enrolled in Wrap-around Milwaukee, a marked increase from the 10% of youth adjudicated of sexual offenses enrolled in the system of care in 1998. This corresponds to a decline in the commitment of adjudicated juvenile sex offenders to correctional institutions from Milwaukee County, down from 19% in 1996 to 10.5% in 2005.

The overall cost per child and family per month for the care of adjudicated juvenile sexual offenders and their families within the Wraparound Milwaukee system of care dropped by 18% between 2000 and 2002 and has remained essentially stable since, despite inflation in service costs. This change can be attributed to the broader implementation and utilization of offense-specific and holistic assessment, the development of effective community-based resources, and a corresponding decrease in reliance on residential treatment as the primary means for treatment and supervision of this population. Of the 109 adjudicated juvenile sexual offenders enrolled in the system of care in 2007, only 22 (20%) were placed within residential treatment centers. The remaining youth resided either at home (39) or within other community-based placements (i.e., 15 in treatment foster care, 18 in group homes).

To ensure appropriate supervision and structure for adjudicated juvenile sexual offenders managed in the community, a range of services are provided, including crisis one-to-one stabilization, parent assistance, treatment foster care, offense-specific individual therapy provided by specialized doctoral-level providers, and in-home family therapy. The services most utilized by high-risk juvenile sex offenders and their families include individual therapy (68%), intensive in-home family therapy (54%), mentoring (46%), group counseling (42%), and crisis one-to-one stabilization and monitoring (41%). Providers in the Wraparound Milwaukee provider network also offer psychoeducational groups that include parent education and support group components. Victims' needs and voices are amplified as part of the collaborative child and family team process. Trauma services for victims are obtained through the provider network, and in some cases, can be paid for through the Wisconsin Crime Victim Compensation Program. This program serves as a payer of last resort if other third party payer resources are exhausted.

Access to residential care remains an option within the Wraparound Milwaukee system of care if deemed appropriate. Residential treatment for these youth occurs only in specialized settings and is preauthorized for no more than 2 months at a time. Outcomes are carefully monitored, and residential treatment lengths of stay have decreased to an average of less than 3 months. Residential providers are part of the child and family team, and they work with family members and community-based providers to ensure a smooth and safe return to the community. Wraparound Milwaukee care coordinators persistently communicate the importance of maintaining a focus on strengths and the development of competencies relevant to risk reduction.

In collaboration with the Milwaukee County Children's Court, juvenile justice outcome data have been collected since 2000 for youth enrolled in Wraparound Milwaukee. Follow-up data for youth served by Wraparound Milwaukee reported at 3- and 5-year intervals revealed an 8% and 12% recidivism rate for sexual offenses, respectively, and a 27% rate for nonsexual delinquency recidivism (Seybold, 2006). A retrospective analysis on youth referred to the court for sexual offenses in 1996 in Milwaukee County, prior to the development of specialized services for this population in Wraparound Milwaukee's system of care, found significantly higher recidivism rates at the time of 5-year follow-up—a 15.5% recidivism rate for sexual offenses and 68% for nonsexual offenses (Driessen, 2002). These data demonstrate the effectiveness of the enhanced system of care in serving this high-risk population of youth.

CONCLUSION

Numerous lessons have been learned from working with high-risk youth, particularly the juvenile sex offender population, that can be shared with other communities. Perhaps the most significant lesson is that the high-risk youth can yield clinical and program outcomes as good as—and sometimes better than—youth who present with fewer risk factors and problematic behaviors.

In working with high-risk populations, trust is crucial among system stakeholders (e.g., child welfare, juvenile justice, and mental health systems; schools; the state Medicaid agency). A consistent, research-based message must be conveyed to all of these partners, stating that high-risk youth can and should be cared for in the community whenever possible. Giving up some turf issues in favor of an integrated, coordinated approach to care planning and delivery for youth and their families is essential to the implementation of a successful system of care.

In serving high-risk populations, the concept of one care plan with one care manager is important to success due to the complexity of the problems of these youth and the likelihood of their involvement with multiple child-serving systems. In addition, flexible funding that allows care coordinators and families to obtain whatever services are needed to assess, treat, monitor, and manage high-risk youth is a critical component of an effective system of care for these youth and their families.

Concerted efforts directed at ensuring community safety are essential requirements for working with high-risk youth. Systems of care must be skilled at properly assessing risk and identifying those factors and problematic situations that may result in a youth engaging in sexual or other high-risk and dangerous behavior. Well thought out, highly individualized crisis safety plans must be developed to address these risks. Without effective strategies for anticipating and responding to dangerous behaviors, children, families, and the entire system of care are placed at great peril.

Creating partnerships among policy-level administrators to strategically plan the implementation and maintenance of recommended practices was a key to overcoming fear and resistance to the expansion of community-based care for high-risk youth, particularly youth adjudicated of sexual offenses. Judges, prosecutors, and probation officers are provided regular updates from the clinical and research literature and from Wraparound Milwaukee's program evaluation, which reinforces the ecologically oriented and community-based wraparound approach to youth with sexual behavior problems and their families.

The credibility of the system of care is another key factor in working with high-risk youth. Credibility is established as courts and other system partners recognize the heightened and detailed attention and effort devoted to designing sound crisis safety plans and utilizing recognized clinical specialists to frequently review the progress and status of each high-risk youth. Confidence in the system of care is built through repeated success on a child-by-child basis and by achieving positive outcomes that can be measured and demonstrated.

Finally, achieving good outcomes for high-risk youth requires the participation, trust, and support of families. Crisis safety plans are only effective if they are understood and implemented well by families and other caregivers. Similarly, families are the experts on the strengths and needs of their children, and they know what resources are necessary to support their children and the family as a whole. It is only with full participation and partnership with families that effective plans of care for high-risk youth can be developed and implemented.

REFERENCES

American Psychiatric Association. (1994). *Diagnostic and statistical manual of mental disorders* (4th ed.). Washington, DC: Author.

Borduin, C.M., & Schaeffer, C.M. (2001). Multisystemic treatment of juvenile sexual offenders: A progress report. *Journal of Psychology & Human Sexuality, 13*(3–4), 25–42.

Bronfenbrenner, U. (1979). *The ecology of human development.* Cambridge, MA: Harvard University Press.

Center for Sex Offender Management. (1999a). *The collaborative approach to sex offender management.* Retrieved October 2000 from http://www.csom.org/pubs/collabortion .html.

Center for Sex Offender Management. (1999b). *The collaborative approach to sex offender management.* Retrieved October 2000 from http://www.csom.org/pubs/collabortion .html

Chaffin, M., & Bonner, B. (1996, June). *Reintegrating juvenile offenders into the family.* Paper presented at the Fourth National Colloquium of the American Professional Society on the Abuse of Children, Chicago.

Contract for services between the Wisconsin Department of Health and Family Services and Milwaukee County. September 2005–June 30, 2007. (2007). Milwaukee: Wisconsin Department of Health and Family Services and Milwaukee County.

Dishion, T.J., McCord, J., & Poulin, F. (1999). When interventions harm: Peer groups and problem behavior. *American Psychologist, 54*(9), 755–764.

Driessen, E.M. (2002). *Characteristics of youth referred for sexual offenses.* Unpublished doctoral dissertation, University of Wisconsin, Milwaukee.

Gilbertson, S.A., Storm, H., & Fischer, E. (2001, November). *Evaluating the families of juvenile sex offenders in Milwaukee County, Wisconsin.* Poster session presented at the annual meeting of the Association for the Treatment of Sexual Abusers, San Antonio, TX.

Henggeler, S.W., Schoenwald, S.K., & Pickrel, S.G. (1995). Multisystemic therapy: Bridging the gap between university- and community-based treatment. *Journal of Consulting and Clinical Psychology, 63*(5), 709–717.

Hunter, J.A., Gilbertson, S.A., Vedros, D., & Morton, M. (2004). Strengthening community-based programming for juvenile sexual offender: Key concepts and paradigm shifts. *Child Maltreatment: Journal of the American Professional Society on the Abuse of Children, 9*(2).

Hunter, J.A., Jr. (2002). *Juvenile sex offender management and treatment: A best practice model*. Final report submitted to the Virginia Department of Criminal Justice Services.

Hunter, J.A., Jr., Figueredo, A.J., Malamuth, N.M., & Becker, J.V. (2003). Juvenile sex offenders: Toward the development of a typology. *Sexual Abuse Journal of Research and Treatment, 15*(1), 27–48.

Hunter, J.A., Jr., & Lexier, L.J. (1998). Ethical and legal issues in the assessment and treatment of juvenile sex offenders. *Child Maltreatment: Journal of the American Professional Society on the Abuse of Children, 3*(4), 339–348.

Kamradt, B. (1999). *The 25 Kid Project: How Milwaukee utilized a pilot project to achieve buy-in among stakeholders in changing the system of care for children with severe emotional problems*. Unpublished monograph.

Malysiak, R. (1997). Exploring the theory and paradigm base for wraparound. *Journal of Child and Family Studies, 6*, 399–408.

Miller, G.E., & Prinz, R.J. (1990). Enhancement of social learning family interventions for childhood conduct disorder. *Psychological Bulletin, 108*(2), 291–307.

National Task Force on Juvenile Sexual Offending. (1993). *Final report: A function of the National Adolescent Perpetration Network*. Boulder, CO: C.H. Kempe National Center, University of Colorado Health Sciences Center.

Planning Council of Milwaukee. (1994). *Study of residential treatment placements in Milwaukee county*. Unpublished study.

Prentky, R., Harris B., Frizzell, K., & Righthand, K., (2000). An actuarial procedure for assessing risk with juvenile sexual offenders. *Sexual Abuse, 12*, 71–93.

President's New Freedom Commission on Mental Health. (2003). *Achieving the promise: Transforming mental health care in America* (Final Report, DHHS Pub. No. SMA-03-3832). Rockville, MD: Author.

Righthand, S., & Welch, C. (2001). *Juveniles who have sexually offended: A review of the professional literature—Office of Juvenile Justice and Delinquency Prevention report*. Washington, DC: U.S. Department of Justice, Office of Justice Programs.

Seybold, E., (2006). *Characteristics and outcomes of youth enrolled in the Wraparound Milwaukee program: Clients enrolled from 1/1/98 to 2/28/06*. Unpublished study.

U.S. Department of Health and Human Services. (1999). *Mental health: A report of the Surgeon General*. Rockville, MD: National Institute of Mental Health, Substance Abuse and Mental Health Services.

Wraparound Milwaukee. (2006). *Annual report for 2005 and 2006*. Unpublished report.

Zigler, E., Taussig, C., & Black, K. (1992). Early childhood intervention: A promising preventative for juvenile delinquency. *American Psychologist, 47*(8), 997–1006.

18

Services for Young Children and Their Families in Systems of Care

Deborah F. Perry, Roxane K. Kaufmann, Sarah Hoover, and Claudia Zundel

---

Much of the work on mental health systems of care has focused on efforts to serve older children with serious emotional disturbances (SEDs) who require services and supports from multiple agencies. Discussions with parents of children diagnosed with SEDs reveal that many of these children manifested behaviors of concern in their first years of life. These concerns were often dismissed by health professionals, who counseled families to be patient and let their children outgrow these behaviors (Nikkel, 2007). Armed with the latest findings about the importance of the first few years for early brain development, a growing chorus of advocates has joined with other stakeholders to encourage systems of care to extend their services to younger children. Many of the principles and strategies articulated throughout this volume are transferable to system building for infants, toddlers, and preschoolers. There are, however, systematic differences in some aspects of systems of care for children who have not yet reached school age. These factors range from how the target population is defined, to a different set of interagency partners and stakeholders that need to be engaged, to how services and supports are planned and delivered. This chapter defines the concept of *early childhood mental health* and articulates a framework for conceptualizing an early childhood mental health system of care. Differences are highlighted in what have been traditionally defined as system of care principles and core components when serving very young children. A case study is presented of an initiative underway in four communities in Colorado to develop a system of care for young children funded by a Substance Abuse and Mental Health Services Administration (SAMHSA) system of care grant. In addition, some of what are considered to be evidence-based practices for young children with or at risk for mental health problems are outlined, and the chapter concludes with a discussion of future challenges and issues to be considered as states and communities move forward in their efforts to serve young children and their families.

WHAT IS EARLY CHILDHOOD MENTAL HEALTH?

Unlike the term *serious emotional disturbance* that drives much of the system of care work undertaken on behalf of school-age youth, early childhood systems focus on a broader construct—the social and emotional well-being of young children and their caregivers. This difference underscores several of the core distinctions in the approaches taken by early childhood professionals and policy makers. First, very few young children are diagnosed with SEDs. This is a product of a complex array of factors. There is widespread reluctance to diagnose mental health problems in very young children, as well as a lack of trained early childhood mental health professionals. Furthermore, there are fewer clinically valid diagnostic tools, a circumstance compounded with concerns about the limited relevance of the prevailing diagnostic classification system to accurately represent the range of mental health concerns that young children may present; the latter concern is also tied up with barriers to getting reimbursement for treatment services without such a billable code. Stigma regarding mental health problems and unnecessary labeling of young children, coupled with the evidence that typical development is self-righting, also lead to caution on the part of well-meaning professionals. Second, early childhood mental health is intimately intertwined with the well-being of caregivers. These two factors lead to early childhood mental health systems necessarily focusing on a broader group of young children and their families, extending beyond those with an established diagnosis to include those at risk for developing mental health problems later.

In this chapter, the term *early childhood mental health* is conceptualized in one of two ways—the first through a developmental/clinical perspective and the second through a system/service delivery lens. The developmental/clinical definition views early childhood mental health as the social, emotional, and behavioral well-being of infants, toddlers, and young children through age 8 and their families, including (ZERO TO THREE, 2002):

- The development of the capacity to experience, regulate, and express emotion

- The ability to form close, secure relationships

- The capacity to explore the environment and learn

A system/service delivery perspective proposed by Knitzer (2000) further defines early childhood mental health as a set of strategies to:

- Promote the emotional and behavioral well-being of all young children

- Strengthen the emotional and behavioral well-being of children whose development is compromised by environmental or biological risk to minimize their risks and enhance the likelihood that they will enter school with the appropriate skills

- Help families of young children address whatever barriers they face to ensure that their children's emotional development is not compromised

- Expand the competencies of nonfamilial caregivers and others to promote the well-being of young children and families, particularly those at risk by virtue of environmental or biological factors

- Ensure that young children experiencing clearly atypical emotional and behavioral development and their families have access to needed services and supports

When combined, these two perspectives articulate the need to adopt a public health framework for early childhood mental health system building, thus laying the infrastructure to support a broad range of services and supports that encourage social and emotional development in all young children, as well as identifying those in need of more targeted assistance due to familial or individual risk factors or current behavioral or social problems.

PUBLIC HEALTH FRAMEWORK

"Early childhood mental health care provides a continuum of services and supports from prevention through intervention. It includes children who will never have a mental health diagnosis, those who may develop a problem at some point, and those who have evident problems early on. It relies on a wide range of both professional helpers and natural helpers— those grandparents, child care workers, neighbors, church members, or others who understand and are willing to support young children and their families. It embraces families as the most important people in their children's mental health development, but it also acknowledges the importance of the quality of relationships that children begin to establish outside the family during their early years." (Edwall, 2005)

Much has been said recently about the need to transform the mental health system in the United States, including the need to adopt a public health framework that extends from promotion through early identification and prevention to treatment (Huang et al., 2005). Such a public health approach is even more essential when building systems of care for young children and their families (Perry, Kaufmann, & Knitzer, 2007). As previously described, early childhood mental health systems are driven by a broad definition of mental health that includes social and emotional well-being. Social and emotional development is built on young children's earliest experiences with caregivers and the attachments that are developed with those who provide consistent, warm, responsive attention. Integral to these processes are the parallel developments of cognitive, motor, and regulatory skills. The distinctions between typical and atypical social and emotional development unfold over time and in the context of these early relationships. Families who are at high risk for having children with serious emotional problems may find that early supportive services alter that probabilistic trajectory. In other families, challenging behaviors may appear in the absence of any observable risk factor. Few families with very young children, however, will present themselves at the mental health system's door—even those whose children may be manifesting clinically significant behaviors. This combination of few children with established mental health diagnoses and many who might benefit from mental health services and supports underscores the importance of including promotion, prevention, and intervention approaches in any system of care for young children (Kaufmann & Hepburn, 2007).

SIMILARITIES AND DIFFERENCES IN SYSTEMS OF CARE FOR YOUNGER CHILDREN

One of the distinctive features of systems of care is that they base their services on core values, specifying that services should be child centered and family focused, community based, and culturally competent. They also maintain a set of guiding principles, including access to a comprehensive array of services; individualized planning and services; least restrictive services; families as full participants in the planning and delivery of services (i.e., family driven and youth guided); integrated and coordinated services with linkages across agencies; case management; early identification and intervention; smooth transitions to adult services; protection of rights and advocacy efforts; and access to services without regard to race, religion, gender, or disability. Many of these core values remain at the heart of early childhood mental health systems as well, but it is important to point out the nuanced differences.

A conceptual model for an early childhood mental health system of care is depicted in Figure 18.1. This model elucidates the common building blocks of a system of care approach for young children, highlighting some of the differences

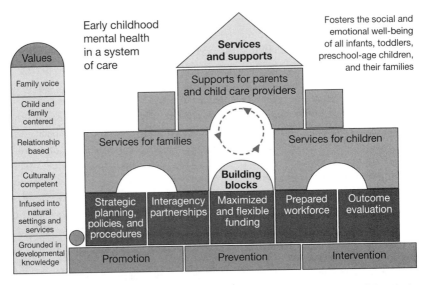

Figure 18.1. Conceptual model. (Designed by Lucia Foley, Hampshire Educational Collaborative.)

in working with infants, toddlers, and preschoolers. These differences focus on the differences for young children in the system of care values and principles of interagency collaboration, cultural and linguistic competence, family-driven and youth-guided services, as well as principles that are unique in systems of care for young children and their families. The unique principles call for systems of care that are grounded in developmental knowledge, infused into natural environments, and relationship based.

Interagency Collaboration

One of the building blocks of a system of care is the need to engage multiple interagency partners in system-building efforts. The public mental health agency at the state or local level has often taken a lead role in creating systems of care. Once children reach school age, the school system is a critical partner in meeting the needs of children with SEDs. These children also often are involved with the child welfare or juvenile justice systems. Medicaid is often an important payer of services rendered through systems of care.

In an early childhood mental health system of care, these interagency partnerships take on different forms. These differences are manifest in: 1) engaging new partners who may not have been involved in system of care work, and 2) asking the traditional partners to provide a different array of services or serve in different roles. Some of the new state-level partners that must be active in early childhood systems of care are the Maternal and Child Health agency, which has the lead responsibility for implementing the Early Childhood Comprehensive Systems (ECCS) grants from the federal Title V authority; the state Child Care Administrator; the Preschool Special Education (619) and Part C Coordinators, both of whom are charged with implementing the early childhood provisions (Part C) of the Individuals with Disabilities Education Act (IDEA) Amendments of 1997 (PL 105-17); the state Head Start/Early Head Start collaboration coordinator; and others involved with the provision of primary health care or home visitation services. All of these stakeholders have community- or county-level representatives who would be relevant for community-level system-building efforts.

It is also necessary to engage traditional partner agencies in new ways for early childhood systems of care. For example, the child welfare system is mandated by the federal Child Abuse Prevention and Treatment Act of 1974 (PL 93-247) to refer infants and toddlers who have substantiated cases of abuse or neglect to the Part C/Early Intervention system for eligibility determination. This can help ensure that the Part C system is addressing the mental health needs of young children with or at risk for other disabilities, something that has been a consistent weakness in many Part C systems. Because very young children themselves will not be the clients of juvenile justice, these systems may assist in innovative efforts to target prevention efforts to the younger siblings and children of adjudicated youth. Adult service systems providing mental health, substance abuse, and domestic violence services for the caregivers of very young children must also be critical allies in system building at the state and community levels.

Cultural and Linguistic Competence

A core value in systems of care is the need to deliver services and supports that are culturally relevant and a match for the families and children they serve. Agencies, programs, and services must be responsive to the cultural, linguistic, racial, and ethnic differences of all the children and families they serve. The United States is growing increasingly diverse, and it is incumbent on agencies to develop policies and procedures that ensure that all children and families have access to services that meet their needs. The workforce in particular requires specialized training in cultural and linguistic competence, and it must expand to include natural healers and cultural brokers. Issues of stigma regarding mental health make this value even more critical.

For agencies and programs serving young children and their families, cultural competence becomes an even more compelling issue. Huang and Isaacs (2007) pointed out that cultural factors stemming from the ethno-cultural heritage of diverse families play a significant role in determining child-rearing practices and expectations of appropriate behavior, influencing salient risk and protective factors. All aspects of early child-rearing are influenced and informed by culture, including sleep and eating habits, expectations about autonomy versus dependence, discipline, trust, early literacy and language acquisition, and health and mental health practices. The programs that serve young children must examine how well they are reaching out to and serving diverse populations and how accessible, relevant, sensitive, and individualized their services are. There is also a need for staff to reflect on how they can communicate about effective parenting practices without implying that there is only one correct way to parent young children. Ongoing training of staff in cultural and linguistic competence and evaluation of program effectiveness will inform and enhance utilization of services.

Family Driven

In many cases, families of children with SEDs experience obstacles when they search for adequate care and services. Stories shared by families express frustration with agencies and providers who do not listen to their concerns, do not individualize services or programs, do not help coordinate services across agencies, and even blame families for their children's disorders (Nikkel, 2007). Families must often advocate and sometimes fight for appropriate services. In an effort to change that negative paradigm, families have banded together to develop advocacy organizations such as the National Alliance on Mental Illness (NAMI) and the Federation of Families for Children's Mental Health. The unified voices of families have challenged and influenced policy at all levels, thus empowering individual families to become drivers of the service planning processes for their own children. Although there is still a long way to go before all children and families have access to the service array that best meets their individual needs, a stronger family movement has emerged to support this process. Existing advocacy organizations, however, have not typically reached out to families of very young children, nor do they always relate to the family support networks engaged with these families. A new approach is required that integrates family support and an understanding of early childhood mental health into early care and education systems through coalition building and education. It can take time for the family of a young child with mental health needs to be ready to join in advocacy efforts. This often begins with families learning to advocate on behalf of services for their own children, and for some families, later adding in the roles of system-level advocacy on behalf of other families with unmet needs.

Youth Guided

The inclusion of youth with emotional or behavioral disorders in the policy and service delivery aspects of systems of care is an important new extension of the value of family-centered care. Older children and youth can shape their own treatment goals, evaluate the effectiveness of services and supports, and inform planning processes in ways that assure compliance and successful outcomes. Policies that are informed by a consumer voice become more relevant and meaningful. Obviously, children younger than the age of 6 years are in no position to inform policy development, and their roles in individualized treatment planning are limited or inappropriate. A 5- or 6-year-old child can share feelings and concerns about peer relationships in ways that might provide some insight into appropriate interventions, but younger children rarely have the language or maturity to be included in team planning processes. Therefore, this construct lacks salience in early childhood system planning.

Grounded in Developmental Knowledge

As the discussion of the relevance of youth-guided services indicates, a developmental perspective is critical in many facets of building an early childhood mental health system of care. Distinguishing between typical and atypical social and emotional development is an essential aspect of determining if a young child's behavior is a cause for concern. This distinction is often a function of the timing, frequency, or intensity of a particular behavior (e.g., temper tantrums), as opposed to the presence or absence of a given behavior. Unfortunately, many early care providers, education specialists, and health care professionals are unaware of the early signs of emotional problems and may not fully understand the importance of consistent early nurturing relationships. Mental health providers often lack an understanding of typical emotional milestones and early development, and they rarely have experience working in group care situations. Families need access to practical information on early brain development, positive discipline, and early social and emotional warning signs.

Infused into Natural Environments

In systems of care for school-age children, services and supports must be delivered in the least restrictive environment. This construct takes on new meaning for very young children. Early childhood mental health services and supports need to be available in the many places where children and families are—their homes; child care settings; pediatric practices; and adult service settings, such as Women, Infants, and Children Program [WIC] offices, homeless shelters, substance abuse clinics, and family courts. This infusion approach requires cross-training of staff from adult- and child-serving systems. Social and emotional curricula for early care and education programs are essential, and practical materials for families on positive parenting, nurturing relationships, and developmental warning signs should be readily available and culturally relevant. Increasingly popular are models of early childhood mental health consultation in which a mental health professional is embedded within a child care setting to provide capacity-building and consultation around young children with challenging behaviors (Cohen & Kaufmann, 2000; Johnston & Brinamen, 2006). Evidence for the effectiveness of these approaches is growing as more rigorous evaluations are being designed and implemented (Brennan, Bradley, Allen, & Perry, 2007; Hepburn et al., 2007).

Relationship Based

At its core, early childhood mental health is about the quality of young children's relationships with significant caregivers, including their parents, grandparents, and child care providers. Effective interventions for young children's mental health are often two-generational, targeting the dyad and directing attention to the individual needs of both the baby and the caregiver. Relationships may also be the focus of psychotherapy with older children with emotional disturbances, but the centrality of this construct in working with young children who have or are at risk for mental health problems cannot be overstated. In serving young children, there are often parallel processes at work in terms of relationships; relationships between staff and families are critical, and they lay the foundation for parallel work between parents and children (Johnston & Brinamen, 2006; Zeanah, 2007).

EVIDENCE-BASED PRACTICES FOR YOUNG CHILDREN

Systems of care focusing on young children and their families must integrate effective interventions and approaches that promote healthy social and emotional development in all young children, prevent the development of mental health problems in young children with known risk factors, and treat young children and families where mental health concerns are identified. The array of programs and practices designed for young children that have reached the highest level of evidence (i.e., through multiple randomized controlled trials) is rather limited, but as the demand for effective early childhood mental health interventions has grown, there has been an increase in the number of effective interventions for older children that are being adapted for use with younger children (see, e.g., Deblinger, Stauffer, & Steer, 2001; Domitrovich, Cortes, & Kusché, 2002).

A review of the literature on effective manualized interventions to promote healthy social-emotional development in young children identified eight curricula that met at least two of nine criteria for scientific rigor (Joseph & Strain, 2003). The criteria were derived from work conducted by the American Psychological Association, and they serve as indicators for the likelihood that prior positive results would be reproduced if interventions were adopted. They included evidence of:

> 1) treatment fidelity; 2) treatment generalization; 3) treatment maintenance; 4) social validity of outcomes; 5) acceptability of interventions; 6) replication across investigators; 7) replication across clinical groups; 8) evidence across ethnic/racially diverse groups; and 9) evidence for replication across settings. (Joseph & Strain, 2003, p. 66)

Of these, only two programs achieved what the reviewers deemed to be a high level of evidence, that is at least seven of nine indicators: *The Incredible Years: Dinosaur School,* developed by Carolyn Webster-Stratton (1990, 2003), and *First Step to Success*, developed by Hill Walker et al. (1998). *The Incredible Years* was initially designed as an intervention to treat young children who were exhibiting conduct problems, but it has since been implemented as a universal intervention to build young children's social skills, problem-solving abilities, and conflict management behaviors. Likewise, *First Step to Success* was developed to address the needs of kindergarten students exhibiting early antisocial behaviors. This program includes a component that screens all young children in classroom settings, as well as school-based and parent-focused interventions.

Although these two evidence-based programs focus on preschool-age children, interventions focused on infants and toddlers have also been developed and tested. Zeanah, Stafford, and Zeanah (2005) conducted a selective review of clinical interventions to enhance infant mental health. Many of these interventions were implemented by trained mental health professionals, although some, including the *Steps Toward Enjoyable Effective Parenting* (STEEP; Erikson, Egeland, Rose, & Simon, 2002), relied on parenting facilitators who conducted home visits that focused on building the skills of new mothers. Some programs were targeted at mothers who were at high risk, such as relational psychotherapy for women who were abusing drugs (Luthar & Sussman, 2000), and these were delivered by a team of providers. Most successful programs have a dyadic focus. For example, an infant/child–parent psychotherapy model was developed for mothers with depression (Cicchetti, Toth, & Rogosh, 1999); the intervention has been expanded to immigrant women who have experienced domestic violence (Lieberman, 2004). These interventions are delivered by trained psychotherapists and take place over a period of 1 year.

Finally, there is growing interest in the role that mental health consultation can play in multiple levels of early childhood systems of care because more states and communities are funding and evaluating these approaches. Early childhood mental health consultation can be used as a strategy to promote positive social-emotional development in young children in a variety of early care and education settings (including family child care homes and child care centers). This approach has been an integral part of Head Start programs since their inception, involving screening young children for problematic behavior and referring those who need more intensive services to mental health practitioners. Mental health consultation can also serve as part of a wraparound strategy for young children identified with significant mental health disorders, helping to build the capacity of preschool teachers to accommodate challenging behaviors. Teaming mental health professionals with paraprofessionals or other home visitors is an approach that has also been implemented for families with young children who are at high risk (Zeanah et al., 2005).

Embedding mental health professionals into early care and education settings to build the capacity of those providers to cope with young children's challenging behaviors has decreased the rate of expulsion from child care (Perry, Dunne, McFadden, & Campbell, 2008). Positive effects on teacher confidence and stress have also been reported (Brennan et al., 2007). Recently, the first two randomized controlled trials of early childhood mental health consultation were conducted, adding to the cumulative evidence from roughly 30 program evaluations that were reviewed by Brennan and her colleagues (2007). Gilliam (2007) conducted a statewide evaluation of the Early Childhood Consultation Partnership, which documented positive effects on children's outcomes, but noted fewer direct effects on teacher-level outcomes. Raver, Jones, Li-Grining, Sardin-Adjei, and Jones-Lewis (2007) reported positive effects on the classroom climate, along with reduced levels of expulsions. Colorado's 2006 survey of licensed child care providers indicated that providers who had access to classroom behavioral consultation had fewer removals from their care and were less likely to remove children from care due to challenging behaviors (Hoover, 2006). In all, a growing evidence base supports the critical role that early childhood mental health consultation can play in systems of care for young children and their families and other caregivers.

COLORADO'S APPROACH TO SYSTEMS OF CARE FOR YOUNG CHILDREN AND FAMILIES

"Project BLOOM's mission is to weave family-centered, culturally competent, and community-based mental health supports and services into a seamless early childhood system of care that promotes healthy social-emotional development, identifies risk factors, intervenes early, and provides high quality services."
—Project BLOOM's Leadership Team (2003)

Background and Infrastructure

Data supporting the need for a deliberate strategy to improve the mental health of young children in Colorado came from various sources. A survey of Colorado child care providers indicated that 15.4 % of children age birth to 8 years in child care settings had behaviors serious enough to disrupt the classroom (Gould, 2000). These data were a wake-up call to many people, including mental health professionals, who were skeptical that children under 6 could have mental health disorders. The study, referred to as the Cost of Failure Study, documented that early childhood mental health services could potentially save public dollars in later years. Several years later, Colorado's Child Health Survey (Colorado Department of Public Health and Environment, 2005) reported that 21% percent of parents with children younger than age 6 had concerns about difficulties with their children's emotions, concentration, behavior, or ability to get along with others; yet of these parents, 79% had never accessed counseling or supports to address these difficulties. The following year, Colorado's state legislature passed a Resolution (i.e., Colorado Senate Joint Resolution 06-015 Concerning Young Children with Challenging Behaviors) authorizing a study on the issue of challenging behavior in children younger than 6 years of age. Study findings revealed that, according to early care and education providers, 11% of all children in their care younger than age 6 had challenging behavior. For all children, 10 of every 1,000 were removed from early care and education settings due to challenging behavior. Of the children whom early care and education providers identified as having challenging behaviors in their programs, 89 of every 1,000 were being removed from care. Combined with earlier data from the Cost of Failure Study (Gould, 2000), the need for a systematic approach for improving the mental health of young children in Colorado seemed clear.

Building on several efforts underway to address the needs of its youngest citizens, state and local leaders in Colorado established Project BLOOM (Building Leveraged Opportunities and Ongoing Mechanisms for children's mental health). Funded in 2002 in large part by a system of care grant from SAMHSA, it was the second such project in the country that focused exclusively on the mental health needs of children from birth to 5 years. Since then, BLOOM has partnered with other child-serving agencies in Colorado to leverage the state ECCS grant from the U.S. Department of Health and Human Services, Health Resources and Services Administration, Maternal Child Health Bureau to integrate mental health into all aspects of the planning and implementation of an early childhood system of care. State and local partners made an intentional decision to focus on integrating mental health into the early childhood system rather than creating a separate mental health system to serve younger children.

The success of Project BLOOM's efforts lies in its unique blend of strong partnerships built at the state level across agencies and systems, as well as in the strength of its ties with community partners. At the state level, core partners are the state Department of Human Services, the Division of Mental Health; JFK Partners (i.e., Colorado's University Center for Excellence in Developmental Disabilities Education, Research, and Service) at the University of Colorado at Denver and Health Sciences Center; the Colorado Children's Campaign; and the Federation of Families for Children's Mental Health. For the SAMHSA grant, Project BLOOM defined its system of care service area by capitalizing on emerging infrastructures in four communities with local Early Childhood Councils—two urban communities (i.e., Aurora and El Paso counties) and two rural communities (i.e., Fremont and Mesa counties). The system-building process provided an opportunity to engage community mental health centers in building collaboration among public sector agencies; higher education institutions; and private and not-for-profit organizations with high potential to affect public policies, preservice education, and in-service professional development as well as the public will to support early childhood mental health efforts. The partners were intentionally chosen for their diverse expertise and their ability to sustain elements of the system of care beyond the grant funding.

Because the primary funding came from the Comprehensive Community Mental Health Services for Children and Their Families Program, with a legislative history and authority that have focused on children with SEDs, an early tension arose between the SAMHSA grant requirements to serve children with SEDs and their families and the communities' desire to build a comprehensive system for *all* young children. The resolution of this conflict emerged through debate and dialogue. The partners in Project BLOOM came to recognize that the system of care is for all young children and that the SAMHSA grant provides an opportunity to develop an infrastructure to serve children who are currently manifesting problematic behaviors, as well as those at risk for developing these behaviors. As one of community director explained, "If we build a bridge for the heavy trucks, all cars will be able to drive on it." Thus, by infusing mental health services and supports into the larger early childhood system in Colorado, the well-being of all young children and their families would be promoted.

This public health approach to integrating mental health into early childhood settings, services, and programs was designed to ensure that all children—including those with the greatest needs—would be served in their homes and communities. Four strategies to develop this system of care were used by BLOOM to address the needs of young children and their families at the levels of promotion, prevention, and intervention: 1) training to develop workforce competencies, 2) developing the infrastructure for an early childhood system, 3) developing the public will to address early childhood mental health, and 4) evaluating processes and outcomes. These strategies, shown on Figure 18.2, cut across the various components of the system (i.e., promotion, prevention, intervention and treatment), ensuring that a continuum of screening, identification, diagnosis, and treatment services would be available in each of the communities and that this continuum would be supported by a state infrastructure that encouraged and supported the use of evidence-based approaches at each of these levels of intervention.

Screening, Assessment, and Diagnosis

In 2004, Project BLOOM developed a screening report with practice recommendations and policy strategies to support the integration of social and emotional screening for young children in three settings—early care and education, Child Find, and primary health care (Stainback-Tracy, 2004). These settings represent the places where young children and their families are most likely to be seen by

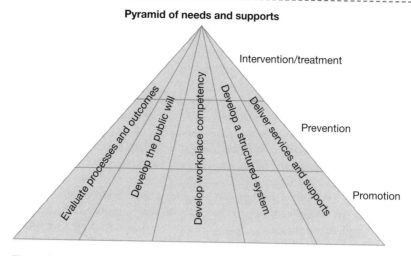

Figure 18.2.   Colorado's pyramid. (Created by Sarah Hoover, 2005.)

service providers and offered a natural place to monitor their well-being and development progress. Counties customized their approaches to integrate screening into these three settings.

In most communities, children in child care settings were screened with tools such as the Devereux Early Childhood Assessment (DECA) program. Fremont County's Child Find system for IDEA had been moving toward universal developmental screening of young children, and by 2005, local providers were able to screen 1,200 children, representing half of the county's population age birth to 5 years. Through participation in Project BLOOM, Fremont County recognized the number of children needing social-emotional support, and, as a result, included the Ages & Stages Questionnaires®: Social- Emotional (ASQ:SE; Squires, Bricker, & Twombly, 2002) as part of these regular screenings. Mesa County also introduced the ASQ:SE in both English and Spanish to the Child Find screening process in their community.

Integrating screening into primary care settings posed different challenges, but it also presented unique opportunities. Initial barriers included the perception that screening for social-emotional development took too much time, concerns about being overwhelmed by the number of children needing services, and not knowing whether community resources existed to meet needs that might be identified through such screening. An Early and Periodic Screening and Diagnosis and Treatment (EPSDT) pilot project, funded by the Colorado Health Foundation, demonstrated that all these barriers could be satisfactorily addressed. Aurora joined with a concurrent developmental surveillance project to introduce ASQ:SE developmental screening into a number of pediatric practices.

Following the lead of Aurora, Project BLOOM sites purchased screening tools for pediatric practices and worked with front office staff to introduce the screening as part of the day-to-day work flow. Screens are typically given at well-child check-ups, particularly at the ages of 9 months and 18 months. Once barriers were addressed and the feasibility and utility of social-emotional screening were demonstrated, pediatric practices were converted, with many pediatricians reporting that the screening helped to organize the well-child visits. Some physicians have become so eager for results that they score the test themselves (Betts, 2006). Efforts are underway to move this project statewide through the state's Assuring Better Child Development (ABCD) technical assistance grant funded by the Commonwealth Fund. As part of sustainability efforts, Project BLOOM is exploring ways to integrate screening for social and emotional health into the state's EPSDT program and Child Health Plan Plus, a low-cost health insurance program for uninsured Colorado children.

If a problem is detected during routine screening, children are referred for comprehensive assessments, which may lead to acquiring mental health diagnoses. An issue that emerged as a major concern was that diagnosing a very young child may lead to a permanent label on that child as he or she grows up. Resistance to assigning diagnoses as a condition for serving children was expressed by many early care and education providers who were more comfortable with a prevention framework that serves children based on their needs rather than their diagnoses. Because children are rapidly growing and developing, any assessment tool used for diagnostic purposes must be developmentally based and consistent with the ways in which social and emotional problems manifest in very young children. Some mental health difficulties in young children may be short lived, whereas others may require ongoing supports and services.

Many of the concerns regarding the diagnosis and labeling of young children were addressed by adopting the Diagnostic Classification of Mental Health and Developmental Disorders of Infancy and Early Childhood: Revised (DC: 0–3R system; ZERO TO THREE, 2005). A developmentally-based system such as the DC: 0–3R recognizes the interrelatedness of the various domains of development and how these emerge over time, while creating a common language that professionals and parents can share in the discussion of approaches to intervention. The DC: 0-3R is a diagnostic system published by ZERO TO THREE (2005) to address the unique developmental and relationship issues of early childhood. It complements rather than replaces more conventional diagnostic systems such as the *Diagnostic and Statistical Manual of Mental Disorders, Fourth Edition, Text Revision* (DSM-IV-TR; American Psychiatric Association, 2000).

To ensure that there was a trained workforce capable of following up on positive screens and applying the DC: 0-3R system in Colorado, a statewide training-of-trainers initiative was undertaken. This training initiative resulted from a partnership between Project BLOOM; the Harris Program for Child Development and Infant Mental Health, a training program for entry-level and mid-career mental health and early childhood professionals located at the University of Colorado at Denver and Health Sciences Center; and JFK Partners, Colorado's University Center for Excellence in Developmental Disabilities Education, Research and Service. Seventeen trainers in six communities have provided training to more than 100 mental health professionals across Colorado. Colorado was the first state in the nation to implement a DC: 0-3R training-of-trainers model.

To support and sustain this investment in workforce development, the DC: 0-3R was incorporated into the infrastructure of several other child-serving systems. The mental health system includes DC: 0-3R as part of its information management system, allowing for a more accurate picture of the number of young children with mental health problems receiving public mental health services. In addition, when funding was available for early childhood specialists to be placed at each of the publicly funded mental health centers, these specialists were required to receive training in DC: 0-3R. This has led to its inclusion in a local electronic records system in Aurora County. Part C has adopted two diagnoses from DC: 0-3R as established conditions under their eligibility definition—*reactive attachment deprivation/maltreatment* and *regulatory disorders*. Work is progressing to fully integrate DC: 0-3R into the Medicaid billing system by creating a crosswalk to ICD-9, as has been accomplished in other states such as Florida and Arizona. In addition, Colorado's use of the DC: 0-3R led to its integration into the national evaluation of federally funded systems of care, laying the groundwork for a cohort of six new system of care sites focusing on young children and their families that were funded in 2005.

The widespread adoption of the DC: 0-3R system for assessing and diagnosing mental health problems in young children has immediate implications for how services and supports are designed in local systems of care. The DC: 0-3R supports recommended practices by encouraging providers to view the child in different settings over three to five sessions. In addition, Axis 2, which focuses on primary caregiving relationships, reminds providers to view this dimension of early childhood development as central to social and emotional health, not simply as context. Clinicians use the information gained from an assessment process using the DC: 0-3R to highlight caregiving issues, including the importance of routines and predictability and consistency for children, as well as to derive specific suggestions for caregivers about techniques or strategies (e.g., to foster language development or understand emotions).

Adapting the Wraparound Process for Young Children and Families

To provide a structured process for service planning and delivery, nationally known trainers in the wraparound approach worked collaboratively with state and community leaders to determine how this process would need to be adapted for very young children in each of the system of care counties. Unlike families with older children who have been diagnosed with SEDs, families of very young children are entering the system for the first time. They may not have experienced frustration with multiple system barriers or even had a need for help in coordinating services. These families are often still trying to understand and accept the diagnoses of SEDs in their young children, and they may want to take small steps toward intervention. Rather than the sense of urgency experienced when an older child is at imminent risk of problems in school or perhaps contact with the juvenile justice system, families of young children may see their problems as developmental and transitory. There may be a sense that child-focused therapy is all that is needed to support the very young child, and a more comprehensive planning process may appear overwhelming or superfluous. Not all families in Project BLOOM see the value of bringing a large team together to discuss the child and family's needs and to plan services. The logistics of caring for a young child with special needs often leads to challenges when it comes to scheduling meetings. Furthermore, the family's needs for child care, a lack of sleep, the challenge of balancing work and baby care, or parent-specific issues such as mental illness and substance abuse often overshadow the presenting child issues and significantly affect the parent's ability to balance both wraparound planning and support of their child's development. In addition to often being overwhelmed with parenting, young families who have children with special needs may still be coping with their own grief related to not having the children they had imagined. When parents are overwhelmed with other struggles, they may have little left to contribute to the relationships that are the vehicles for the wraparound process and associated interventions.

Another difference is that children at young ages have fewer outside resources to draw on. With older children, fostering youth voice and working toward some independence are important goals, and in many cases, peer support or outside mentors can be engaged in the process. These resources are not appropriate for young children. Young children are still learning social skills, and they are dependent on caregivers in many ways such as helping them to learn emotional regulation. Accordingly, interventions for young children and their families occur at multiple levels (e.g., the child, the parent, the parent–child relationship), making the wraparound process with young children more complex. These differences must be carefully considered as the wraparound process is adapted to serve young children and their families.

As the early childhood system of care communities began to adopt the wraparound approach, many chose wraparound facilitators connected with other systems. Facilitators are generally employed by mental health centers, Part C of IDEA, Head Start, the child welfare system, and school districts. Time for personnel to implement the wraparound approach was garnered through memoranda of understanding with the host agency. It was deemed essential to embed this process into the fabric of each of these existing early childhood programs. Communities reached consensus on the essential elements of wraparound and undertook a comprehensive analysis of how these core wraparound components compared with other planning processes such as the Individualized Family Service Plan (IFSP) of the Part C program of IDEA and several plans used in the child welfare system to support the Family to Family program. Integration of community-specific results occurred at a state-sponsored day-long work session. Through this process, stakeholders discovered that the IFSP of Part C had the most similarities to the core elements of wraparound. The major missing components were a crisis plan and a strengths, needs, and culture discovery process.

Communities designed a wraparound planning protocol that includes a crisis plan and enhances the strengths, needs, and culture discovery process. Once these conceptual issues were resolved, questions about how to fund this process were raised; state-level staff permitted wraparound to qualify as *intensive service coordination,* which could be listed as a service on the IFSP, thereby generating one potential funding source. In addition, Colorado's Part C program renamed *social work services* on their service list as *social-emotional interventions,* thereby providing a funding source for some services identified in the wraparound plan (e.g., mental health consultation) that are not covered by another funding source.

The wraparound approach used in Project BLOOM's communities involves creating a child and family team typically comprising the child's parent(s), other family members as desired, family friends, service and support providers, and other community members as identified by the family (e.g., church clergy, a neighbor, a child care provider). With assistance from the trained wraparound facilitator, the team proceeds to undertake an assessment of the strengths, needs, and culture of the family and to develop a service plan that addresses these areas. Families may be addressing such issues as how to find child care with adequate supports for their child, how to parent a child with mental health issues, or how to stabilize the home living situation.

Service Delivery

An ongoing issue in developing an early childhood mental health system of care is the need to adopt and adapt evidence-based and promising practices for young children and families. In addition, as communities seek to implement these evidence-based interventions, adaptations for local context and the specific populations served need to be undertaken in a deliberate and data-driven manner. Project BLOOM has addressed this complex concern by adopting the Teaching Pyramid, a comprehensive model that incorporates both professional development and the public health framework to guide service delivery. Using this model as a guide, each local system of care selected an array of scientifically-based strategies to incorporate into their array of services and supports.

The Teaching Pyramid Model   Colorado has adopted the Teaching Pyramid model, a conceptual framework that supports early care and education providers in enhancing the social and emotional competency of children ages birth to 5 years by teaching staff to promote social-emotional development, provide support for children's appropriate behavior, and prevent challenging behavior. As shown on Figure 18.3, the model provides a framework for addressing the needs of all children, including those with persistent challenging behavior.

A consortium of universities and organizations was funded by the Office of Head Start and the Child Care Bureau of the Administration on Children, Youth, and Families at the U.S. Department of Health and Human Services to develop a national center, the Center on the Social and Emotional Foundations for Early Learning (CSEFEL; http://www.vanderbilt.edu/csefel/). The consortium includes

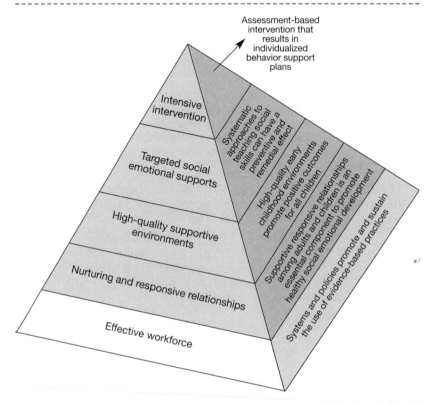

Figure 18.3. CSEFEL pyramid. (*Sources:* Center on the Social and Emotional Foundations for Early Learning, n.d.; Fox, Dunlap, Hemmeter, Joseph, & Strain, 2003.)

Vanderbilt University, the University of Illinois at Urbana-Champaign, the University of Colorado at Denver and Health Sciences Center, the University of South Florida, ZERO TO THREE, and the Georgetown University Center for Child and Human Development. CSEFEL is intended to promote the social-emotional outcomes and enhance the school readiness of children ages birth to 5 years and to serve as a national resource center for disseminating research and evidence-based practices. CSEFEL faculty provide training and technical assistance on the Teaching Pyramid modules to trainers and coaches in a number of states, including Colorado. CSEFEL staff are also facilitating a planning process in a selected group of states focusing on the development of sustainability plans for continuing the capacity-building into the future. Colorado partners selected the Teaching Pyramid training (see Figure 18.3) because it complements their early childhood mental health system of care in several important ways such as:

- Providing a comprehensive, evidence-based conceptual framework that programs and professionals can use to enhance young children's social and emotional development and behavior

- Providing a conceptual framework and common language across disciplines and among trainers and programs

- Providing an inventory of competencies that can be used for self-assessing training, support, and organizational needs

This model describes three interrelated levels of practice that address the social and emotional development of all children. The foundational levels of the pyramid depict universal mental health promotion that addresses the needs that all children have for nurturing, positive, and responsive relationships, as well as high quality environments. The next level targets preventive practices in natural environments that promote systematic, positive teaching and parenting strategies, social skills development, emotional literacy, and environmental adaptations, primarily addressing and attempting to mitigate risk factors for the development of mental health problems. For those children needing more intensive interventions, the model calls for individualized, assessment-based interventions. At the base of the pyramid, supporting the interventions is the need for an infrastructure to plan, evaluate, and sustain the CSEFEL model. CSEFEL was embraced by Colorado because of the compatibility with the early childhood planning, system of care development, and the new focus on early childhood mental health competencies.

Array of Services and Supports   The systems of care in Project BLOOM communities include a broad array of services and supports, including individual, family, and group therapy; medical and medication management; home visitation and home-based services; crisis services; behavior management skills training; care coordination; respite services; family support and education; and mental health consultation. In addition, Project BLOOM communities chose empirically supported practices to include in their array of services depending on the needs of the community.

Implementing approaches that are evidence based involves an investment of both time and money because specific training and supervision are required to ensure adherence to a protocol. Thus, it is important that communities carefully choose interventions and avoid adopting the latest approach without considering the needs of the community or the children to be served.

Each Project BLOOM community chose specific interventions for different reasons. Two communities chose interventions that would be appropriate for settings that they wanted to include in their systems of care. Mesa County chose to implement *The Incredible Years* (Webster-Stratton, 1990, 2003) to address the needs of children within child care settings and to focus on the transition to elementary school. The county comprehensively implemented this intervention throughout numerous child care settings. Support and training was provided by Invest in Kids, a nonprofit organization in Colorado. El Paso County, a larger urban area, wanted to include interventions within medical settings in its service array. *Touch Points*, an approach created by T. Berry Brazelton, M.D. (1994), was implemented to help pediatricians and other health practitioners provide anticipatory guidance to parents at critical periods of their children's development. In 2006, El Paso County hosted Dr. Brazelton to provide training in this approach. El Paso County is developing a cadre of local trainers who will work with primary care offices to help pediatricians become more knowledgeable about children's development, including social and emotional development. This effort will complement the ASQ:SE screening efforts.

The communities also chose interventions because they identified some children who were not responding well to current practices. Data from Project BLOOM children showed that half of the children enrolled had witnessed domestic violence; 65% of their families showed evidence of substance abuse problems; and 9 out of 10 children had family members with serious mental illnesses such as depression. One third of the children were involved in the child welfare system at the time of intake. Clinicians needed robust interventions that could work in a short time to enable successful engagement between parents and children. Consultation was sought to identify effective approaches for working with families at high risk. This resulted in the implementation of several interventions, including Dialectical Behavior Therapy, which has a parenting focus (Linehan, 1993). This intervention is based largely in behavior theory, along with the addition of elements of cognitive therapy, and consists of both individual and group sessions. Child therapists in Project BLOOM communities were trained in this approach and use the groups to help parents manage their own emotions. Parents are then able to attend to the parent–child relationship by applying the same skills to parenting. Training and ongoing clinical coaching are provided by the Community Infant Program in Boulder, Colorado.

To further develop the array of early childhood mental health services and supports, Project BLOOM surveyed early childhood therapists to identify what interventions they were using, which interventions they considered effective, and their level of expertise in utilizing specific interventions. This survey was used to identify service gaps and the need for investment of targeted resources to adopt additional interventions or protocols within the community systems of care. Through this process, four approaches emerged as practices in which therapists wanted to gain expertise—*Circle of Security, Parent–Child Interaction Therapy, Trauma-Focused Cognitive Behavioral Therapy,* and *Child–Parent Psychotherapy for Family Violence*—all of which include strategies to strengthen the parent–child relationship, a critical component of early childhood mental health therapy.

Two of these approaches—*Circle of Security* and *Parent–Child Interaction Therapy*—were subsequently implemented in Project BLOOM communities. Fremont County had been providing early childhood mental health services for some time and had invested in training several early childhood mental health specialists. The specialists noted that a number of children and families did not seem to respond to therapeutic interventions; these families were often involved in the child welfare system and had highly disturbed parent–child relationships. *Circle of Security* was embraced as a model to address the treatment needs of these children and families (Marvin, Cooper, Hoffman, & Powell, 2002). The approach seeks to strengthen parents' ability to observe and improve their own caregiving capacity by identifying their unique challenges with the attachment cycle and developing individualized intervention strategies. The developers of this approach used 50 years of attachment research to create a video-based intervention. In an extremely supportive environment, videotapes are reviewed that help parents see their behavior and their children's reactions. Although research on the practice is not as yet extensive, initial results have been promising (Marvin et al., 2002). Fremont County has been supporting one of its therapists to become certified in this approach and has also been working with the developers to create a module specifically for home visiting programs. This module will ultimately be included in Parents and Teachers, the county's existing home visiting program.

Parent–Child Interaction Therapy is an evidence-based practice designed to teach parents of children ages 2–8 years how to manage their children's behavior by developing warm and responsive relationships (Herschell, Calzada, Eyberg, & McNeil, 2002). This empirically supported approach is designed to treat conduct disorders by improving the quality of parent–child relationships and changing parent–child interaction patterns through a highly structured intervention. Aurora County has implemented this practice extensively in its early childhood system of care.

CURRENT CHALLENGES AND FUTURE DIRECTIONS

As policy makers and advocates have advanced system of care work at the federal, state, and local levels on behalf of children with SEDs, there has been a growing emphasis on efforts to extend this framework to younger children with and at risk for mental health disorders. In some states and communities, this extension builds on other early childhood system efforts such as those funded by the federal Maternal and Child Health Bureau through their ECCS initiative or the Part C/Early Intervention programs funded by the U.S. Department of Education. In other jurisdictions, the focus on young children and their caregivers has been led by professionals with clinical expertise in infant mental health seeking to integrate a more intentional focus on these issues for families at higher risk. In the SAMHSA-funded system of care grants funded in 2005, six sites chose to focus their efforts on children younger than the age of 10 years, adding volumes to the lessons learned from Colorado and Vermont. Vermont was the first system of care grantee to focus on early childhood mental health and the only grantee to develop a statewide system of care for very young children. The experience of all of these sites in building early childhood mental health systems of care underscores the need to integrate mental health into the existing array of services and settings where young children and families live and visit. Their experience has also pointed to the many system barriers that continue to hinder attempts to effectively meet the mental health needs of infants, toddlers, preschoolers, and their caregivers.

At the federal level, there continues to be a lack of consensus on how to integrate mental health promotion and prevention into system of care language and frameworks. There is a noted tension between those who believe that the federal legislation that authorizes the system of care grant program should remain focused on those children who have SEDs and those who would like the focus of these efforts to broaden to include those who are at risk for mental health disorders. There are arguably too few resources devoted to meeting the mental health needs of children with SEDs and their families, and categorical programs exist to ensure that the most vulnerable populations retain some share of the limited resources available at the federal level. The continued reliance on a siloed approach to funding systems of care, however, flies in the face of many of the tenets that underlie this framework. A system of care construct could easily lend itself to integrated funding from multiple federal agencies to promote a developmental or public health approach to mental health.

The policy barriers to effective system building for young children with or at risk for mental health challenges are driven in large part by the unique developmental demands of this population. The current public mental health system requires the assignment of a DSM-IV-TR diagnosis to authorize and pay for mental health services, something few clinicians who work with young children are willing to do. Furthermore, the dyadic, multigenerational, or consultative approaches that are recommended practice in working with young children and their caregivers are not easily reimbursed under current policies that typically require a face-to-face contact with a single identified patient. The EPSDT program's promise to pay for any and all services that a child enrolled in Medicaid might need, once such a need is determined through a screening visit, remains far out of reach for most impoverished children in the United States. The failure to conduct routine mental health screening for young children, coupled with a serious lack of mental health practitioners with expertise in the DC: 0-3R and evidence-based treatment modalities for this age group, results in few infants and young children receiving publicly funded mental health services. Even in the Part C/Early Intervention and child welfare systems, where vulnerable infants, toddlers, and preschoolers have already been identified, far too few are receiving the mental health services and supports needed to address these vulnerabilities.

The challenges in integrating effective mental health promotion, prevention, and intervention strategies into early childhood settings is made even more difficult by the fact that there is no system of early childhood services and supports. Young children and their families obtain formal services and informal supports through a largely voluntary process until they reach mandatory school age. Parents can choose from an array of publicly funded and privately offered services, and they often make ample use of informal community-based resources from kin and neighbors during the early years of their children's lives. The child care network is a similar patchwork of public, private, and kin options that is loosely regulated and relies on a workforce that is poorly compensated and often highly stressed. There are specially focused programs for families where additional support might be helpful, including those targeted to single mothers, adolescent mothers, and first-time mothers, but many do not have mental health professionals as partners in program or curriculum design or implementation.

CONCLUSION

As policy makers, practitioners, program managers, and advocates address the complex challenges of designing, implementing, and evaluating early childhood mental health systems of care, it is important to remember that the unique needs of young children (e.g., their dependence on other caregivers for meeting their social-emotional needs, the qualitative differences in what is classified as a mental health disorder, the dyadic approaches to ameliorating mental health problems that may arise, the new array of partners who need to be engaged) must be central. To truly be effective, policy makers should not seek to build a mental health system for young children, but should instead integrate the best scientifically valid mental health services and supports into the early childhood continuum.

REFERENCES

American Psychiatric Association. (2000). *Diagnostic and statistical manual of mental disorders* (4th ed., text rev.). Washington, DC: Author.

Betts, W. (2006). *Early childhood mental health screening pilot project final report.* Report submitted to The Colorado Health Foundation (formerly HealthONE Alliance), Denver, CO.

Brazelton, T.B. (1994). *Touchpoints 0 to 3: Your child's emotional and behavioral development.* Cambridge: Da Capo Press.

Brennan, E.M., Bradley, J.R., Allen, M.D., & Perry, D.F. (2007). *The evidence base for mental health consultation in early childhood settings: Research synthesis addressing staff and program outcomes.* Manuscript submitted for publication.

Center on the Social and Emotional Foundations for Early Learning. (n.d.). *The pyramid model for promoting the social and emotional development of infants and young children: A Colorado Collaborative Initiative.* Available online at http://www.vanderbilt.edu/csefel/CO.CSEFELPartnership.pdf

Child Abuse Prevention and Treatment Act of 1974, PL 93-247, 42 U.S.C. §§ 5101 *et seq.*

Cicchetti, D., Toth, S.L., & Rogosch, F.A. (1999). The efficacy of toddler parent psychotherapy to increase attachment security in offspring of depressed mothers. *Attachment Human Development, 1,* 34–66.

Cohen, E., & Kaufmann, R. (2000). *Early childhood mental health consultation.* Washington, DC: Center for Mental Health Services of the Substance Abuse and Mental Health Services Administration and the Georgetown University Child Development Center.

Colorado Department of Public Health and Environment. (2005). Health statistics section. *Colorado Child Health Survey 2005 dataset.* Denver: Author.

Deblinger, E., Stauffer, L., & Steer, R. (2001). Comparative efficacies of supportive and cognitive behavioral group therapies for children who were sexually abused and their nonoffending mothers. *Child Maltreatment, 6*(4), 332–343.

Domitrovich, C.E., Cortes, R.C., & Kusché, C.A. (2002, May). *PATHS Preschool: Promoting social and emotional competence in young children.* Paper presented at the Society for Prevention Research, Seattle.

Edwall, G. (2005). *Early childhood mental health: The continuum.* St. Paul: Minnesota Association for Children's Mental Health. Available online at http://www.macmh.org/info_resources/articles/glenace_article.php

Erikson, M.F., Egeland, B., Rose, T.K., & Simon, J. (2002). *STEEP facilitator's guide.* Minneapolis: Regents of the University of Minnesota.

Fox, L., Dunlap, G., Hemmeter, M.L., Joseph, G.E., & Strain, P.S. (2003, July). *The Teaching Pyramid: A model for supporting social competence and preventing challenging behavior in young children.* Available online at http://www.vanderbilt.edu/csefel/modules/module4/handout7.pdf

Gilliam, W.S. (2007, March). *Findings from a random controlled trial of a statewide early childhood mental health consultation system.* Paper presented at the 20th Annual Research Conference: A System of Care for Children's Mental Health: Expanding the Research Base, Tampa, FL.

Gould, M. (2000). *Summary of findings from the Colorado survey of incidence of mental health problems among young children in early childhood programs.* Report submitted to the Colorado Department of Human Services.

Hepburn, K.S., Kaufmann, R.K., Perry, D.F., Allen, M.D., Brennan, E.M., & Green, B.L. (2007). *Early childhood mental health consultation: An evaluation tool kit.* Portland, OR: Research and Training Center on Family Support and Children's Mental Health, and Georgetown University, National Technical Assistance Center for Children's Mental Health.

Herschell, A., Calzada, E., Eyberg, S.M., & McNeil, C.B. (2002) Parent–child interaction therapy: New directions in research. *Cognitive and Behavioral Practice, 9,* 9–16.

Hoover, S. (2006, June). *Study of current status of children with social, emotional, and behavioral concerns and the providers who support them.* Report submitted to the Colorado Department of Human Services, Division of Childcare, Denver.

Huang, L.N., & Isaacs, M.R. (2007). Early childhood mental health: A focus on culture and context. In B.A. Stroul & R.M. Friedman (Series Eds.) & D.F. Perry, R.K Kaufman, & J. Knitzer (Vol. Eds.), *Systems of care for children's mental health series: Social and emotional health in early childhood: Building bridges between services and systems* (pp. 37–62). Baltimore: Paul H. Brookes Publishing Co.

Huang, L, Stroul, B., Friedman, R., et al. (2005). Transforming mental health care for children and their families. *American Psychologist, 60*(6), 615–627.

Individuals with Disabilities Education Act (IDEA) Amendments of 1997, PL 105-17, 20 U.S.C. §§ 1400 *et seq.*

Johnston, K., & Brinamen, C. (2006). *Mental health consultation in childcare: Transforming relationships among directors, staff, and families.* Washington, DC: ZERO TO THREE.

Joseph, G.E., & Strain, P.S. (2003). Comprehensive evidence-based social-emotional curricula for young children: An analysis of efficacious adoption potential. *Topics in Early Childhood Special Education, 23*(2), 65–76.

Kaufmann, R., & Hepburn, K. (2007). In B.A. Stroul & R.M. Friedman (Series Eds.) & D.F. Perry, R.K Kaufman, & J. Knitzer (Vol. Eds.), *Systems of care for children's mental health series: Social and emotional health in early childhood: Building bridges between services and systems* (pp. 121–146). Baltimore: Paul H. Brookes Publishing Co.

Knitzer, J. (2000). Early childhood mental health services: A policy and systems perspective. In J.P. Shonkoff & S.J. Meisels (Eds.), *Handbook of early childhood intervention* (pp. 416–438). New York: Cambridge University Press.

Lieberman, A.F. (2004). Child–parent psychotherapy: A relationship-based approach to the treatment of mental health disorders in infancy and childhood. In A.J. Sameroff, S.C. McDonough, & K.L. Rosenblum (Eds.), *Treating parent infant relationships problems: strategies for intervention* (pp. 97–122). New York: Guilford Press

Linehan M.M. (1993). *Cognitive-behavioral treatment of borderline personality disorder.* New York: Guilford Press.

Luthar, S.S., & Sussman, N.E. (2000). Relational psychotherapy mothers' group: A developmentally informed intervention for at-risk mothers. *Developmental Psychopathology, 12,* 235–253.

Marvin, R., Cooper, G., Hoffman, K., & Powell, B. (2002). The Circle of Security Project: Attachment-based intervention with caregiver–preschool child dyads. *Attachment and Human Development, 4*(1), 107–124.

Nikkel, P. (2007). Building partnerships with families. In B.A. Stroul & R.M. Friedman (Series Eds.) & D.F. Perry, R.K Kaufman, & J. Knitzer (Vol. Eds.), *Systems of care for children's mental health series: Social and emotional health in early childhood: Building bridges between services and systems* (pp. 147–168). Baltimore: Paul H. Brookes Publishing Co.

Perry, D.F., Dunne, M.C., McFadden, L., & Campbell, D. (2008). Reducing the risk for preschool expulsion: Mental health consultation for young children with challenging behavior. *Journal of Child and Family Studies, 17,* 44–54.

Perry, D.F., Kaufmann, R.K., & Knitzer, J. (Vol. Eds.). (2007). *Systems of care for children's mental health series: Social and emotional health in early childhood: Building bridges between services and systems.* Baltimore: Paul H. Brookes Publishing Co.

Raver, C.C., Jones, S., Li-Grining, C., Sardin-Adjei, L., & Jones-Lewis, D. (2007, March). *Mental health consultation as a pathway to improving preschool classroom processes: Preliminary findings from a randomized trial implemented in Head Start settings.* Paper presented at the 20th Annual Research Conference: A System of Care for Children's Mental Health: Expanding the Research Base, Tampa, FL.

Squires, J., Bricker, D., & Twombly, E. (with Yockelson, S., Davis, M.S., & Kim, Y.). (2002). *Ages & Stages Questionnaires®: Social-Emotional (ASQ:SE): A parent-completed, child-monitoring system for social-emotional behaviors.* Baltimore: Paul H. Brookes Publishing Co.

Stainback-Tracy, K. (Ed.). (2004). *Social and emotional screening for infants, toddlers, and preschoolers in Colorado: Summary of recommendations from Colorado workgroups.* Unpublished manuscript.

Walker, H.M., Kavanagh, K., Stiller, B., Golly, A., Herbert, H., & Feil, E.G. (1998). First step to success: An early intervention approach for preventing school antisocial behavior. *Journal of Emotional and Behavioral Disorders, 6,* 66–81.

Webster-Stratton, C. (1990). *The teacher's and children's videotape series: Dina Dinosaur's social skills and problem-solving curriculum.* Seattle: University of Washington Press.

Webster-Stratton, C., & Reid, M.J. (2003) Treating conduct problems and strengthening social and emotional competence in young children: The Dina Dinosaur Treatment Program. *Journal of Emotional and Behavioral Disorders, 11,* 130–143.

Zeanah, C. (2007). *Handbook of infant mental health* (2nd ed., p. 11). New York: The Guilford Press.

Zeanah, P.D., Stafford, B., & Zeanah, C.H. (2005). *Clinical interventions to enhance infant mental health: A selective review.* Los Angeles: National Center for Infant and Early Childhood Healthy Policy at UCLA.

ZERO TO THREE. (2002). *Definition of infant mental health.* Unpublished manuscript.

ZERO TO THREE. (2005). *Diagnostic classification of mental health and developmental disorders of infancy and early childhood* (Rev. ed.). Washington DC: Author.

19

Services for Youth in Transition to Adulthood in Systems of Care

Hewitt B. "Rusty" Clark, Nicole Deschênes,
DeDe Sieler, Melanie E. Green, Gwendolyn White, and Diane L. Sondheimer

---

"It is our hope that every youth who participates in our program will leave with a renewed sense of self and that they will be healthy, confident, capable, and empowered."
—Melanie Green, Youth Coordinator, Options

Young adults experience dramatic changes across all areas of development during their transition to adulthood. Young people's decisions, choices, and associated experiences set a foundation for their transition to future adult roles in the domains of employment, education, living situation, and community-life functioning. This period of transition is especially challenging for the more than 3 million youth and young adults with serious emotional disturbances or serious mental illness (SED/SMI) (Clark & Davis, 2000; Vander Stoep, Bersford, et al., 2000). This population of young people has a higher secondary school dropout rate, higher arrest and unemployment rates, and a lower independent living rate compared with their peers without disabilities (Davis & Vander Stoep, 1997; Wagner, 2005).

In a community-based study, young adults with severe psychiatric disorders were nearly 14 times less likely to complete secondary school compared with their peers without disabilities, and 44% of the failure to complete school was attributed to their disorders (Vander Stoep, Bersford, et al., 2000; Vander Stoep, Weiss, Saldana Kuo, Cheney, & Cohen, 2003). In addition, young adults with SED/SMI have significantly higher unemployment rates (34%–82%) after exiting high school in contrast to their peers without disabilities. This difference is largely attributed to the lack of social skills necessary to maintain a given job (Bullis & Fredericks, 2002; Carter & Wehby, 2003; Chadsey & Beyer, 2001; Gresham, Sugai, & Horner, 2001; Rylance, 1998). Fragmented services, varying eligibility criteria, different funding mechanisms, and distinctly different philosophies across the child and adult mental health systems further complicate the situation for young people with SED/SMI by making their transition to the adult mental health system and their ability to obtain appropriate services and supports challenging endeavors.

The Partnerships for Youth Transition (PYT) initiative provided an opportunity for the establishment of five demonstration community sites to examine ways to improve the outcomes of transition-age youth with SED/SMI. In 2002, the Substance Abuse and Mental Health Services Administration (SAMHSA) of the U.S. Department of Health and Human Services and the U.S. Department of Education, Office of Special Education and Rehabilitative Services awarded approximately $2.5 million annually for 4 years to fund five cooperative agreements to develop the PYT initiative. The cooperative agreement programs were created to allow competitively selected communities and counties to develop, implement, stabilize, and document models of comprehensive transition systems to improve outcomes for youth and young adults ages 14–25 with SED/SMI as they enter the period of emerging adulthood. To influence policy at the national level, SAMHSA leadership involved several national partners for this initiative. Some of these included the U.S. Department of Education, the Jim Casey Youth Opportunities Initiative, the National Center on Youth Transition (NCYT), and the Annie E. Casey Foundation. Representatives from these and other organizations became a part of the community of learning that emerged from the PYT initiative.

To achieve the goal of developing transition systems for youth and young adults, each of the PYT sites in Washington, Pennsylvania, Maine, Minnesota, and Utah undertook efforts to provide community-based transition services and supports to this population of youth and their families in a manner consistent with the community culture, accepted models, and state and local policy. Although the federal funding for these sites ended in September 2006, as of 1 year later, four of the five communities (i.e., Washington, Pennsylvania, Minnesota, Utah) have sustained all, or at least a substantial portion, of their transition services and supports for serving youth and young adults with SED/SMI and their families.

This chapter highlights the development, implementation, and preliminary evaluation of the transition systems developed by the PYT sites. Specifically, this chapter provides: 1) an overview of the PYT initiative and delineation of the age-appropriate interventions and support services that were common across the majority of the sites; 2) an overview of the Transition to Independence Process (TIP) model framework, including an outline of the transition domains of employment and career, education, living situations, and community-life functioning; 3) brief descriptions of the community transition systems implemented at the five PYT sites, with particular attention to the involvement of youth, family, and local and state partners; 4) preliminary PYT evaluation outcome findings; and 5) lessons learned at the practice, system, and policy levels. Thus, this chapter is designed to provide the reader with promising practices and lessons learned related to planning, implementing, and sustaining community transition systems for youth and young adults with SED/SMI and their families.

OVERVIEW OF THE PARTNERSHIPS
FOR YOUTH TRANSITION INITIATIVE

Under the cooperative funding agreement, the PYT sites were required to conduct planning with community stakeholders to review, adapt, and adopt promising models of transition to adulthood systems to address the strengths and needs of the community as related to transition-age youth and young adults with SED/SMI and their families. The capacity to offer an array of relevant services was achieved through partnering with community agencies and organizations; developing new services; and employing the creative work of young people, families, and other informal and formal stakeholders in the community who were willing to provide necessary and appropriate services and supports.

Young people and family representatives were involved in the planning, design, and selection of services and supports provided within the PYT initiative. In collaboration with youth, families, and other PYT partners and stakeholders, a theory-based logic model was developed for each PYT community site to visually illustrate the underlying assumptions and service delivery strategies being designed and incorporated into their systems as active ingredients in working with this population of young people and their families. Table 19.1 provides an overview of the expectations for PYT sites, including the primary activities to be accomplished, the program elements to be implemented, and the desired results and products to be completed within each site over each of the 4 years.

The NCYT at the University of South Florida served as the training and technical assistance partner to assist the PYT community sites in their efforts across all of the required activities and products (see the NCYT web site for additional information about its programmatic, systemic, and evaluation services at http://ncyt.fmhi.usf.edu). The leadership of the NCYT worked with the communities and state leaders through site-specific consultation, training, cross-site teleconferencing, and biannual PYT cross-site forums. The teleconferences and PYT forums focused on themes that the sites and national partners established as priorities during the evolution of their programs (e.g., youth engagement, employment, educational opportunities). The PYT forums and cross-site teleconferences served to develop a community of learning, fostering an ongoing exchange of information about the issues that sites were wrestling with, challenged by, and succeeding with.

A major assumption underlying the PYT initiative was that communities could expand their collaborative efforts to tap into an additional array of relevant services and supports for these youth and young adults and their families. The PYT community sites were to consider the following features as they developed and implemented their transition service systems:

- Outreach and engagement

- Assessment of individual strengths and needs

- Age-appropriate mental health care, including transition from the child to adult mental health system where appropriate

Table 19.1. Partnerships for youth transition: Summary of program activities

Year	Primary activity	Program elements	Desired results/ products
1	Collaborative strategic planning process *Goal*: To build upon the model comprehensive youth transition program proposed in the grant application by determining details for implementation.	Engage all relevant partner organizations in collaborative strategic planning that includes: • Mental health services • Substance abuse services • Foster care and/or child welfare • Corporate/business community • Criminal justice/juvenile justice • Education and/or special education • Community-based organizations representing the ethnic, racial, and cultural diversity of the geographic region in which the model will be implemented • Young people and their families	1. Theory-based logic model (to link the design of the transition program with implementation involving all community partner organizations) 2. Written action plan 3. Process evaluation (to document the strategic planning process)
2	Implementation of the program model *Goal*: To implement the transition program.	Enhance existing programming to fill gaps in the model comprehensive youth transition program Align resources and coordinate services Train staff Execute/renew needed interagency partnerships Collect quality assurance data	1. Document the final operational transition system into a program manual. 2. Enroll and serve young people, collect demographic and other data based on the logic model. 3. Complete a process evaluation to examine how implementation occurred. 4. The comprehensive youth transition program is addressing all specific domains and additional ones based on the logic model. 5. A structure for the comprehensive youth transition program exists and coordinates and integrates services. 6. Identify and define measurable short-term outcomes.

Year	Primary activity	Program elements	Desired results/products
3–4	Stabilization of the Comprehensive Youth Transition Program *Goal*: To ensure that service delivery is consistent and of high quality.	Update sections of the written action plan regarding sustainability Conduct annual process evaluations Develop an integrated management information system that will allow cross-site evaluation Report outcomes annually to CMHS/SAMHSA	1. Draft sustainability plan 2. Process evaluation 3. Outcomes/data 4. Develop fidelity measures

Key: CMHS, Center for Mental Health Services; SAMHSA, Substance Abuse and Mental Health Services Administration.

- Substance abuse services

- Assistance with housing needs

- Vocational training, career development, and employment support services

- Educational support services

- Services to help develop and nurture instrumental living skills and proper socialization

- Family and peer supports

- Care management or service coordination

In their proposals, applicants were required to describe a model or framework for a Comprehensive Youth Transition Program they planned to implement under the PYT initiative. Applicants were to tie their proposed transition systems to previously existing literature on recommended practices and strategies for providing services to youth with SED/SMI. Most PYT sites developed a transition system that incorporated most, if not all, of the principles of the TIP model (Clark, Deschênes, & Jones, 2000; Clark & Foster-Johnson, 1996).

OVERVIEW OF THE TRANSITION TO INDEPENDENCE PROCESS MODEL

The TIP system prepares youth and young adults for their movement into adult roles through an individualized process that engages them in their own futures planning process and provides them with developmentally appropriate services and supports. The TIP model involves youth and young adults, their families, and other informal key players in a process that facilitates their movement toward greater self-sufficiency and successful achievement of their goals related to each of the transition domains: employment and career, education, living situation, and community-life functioning, which is composed of subdomains such as daily living skills; friends, family, and other social supports; emotional adjustment and well-being; leisure time skills; physical health; and parenting. The TIP system is operationalized through seven guidelines that drive practice-level activities with young people and also provides a framework for program and community systems to support and facilitate this effort. These guidelines, refined from those published by Clark and Foster-Johnson (1996), are listed in Table 19.2.

The TIP guidelines synthesize the current research and practice knowledge base for transition facilitation with youth and young adults with SED/SMI and their families. The TIP model is a *practice model*, meaning that it can be delivered by personnel within different service delivery platforms such as care management or a team format (e.g., Assertive Community Treatment [ACT]). At the heart of the TIP practice model are proactive care managers with small caseloads (i.e., transition facilitators such as life coaches, transition specialists, or coaches that serve 15 or fewer youth or young adults). In operationalizing their transition systems, the five PYT sites either fully implemented the TIP model or adopted many of the guidelines. Each site was required to develop a logic model to provide a visual display of their transition system. A generic logic model for the TIP model is provided in Figure 19.1 to illustrate the TIP system components, some of the community contextual factors to be considered in implementation, and indicators of the planned outcomes or impact from the transition system.

Table 19.2.   Seven Transition to Independence Process (TIP) system guidelines

---

Engage young people through relationship development, person-centered planning, and a focus on their futures.

Tailor services and supports to be accessible, coordinated, developmentally-appropriate, and build on strengths to enable the young people to pursue their goals across all transition domains.

Acknowledge and develop personal choice and social responsibility with young people.

Ensure a safety-net of support by involving a young person's parents, family members, and other informal and formal key players.

Enhance young persons' competencies to assist them in achieving greater self-sufficiency and confidence.

Maintain an outcome focus in the TIP system at the young person, program, and community levels.

Involve young people, parents, and other community partners in the TIP system at the practice, program, and community levels.

Reprinted from Transition to Independence Process web site, http://tip.fmhi.usf.edu.

Note: For more detail regarding the TIP model and its guidelines and associated practices, refer to the TIP System Development and Operation Manual at the TIP web site: http://tip.fmhi.usf.edu.

PARTNERSHIPS FOR YOUTH TRANSITION COMMUNITY SITES

The key features of the transition systems developed by each of the PYT sites are summarized in Table 19.3, which provides a cross-site view of the variation in target populations and activities across communities.

Clark County, Washington: Options Program

As part of the Washington State mental health managed care system, the Clark County Regional Support Network was initially the mental health provider for all of Clark County. Since the 1990s, Clark County has built a family-driven system of care based on the principles of individualized and tailored care. Through the PYT initiative, Clark County built on its system base to create a comprehensive, integrated system for transition-age youth and young adults with SED/SMI through the: 1) adoption of the TIP model; 2) use of an ACT team involving a service delivery model in which treatment is provided by a team of professionals such as mental health care managers, a psychiatrist, a nurse, a substance use specialist, and a vocational rehabilitation counselor (Bridgeo, Davis, & Florida, 2000); and 3) an emphasis on the supported employment approach as a key component of the PYT program.

During the strategic planning process, PYT stakeholders and partners, including young people and family members, developed a unified PYT vision, clarified the strengths and challenges of the service system, and developed a theory-based logic model for its planned transition system. The initial priority target population of the transition system was youth with SED/SMI exiting the juvenile justice system.

From the start of the Clark County PYT planning process, the voice of youth and young adults was viewed as essential in the development and implementation of the innovative transition system. Young people were active participants on the Community Transition Steering Committee, and they led the process in establishing the name for the program—Options. During the planning phase of the PYT initiative, young people insisted that, to be effective, outreach and activities needed to occur in youth-friendly locations that had no overt affiliation with any of the public mental health facilities. The PYT leaders listened to young people's suggestions, and they were ultimately successful in locating the Options personnel in a beautiful Victorian house in the community known as the Youth House. The mission of the Youth House, as articulated by young people, is to encourage positive youth development through strengthening youth and adult relationships and to support efforts by and for youth. It is an inclusive, youth-friendly location that honors diversity and operates with joy.

Young people helped to develop the space within the Youth House, including some areas that adults can only enter when accompanied by young people. The Youth House provides other youth services, including a TeenTalk "warm line" phone support service and the Clark County Youth Advisory Commission for the County Commissioners. Thus, there is no stigma associated with young

TIP General Logic Model

The mission of the Transition to Independence Process (TIP) system is to assist young people with SED/SMI in making a successful transition into adulthood, with all young persons achieving, within their potential, their goals in the transition domains of employment, education, living situation, personal effectiveness/well-being, and community-life functioning.

Situation Where we are	Activities What we do	Who Who is involved	Outcomes-Impact What the impacts will be long-term
Youth *Challenges:* Poor outcomes in: Education (e.g., high drop out rates, difficulties related to accessing specialized training or higher education programs) Employment (e.g., unstable employment) Living situation (e.g., homeless) Community life (e.g., involvement with juvenile justice, mental health, co-morbidity, adolescent pregnancy) *Assets:* Individual strengths & good will **Family** *Challenges:* Difficulties relating/communicating with young person leading to conflicts	• Engage young people through relationship development, person-centered planning, and a focus on their futures. • Tailor services and supports to be accessible, coordinated, developmentally-appropriate, and built on strengths to enable the young people to pursue their goals across all transition domains. • Acknowledge and develop personal choice and social responsibility with young people.	• Young people/young adults • Youth councils • Families & family advocates • Natural supports • Peers/mentors • Schools (e.g., teachers, social workers, nurses, principals, guidance counselors, administrators, in-service/ training personnel) • Vocational schools & institutions of higher education • Formal providers (e.g., transition facilitators/ specialists, children & adult mental health,	**Youth** Goal attainment & positive engagement in: *Education* (e.g.,⇑ graduate and school completers, successful entry to post-secondary education programs—college, vocational technical school) *Employment* (e.g., obtain and retain valued employment; access to positions with advancement possibilities & benefits; sufficient income to support self) *Living situation* (e.g., access to safe, stable and affordable community living arrangement, stability in living with a preferred person or alone/independently, access to transportation, satisfaction with living arrangement) *Community life* (e.g., engagement & participation in community life/activities; access to community-based/integrated leisure/activities; access to needed support services; affordable health care; ⇓ adolescent pregnancy; ⇓ JJ involvement; ⇑ social, physical and

Feeling young person is vulnerable/needs to be protected (e.g., how to let go, yet be supportive)

Assets:
Family strengths

System & community
Challenges:
Ignorance of needs (e.g., health insurance, access to community-based services, self-advocacy skills)

Stigma & segregation (e.g., SED centers, jail)

Gap of services (e.g., no low-cost housing available, different eligibility criteria)

Lack of coordination & flexibility (e.g., between youth serving agencies and adult systems, co-morbidity)

Lack of knowledge/training (e.g., how to empower youth while being family-centered/focused)

Assets:
Dedicated staff
Awareness of challenge
Neighborhood resources
Increasing levels of inter-agency collaboration
Legislation
Funding

- Ensure a safety-net of support by involving a young person's parents, family members, and other informal and formal key players.
- Enhance young persons' competencies to assist them in achieving greater self-sufficiency and confidence.
- Maintain an outcome focus in the TIP system at the young person, program, and community levels.
- Involve young people, parents, and other natural and community partners in the TIP system at the practice, program, and community levels.

health clinics & physicians, probation officers)
- Private agencies/practitioners
- Employers
- Housing
- Parks & recreation
- Media
- Community/resources development
- Justice representatives/police
- Government representatives—local, state and federal
- Legislators/political representatives
- Foundations/grants initiatives

---

emotional well-being; ⇑ supportive relationships and life long family-like connections)

Family
⇑ Competency for family members/representatives (e.g., self-efficacy)
⇑ Social support (e.g., maintenance of positive relationship with young person and others)
⇑ Positive relationship with young person & others
⇑ Involvement/engagement in planning, implementing, evaluating activities at youth & system levels.

System & community
⇑ Number of transitioning youth accessed and engaged
⇑ Linkages between youth, families, providers and community (e.g., flexible infrastructure/partnerships, data sharing)
⇑ Training and support for youth, family, providers and community (e.g., expanded eligibility to programs; development of required community-based supports and services)
⇑ Public support & practices fostering opportunities for young people to succeed in 4 transition domains (e.g., flexible funding arrangements; inclusive policies and legislation)

Figure 19.1. Transition to Independence Process (TIP) generic logic model. (Reprinted from Transition to Independence Process web site, http://tip.fmhi.usf.edu) (Key: JJ, juvenile justice; SED, serious emotional disturbances; SMI, serious mental illness.)

Table 19.3. Overview and highlights of the transition systems in the Partnerships for Youth Transition sites

Site	Target population	Goal	Program characteristics and activities
Clark County Department of Community Services in Vancouver, Washington (Options)	Youth and young adults ages 14–21 with serious emotional disturbances (SED) or serious mental illness (SMI), and then may continue serving up to age 25 Emphasis on youth who are in, or at imminent risk of, an out-of-home placement (e.g., incarceration, hospitalization, homelessness) Most were initially involved with an established wraparound team in juvenile justice system	Develop an effective approach to supporting youth with complex needs and their families as they complete their transformation to adulthood, based on an investigation of best practices.	Theory-based logic model Adoption and adaptation of the Transition to Independence Process (TIP) system to their community Strong commitment to implementing positive youth development principles and practices Options services and supports provided by TIP team operating out of a Victorian Community Youth House TIP model and supported employment Continuous quality improvement—using data to inform their management and broader decision-making
Allegheny County Department of Human Services, Pennsylvania (PYT-SOCI sites)	Youth and young adults ages 14 to 21 with SED or SMI, and then may continue serving up to age 25 Priority given to serving their families in the communities of Sto-Rox and Wilkinsburg, two municipalities with economic challenges that border the City of Pittsburgh	Obtain productive employment, safe living situations, community involvement, including satisfying social relationships, and cultural and ethnic integration.	Two distinct programs, each located in a community setting with support and oversight from one central office Integration of the TIP and system of care (SOC) principles to create a developmentally appropriate system of supports and services for these young people

Program	Population served	Goal	Key features
Department of Behavioral and Development Services and Maine Medical Center, Portland, Maine (Odyssey)	Youth and young adults ages 14–21 with SED or SMI, and then may continue serving up to age 25 Selection of those with first-time hospitalization in a psychiatric treatment facility	Increasing educational achievement and employment for youth is a desired result for young people because of the rationale that work plays a central role in the lives of adults.	Authentic community-driven practice: youth, family, community, and system partnerships Value-based service delivery process Connecting to and strengthening of community resources Youth involvement, including paid positions for young people at the community and administrative levels Continuous quality improvement Multidisciplinary team of professionals Located at the Career Center Early identification of needs Linkages with medical services Transition Linkage Coalition (TLC) Supported employment Educational component: mentors and anatomy of leadership. Support/services offered to family members Implemented in four rural counties (three community mental health centers)
PACT-4 Families Collaborative in Willmar, Minnesota (PRIDE-4)	Youth and young adults ages 14 to 21 with SED or SMI, and then may continue serving up to age 25	Assist youth and young adults with mental health needs to successfully transition into adulthood.	

(continued)

Table 19.3. *(Continued)*

Site	Target population	Goal	Program characteristics and activities
PACT-4 *(continued)*	Served across a four county rural area Priority given to youth who need to complete their high school education requirements or are in immediate need of a place to live		Adaptation of SOC and TIP system guidelines Family liaison—family involvement staff—assists parents of program participants in obtaining information and support Youth involvement Collaborative of more than 100 agencies
Utah Department of Human Services (RECONNECT)	Youth and young adults ages 14–21 with SED or SMI, and then may continue serving up to age 25 Priority on three subgroups: 1. Traditional community mental health center (CMHC) clients (Medicaid eligible, youth in custody) 2. Nontraditional CMHC clients: (GLBTQ, homeless, physical disabilities) 3. Underserved (currently receiving services at CMHCs, but at an inadequate level—ethnic/racial minorities, refugees, deaf/hearing impaired, and youth as parents)	Mobilize and coordinate community resources to assist youth to successfully transition to adulthood and achieve full potential in life.	Implemented in five community mental health centers serving an 11-county catchment area Adaptation of SOC and TIP system guidelines Transition Facilitators were also trained as job coaches Use of Ansell-Casey Life Skills Assessment Youth Action Council (YAC) "Growing Up Without Growing Apart" curriculum for parents and family members Plan is for the demonstration to lead to the application of the transition system in communities throughout the state. This replication is occurring.

Key: GLBTQ, gay, lesbian, bisexual, transgender, or questioning youth.

people entering this facility. The Options' team includes a project manager, a youth coordinator, transition facilitators, and a job developer to assist youth in establishing and achieving goals across the transition domains of employment and career, educational opportunities, living situation, and community-life functioning.

As noted, the Options transition system was originally based on the three foundations—the TIP model, ACT, and supported employment. Over the course of system implementation, it was found that the TIP model, with its employment-oriented transition facilitators, was the most effective and economically feasible model to sustain. A job developer was maintained, and an employment specialist position was converted to create another transition facilitator position. The Options leadership and stakeholders also determined that the TIP model delivered through a care management platform (i.e., each transition facilitator being assigned a specific set of youth) was more compatible with serving the targeted youth population than through an ACT model platform (i.e., the treatment team care managers serve all of the youth and the team also includes a psychiatrist and nurse). The leadership and stakeholders determined that they wanted the TIP practices delivered through a platform that maximized the relationship features of the transition facilitator–youth dyad.

The Options transition system is guided heavily by youth voice, and as such, the system continues to be engaging and nonstigmatizing for youth and young adults with SED/SMI as they pursue their transition goals. An illustration of the types of services and supports provided through Options and the other transition sites is provided in the story of Kendra in Box 19.1.

Allegheny County, Pennsylvania: Partnerships for Youth Transition–System of Care Initiative Sites

Having developed a system of care for children and families under a previous SAMHSA grant, Allegheny County leaders were eager to demonstrate that some of the features of their system of care initiative (SOCI) could be used to benefit young adults with SED/SMI as they made the transition to adulthood. They focused on three primary features of their SOCI: 1) youth, family, community, and system partnership; 2) the value-based service delivery process; and 3) continuous quality improvement. During the planning phase of their PYT-SOCI, focus groups were conducted with young people who endorsed aspects of the SOCI and advocated for elements of the TIP model. The planning process with the youth and young adults, as well as other stakeholders, lead to the integration of TIP and SOCI values and practices to create a developmentally appropriate transition system capable of meeting the diverse needs of this population of young people and their families.

The Allegheny County PYT-SOCI was implemented in two communities with economic challenges that border the City of Pittsburgh, namely the neighborhoods of Sto-Rox and Wilkinsburg. Young people ages 14–21 with SED/SMI were enrolled in the PYT-SOCI programs with proactive support and services also offered to their families. Service could be continued to age 25 for those who were still in need.

Box 19.1. Description of a young person, illustrating how a transition system functions

Kendra, a 17-year-old-girl diagnosed with bipolar disorder, refused to take her prescribed medications. Her use of street drugs may have been her way of self-medicating. Although she was in high school, her attendance, disciplinary record, and grades were all on the edge. Ronda, Kendra's transition facilitator, began meeting with her in comfortable settings such as Starbucks and neighborhood parks. As they took walks together, Ronda began conducting informal strength discovery assessments and person-centered planning. During the first 6 weeks, Ronda was earning Kendra's trust and learning about her interests, strengths, needs, resources, challenges, dreams, and social connections by speaking to her and to her mother and an older sister, who also lived at home. During this period, Ronda was also prompting, cajoling, and supporting school attendance, as well as teaching Kendra ways to manage her anger when she was faced with someone who was intimidating or teasing her.

School remained a major challenge, and Kendra continued to use drugs on occasion. She also experienced episodes of severe depression. Although she seemed to be developing more of a trusting relationship with Ronda, Kendra refused to attend any therapy or medication reviews. Ronda continued to reach out to her, and after about to two-and-a-half months, Kendra revealed that the loss of her grandmother a year earlier had been devastating to her because she was the only family member who Kendra found to ever express that she loved her. Ronda also learned through the informal strength discovery conversations that Kendra dreamed of being a nurse, as her grandmother had been.

Based on this new information, Ronda worked with Kendra to explore how she could improve her sense of family with her mother and her older sister, as well as explore the options she'd have in the nursing profession. Ronda arranged for Kendra to visit the community college program for nursing and meet with the program coordinator. The program coordinator gave Kendra a tour, discussed program options, and arranged for Kendra to sit in on some classes to get a feel for the subjects being studied and to meet some of the students. Kendra was very inspired by what she experienced and learned about the associate's degree program option.

Concurrently, Ronda and Kendra met with a mental health therapist to see if Kendra would be willing to engage in individual therapy and try a new type of medication that might not have the side effects that she had experienced previously. She reluctantly began attending individual therapy twice per week, often asking Ronda to attend with her. Over the course of the next month, Kendra was stabilized on a new medication and decided to expand her therapy to include her mother and sister in an attempt to create a sense of family.

Ronda worked with Kendra on composing a résumé and developing interview skills so that she might obtain a receptionist position at a doctor's office for the summer. Ronda had also learned from conversations with Kendra and her mother and sister that Kendra and her sister used to enjoy roller skating when they were younger. Ronda asked Kendra and her sister if they wanted to do some in-line skating at the local rink. The two sisters enjoyed their time together at the rink and began to spend more time together.

Now in her senior year of high school, Kendra is working, making good progress toward completing high school, taking one class at the community college, making some new friends there, and living with a better sense of family. Ronda facilitated this through informal strength assessments and person-centered planning that engaged Kendra and revealed her strengths, needs, and dreams. Ronda then provided tailored supports and services to assist Kendra in addressing her needs and achieving her goals. This process has allowed Kendra to find a new trajectory for her life and future.

The SOCI central office team and teams from the two partner communities developed an authentic community-driven partnership with youth, families, parent advocates, and representatives from community and faith-based organizations, as well as from the formal systems of education and special education, vocational rehabilitation, housing, child welfare, and child and adult behavioral health, including the area's managed care organization. Both of these communities are ethnically diverse and economically challenged. This community-driven partnership works to carry out a common vision and build on the SOCI infrastructure and the TIP model to support youth and young adults in meeting their goals of productive employment, career education, safe living situations, and community involvement, including satisfying social relationships.

The PYT-SOCI transition systems in both Sto-Rox and Wilkinsburg are designed to facilitate access to transition-relevant services and supports for young people and families in the communities where they live. Informal networks of support are essential in these communities, as formal services there are in need of better coordination and not trusted by many youth and adult residents. Thus, the PYT-SOCI supports and services provided include:

- Strengths, needs, and cultural discovery assessments

- Support and assistance in the development and maintenance of a consumer and family support team

- Consumer-directed service and support planning, coordination, and implementation

- Transition planning and goal setting

- Crisis and safety planning

- Support and assistance with housing and other needs (e.g., health insurance, food, clothing, transportation)

- Support and assistance with vocational and educational needs (e.g., college and financial aid applications, linkage to vocational training)

- Support and assistance with employment needs (e.g., assistance with résumés, job coaching, training, career counseling)

- Linkage to appropriate mental health services and supports (e.g., evaluations, psychiatric services, counseling)

- Monitoring mental health services and supports and progress

- Social connection and informal supports through youth and young adult peer support groups, mentoring, recreational activities, and linkage to community resources and natural supports for youth and families (e.g., YMCA, church groups, community organizations)

Commitment to youth involvement is evident at all levels of the Allegheny County PYT-SOCI. Two extremely powerful youth features evolved out of the community planning process that encouraged youth voice and leadership. A young adult from the community who was actively involved in the planning process emerged as a leader. During the second year, this young person was hired as the Youth Support Coordinator for the PYT-SOCI sites and also as the NCYT Youth Representative to increase the youth perspective on a national level. The PYT-SOCI also promotes youth leadership through the Youth Outreach Union (Y.O.U.). Y.O.U. grew out of the planning process for this initiative. It was formed by young people to utilize the strengths and experiences of youth leaders within the mental health system to assure that current and future generations in Allegheny County could obtain the information and support needed to become successful adults. The goal of Y.O.U. is to create opportunities for young people to socialize, discuss mental health concerns and issues, organize recreational and educational activities, and serve as leaders in their communities. The PYT-SOCI transition facilitators and youth support specialists in Sto-Rox and Wilkinsburg work closely with young people to secure their voice in guiding and refining all aspects of the transition system.

Accountability and quality assurance within the Allegheny County PYT-SOCI is evident in its structure, as well as in its use of evaluation tools and measures. Structurally, the PYT-SOCI was designed for accountability by hiring young people and family members as staff members, as well as by ensuring that young people and family members participate in decisions about operations, programming, and fiscal management. Furthermore, both the Sto-Rox and Wilkinsburg offices made a commitment to recruit and hire qualified individuals from these communities. By virtue of living and working in these communities, the PYT-SOCI teams are held accountable by their fellow community members, as well as by the continuing quality improvement features of the initiative.

Throughout the years of the cooperative agreement, those involved with the PYT-SOCI program developed and conducted a variety of user-friendly assessments that reflect the youth and family members' point of view. To make these assessments and related instruments accessible to and relevant for program participants, the PYT-SOCI involved young people and family members in the development and modification of instruments by engaging them to serve on the Youth Think Tank Quality Improvement Committee and by compensating them as partners in the development of these tools. Young people and family members were also compensated for their contributions when completing optional assessments that were used to evaluate programmatic outcomes.

In collaboration with the developer of the Child and Adolescent Needs and Strengths (CANS; Lyons, Sokol, & Lee, 1999), the site evaluator and the Youth Think Tank modified the CANS to create an assessment tailored to transition-age youth. The instrument is referred to as the Young Adult Needs and Strengths Assessment (YANSA). A link to the YANSA is available through the NCYT web site at http://ncyt.fmhi.usf.edu.

The Allegheny PYT-SOCI periodically publishes reports to illustrate the challenges, successes, and impact of the program. One such publication is the biannual outcome report entitled *Making Waves,* featuring progress on PYT-

SOCI milestones and outcomes. This PYT-SOCI has established a recommended practice of consulting with young people and families in the development of such reports, giving them the opportunity to share personal stories that enhance the interpretation of the data and to provide valuable insight into the design of youth and family-friendly publications.

Portland, Maine: The Odyssey Program

The Odyssey program focuses on a group of young people who are most difficult to serve—those between the ages of 14 and 21 with SED/SMI at the point of their first hospitalization. The goal of this PYT program is to increase the number of graduates from high school and college, increase employment rates for this population of young people, and decrease homelessness, substance abuse, and criminal activity. By targeting youth and young adults experiencing a first hospitalization, the Odyssey program is able to intervene early and track outcomes within a particularly vulnerable group of young people as they transfer back to school, work, and family life.

To increase opportunities for these young people, the project operates at both the programmatic and systemic levels. At the programmatic level, the Odyssey program focuses on inspiring and supporting young people to achieve their education and career goals. The program promotes the message that hopes and dreams can be realized beyond hospitalization. To assist program participants, the Odyssey team applies a comprehensive set of strategies that include multidisciplinary assessment; futures planning; referrals to relevant services; and transition supports and services focused on mental health treatment, education, employment, independent living, and social support.

At the heart of the Odyssey program are transition specialists to whom each young person and his or her family are assigned. The Odyssey team also includes an interdisciplinary group of professionals with expertise in employment, social work, psychiatry, psychiatric nursing, occupational therapy, and education. The team is structured to meet regularly to share information on each young person and his or her family and on available community resources. The team assists participating youth and their families in gaining access to needed resources such as employment opportunities and housing.

At the systemic level, the Odyssey program builds on existing resources to develop a comprehensive program for this population of young people and their families. An array of services offered through this PYT initiative allows these individuals maximum access to community supports, which minimizes their penetration into the mental health system. The Odyssey team is located in a local career center to minimize stigma and to allow easy access to personnel who provide employment-related services and who know how to maneuver the arena of vocational rehabilitation services, funding, and supports. A Mental Health Employer Consortium was established that meets on a quarterly basis to generate education, work, and career opportunities for program participants. The Odyssey program also taps into existing high school programs to secure services relevant to participants, including a student mentoring program and services offered through the Office of Multilingual and Multicultural Programs, the Anatomy of Leadership program, and Jobs for Maine's Graduates.

The Odyssey team works with representatives from various transition-related agencies by participating on the Transition Linkage Coalition (TLC). The TLC community forum was created to enable service providers to collaborate to improve and better integrate service delivery. It enables community agencies and organizations to identify solutions to existing and perceived barriers to service delivery for transition-age youth. The group meets regularly to secure information regarding barriers at the practice, program, or system levels. Priority issues are assigned to different time-limited subcommittees known as solution teams. Each solution team meets monthly to define a target issue, learn more about the specifics of the issue, and formulate a proposed action plan to address this priority issue at the practice, funding, policy, or system level. The TLC forum then determines which of these action plans, or parts therein, to implement immediately and which to implement on a long-term basis.

Minnesota: PRIDE-4

The Putting All Communities Together (PACT) 4 Families Collaborative is a system of care serving four rural counties in Minnesota. When the opportunity arose to apply for federal funding, family members persuaded PACT leaders and staff members that services and supports for young people ages 14–21 were desperately needed. With the PYT grant funds, Minnesota's PACT-4 Families Collaborative—comprising 110 organizations, agencies, and community partners—created a transition program to serve their four-county rural area. They named their initiative Persons Realizing Independence and Developing Empowerment (PRIDE-4), a name created by a young man who contributed to the design of the program. With the addition of this initiative, the PACT-4 Collaborative offers an array of mental health services spanning from birth to adulthood, an unusual accomplishment for a rural area.

PRIDE-4 was the first PYT site to draft a logic model to encompass the area's vision of fostering healthy and safe communities where individuals, families, and youth care and support one another. As can be seen in their logic model shown in Figure 19.2, PRIDE-4 encompasses elements of the TIP system and features young people surrounded by layers of nurturing and supportive opportunities that begin with the family and then circle wider to include the broader community and other service systems. The logic model also reflects a commitment to assist youth and young adults across all of the transition domains of employment and career, educational opportunities, living situation, and community-life functioning.

PRIDE-4's logic model is brought to life by pairing every young person with a transition facilitator referred to as a coach. The coaches, along with other PRIDE-4 staff members (i.e., project coordinator, clinical supervisor, family liaison), support each young person in identifying his or her transition goals and coordinating the community supports and resources needed to meet the needs and challenges identified through the individualized service planning process.

As the TIP guidelines indicate, coaches engage young people through relationship development, person-centered planning, and a focus on their futures by meeting with young people individually, conducting strength discovery assessments, assisting them in setting short- and long-term goals, and coordinating services and supports accordingly. The coaches act as hubs for a wheel of opportunities and resources. Being in rural areas with few formal services, each coach works with 12–15 young people to determine an appropriate set of activities and interventions for assisting each in learning new skills and achieving his or her desired goals. These interventions may include teaching improved social skills, guiding young people through the process of securing their driver's licenses, helping young people prepare for and attend the high school prom, creating occasions for young people to get together and socialize at the bowling alley, and securing and maintaining their first jobs. Mental health services and supports are provided by local mental health service providers.

Through this PYT initiative, PRIDE-4 made connections with system partners that resulted in many new opportunities for young people to make successful transitions to adulthood. For example, in conjunction with Goodwill Industries, PRIDE-4 formed a Job Club that provides opportunities for young people to acquire job readiness skills such as interviewing techniques, résumé writing, and job searching. PRIDE-4 also partnered with other agencies and organizations to improve transition opportunities by securing funding to provide new housing options for young adults in the form of scattered-site apartments. PRIDE-4 also partnered with the juvenile justice system on a restorative justice initiative called Community Sentencing Circles. Through this effort, which involves the County Attorney's Office, the local police departments, the District Court, the Public Defenders Office, and the PACT-4 Families Collaborative, judges remand young people to PRIDE-4 as a sentencing option. This alternative system reports a zero recidivism rate.

PRIDE-4's implementation of the TIP model includes a family liaison position in addition to the coaches. The role of the family liaison is to support young people's family members in their understanding of the transition process and to assist them in securing other services that the family might need, such as employment or substance abuse treatment. The coaches and the family liaison coordinate their activities as necessary to ensure continuity for the young person and other family members.

Utah: Project RECONNECT

Project RECONNECT was named through a youth-driven contest and stands for Responsibilities, Education, Competency, Opportunities, Networking, Neighborhood, Employment, and Collaboration for Transition. Project RECONNECT is a statewide initiative that was initially implemented across five community mental health centers (CMHCs), serving 11 counties in the Greater Salt Lake metropolitan area and associated rural communities. Most of the young people served are between the ages of 16 and 21 and come from culturally and

Mission: Pride-4 will work at multiple levels to further the PACT-4 Families version of "healthy and safe communities where individuals, families, and youth care and support each other" by assisting youth and young adults with mental health needs to successfully transition into adulthood.

Context	Strategies		Outcomes

Context

Youth in transition

45–50 youth/year

16–21 years old with mental health issues

Emphasis on dropouts, those in dire need of housing

Or about to age out of the youth support system

Challenges

Individual level

Individuals have limited knowledge of resources and support staff have limited expertise on the developmental needs of youth

Values

1. Our shared vision will be strength based and outcome driven.

2. All youth and families are valued and treated with respect.

Strategies

Theory of change: By implementing multilevel service development strategies that are grounded in a set of values and principles and directed by a set of goals, young adults with mental health issues will successfully increase their skills for living as adults.

1. Be tailored for individuals and communities

Services and supports will

Community goal
Community is more aware of transition challenges for these youth.

System goal
Youth and adult service providers learn and practice person-centered approaches in serving transitioning youth.

Family goal
Family members are assisted in supporting their youth with mental health issues through the transition process

Youth goal
Identified youth and adults with mental health issues are supported in their transition from adolescence to adulthood

Youth

Families

Systems

Communities

Outcomes

Increased skills and success for young adults with mental health issues

Supportive and relieved family members

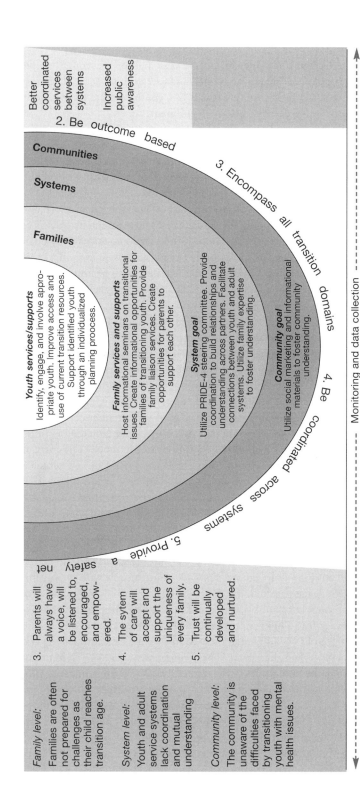

Figure 19.2. PRIDE-4 theory-based framework.

ethnically diverse backgrounds. In addition, at least half of the young people served are from populations that are typically underserved and overlooked (i.e., homeless youth, children from immigrant families, youth who are state custody dependents, or very young parents with small children).

Transition facilitators and their supervisors received training to implement the TIP model. The transition facilitators were also trained and certified as job coaches to help strengthen their employment support expertise. They serve as a young person's primary contact, and in their roles as resource brokers, they help to ensure that services, supports, and informational resources are coordinated. The transition facilitators use informal assessments such as strength discovery (Blase, Wagner, & Clark, 2007) and the Ansell-Casey Life Skills Assessment (Ansell & Casey Family Programs, 2000) to assist youth in the development of individualized plans based on their strengths and needs (e.g., finding safe and affordable housing, securing jobs, learning to manage anger, dealing with feelings of loneliness, completing paperwork for U.S. citizenship to pursue postsecondary education and employment opportunities in this country).

To support this youth-centered approach to transition, Project RECONNECT has an active Family Council led by Allies with Families, Utah's chapter of the Federation of Families for Children's Mental Health. Through Allies with Families, parents and family members participate in educational workshops and retreats. In addition, Allies with Families offers support to family members affected by their youths' mental health concerns, even if the young people in their lives are not officially involved in Project RECONNECT. Another contribution of Allies with Families was the development of a curriculum aimed at assisting families and parents during their children's transitions to adulthood. The curriculum provides classes on topics ranging from guardianship and person-centered planning to developmental issues and milestones associated with the transition period. The curriculum entitled *Growing Up Without Growing Apart* is available through the NCYT web site at http://ncyt.fmhi.usf.edu/partnerships/index.htm.

Project RECONNECT also brings young people together, depending on their interests and time availability, through Community Youth Action Councils (CYAC) convened by each of the four CMHCs and a statewide Youth Action Council (YAC). The community councils provide young people with opportunities to participate in leadership training, learn life skills, expand their network of peer supports, carry out community service and fundraising projects, take on collective action projects, and otherwise pursue their interests individually and in groups. One example of how influential these councils are is demonstrated by two enterprising young men and their peers. These young men conducted a 3-month community resource mapping project, which led them to draft a business proposal with a local foundation to purchase two real estate properties to create housing options for young people. The foundation funded the proposal, and the properties were purchased, renovated, and converted into housing complexes for young people. The statewide YAC brought great visibility to many issues related to transition-age young people. The governor established a Transition to Adult Living initiative led by the Department of Human Services and Project RECONNECT, which also involved various statewide task groups focused on recommendations regarding the development of living skills, physical and mental health, mentoring, employment, and housing. The governor's initiative, in conjunction with the statewide and local councils, made numerous recommendations regarding practices, funding, and policy during the course of this initiative.

Project RECONNECT is approaching sustainability of this transition initiative by building on and enhancing the relationships within and outside the existing mental health infrastructure across its communities and counties. The TIP model laid the framework for Project RECONNECT to build and expand partnerships across the mental health system and other public and private provider agencies and organizations. Allies with Families enhances family involvement during this transition to adulthood period. The Project RECONNECT transition initiative developed through the PYT initiative in Utah is transformative in its approach and enhances the delivery of child- and adult-serving services at the practice, program, and policy levels.

COMMUNITY TRANSITION SYSTEMS: FINDINGS AND LESSONS LEARNED

Preliminary Findings

The NCYT team conducted a cross-site analysis of the PYT projects. The preliminary findings from a group of 192 young people who were involved with their sites for at least 1 year are encouraging (Clark, Karpur, Deschênes, Gamache, & Haber, 2008). Initial findings revealed that an increasing proportion of the transition-age youth improved over time in six major outcome areas. The young people were more likely to be employed and more likely to be pursuing high school or postsecondary education. They were less likely to have dropped out of high school, less likely to experience interference in their lives from their mental health conditions, and less likely to experience interference from drug or alcohol use. These improvement trends were statistically significant across the year of enrollment in the PYT programs. Although involvement in the criminal justice system showed a slight decrease from the initial assessment, this trend over all of the assessments was not statistically significant.

These improvements across the transition progress indicators are illustrated in Figure 19.3 for the first five assessments (i.e., Initial Baseline at intake through Quarter 4 assessment) conducted on each participant. The asterisks on the outcome legends indicate that these are statistically significant trends.

Young adults with SED/SMI have the poorest outcomes of all people with disabilities as they enter adulthood. Still, these PYT findings, as well as others (e.g., Karpur, Clark, Caproni, & Sterner, 2005), have shown that outcomes for these young people can improve with futures planning that builds on their strengths, interests, and goals. Developmentally appropriate services and supports tailored to help this population of young people can facilitate goal achievement, enhance their social and life skills, and strengthen their connections to important people in their lives. Additional information on progress and outcome studies can be found in the Theory and Research Section of the TIP web site at http://

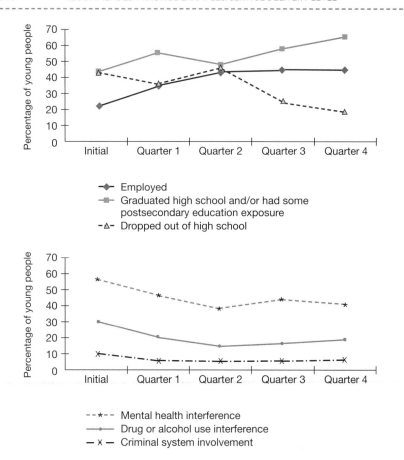

Figure 19.3. The percent of young people exposed to each of six outcome indicators of progress at the initial baseline assessment prior to entry to a transition program and the trends across the four 90-day assessments after entry. (From Clark, H.B., Karpur, A., Deschênes, N., Gamache, P., & Haber, M. [2008]. Partnerships for Youth Transition [PYT]: Overview of community initiatives and preliminary findings on transition to adulthood for youth and young adults with mental health challenges. In C. Newman, C. Liberton, K. Kutash, & R.M. Friedman [Eds.], *The 20th annual research conference proceedings: A system of care for children's mental health: Expanding the research base* [pp. 329–332]. Tampa: University of South Florida, The Louis de la Parte Florida Mental Health Institute, Research and Training Center for Children's Mental Health; reprinted by permission.)

tip.fmhi.usf.edu. In addition, the NCYT has developed the Fidelity Protocol for Continuing Improvement of Transition Systems (Deschênes, Clark, & Herrygers, 2008); a description of this protocol and its process is provided on the NCYT web site at http://ncyt.fmhi.usf.edu.

Lessons Learned from the PYT Initiative

Many lessons have been learned from the experience and evaluation related to the PYT initiative, providing valuable guidance for communities and states seeking to improve services for youth and young adults in transition to adulthood:

- Young people with SED/SMI can be engaged through relationship development, person-centered planning, and a focus on their futures.

- Transition facilitators and other program personnel who use informal strength-based assessments rather than traditional formal assessments that tend to be deficit-based are more likely to engage a young people.

- Services must be provided in youth-friendly, nonstigmatizing community environments (e.g., at home, over lunch, in school, in a park).

- Young people with SED/SMI have many dreams as they make the transition to adulthood. With informal and formal supports, young people can develop goals and become successful in the transition domains of employment and career, educational opportunities, living situations, and community-life functioning.

- The period of transition to adulthood is one of discovery, one where many young people tend to take risks. Young people are capable of being strong, responsible community members. Competency-building approaches allow them to make wiser choices and help them to achieve greater self-sufficiency and confidence.

- Young people can be instrumental in assisting in the planning and implementation phases of community transition initiatives that are relevant to them. Involvement of young people in these processes requires the use of youth-friendly strategies. Some of these strategies include stipends for their services and understanding that youth might not be willing to sit through 2-hour meetings. They will, however, be actively involved for the first hour with the agenda shifted to include the youth-relevant items early on. Of course, pizza always helps!

- The development and implementation of community-based transition systems can inform already existing practices and policies that support the belief that young people with SED/SMI are able to discover and recover.

- Advancing the PYT initiatives required champions. Some of these people were adults and others were young people, but they were all transformative.

- Sometimes system barriers are myths that are not grounded in reality. For example, in one of the PYT sites, a barrier to services was that the bureaucracy consistently indicated that a particular set of funds was only available to serve a certain age group. This proved to be a myth due to changes in state law that had been put into place a number of years prior, but had seemingly gone unnoticed by the bureaucrats and system providers. Thus, funding was available up to 21 years of age and not terminated at 18.

- Younger teens between the ages of 14 and 16 seem to require activities that differ from those implemented for the greater majority of young people between the ages of 16 and 21. As the PYT initiative unfolded, it became apparent that the process and types of activities selected by more mature young adults were less appropriate and beneficial for younger adolescents. Systems of care should consider implementing a different set of transition strategies for young people ages 14–16 such as greater family involvement or enhanced efforts of high schools to address transition issues (e.g., daily living skills, budgeting).

CONCLUSION

The PYT initiative provided a rich learning experience both for community stakeholders and national partners. There were many examples of the significance of youth voice in the planning, implementation, and sustaining phases of the PYT experience. Site stakeholders also found that the transition arena was inherently transformative to their child- and adult-serving systems in that it was typically the first time that they had ever confronted and coordinated activities across both sectors. Community leaders and stakeholders, however, should understand that developing a meaningful and effective transition system is an extremely challenging task, but one that holds great rewards for all if a collective, serious, and explicit commitment is made to the needs of young people and to ensure the presence of their voice in system planning and service delivery.

REFERENCES

Ansell, D.I., & Casey Family Programs. (2000). *Ansell-Casey Life Skills Assessment*. Retrieved August 15, 2007, from http://www.caseylifeskills.org

Blase, K., Wagner, R., & Clark, H.B. (2007). *Strength discovery assessment process for working with transition-aged youth and young adults*. Tampa: University of South Florida, Louis de la Parte Florida Mental Health Institute.

Bridgeo, D., Davis, M., & Florida, Y., (2000). Transition coordination: Helping youth and young adults put it all together. In B.A. Stroul & R.M. Friedman (Series Eds.) & H.B. Clark & M. Davis (Vol. Eds.), *Systems of care for children's mental health series: Transition to adulthood: A resource for assisting young people with emotional or behavioral difficulties* (pp. 155–178). Baltimore: Paul H. Brookes Publishing Co.

Bullis, M., & Fredericks, H.D. (2002). *Vocational and transition services for adolescents with emotional and behavioral disorders: Strategies and best practices*. Champaign, IL: Research Press.

Carter, E.W., & Wehby, J.H. (2003). Job performance of transition-age youth with emotional and behavioral disorders. *Exceptional Children, 69*(4), 449–465.

Chadsey, J., & Beyer, S. (2001). Social relationships in the workplace. *Mental Retardation and Developmental Disabilities Research Reviews, 7*(2), 128–133.

Clark, H.B., & Davis, M. (Vol. Eds.). (2000). *Systems of care for children's mental health series: Transition to adulthood: A resource for assisting young people with emotional or behavioral difficulties*. Baltimore: Paul H. Brookes Publishing Co.

Clark, H.B., Deschênes, N., & Jones, J. (2000). A framework for the development and operation of a transition system. In B.A. Stroul & R.M. Friedman (Series Eds.) & H.B. Clark & M. Davis (Vol. Eds.), *Systems of care for children's mental health series: Transition to adulthood: A resource for assisting young people with emotional or behavioral difficulties* (pp. 29–51). Baltimore: Paul H. Brookes Publishing Co.

Clark, H.B., & Foster-Johnson, L. (1996). Serving youth in transition into adulthood. In B.A. Stroul & R.M. Friedman (Series Eds.) & B.A. Stroul (Vol. Ed.), *Systems of care for children's mental health series: Children's mental health: Creating systems of care in a changing society* (pp. 533–551). Baltimore: Paul H. Brookes Publishing Co.

Clark, H.B., Karpur, A., Deschênes, N., Gamache, P., & Haber, M. (2008). Partnerships for Youth Transition (PYT): Overview of community initiatives and preliminary findings on transition to adulthood for youth and young adults with mental health challenges. In C. Newman, C. Liberton, K. Kutash, & R.M. Friedman (Eds.), *The 20th Annual Research Conference Proceedings: A system of care for children's mental health: Expanding the research base.* (pp. 329–332). Tampa: University of South Florida, Louis de la Parte Florida Mental Health Institute.

Davis, M., & Vander Stoep, A. (1997). The transition to adulthood for youth who have serious emotional disturbance: Development transition and young adult outcomes. *Journal of Mental Health Administration, 24,* 400–427.

Deschênes, N., Clark, H.B., & Herrygers, J. (2008). The development of fidelity measures for youth transition programs. In C. Newman, C. Liberton, K. Kutash, & R.M. Friedman. (Eds.), *The 20th Annual Research Conference Proceedings: A system of care for children's mental health: Expanding the research base.* (pp. 333–338). Tampa: University of South Florida, Louis de la Parte Florida Mental Health Institute.

Gresham, F.M., Sugai, G., & Horner, R.H. (2001). Interpreting outcomes of social skills training for students with high-incidence disabilities. *Exceptional Children, 67,* 331–344.

Karpur, A., Clark, H.B., Caproni, P., & Sterner, H. (2005). Transition to adult roles for students with emotional/behavioral disturbances: A follow-up study of student exiters from Steps-to-Success. *Career Development for Exceptional Individuals, 28*(1), 36–46.

Lyons, J.L., Sokol, P.T., & Lee, M., (1999). *Child and adolescent needs and strengths: For children and adolescents with mental health challenges (CANS-MH).* Retrieved November 2007 from http://www.buddinpraed.org

Rylance, B.J. (1998). Predictors of posthigh school employment for youth identified as severely emotionally disturbed. *Journal of Special Education, 32,* 184–192.

Vander Stoep, A., Bersford, S., Weiss, N.S., McKnight, B., Cauce, A.M., & Cohen, P. (2000). Community-based study of the transition to adulthood for adolescents with psychiatric disorder. *American Journal of Epidemiology, 152,* 353–362.

Vander Stoep, A., Davis, M., & Collins, D. (2000). Transition: A time of developmental and institutional clashes. In B.A. Stroul & R.M. Friedman (Series Eds.) & H.B. Clark & M. Davis (Vol. Eds.), *Systems of care for children's mental health series: Transition of youth and young adults with emotional or behavioral difficulties into adulthood: Handbook for practitioners, educators, parents, and administrators.* Baltimore: Paul H. Brookes Publishing Co.

Vander Stoep, A., Weiss, N.S., Saldana Kuo, E., Cheney, D., & Cohen, P. (2003). What proportion of failure to complete secondary school in the U.S. population is attributable to adolescent psychiatric disorder? *Journal of Behavioral Health Services and Research, 30*(1), 119–124.

Wagner, M. (2005). Moving on. In M. Wagner, L. Newman, R. Cameto, N. Garza, & P. Levine (Eds.), *Life outside the classroom for youth with disabilities. A report from the National Longitudinal Transition Study–2 (NLTS).* Menlo Park, CA: SRI International.

20

School-Based Mental Health Services in Systems of Care

KRISTA KUTASH, ALBERT J. DUCHNOWSKI,
VESTENA ROBBINS, AND SANDRA KEENAN

I n the first decade of the new millennium, there is increasing concern about the growing number of children and adolescents who experience difficulties facing the challenges of development and the effects of emotional disturbance. This concern occurs in a context of system transformation efforts aimed at improving the effectiveness of services and increasing the capacity to serve all children in need. An important strategy to help to achieve this transformation is the proposed development of effective and integrated school-based mental health (SBMH) services. The 1999 *Report of the Surgeon General on the Mental Health of the Nation* (U.S. Department of Health and Human Services [US DHHS], 1999), the No Child Left Behind Act of 2001 (PL 107-110), and the President's New Freedom Commission on Mental Health (2003) all focused attention on the potential of SBMH services to improve the emotional well-being and academic achievement of all children. This chapter summarizes the current status of SBMH, outlines effective strategies, provides an example of a comprehensive model of SBMH, outlines recommendations on implementing SBMH initiatives, and presents a future vision of SBMH as part of comprehensive systems of care based on the public health model.

There is a long history in this country, dating back to the end of the 19th century, of providing mental health services to children in schools. In the 21st century, there is increased interest in SBMH and hope that SBMH services may play a larger role in better meeting the needs of the millions of children who have emotional disturbances and need mental health intervention. Through more effective implementation of these services, the academic and social/emotional outcomes for these children can improve, leading to a healthier adulthood and a better quality of life.

Examination of the literature base describing SBMH services and program models reveals that the field can be characterized at present as fragmented, underdeveloped, and influenced by diverse and sometimes conflicting models (Adelman

& Taylor, 1998; Kutash, Duchnowski, & Lynn, 2006; Weist, Goldstein, Morris, & Bryant, 2003). In addition, confusion is created by the different languages and terminologies used by the various agencies providing SBMH, especially the education and mental health systems. This is not to say that the field lacks areas of strength. There is a strong multidisciplinary and multiagency presence in the field, a growing evidence base for specific programs, and a growing recognition of the need for a comprehensive, integrated approach to scale up emerging localized successes to a level that will have significant national impact.

Examination of the literature also reveals that the term *school-based mental health* has no agreed-on definition or parameters. It is generally used to describe any mental health service delivered in a school setting or any mental health service linked with schools. It has also been broadly used to describe any skill-building activities or services delivered in schools to help youth regulate their emotions, moods, or behavior. Several factors reflect the complexity involved in narrowing the scope and definition of SBMH. First, there is a wide range of educational environments in which mental health services can be delivered, ranging from neighborhood schools to programs in hospitals and juvenile justice facilities administered by public school districts. Therefore, the term *school* in *school-based mental health* can reflect a variety of settings. Another factor influencing the conceptualization of SBMH is the history of mental health services in schools. Historically, mental health services and supports have been delivered by staff employed by schools through the special education program for students with emotional disturbances.

Perhaps one of the most important characteristics affecting the concept of SBMH is the history of uneven collaboration between mental health systems and schools systems. The passage of the Education of All Handicapped Children Act of 1975 (PL 94-142), later reauthorized as the Individuals with Disabilities Education Act (IDEA) of 1990 (PL 101-476), placed an increased responsibility on the education system to meet the mental health needs of youth with emotional disturbances. This legislation was viewed by many mental health leaders as a mandate for schools to pay for mental health services that were underfunded within community mental health centers. Educational leaders, however, viewed the legislation as an unfunded mandate. The result was a blurred responsibility for the delivery of mental health services combined with confusion about which youth were to be served by which agency and which services were to be delivered.

The current conceptualization of SBMH acknowledges that schools have the responsibility for providing services to all children with mental health needs ranging from acute to profound when these needs interfere with learning. Mental health providers can be partners with schools when educational outcomes are a shared goal between the two systems. This conceptualization has resulted in a three-tiered model that emphasizes the range of the severity of mental health challenges when planning for all children, as well as the range of services and educational supports needed to effectively meet these needs (Sugai & Horner, 2002). This model builds on previous prevention models (Mrazek & Haggerty, 1994) and includes universal strategies targeted to the general school population, selec-

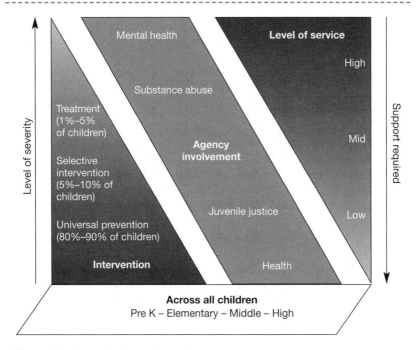

Figure 20.1. Comprehensive service continuum.

tive interventions aimed at those youth who are at risk of developing mental health disorders, and indicated interventions targeted at those youth who are expected to meet diagnostic criteria for mental health disorders (Figure 20.1).

EMPIRICAL BASE FOR SCHOOL-BASED MENTAL HEALTH SERVICES

The empirical base for SBMH can be categorized into three major areas: 1) the structure and organization of SBMH, 2) evidence-based programs and interventions to improve the mental health of youth, and 3) the implementation of Positive Behavior Support systems in schools to manage behavior. There are other issues to consider in examining SBMH, but these particular areas provide a focused context for discussion.

Organization of School-Based Mental Health Services

Two recent surveys—The School Health Policies and Programs Study (SHPPS), 2000 (Brener, Martindale, & Weist, 2001) and School Mental Health Services in the United States, 2002–2003 (Foster et al., 2005)—reported on the organization of SBMH services using a nationally representative sample of schools and districts or states. Both surveys yielded similar results and documented the immense ef-

forts made by schools to supply mental health services by using both school resources and by contracting with community organizations such as mental health
agencies. These efforts, however, are not uniformly implemented and may differ
by region (Slade, 2003).

Both surveys documented that the majority of schools offer some type of
mental health or social service support to students, with 20% of all students receiving some type of school-supported mental health service. Foster et al. (2005) found
that most schools provide individual counseling (76%), case management (71%),
or group counseling (68%) to their students. The service most frequently reported
as being difficult to provide was family support, a finding supported by multiple
studies (see Wagner et al, 2006). For those schools delivering mental health services, most (96%) reported that at least one staff member has the responsibility of
providing mental health services to students; most schools reported having between two and five staff members delivering these services (Foster et al., 2005).

The most common administrative arrangement for the delivery of SBMH
services is for schools to have their own staff provide mental health services and to
augment these services through contracts with local community mental health
providers. Approximately half of all schools have a contract with a local provider
to supply mental health services on school grounds (Brener et al., 2001).

Evidence-Based Programs and Interventions for Improving the Mental Health of Youth

Zins, Weissberg, Wang, and Walberg (2004) reported that a typical school delivers an average of 14 separate programs that broadly address social and emotional
issues. Most of these programs, however, are not empirically based. In addition,
there is little evidence of a systematic deployment of these programs. Instead, they
tend to emerge in response to immediate pressures or trends.

A review of five popular compendiums of evidence-based mental health programs for children revealed a total of 92 programs or interventions promoted as
being evidence-based (Kutash et al., 2006). Approximately one third of the programs included on these lists target substance abuse, trauma, or health problems,
and the remaining two thirds address the regulation of emotional or social functioning. Overall, these evidence-based mental health interventions focus equally
at the universal level of prevention (53%, or 48 of 90 programs) and the selec-
tive/indicated levels of prevention (47%, or 42 of 90 programs). Most of the evidence-based programs (58%) listed in these compendiums take place in schools
or in both the school and the community (16%), making it clear that the delivery
of evidence-based mental health interventions is dependent on cooperation with
school systems.

Examples of universal programs implemented in the school setting include
Promoting Alternative Thinking Strategies (PATHS; Greenberg, Kusché, Cook,
& Quamma, 1995) for children 5–12 years of age and Life Skills Training
(Botvin, Griffin, Paul, & Macaulay, 2003) for older youth, 11–16 years of age.
Selective programs include the Olweus Bullying Prevention Program (Olweus,

1991) and the Children in the Middle Program (Arbuthnot & Gordon, 1996), an intervention that targets children whose parents are experiencing divorce. Examples at the indicated/selective level include the Incredible Years for children 2–8 years of age (Webster-Stratton & Taylor, 2001) and Multidimensional Family Therapy (Liddle, 1998) for youth between 11 and 18 years of age.

Overall, the empirically based interventions contain a limited number of comprehensive strategies and typically include either a skill development curriculum or a therapeutic approach involving either behavior management or Cognitive-Behavioral Therapy. The primary differences among these interventions concern teachers and parents, including the amount of time they are involved, the type of involvement, and their respective roles. Universal prevention programs are more likely to involve parents and teachers in delivering and reinforcing a skills curriculum, and parents may be recipients of skill-building curricula such as training in parenting skills. As programs move to the selective and indicated levels of prevention, skill-building curricula are typically delivered to only a select group of students, and parents are involved in the therapeutic process or as providers of skill-building curricula, or both. Although it appears that there are many options of evidence-based interventions for SBMH, there is no perfect match between the array of problems presented by youth covering the entire developmental continuum and empirically supported approaches. Furthermore, it is widely recognized that many youth have multiple or co-occurring problems that are not adequately addressed by the available selection of interventions.

Implementation of Positive Behavior Support Systems in Schools

Positive Behavior Support (PBS; Horner, 1999), a standardized approach to managing behavior that has been extensively supported by federal funding, offers a comprehensive framework for SBMH. PBS was developed initially as an alternative to aversive interventions for youth with severe disabilities who engaged in self-injurious and aggressive acts (Durand & Carr, 1985). The approach has since extended from a focus on individual children and youth to a systemwide intervention approach for schools (Dwyer & Osher, 2000; Scott & Hunter, 2001). PBS is a proactive data-based approach that focuses on providing multiple levels of intervention and support to address the academic and behavioral needs of all youth, not just those with the most challenging behaviors. The assumption underlying PBS is that a continuum of positive behavior supports is required to meet the needs of all students in a school (Sugai, Sprague, Horner, & Walker, 2000). Modeled after the public health approach, PBS offers a consistent research-based approach for promoting prosocial behavior in students without chronic problems (i.e., universal prevention) and in students at risk for problem behavior (i.e., selective prevention), as well as those with intensive behavioral needs (i.e., indicated prevention).

The success of PBS with individual cases of problem behavior in children is supported by the requirements in the 1997 amendments to IDEA (PL 105-17) mandating that PBS and functional behavioral assessments be used to reduce challenging behaviors in students with disabilities (Sugai & Horner, 2002). Research is beginning to emerge supporting the effectiveness of PBS at the system level, particularly as a schoolwide prevention intervention to reduce the incidence of problem behaviors and increase student learning (see Nelson, Martella, & Marchand-Martella, 2002). In addition, there is a growing body of literature describing the integration of PBS with system of care principles and wraparound in school settings at the selective and indicated levels. Experience in Kentucky illustrates how positive behavior supports can be implemented within the overall framework of a system of care to provide SBMH services and supports.

IMPLEMENTING SCHOOL-BASED MENTAL HEALTH SERVICES IN KENTUCKY

Kentucky has implemented a variety of SBMH service delivery mechanisms to address the mental health needs of students across the state. These delivery mechanisms range from school-financed student support services (e.g., school psychologists), to formal partnerships with regional community mental health centers to provide school-based therapy and wraparound, to the colocation of community mental health center staff in schools to assist in the implementation of schoolwide PBS systems. Calls for the adoption of a public health approach, the emerging evidence base supporting schoolwide PBS, and the complementary nature of the system of care philosophy and a schoolwide system of PBS led to Kentucky's efforts to integrate PBS into its existing system of care.

Kentucky's focus on designing and implementing systems of care for youth with serious mental health conditions and their families dates back to 1986. In 1998, the Kentucky Department of Mental Health and Mental Retardation Services (KDMHMRS) received funds from the Center for Mental Health Services through the Comprehensive Community Mental Health Services for Children and Their Families Program to expand its evolving system of care for youth with serious mental health conditions in three Appalachian regions in the state. Acknowledging schools as critical partners in system of care efforts, as well as the challenges and opportunities underlying their effective inclusion, the primary feature of this mental health initiative, called the Bridges Project, was to design, implement, and evaluate a schoolwide PBS approach, including the use of school-based wraparound for students and families whose needs required intensive services and supports (Eber, 2003; Eber, Nelson, & Miles, 1997; Kutash & Rivera, 1996). This model extended SBMH services beyond traditional mental health therapy and consultation to a schoolwide system of PBS for all students. The goal was to link mental health staff with school staff to build capacity for school personnel to become more confident and effective in implementing schoolwide prevention efforts and interventions for students with or at risk for mental health challenges. The Bridges Project has served as the basis for the development of an integrated model of SBMH services and supports throughout the state of Kentucky.

Staffing Structure

The delivery of SBMH services is accomplished through a partnership among mental health agencies, schools, and families. Services are delivered through student care teams made up of service coordinators, family liaisons, and child and family intervention specialists, all of whom are employees of a regional mental health center but are colocated on school campuses. These individuals serve on different teams throughout the school and also coordinate with one another to help ensure the efficient use of services and supports. The service coordinator serves as a case manager for students identified with serious mental health challenges by facilitating school-based wraparound team meetings and linking families with formal community resources and natural supports. These individuals are bachelor's-level service providers who receive training in service coordination and team facilitation strategies. The family liaison, required to be a parent of a child or youth with serious emotional or behavioral challenges, serves in a professional role by providing peer-to-peer support to other family members and by building local and regional family support networks. There are no formal educational requirements for the family liaison position; however, these individuals complete a certification process through Opportunities for Family Leadership, the state office for family leadership within the KDMHMRS. The child and family intervention specialist is a mental health clinician who receives additional training in functional behavioral assessment and the development of behavior intervention plans and school-based supports. Through a partnership with the Division of Exceptional Children Services within the Kentucky Department of Education, each school also has access to a regional behavior consultant who provides training, coaching, and other technical assistance to school staff to facilitate the implementation of schoolwide strategies and supports, as well as consultation on individual and group behavioral interventions.

Positive Behavior Supports

As noted, PBS involves the provision of a continuum of positive behavior supports to meet the needs of all students. Following the public health approach, PBS universal, selective, and indicated interventions are implemented throughout the school.

Universal Interventions and Supports   Universal interventions constitute a form of primary prevention and focus on promoting prosocial behavior among all students. Universal approaches are typically effective at preventing problem behavior for the majority (80%–90%) of students (Sugai & Horner, 2002). These prevention strategies focus on enhancing protective factors in the school, home, and community while preventing the development of problems through the efforts of all school personnel and caregivers. Essentially, universal interventions focus on creating a positive school climate that increases school safety and promotes positive student–adult relationships.

In Kentucky, coordination and oversight of universal interventions and supports rests with the PBS team, which includes full representation of school personnel (i.e., administration, all grade level teachers, and specialized support staff), as well as community members (e.g., mental health agency staff) and family members. The PBS team receives ongoing training from regional behavior consultants who also coach teams as they plan, implement, monitor, and maintain schoolwide efforts.

Examples of universal interventions and supports include developing a set of clearly defined schoolwide behavioral expectations; establishing schoolwide approaches for teaching and reinforcing expected prosocial behaviors; and redesigning routines, schedules, and environments to prevent, minimize, or eliminate disruptive behavior (see Box 20.1). Schoolwide initiatives to prevent mental health and substance abuse problems include education and awareness activities (e.g., the inclusion of a mental health column in the school newsletter, participation in substance abuse prevention activities such as the Red Ribbon Week, participation in Child Abuse Prevention Month activities), suicide prevention programs, substance abuse prevention curricula, parent networking, and parent education opportunities.

Selective Interventions and Supports   The implementation of effective universal strategies and supports is likely to result in a significant reduction in problem behavior. Not all students, however, are responsive to schoolwide strategies, and an estimated 5%–10% of students require interventions targeted specifically to their unique needs. Selective interventions are designed for youth who

---

Box 20.1.   Building the foundation for student success: Example of a schoolwide intervention

A small elementary (K–5) school that participated in the Bridges Project met with success in planning, designing, and implementing schoolwide academic and mental health interventions to improve the school climate and overcome barriers to student success. The Positive Behavior Support team created the following mission statement to guide the actions of the team: "We, the staff, are committed to providing a positive learning environment where students are encouraged to reach their full potential." The following behavioral expectations were established to meet the mission: *Be responsible, always try, do your best, cooperate with others, and treat everyone with dignity and respect*. These guidelines were posted throughout the school, and lesson plans were developed to teach students the necessary skills to behave in accordance with the behavioral expectations. For example, a schoolwide kick-off was held in which students and staff designed and performed skits illustrating each expectation. Students were reinforced for following the expectations through activities such as *Caught Ya Being Good* tickets that could be exchanged for incentive items at the school store. The Positive Behavior Support team met monthly to review existing interventions, make needed revisions, and review office discipline referral and other data to guide decisions about additional schoolwide strategies and supports.

Note: Adapted from Robbins, V., and Armstrong, B.J., The Bridges Project: Description and Evaluation of a School-Based Mental Health Program in Eastern Kentucky. In M.H. Epstein, K. Kutash, and A.J. Duchnowski (Eds.), *Outcomes for Children with Emotional and Behavioral Disorders and Their Families: Programs and Evaluation Best Practices* 2nd ed., (pp. 355–373), 2005, Austin, TX: PRO-ED. Copyright 2005 by PRO-ED, Inc. Adapted with permission.

are at risk or who are beginning to exhibit signs of emotional or behavioral problems. Such interventions are more specialized than universal approaches and are administered individually or in small groups (Sprague, Sugai, & Walker, 1998).

The design, implementation, and monitoring of individual or small group selective interventions and supports in Kentucky is the responsibility of the problem solving team. The composition of this team varies from school to school, depending on the level of behavioral expertise of individual members, but the team typically includes a school administrator, a special educator, student support personnel (school counselor or school social worker), a family liaison, and a child and family intervention specialist from the student care team. The problem solving team meets on an as-needed basis to review referral information, collect additional data (e.g., behavioral observations, record reviews), and develop a behavior support or treatment plan to target the identified problem area. Caregivers and youth, as appropriate, as well as the referring teacher, participate in the problem-solving process. Examples of these interventions and supports include mentoring, academic tutoring and support, and check and connect programs, in which a school staff member is assigned to check in with a student on a regular basis and connect the student and his or her family with services and supports. Short-term individual and group therapies also are used (see Box 20.2).

Indicated Interventions and Supports   Approximately 1%–5% of students require more than primary and secondary interventions and supports to succeed. These students have serious and complex emotional and behavioral needs that span across home, school, and community settings and require a comprehensive multiagency treatment approach. Similar to other communities imple-

---

Box 20.2.   A secondary (targeted) intervention in action:
Homework helpers

A review of referrals to the problem solving team revealed a group of five elementary school–age boys who were having difficulty with homework completion. Through a strengths-based problem-solving process, the team determined that a small group intervention would be implemented as a first step to address this issue. The intervention specialist sent caregivers an information packet that included tips for setting up an effective study environment at home and assisting students with homework. On Monday mornings, the students met with the intervention specialist to receive their weekly homework tracking form and participate in skill-building sessions related to organization, study habits, and goal setting. On Fridays, students met again with the intervention specialist to conduct a progress check of homework completion, celebrate successes, and assist those who did not meet their goals. Anecdotal evidence suggests that for some students, participation in the Homework Helpers group led to improved grades, improved self-confidence, and increased parent satisfaction with student progress.

Note: Adapted from Robbins, V., and Armstrong, B.J., The Bridges Project: Description and Evaluation of a School-Based Mental Health Program in Eastern Kentucky. In M.H. Epstein, K. Kutash, and A.J. Duchnowski (Eds.), *Outcomes for Children with Emotional and Behavioral Disorders and Their Families: Programs and Evaluation Best Practices* 2nd ed., (pp. 355–373), 2005, Austin, TX: PRO-ED. Copyright 2005 by PRO-ED, Inc. Adapted with permission.

menting system of care initiatives, the Bridges Project decided to apply the wraparound process to design and implement individualized service plans (Burns & Goldman, 1999; Eber & Nelson, 1997). Wraparound, a promising practice for improving outcomes for youth with the most challenging needs (Burns & Goldman, 1999; Burns & Hoagwood, 2002), incorporates a family-centered and strength-based philosophy of care to guide the individualized service planning process. The service coordinator facilitates the development of an individualized child and family wraparound team composed of the youth, his or her family, and other members selected by the youth and family. Other team members typically include school personnel, community agency service providers, and natural community supports (e.g., extended family members, clergy, neighbors, friends).

Following a defined eight-step process, the team begins by identifying the strengths, resources, and barriers that exist across the youth's life domains. The team then prioritizes the needs and identifies or designs individualized interventions using a blend of formal (e.g., respite, counseling, behavior supports) and informal services and supports (e.g., recreational or sports activities, church activities, support groups). The wraparound planning process is used to build trust and consensus within the team of family members, professionals, and natural support providers to improve the effectiveness and relevance of services and supports developed for the youth and family (Eber, Smith, Sugai, & Scott, 2002). Careful monitoring of implementation and outcomes across multiple life domains (e.g., social/emotional, medical, basic needs, academic, living environment) is an integral part of the process.

As the service coordinator facilitates the wraparound planning process, the responsibility for its consistent implementation, monitoring, and evaluation rests with all members of the team (see Box 20.3). The wraparound process is a key component of the full continuum of PBS because it is the mechanism for ensuring that proactive, outcome-based interventions for students with the most intensive needs and their families are developed in a creative yet efficient manner. Likewise, evidence from Illinois suggests that implementing the wraparound process within the context of PBS increases school personnel's confidence and ability to effectively educate students with the most challenging emotional and behavioral problems. Lewis-Palmer, Horner, Sugai, and Eber (2002) found that schools implementing universal strategies reported greater effectiveness of their wraparound processes when compared with schools that were not fully implementing universal strategies.

Evaluation results from the implementation of a school-based wraparound process within the context of PBS have documented positive outcomes for youth served through the Bridges Project, including lower levels of problem behavior and functional impairment, improved grades, and decreased office disciplinary actions (Armstrong, Robbins, Collins, & Eber, 2004; Robbins & Armstrong, 2005; Robbins, Armstrong, & Collins, 2002). The impact of school-based wraparound on substance use was not as readily evident (Robbins, Collins, & Marcum, 2004). The success of the Bridges Project paved the way for a second grant from the federal Comprehensive Community Mental Health Services for Children and Their Families Program, awarded to Kentucky in 2004. Using lessons

Box 20.3.   School-Based Wraparound: Jake's story

Jake, a 13-year-old middle school student, lived with his maternal grandmother. By the beginning of his fifth-grade year, Jake had been enrolled in five schools in three states. Jake's family changed schools frequently as a result of an inability to address his behavior within the school system. Currently, Jake attends a school implementing schoolwide Positive Behavior Support, including school-based wraparound. Since enrolling in the school 2 years ago, Jake has had a total of three office referrals. In the past, he averaged three office referrals per week.

Jake's initial involvement with the Bridges Project began when his school was selected to participate in the project. Prior to that time, Jake and his family received service coordination through Kentucky IMPACT, a community-based interagency service coordination program. Because most of his difficulties occurred in the school setting, his IMPACT team determined that the Bridges Project would more comprehensively serve his needs. Jake's school-based wraparound team includes his grandmother, service coordinator, intervention specialist, two teachers, and the school principal. Extended team members include his aunt, a family friend, and his coach. Initial conversations revealed that Jake is bright, motivated, wants to succeed, and enjoys positive adult attention.

Given Jake's history and identified strengths, his wraparound team developed the following mission statement: "Jake will interact successfully with peers and succeed in the classroom." The majority of needs identified by Jake's team fell into the educational/vocational and social/recreational life domains. Due to the severity of school-related problems, the team chose to prioritize needs in the educational/vocational domain. The needs centered on classroom behavior problems and Jake's difficulty with completion of schoolwork. The primary action was the development and implementation of a 504 modification plan that listed the accommodations necessary to meet the educational needs of a student with a disability. All core team members accepted responsibility for ensuring that the plan was implemented as written and modified as needed to meet Jake's behavioral and academic needs.

Before his involvement in school-based wraparound, Jake tried hard to finish his homework, working from the time he got home until bedtime, but he was still failing most of his classes. His family was told he would be in reform school by the time he was 12. He now completes his homework quickly in the evening, and he consistently receives As and Bs.

Jake's grandmother describes past school and mental health services as disjointed and prescriptive. Professionals encouraged Jake's family to put him on medication, but they did not discuss the importance of other supportive services. Due to the coordinated supports provided to Jake and his family by school and mental health personnel through the Bridges Project, Jake's grandmother receives fewer calls from the school, and she can now focus on supporting her family without having to leave work to meet with school personnel. She is now working in partnership with school personnel rather than fighting against them.

Through her family's involvement in Kentucky's system of care, Jake's grandmother has learned how to live with his disability. She is always getting ideas about new things to try and how to modify them if they don't work. She has called it a "life-changing experience." Jake and his grandmother now present at state and national conferences to share his success story with other families and professionals. The improvements in the family's quality of life testify to the importance of providing coordinated services, focusing on strengths rather than deficits, and including family members as equal partners at all levels of decision making.

(continued)

Box 20.3.   *(continued)*

> As Jake met with success at school, as evidenced through a reduction in office referrals and improved grades, the team reconvened and determined that the next priority was to improve his peer-interaction skills. To meet this need, Jake began participating in a highly structured after-school program with an emphasis on prosocial development. Building on his strength of responding well to adult attention, Jake has also begun assisting Bridges Project staff with implementation of an experiential curriculum in a third grade classroom. Currently, Jake is working with his intervention specialist to appropriately apply the skills he learned in the after-school program to school and classroom settings. Jake and his team will continue to meet to address identified needs and modify his plan toward the achievement of the team's mission statement.
>
> ---
>
> *Note:* Adapted from Robbins, V., and Armstrong, B.J., The Bridges Project: Description and Evaluation of a School-Based Mental Health Program in Eastern Kentucky. In M.H. Epstein, K. Kutash, and A.J. Duchnowski (Eds.), *Outcomes for Children with Emotional and Behavioral Disorders and Their Families: Programs and Evaluation Best Practices* 2nd ed., (pp. 355–373), 2005, Austin, TX: PRO-ED. Copyright 2005 by PRO-ED, Inc. Adapted with permission.

learned from the Bridges Project, the Kentuckians Encouraging Youth to Succeed (KEYS) system of care initiative includes continued implementation of the schoolwide PBS model, but with a specific emphasis on the use of evidence-based assessment and treatment approaches to address the needs of youth with co-occurring mental health and substance use challenges.

Addressing Common Barriers

Despite policy and legal support, as well as data illustrating the effectiveness of specific SBMH models (Atkins, Abdul-Adil, Jackson, Talbott, & Bell, 2001; Catron, Harris, & Weiss, 1988; Vernberg, Jacobs, Nyre, Puddy, & Roberts, 2004; Weist, Sander, Lowie, & Christodulu, 2002), the field continues to struggle with the operationalization of comprehensive SBMH programming (Eber & Keenan, 2004). A myriad of barriers affect implementation of SBMH services, and empirically-based strategies for addressing these barriers are sparse. The experience of implementing SBMH services and supports in Kentucky has yielded important lessons about effective strategies for addressing common barriers (VanTreuren, Robbins, & Armstrong, 2006).

Addressing Perceived Mission Disparity   One of the most commonly cited barriers to collaboration between school and mental health systems is the perceived difference in mission. The goal of education is to promote academic success, whereas the mental health profession is designed to address social, emotional, and behavioral challenges. Despite perceived disparities in their missions, consensus is emerging regarding the potential role of mental health in promoting educational aims by addressing nonacademic barriers to learning (Hunter et al.,

2005; UCLA School Mental Health Project, 2005). This consensus, however, exists primarily at the national level and is less apparent at state and local community levels.

The Bridges Project afforded an opportunity to pilot practical strategies for reducing perceived mission disparities at the local level. One of the most successful strategies for addressing mission disparity was the collection and review of academic and psychological outcome data by both education and mental health staff. The positive mental health and educational outcomes of youth receiving school-based wraparound suggested that by utilizing a comprehensive approach to SBMH, both academic and nonacademic barriers to learning can be addressed, allowing educators and mental health staff alike to realize achievement of their respective missions. A second local strategy to address perceived mission disparity involved the examination of goals in school improvement plans. Aligning mental health prevention and treatment services and supports with school improvement goals (e.g., family involvement, improved school culture and climate) led to increased buy-in by school staff and helped mental health professionals to better understand their role in promoting the educational success of students.

Understanding School and Agency Culture The concept of cultural differences must extend beyond traditional racial and ethnic mindsets to encompass agency culture. When mental health professionals begin providing services in schools, oftentimes the unfamiliarity with the culture of the school inhibits success in implementing comprehensive services and supports. Anecdotal data from the Bridges Project highlighted some key strategies in understanding school culture:

- *Recognizing the importance of the tone set by the building principal*—The principal's attitude toward implementing and sustaining innovative programming can make or break SBMH programs.

- *Identifying and connecting with a key contact in schools*—This may or may not be the building administrator. This person has credibility among his or her peers and advocates for the integration of SBMH initiatives into the school culture.

- *Realizing that schools have a rhythm of their own*—Educators are aware of the patterns within the school, be they seasonally related or a result of district deadlines. Learning about these rhythms and associated expectations is vital to the partnership.

- *Understanding the climate of the school*—A given school may have a collective attitude that is positive and proactive or one that is negative and reactive. This climate can set the stage for whether or not innovative programs will succeed or fail, and it is often a gauge for the degree of work needed to successfully implement a comprehensive spectrum of mental health services and supports.

Regulatory Limitations   Regulatory limitations have been cited as barriers to providing mental health services in schools (Hunter et al., 2005). One such regulatory limitation is encompassed in Medicaid regulations in some states that require outpatient services to be provided in clinic settings and prohibit Medicaid reimbursement for services provided off-site of a mental health provider (i.e., at a school). Kentucky addressed and resolved this issue during the late 1980s when it developed its plan for a statewide system of care. At that time, the Mental Health Commissioner and Medicaid Director assessed how the Medicaid Rehabilitation Option might be applied to children's behavioral health services and ultimately collaborated to support adoption of the Medicaid Rehabilitation Option. This change made it possible for providers to bill Medicaid for services delivered either on-site, which was defined as the Community Mental Health Centers' leased or donated space, or off-site, which includes "the client's home, congregate living facility . . . , school or day care center, . . . and Family Resource and Youth Center" (Kentucky Cabinet for Human Resources, 1993, p. 4.2). This change, which in many ways is the backbone of school-based mental health services in Kentucky, came as a result of a shared vision at the state level between mental health and Medicaid agency leadership (Biebel, Katz-Leavy, Nicholson, & Williams, 2005).

Funding and Sustainability   Services in schools are becoming less dependent on fee-for-service models and more reliant on grant-funded or school-subsidized approaches (VanTreuren et al., 2006). Fee-for-service models are traditional in mental health. There is vast experience in stretching dollars to maximize services, but the current disadvantage is that reimbursement rates are either frozen or in decline. At the same time, cost pressures are increasing. School-based programs operating in a fee-for-service environment are forced to either cut costs (i.e., reduce staffing levels, number of schools served, or the amount of services to students) or look for additional funding.

School districts can play a valuable role in financing and sustaining effective mental health services. The President's New Freedom Commission on Mental Health (2003) report highlights the relationship between schools and mental health. The connection is obvious—schools and mental health agencies serve the same children whose families live and work in the community. The dilemma, however, is that like mental health, funding for behavioral initiatives in education is shrinking. Existing dollars are increasingly earmarked for reform programs aimed at improving academic performance. Schools that recognize the value of mental health partnerships have invested their limited resources to incorporate the full spectrum of mental health services and supports. Investments take different forms, including human resources to collaborate on grants, confidential space for mental health practitioners to meet with students, and budgeted dollars. Few schools have the luxury of hiring their own mental health professionals, and those that do often contract for services that they cannot provide in their array (e.g., psychiatric medication management, psychological testing for diagnostic purposes). Some schools elect to offset the cost of service provision by providing a stipend or retainer for mental health providers. Alternatively, school districts may contract with mental health providers on a flexible basis. In these arrangements, schools may agree to offset the cost of downtime for mental health providers, meaning they agree to a negotiated rate for hours that cannot be billed to a third party payer such as Medicaid or private insurance. In this way, both the mental health provider and the school district share the risk in order to achieve the goal of assisting the school community in maximizing the educational potential for all students.

Reliance on third-party payers such as Medicaid was evident in the Bridges Project. Grant funds were initially used to support child and family intervention specialists and service coordinators until a sufficient case load was attained so that third-party reimbursement could cover the cost of these staff. Unfortunately, no third-party reimbursement mechanism such as Medicaid or a private insurance carrier exists for the services and supports provided by the family liaisons, and thus state funds are used to cover these costs. Given their critical role in building school, family, and community partnerships, Kentucky is undertaking an effort to build the evidence base to support family-to-family and youth-to-youth support services to establish a basis for funding these services through Medicaid or other third-party payers. Along with plans for an extensive study, the current certification program for family liaisons is being redesigned to increase alignment with the family-driven philosophy. Regional youth councils have been created across the state, and youth liaisons are being hired in some areas to provide youth-to-youth support services and to build a youth support network. A certification program is planned for youth liaisons similar to the certification program for family liaisons. These efforts will culminate in a change in Medicaid regulations to allow family-to-family and youth-to-youth support to become billable services. The sustainability of the family and youth liaison positions is critical to the success of the school-based wraparound process as well as system of care transformation efforts.

STRATEGIES FOR FAMILY AND YOUTH INVOLVEMENT

School reform initiatives, new legislation, and recent governmental reports emphasize the need to increase family involvement in the education and mental health treatment of their children, but families of children who have emotional disturbances have traditionally been, and continue to be, the least engaged families (Singer & Butler, 1987; U.S. Public Health Service, 2000). Parent involvement is considered to be a key factor in the academic achievement and emotional functioning of children (Comer & Haynes, 1991; Keith et al., 1993), but there is a paucity of evidence demonstrating effective approaches for increasing the involvement of families who have children with emotional disorders (Kutash, Duchnowski, Sumi, Rudo, & Harris, 2002).

Although the reasons for the lack of effective parent involvement are complex, the perceptions by professionals of families who have children with emotional problems have contributed to the situation. In particular, professionals in both the education and mental health fields were influenced in the past by unsupported theories and biased studies that cast parents in a negative role as the major cause of their children's problems (Duchnowski, Berg, & Kutash, 1995). Fortunately, these perceptions have changed over time, and new system reform initiatives have called for new roles for parents that reflect their strengths and emphasize their role as partners with professionals.

New Rules for Families and Youth

This new paradigm is reflected in Kentucky's work. Within the SBMH services and supports provided in Kentucky, parents are equal partners. They serve in a professional role by providing peer-to-peer support to family members and building support networks. They are also equal decision makers as reflected in their integral role on the school-based wraparound teams for their own children. Although this demonstrates what can be accomplished, parent involvement and support in schools is not as yet widespread. In a recent study using a nationally representative sample of parents whose children were served in special education programs due to emotional disturbances, parents reported that the least available and hardest service to obtain was parent support services (Wagner et al., 2006).

The positive examples from Kentucky, coupled with the disappointing reality found by Wagner and her colleagues (2006), underscore the need to more fully capitalize on the potential of families to provide support to other families in need. In moving to family-driven systems of care, policy makers and administrators should be aware of the potential to increase service capacity by including families as partners in service provision, particularly in providing family support. Kentucky's approaches offer a good starting point.

The strength of the family movement has paved the way for a similar national effort to empower youth to become full partners at all levels within systems of care. Based on the components of positive youth development—having a sense of competence, usefulness, belonging, and power (National Clearinghouse on Families and Youth, 1996)—this movement is aimed at involving youth with serious mental health conditions more fully in their own care, as well as in system transformation efforts. In their guide to youth empowerment, Matarese, McGinnis, and Mora (2005) describe the values underlying the youth movement and share concrete strategies for engaging and involving youth in various ways within the system, for example, serving on governance boards and committees, assisting with research and evaluation efforts, and serving as social marketers.

Schools can be major facilitators of youth involvement in a variety of ways, including providing training opportunities in youth leadership, partnering with youth when conducting staff development training, and assisting youth in establishing support groups in schools and other community settings. A useful planning tool for school staff to increase youth involvement is *Planning for Youth Success* (Dorfman et al., 2001), a resource that outlines a process for positive youth development. The process involves: 1) identifying characteristics of youth thought to be important for success; 2) generating strategies to determine if students are developing these characteristics; 3) identifying resources and assets in the community that will help youth develop these characteristics; and 4) planning and implementing a project to promote the characteristics, evaluate the effectiveness of the project, and communicate the results to the public.

Increasing Involvement Through Cultural Competency

Since the inception of the system of care concept (Stroul & Friedman, 1986), the need for services and organizations that are culturally sensitive and competent has been a foundational value. This value permeates the entire service system for children who have emotional disturbances, including schools. There is encouraging research on the implementation of evidence-based practices, indicating that the superiority of these practices is not reduced by the inclusion of minority youths (Weisz, Jensen-Doss, & Hawley, 2006). School staff, therefore, can feel secure in promoting evidence-based services when they are located in communities that have service populations with a high degree of cultural and ethnic diversity. There is also encouraging research on how to increase the cultural competency of schools in their efforts to engage families that are culturally and linguistically diverse. In a national survey of school staff conducted by the Center for Health and Health Care in Schools (2004), 87% of the respondents reported that cross-cultural issues had affected the way in which they responded to students and families. Respondents provided the following recommendations for increasing cultural and linguistic competency in schools:

1. Provide written materials in all appropriate languages and literacy levels.

2. Hire staff members who reflect the community served.

3. Collaborate with interpreter services to assist with important conversations with parents.

4. Develop a parent/community advisory committee to provide feedback and suggestions.

5. Develop training sessions for staff.

6. Use outreach workers to connect with new communities.

In their efforts to increase family and youth involvement, schools must be aware of the importance of addressing issues related to the diversity of the families they serve. Recommendations that have emerged from the research and practice communities, including those previously cited, can assist schools in this endeavor.

FUTURE DIRECTIONS FOR SCHOOL-BASED MENTAL HEALTH: A PUBLIC HEALTH APPROACH

Although the empirical knowledge base describing SBMH is still evolving (Rones & Hoagwood, 2000), a number of federal policies and reports are promoting the potential of SBMH to reduce the gap between the need for and receipt of mental health services by children (Kutash et al., 2006). *The Surgeon General's Report on*

Mental Health (U.S. DHHS, 1999), the report from the President's Commission on Excellence in Special Education (U.S. Department of Education, 2002), and the President's New Freedom Commission on Mental Health (2003) all noted the value of enhancing the provision of mental health services for children in schools. Furthermore, these reports also recommended the implementation of the public health model to increase the capacity of the service delivery system in communities.

The public health model may be conceived of as having four components or steps (see Figure 20.2). Each component is outlined below, with a specific focus on how a community may use this model to develop and implement a comprehensive system of SBMH services.

Focus on the Population

When a community decides to use a public health model to guide the implementation of SBMH services for its school-age children and youth, the first step involves surveillance. The community will seek answers to the question, "What is the problem in our community?" Surveillance entails systematic data collection to produce information for action. The community will want to know the degree to which the mental health needs of its children are being met, the gaps that exist in

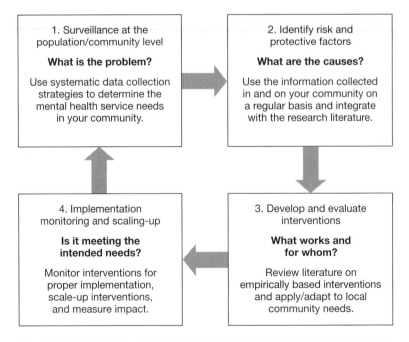

Figure 20.2. Implementing school-based mental health systems using a public health approach. (Adapted from Kutash, K., Duchnowski, A.J., & Lynn, N. [2006]. *School-based mental health: An empirical guide for decision-makers* [p. 75]. Tampa: University of South Florida, Louis de la Parte Florida Mental Health Institute, Department of Child and Family Studies.)

service delivery, and the potential for effective SBMH services to contribute to meeting the needs. In a public health approach, the focus is on all school-age children, not just those with the most severe emotional disturbances or who may be at risk for suicide. Consequently, the school district is a major player in the surveillance process, as opposed to individual schools or classrooms. Surveillance information can be derived from districtwide data, census information, county health department data, and other similar databases. This information will help not only by producing estimates of the magnitude of the problem and possible geographic and demographic relationships, but it will also lead to the development of strategies for improved outcomes. High-quality surveillance in a community will facilitate progress to the next step—attempting to identify the risk and protective factors that contribute to the manifestation of undesirable conditions.

Analyze Risk and Protective Factors

In the public health model, potential causes of problems are identified through analysis of risk and protective factors. Risk and protective factors are not causes or cures themselves, but rather are statistical predictors that have a theoretical and empirical base. *Risk factors* are personal characteristics or environmental conditions that have been empirically demonstrated to increase the likelihood of problem behavior. Some examples of risk factors are gender, family history, a lack of social support, reading disabilities, and exposure to bullying. These factors vary in terms of their malleability to change. *Protective factors* are personal characteristics or environmental conditions that have been empirically established to interact with risk factors to reduce the likelihood of the occurrence of problem behavior. Examples of protective factors include caring parents and teachers, social competence and problem solving skills, schools that establish high expectations for all students and supply the supports necessary for all students to achieve these expectations, and opportunities to participate in positive activities in school and in the community. As in the case of risk factors, these protective factors vary in the degree to which schools and child-serving agencies can promote them, but they all have been empirically demonstrated to reduce the effects of risk factors. As the research base on risk and protective factors expands, it is becoming clear that there must be a balance in addressing the reduction of risk factors (i.e., a deficit approach) and promoting protective factors (i.e., a strengths-based approach).

Develop and Evaluate Interventions

A plethora of innovative and empirically based interventions have been developed over the past several decades to meet the emotional and behavioral needs of youth. The implementation of effective, community-based systems of care may play an important facilitating role in the implementation of these evidence-based practices. In combination with a public health orientation, the two approaches may provide the kind of host environment proposed by Zins and Ponti (1990) necessary to facilitate the implementation of evidence-based practices at a sustainable and scaled-up level. Communities that desire to implement a public health model may find that the existence of a system of care in the community provides a level of interagency collaboration, as well as the shared values and vision necessary to implement state-of-the-art evidence-based interventions for their children and youth.

Many of the effective strategies promoted as evidence-based, however, are not being widely implemented, particularly in the area of universal prevention. Prevention is an area in which there is a long history of empirical support, as outlined in *Neurons to Neighborhoods* (National Research Council and Institute of Medicine, 2000) and in the work of Greenberg and colleagues (2003). Two school-based universal programs—PATHS (Greenberg, Domitrovich, & Bumbarger, 2000) and schoolwide use of PBS (Horner, 1999)—are increasingly being implemented in schools nationwide. The use of these strategies and their effectiveness in various types of communities should be carefully assessed and documented.

Another challenge is to integrate empirically supported selective and indicated programs into schools. Communities are creating interesting strategies to increase awareness of the various empirically supported programs. Work groups were formed in Hawaii to study empirically based programs and to determine which interventions would be most applicable to their populations (Chorpita & Taylor, 2001; Chorpita et al., 2002). Ohio has a statewide initiative to increase awareness of evidence-based practices (Ohio Department of Mental Health, 2001), as well as an initiative to increase the empowerment of teachers in delivering SBMH services (Paternite, 2004). A growing literature shows that many communities nationwide are active in building SBMH services (Vernberg et al., 2004).

What is typically missing is the evaluation of these SBMH services and documentation of the student outcomes resulting from these services. This type of information is critical to informing future policy and practice. Evaluation is especially needed with respect to services for students with emotional disturbances who are served in special education settings. This population of students continues to experience low levels of academic achievement and high drop-out rates, and receives few support services (Wagner & Sumi, 2006; Wagner, Kutash, Duchnowski, Epstein, & Sumi, 2005).

An additional challenge inherent in the delivery of SBMH services is the need to direct attention to improving academic outcomes for students with emotional disturbances. The lack of attention may be partly due to teacher preparation programs focusing predominantly on the social and behavioral characteristics and needs of this population, along with the misconception held by many educators that students must behave properly before academic learning is possible. Research suggests that, in some instances, students may act out to avoid aversive academic tasks that do not match their skill levels because they are either too easy or too difficult (Lane, 2004). Other research is exploring the existence of a reciprocal relationship between academic success and decreases in negative behavior. There is a growing body of research indicating that academic success is associated with a decrease in problem behavior (Gottfredson, Gottfredson, &

Skroban, 1996; Lane, O'Shaughnessy, Lambros, Graham, & Beebe-Franken-berger, 2001; Lane, Wehby, Menzies, Gregg, Doukas, & Munton, 2002). This research suggests that mental health professionals may need to support classroom teachers in instructional activities and classroom management to a greater degree than previously recognized.

Implementation Monitoring and Scaling-Up

The final step in the public health model addresses the issue of implementation. Numerous efforts have been initiated to better understand the factors associated with the successful implementation of evidence-based practices in community-based settings, and the complexity of scaling-up innovative interventions for wide-scale community adoption is becoming apparent. Both the National Implementa-tion Research Network (Fixsen, Naoom, Blase, Friedman, & Wallace, 2005) and the Prevention Research Center for the Promotion of Human Development at Penn State University (Greenberg, Domitrovich, Graczyk, & Zins, 2004) have conducted extensive reviews of the literature in this area and have reached similar conclusions. First, providing training on innovative techniques to staff without adequate follow-up (e.g., coaching, supervision) is not effective and will result in flawed implementation and outcomes that do not match those achieved by pro-gram developers. Although most program developers provide manuals and initial training sessions for their programs, very few offer mechanisms for the ongoing monitoring of implementation quality. Without continued support of staff as they implement these new approaches, and without the ongoing monitoring of imple-mentation, most programs will not be implemented as planned, and thus the promised outcomes will not materialize. Fixsen and colleagues (2005) suggested the key to successful implementation is a combination of supportive policies, community involvement, and an organizational infrastructure able to supply post-training support and conduct process and outcome evaluations.

In addition, for innovations implemented in schools, factors at the school, district, and community level influence the quality of program delivery (Green-berg et al., 2004). Without support and active involvement of the community and district, most innovations adopted at the school level will not succeed. In ad-dition, along with collecting information on the level of implementation of an in-novation, school personnel and practitioners should examine and record factors that substantially affect the quality of implementation in their setting and share this information with the developers of the program and the field. It is through the collection and dissemination of information on implementation in a variety of schools that the field will move forward. Daleiden and Chorpita (2005) pre-sented an extended discussion of how evidence-based services have been inte-grated into information systems, performance measurement, and feedback tools, providing an excellent framework for schools and communities.

Figure 20.3 illustrates how a community can proceed to implement a public health approach to address the mental health needs of its children and focus the delivery of services in the schools. Communities that have established or emerg-ing systems of care will have already developed many of the collaborative mecha-

1. Surveillance at the population/community level	2. Identify risk and protective factors
What is the problem?	**What are the causes?**
Use systematic data collection strategies to determine the mental health service needs in your community.	Use the information collected in and on your community on a regular basis and integrate with the research literature.
Steps to identify priority problems through surveillance	**Steps to identify risk and protective factors**

• Establish a task force that includes representatives from schools and has resources and authority for engaging in decision making for service planning.
 	
• Use existing data (especially from schools) to create a composite picture of the mental health challenges in the community.
 	
• Existing data should be examined for indicators of mental health functioning in youth in your community and will help direct action.
 	
• Examples:
  • What is the youth suicide rate in your community?
  • What is the rate of involuntary psychiatric hospitalizations in your community?
  • What are some indicators of substance abuse problems among the youth in your community?
  • Do existing data point to mental health problems of youth in the juvenile justice system?
  • What are the rates of suspensions and dropping out of school in your community?
  • What are the rates of young children entering school who are not ready to learn?
 	
• Prioritize the problems to be addressed.
	• Identify risk and protective factors for each prioritized problem. Risk factors are those conditions that increase the likelihood of a negative outcome for children. Protective factors are conditions that reduce the probability of the negative outcome.
	
	• Examine the empirical literature and condense the information to identify the risk and protective factors associated with the priority problem.
	
	• Examples:
	  • Depression is a well-documented risk factor for suicide. Possessing adequate coping skills to deal with stress is an effective protective factor against depression and, subsequently, suicide.
	  • A common risk factor associated with the problems of aggression and substance use is negative peer influence. For both, protective factors are increased social competence and communication skills.
	  • A common risk factor for early school failure is a lack of preschool academic skill development. The protective factors include an academic environment that engages in screening and early intervention for students with academic deficits.
	
	• Integrate the community data with the research literature to identify and prioritize risk and protective factors needing to be addressed in your community.

Figure 20.3. An example of the components in implementing a public health model for school-based mental health services. (Adapted from Kutash, K., Duchnowski, A.J., & Lynn, N. [2006]. *School-based mental health: An empirical guide for decision-makers* [p. 114]. Tampa: University of South Florida, Louis de la Parte Florida Mental Health Institute, Department of Child and Family Studies.)

3. Develop and evaluate
interventions

What works and for whom?

Review literature on
empirically based interventions
and apply/adapt to local
community needs.

**Steps to implement evidence-based
programs and practices**

- Use the research literature to identify
evidence-based programs and practices
that are appropriate for addressing the
prioritized risk and protective factors in
your community.

- Communities need to be aware of the
need to integrate and balance the implementation of universal, selective, and
indicated interventions. After universal
interventions have been established, the
effectiveness of implementing selective and
indicated interventions will be facilitated.

- The Task Force must also investigate the
feasibility of implementing the selected
evidence-based program for issues such
as cost of the program, staff training
necessary for implementation, and cultural relevance. In addition, Task Force
members should outline the resources
needed to support the implementation of
the selected intervention over the life of
the program.

- Example: A Task Force that prioritizes depression, aggression and substance
abuse for possible action could examine
the feasibility of implementing the following programs:

  - *For depression*—The Coping with
  Stress Course is a selective inter-
  vention that involves Cognitive-
  Behavioral Therapy in a group setting.

  - *For aggression*—The PATHS Program
  (Promoting Alternative Thinking
  Strategies) is a universal prevention
  program that teaches skills such as
  self-control, social competence, and
  interpersonal problem-solving skills.
  An example of an indicated intervention is the Anger Coping Program,
  which uses a group setting to reduce
  antisocial behavior.

  - *For substance use*—The Midwestern
  Prevention Project focuses on drug
  abuse prevention with classroom-based
  sessions and parent involvement.

4. Implementation
monitoring and scaling-up

**Is it meeting the
intended needs?**

Monitor interventions for
proper implementation,
scale-up interventions,
and measure impact.

**Steps for implementation,
monitoring, and
scaling-up**

- Create infrastructure to
examine and monitor
youth and community
outcomes to determine
the effectiveness of
efforts.

- Create quality assurance
standards and training
opportunities to support
the dissemination and
widespread adoption of
successful efforts.

nisms needed to achieve such a system. For communities that are just beginning, this model can serve as a framework that will facilitate the complex task of meeting the mental health needs of the community's children.

CONCLUSION

The current climate of transformation and reform may provide an opportune time to implement SBMH services with new tools and perspectives. The public health model provides a framework for SBMH services that can span the vast age groups and problems encountered in public schools today.

It also is important to note that in this era of accountability and school reform, the mental health community should be aware that its interventions must align with the major concern of the schools, which is academic achievement. Likewise, the education community must be aware that mental health professionals have strategies for improving instruction and achievement, as well as for improving social and emotional functioning in children. The convergence of these two perspectives is the hallmark of SBMH.

REFERENCES

Adelman, H.S., & Taylor, L. (1998). Mental health in schools: Moving forward. *School Psychology Review, 27,* 175–190.

Arbuthnot, J., & Gordon, D.A. (1996). Does mandatory divorce education work? A six-month outcome evaluation. *Family and Conciliation Courts Review, 34,* 60–81.

Armstrong, B.J., Robbins, V., Collins, K., & Eber, L. (2004). The Bridges Project: Meeting the academic and mental health needs of children through a continuum of positive supports. In K.E. Robinson (Ed.), *Advances in school mental health interventions: Best practices and program models* (pp. 15–22). Kingston, NJ: Civic Research Institute.

Atkins, M.S., Abdul-Adil, J., Jackson, M., Talbott, E., & Bell, C.C. (2001). PALS: An ecological approach to school-based mental health services in urban schools. *Emotional and Behavioral Disorders in Youth, 1*(4), 75–76, 91–92.

Biebel, K., Katz-Leavy, J., Nicholson, J., & Williams, V. (2005). *Using Medicaid effectively for children with serious emotional disturbances.* Rockville, MD: Center for Mental Health Services, Substance Abuse and Mental Health Services Administration.

Botvin, G.J., Griffin, K.W., Paul, E., & Macaulay, A.P. (2003). Preventing tobacco and alcohol use among elementary school students through Life Skills Training. *Journal of Child and Adolescent Substance Abuse, 12,* 1–18.

Brener, N.D., Martindale, H., & Weist, M.D. (2001). Mental health and social services: Results from the School Health Policies and Programs Study 2000. *Journal of School Health, 71*(7), 305–312.

Burns, B.J., & Goldman, S.K. (1999). *Promising practices in wraparound for children with serious emotional disturbances and their families: Vol. IV. Systems of care: Promising practices in children's mental health.* Washington, DC: Center for Effective Collaboration and Practice, American Institutes for Research.

Burns, B.J., & Hoagwood, K.J. (2002). *Community treatment for youth: Evidence-based interventions for severe emotional and behavioral disorders.* New York: Oxford University Press.

Catron, T., Harris, V., & Weiss, B. (1998). Post-treatment results after 2 years of services in the Vanderbilt School-Based Counseling Project. In M.H. Epstein, K. Kutash, & A.J. Duchnowski (Eds.), *Outcomes for children with emotional and behavioral disorders and their families: Programs and evaluation best practices* (pp. 633–653). Austin, TX: PRO-ED.

Center for Health and Health Care in Schools. (2004). *Caring across cultures: Achieving cultural competence in health programs at school: Survey results.* Washington, DC: Author.

Chorpita, B.F., & Taylor, A.A. (2001). Building bridges between the lab and the clinic: Hawaii's experience using research to inform practice policy. *Emotional and Behavioral Disorders in Youth, 2,* 53–56.

Chorpita, B.F., Yim, L.M., Donkervoet, J.C., Arensdorf, A., Amundsen, M.J., McGee, C., et al. (2002). Toward large-scale implementation of empirically supported treatments for children: A review and observations by the Hawaii Empirical Basis to Services Task Force. *Clinical Psychology: Science and Practice, 9,* 165–190.

Comer, J.P., & Haynes, N.M. (1991). Parent involvement in schools: An ecological approach. *The Elementary School Journal, 91*(3), 271–277.

Daleiden, E.L., & Chorpita, B.F. (2005). From data to wisdom: Quality improvements strategies supporting large-scale implementation of evidence based services. *Child and Adolescent Psychiatric Clinics of North America, 14,* 329–349.

Dorfman, D., Douglas, R., Ellis, D. Fisher, A., Geiger, E., Hughes, K., et al. (2001). *Planning for youth success: Resource and training manual.* Portland OR: Northwest Regional Educational Laboratory.

Duchnowski, A.J., Berg, K., & Kutash, K. (1995). Parent participation in and perception of placement decisions. In J.M. Kauffman, J.W. Lloyd, D.P. Hallahan, & T.A. Astuto (Eds.), *Issues in educational placement of pupils with emotional or behavioral disorders* (pp. 183–196). Mahwah, NJ: Lawrence Erlbaum Associates.

Durand, M.V., & Carr, E.G. (1985). Self-injurious behavior: Motivating conditions and guidelines for treatment. *School Psychology Review, 14,* 171–176.

Dwyer, K., & Osher, D. (2000). *Safeguarding our children: An action guide.* Washington, DC: U.S. Departments of Education and Justice, American Institutes for Research.

Eber, L. (2003). *The art and science of wraparound: Completing the continuum of schoolwide behavioral support.* Bloomington, IN: Forum on Education at Indiana University.

Eber, L., & Keenan, S. (2004). Collaboration with other agencies: Wraparound and systems of care for children and youth with EBD. In R. Rutherford, M.M. Quinn, & M. Sarup (Eds.), *Handbook of research in emotional and behavioral disorders* (pp. 502–521). New York: Guilford Press.

Eber, L., & Nelson, C.M. (1997). School-based wraparound planning: Integrating services for students with emotional and behavioral needs. *American Journal of Orthopsychiatry, 67*(3), 385–395.

Eber, L., Nelson, C.M., & Miles, P. (1997). School-based wraparound for students with emotional and behavioral challenges. *Exceptional Children, 63,* 539–555.

Eber. L., Smith, C., Sugai, G., & Scott, T. (2002). Wraparound and positive behavioral interventions and supports in schools. *Journal of Emotional and Behavioral Disorders, 10*(3), 171–180.

Education for All Handicapped Children Act of 1975, PL 94-142, 20 U.S.C. §§ 1400 *et seq.*

Fixsen, D.L., Naoom, S.F., Blase, K.A., Friedman, R.M., & Wallace, F. (2005). *Implementation research: A synthesis of the literature* (FMHI Publication #231). Tampa: University of South Florida, Louis de la Parte Florida Mental Health Institute, National Implementation Research Network.

Foster, S., Rollefson, M., Doksum, T., Noonan, D., Robinson, G., & Teich, J. (2005). *School mental health services in the United States, 2002–2003* (DHHS Publication No. SMA 05-4068). Rockville, MD: Center for Mental Health Services, Substance Abuse and Mental Health Services Administration.

Gottfredson, D.C., Gottfredson, G.D., & Skroban, S. (1996). A multi-model school-based prevention demonstration. *Journal of Adolescent Research, 11,* 97–115.

Greenberg, M.T., Domitrovich, C., & Bumbarger, B. (2000). *Preventing mental disorders in school-age children: A review of the effectiveness of prevention programs.* Prevention Research Center for the Promotion of Human Development, College of Health and Human Development, Pennsylvania State University. Retrieved March 6, 2006, from http://www.prevention.psu.edu/pubs/docs/CMHS.pdf

Greenberg, M.T., Domitrovich, C.E., Graczyk, P.A., & Zins, J.E. (2004). *The study of implementation in school-based preventive interventions: Theory, research, and practice.* Washington, DC: U.S. Department of Health and Human Services, Substance Abuse and Mental Health Services Administration, Center for Mental Health Services.

Greenberg, M.T., Kusché, C.A., Cook, E.T., & Quamma, J.P. (1995). Promoting emotional competence in school-aged children: The effects of the PATHS curriculum. *Developmental Research and Psychopathology, 7,* 117–136.

Greenberg, M.T., Weissberg, R.P., O'Brien, M.E., Zins, J.E., Fredericks, L., Resnik, H., et al. (2003). Enhancing school-based prevention and youth development through coordinated social, emotional, and academic learning. *American Psychologist, 58,* 466–474.

Horner, R.H. (1999). Positive behavior supports. In M. Wehmeyer & J. Patton (Eds.), *Mental retardation in the 21st century* (pp. 181–196). Austin, TX: PRO-ED.

Hunter, L., Hoagwood, K., Evans, S., Weist, M., Smith, C., Paternite, C., et al. (2005). *Working together to promote academic performance, social and emotional learning, and mental health for all children.* New York: Center for the Advancement of Children's Mental Health at Columbia University.

Individuals with Disabilities Education Act Amendments (IDEA) of 1997, PL 105-17, 20 U.S.C. §§ 1400 *et seq.*

Individuals with Disabilities Education Act (IDEA) of 1990, PL 101-476, 20 U.S.C. §§ 1400 *et seq.*

Keith, I.Z., Keith, P.B., Troutman, G.C., Bickley, P.G., Trivette, P.S., & Singh, K. (1993). Does parental involvement affect eighth grade student achievement? Structural analysis of national data. *School Psychology Review, 2,* 474–496.

Kentucky Cabinet for Human Resources. (1993). *Kentucky Medicaid Program: Community mental health manual policies and procedures.* Frankfort, KY: Author.

Kutash, K., Duchnowski, A.J., & Lynn, N., (2006). *School-based mental health: An empirical guide for decision makers.* Tampa: University of South Florida, Louis de la Parte Florida Mental Health Institute, Department of Child and Family Studies, Research and Training Center for Children's Mental Health.

Kutash, K., Duchnowski, A.J., Sumi, W.C., Rudo, Z., & Harris, K.M. (2002). A school, family, and community collaborative program for children who have emotional disturbances. *Journal of Emotional and Behavioral Disorders, 10*(2), 99–107.

Kutash, K., & Rivera, V.R. (1996). *Systems of care in children's mental health series: What works in children's mental health: Uncovering answers to critical questions.* Baltimore: Paul H. Brookes Publishing Co.

Lane, K.L. (2004). Academic instruction and tutoring interventions for students with emotional and behavioral disorders: 1990 to present. In R.B. Rutherford, M.M. Quinn, & S.R. Mathur (Eds.), *Handbook of research in emotional and behavioral disorders* (pp. 462–486). New York: Guilford Press.

Lane, K.L., O'Shaughnessy, T.E., Lambros, K.M., Graham, F.M., & Beebe-Frankenberger, M.E. (2001). The efficacy of phonological awareness training with first-graders who have behavior problems and reading difficulties. *Journal of Emotional and Behavioral Disorders, 9,* 219–231.

Lane, K.L., Wehby, J.H., Menzies, H.M., Gregg, R.M., Doukas, G.L., & Munton, S.M. (2002). Early literacy instruction for first-grade students at-risk for antisocial behavior. *Education and Treatment of Children, 25,* 438–458.

Lewis-Palmer, T., Horner, R.H., Sugai, G., & Eber, L. (2002). *An end-of-year progress report for the Illinois PBIS initiative.* Available at http://www.ebdnetwork-il.org

Liddle, H.A. (1998). *Multidimensional family therapy treatment manual.* Miami: University of Miami School of Medicine, Center for Treatment Research on Adolescent Drug Abuse.

Matarese, M., McGinnis, L., & Mora, M. (2005). *Youth involvement in systems of care: A guide to empowerment.* Washington, DC: American Institutes for Research.

Mrazek, P.J., & Haggerty, R.J. (Eds.). (1994). *Reducing risks for mental disorders: Frontiers for preventive intervention research.* Washington, DC: National Academies Press.

National Clearinghouse on Families and Youth. (1996). *Reconnecting youth and community: A youth development approach.* Silver Spring, MD: U.S. Department of Health and Human Services, Administration for Children and Families, Administration on Children, Youth and Families, Family and Youth Services Bureau.

National Research Council and Institute of Medicine. (2000). *From neurons to neighborhoods: The science of early childhood development.* Washington, DC: National Academies Press.

Nelson, J.R., Martella, R.M., & Marchand-Martella, N. (2002). Maximizing student learning: The effects of a school-based program for preventing problem behavior. *Journal of Emotional and Behavioral Disorders, 10*(1), 136–148.

No Child Left Behind Act of 2001, PL 107-110, 115 Stat. 1425, 20 U.S.C. §§ 6301 *et seq.*

Olweus, D. (1991). Bully/victim problems among schoolchildren: Basic facts and effects of a school based intervention program. In D.J. Pepler & K.H. Rubin (Eds.), *The development and treatment of childhood aggression* (pp. 411–448). Mahwah, NJ: Lawrence Erlbaum Associates.

Ohio Department of Mental Health. (2001). *Ohio Mental Health/Alternative Education Network Strategic Plan, 2001–2002.* Columbus, OH: Author

Paternite, C.E. (2004). Involving educators in school-based mental health programs. In K.E. Robinson (Ed.), *School-based mental health: Best practices and program models* (pp. 1–21). Kingston, NJ: Civic Research Institute.

President's New Freedom Commission on Mental Health. (2003). *Achieving the promise: Transforming mental health care in America. Final report* (DHHS Publication No. SMA-03-3832). Rockville, MD: U.S. Department of Health and Human Services.

Robbins, V., & Armstrong, B.J. (2005). The Bridges Project: Description and evaluation of a school-based mental health program in Eastern Kentucky. In K. Kutash, A.J. Duchnowski, & M. Epstein (Eds.), *Outcomes for children and youth with emotional disorders and their families: Programs and evaluation best practices* (2nd ed., pp. 355–373). Austin, TX: PRO-ED.

Robbins, V., Armstrong, B.J., & Collins, K. (2002). The Bridges Project: Closing the gap between schools, families, and mental health services for all children and youth. *Community Mental Health Report, 79*, 67–70.

Robbins, V., Collins, K., & Marcum, L. (2004). Adolescents with substance abuse comorbidity in Eastern Kentucky: Characteristics and patterns of use. In C. Newman, C. Liberton, K. Kutash, & R.M. Friedman (Eds.), *The 16th Annual Research Conference proceedings: A system of care for children's mental health: Expanding the research base* (pp. 60–62). Tampa: University of South Florida, Louis de la Parte Florida Mental Health Institute, Research and Training Center for Children's Mental Health.

Rones, M., & Hoagwood, K. (2000). School-based mental health services: A research review. *Clinical Child and Family Psychology Review, 3*(4), 223–241.

Scott, T.M., & Hunter, J. (2001). Initiating school-wide support systems: An administrator's guide to the process. *Beyond Behavior, 11*(1), 13–15.

Singer, J.D., & Butler, J.A. (1987). The Education for All Handicapped Children Act: Schools as agents of social reform. *Harvard Educational Review, 57*, 25–152.

Slade, E.P. (2003). The relationship between school characteristics and the availability of mental health and related health services in middle and high schools in the United States. *Journal of Behavioral Health Services & Research, 30*(4), 382–392.

Sprague, J., Sugai, G., & Walker, H. (1998). Antisocial behavior in schools. In S. Watson & F. Gresham (Eds.), *Child behavior therapy: Ecological considerations in assessment, treatment, and evaluation* (pp. 451–474). New York: Plenum Press.

Stroul, B.A., & Friedman, R.M. (1986). *A system of care for children and adolescents with severe emotional disturbance.* Washington, DC: National Technical Assistance Center for Child Mental Health, Georgetown University Child Development Center.

Sugai, G., & Horner, R.H. (2002). Introduction to the special series on positive behavior support in schools. *Journal of Emotional and Behavioral Disorders, 10*(1), 130–135.

Sugai, G., Sprague, J., Horner, R., & Walker, H. (2000). Preventing school violence: The use of office discipline referral data to assess and monitor school-wide discipline interventions. *Journal of Emotional and Behavioral Disorders, 8*(2), 94–101.

UCLA School Mental Health Project. (2005). *Addressing Barriers to Learning, 19*(4), 1–12.

U.S. Department of Education, Office of Special Education and Rehabilitative Services. (2002). *A new era: Revitalizing special education for children and their families.* Washington, DC: Author.

U.S. Department of Health and Human Services (U.S. DHHS). (1999). *Mental health: A report of the Surgeon General.* Rockville, MD: Substance Abuse and Mental Health Services Administration, Center for Mental Health Services.

U.S. Public Health Service. (2000). *Report of the Surgeon General's conference on children's mental health: A national action agenda.* Washington, DC: Author.

VanTreuren, R., Robbins, V., & Amstrong, B.J. (2006, Winter). Developing evidence-based practice in schools: Strategies and components to sustain positive mental health and academic outcomes. *Emotional and Behavioral Disorders in Youth, 8*(10), 16–18.

Vernberg, E.M., Jacobs, A.K., Nyre, J.E., Puddy, R.W., & Roberts, M.C. (2004). Innovative treatments for children with serious emotional disturbance: Preliminary outcomes for a school-based intensive mental health program. *Journal of Clinical Child and Adolescent Psychology, 33*(2), 359–365.

Wagner, M., Friend, M., Bursuck, W., Kutash, K., Duchnowski, A.J. Sumi, W.C., et al. (2006). Educating students with emotional disturbances: A national perspective on programs and services. *Journal of Emotional and Behavioral Disorders, 14*, 12–30.

Wagner, M., Kutash, K., Duchnowski, A.J., Epstein, M.H., & Sumi, W. (2005). The children and youth we serve: A national picture of the characteristics of students with emotional disturbances receiving special education. *Journal of Emotional and Behavioral Disorders, 13*(2), 79–96.

Wagner, M., & Sumi W.C. (2006, February). *A national overview of current school-based mental health services, the evidence base, and efforts to sustain good practice.* Paper presented at the meeting of the Research and Training Center for Children's Mental Health, Tampa, FL.

Webster-Stratton, C., & Taylor, T. (2001). Nipping early risk factors in the bud: Preventing substance abuse, delinquency, and violence in adolescence through interventions targeted at young children (0–8 years). *Prevention Science, 2*(3), 165–192.

Weist, M.D., Goldstein, A., Morris, L., & Bryant, T. (2003). Integrating expanded school mental health programs and school-based health centers. *Psychology in the Schools, 40*(3), 297–308.

Weist, M.D., Sander, M., Lowie, J.A., & Christodulu, K. (2002). The expanded school mental health framework. *Childhood Education, 78*, 269–273.

Weisz, J.R., Jensen-Doss, A., & Hawley, K.M. (2006). Evidence-based youth psychotherapies versus usual clinical care: A meta-analysis of direct comparisons. *American Psychologist, 61*, 671–689.

Zins, J.E., & Ponti, C.R. (1990). Best practices in school-based consultation. In A. Thomas & J. Grimes (Eds.), *Best practices in school psychology* (Vol. II, pp. 673–694). Washington, DC: National Association of School Psychologists.

Zins, J.E., Weissberg, R.P., Wang, M.C., & Walberg, H.J. (Eds.). (2004). *Building academic success on social and emotional learning: What does the research say?* New York: Teachers College Press.

21

Services for Youth in the Juvenile Justice System in Systems of Care

Joseph J. Cocozza, Kathleen R. Skowyra,
Joyce L. Burrell, Timothy P. Dollard, and Jacqueline P. Scales

As of 1992, the federal government has provided funding for children's mental health services through the Comprehensive Community Mental Health Services for Children and Their Families Program, referred to as the *system of care initiative* (Substance Abuse and Mental Health Services Administration [SAMHSA], 2005). The system of care philosophy emphasizes community-based, comprehensive, culturally competent, coordinated services provided in the least restrictive environments and with the full participation of children's families (Stroul & Friedman, 1986). Recent changes require system of care initiatives to integrate a family-driven and youth-guided perspective. Although systems of care are configured differently in different states and communities, all are based on a philosophy that embraces an individualized wraparound approach to service planning and delivery and includes the following principles:

- Mental health services should be driven by the needs and preferences of the child and family and should address these needs through a strength-based approach.

- The focus and management of services should occur within a multiagency collaborative environment and be grounded in a strong community base.

- The services offered, the agencies participating, and the programs generated should be responsive to the cultural and linguistic context and characteristics of the populations served.

- Families and youth should be partners in the planning, implementation, and evaluation of systems of care.

All system of care grantees are required to engage in an extensive interagency planning process with other child-serving systems and family members within the community to help plan and implement their systems of care. The juvenile justice system has been identified as a critically important component in the planning process (SAMHSA, 2000), and the federal Center for Mental Health Services enacted a policy change resulting in the identification of juvenile justice youth as a priority population in their 2005 Guidance for Applicants to support new system of care sites. Despite the significant financial investment in the program and the stated emphasis on interagency involvement and the juvenile justice system, the focus on serving youth involved with the justice system varies widely across funded sites, and for most sites, the juvenile justice population has not been considered a priority population.

Other than a few classic examples, such as Wraparound Milwaukee, Project Hope in Rhode Island, or the Dawn Project in Indiana, very few systems of care or wraparound programs focus on juvenile justice youth (Pullman et al., 2006). Data collected as part of the national cross-site evaluation of the system of care initiative found that only 15% of all referrals come from the juvenile justice system and that half of all sites receive less than 5% of their referrals from the juvenile justice system (Cocozza, 2004). This suggests that only a handful of the federally funded system of care communities are serving youth referred from the juvenile justice system.

WHY FOCUS ON JUVENILE JUSTICE?

The lack of focus on the mental health needs of youth in the juvenile justice system stands in contrast with what research has confirmed about these youth. Data has shown the high prevalence of mental health problems among youth involved in the juvenile justice system and the lack of services available to them. Significant findings include the following:

1. **Research studies are consistently identifying high rates of mental health disorders among the juvenile justice population.**

Many of the earlier mental health prevalence studies conducted among the juvenile justice population were found to be too flawed in their methodological design to yield meaningful results (Cocozza, 1992). Fortunately, most of the limitations of the earlier research have been addressed through the development of carefully designed, scientifically sound, and thoughtfully executed studies (Shufelt & Cocozza, 2006). This research has resulted in new data that expands the field's collective knowledge and understanding of the nature and prevalence of mental health disorders among the juvenile justice population and provides unequivocal documentation of the problem. As a result, it has become firmly established that the majority of youth involved with the juvenile justice system in the United States have mental health disorders. Findings from a number of recent studies conducted within various types of juvenile justice residential settings (e.g., community-based, detention, correctional) are remarkably similar. Anywhere from 65% to 70% of youth in the juvenile justice system have a diagnosable mental health disorder (Shufelt & Cocozza, 2006; Teplin, Abram, McClelland, Dulcan, & Mericle, 2002; Wasserman, Ko, & McReynolds, 2004; Wasserman, McReynolds, Lucas, Fisher, & Santos,

2002). The most recent study completed by the National Center for Mental Health and Juvenile Justice found that (Shufelt & Cocozza, 2006):

- More than half of youth (55.6%) met criteria for at least two diagnoses.

- Of the youth with mental health disorders, 60.8% also had substance use disorders.

- Approximately 27% of youth experience disorders so severe that their ability to function is severely impaired, and they require significant and immediate treatment.

2. Youth are frequently placed in the juvenile justice system because of a lack of community-based mental health services.

Many youth are detained or placed in the juvenile justice system for relatively minor, nonviolent offenses because of a lack of community-based treatment options. A review in Louisiana by the Annie E. Casey Foundation (2003) found that more than 75% of Louisiana's incarcerated youth were locked up for nonviolent and drug offenses. A review by the Congressional Committee on Government Reform (U.S. House of Representatives, 2004) found that two thirds of juvenile detention facilities reported holding youth in custody unnecessarily simply because of a lack of available services. Furthermore, in a study of mental health prevalence among youth in the juvenile justice system, researchers found that only 23.5% of youth with mental health diagnoses had committed a violent offense as their most serious offense, with the majority of youth involved with the system for property offenses and probation or parole violations (Shufelt & Cocozza, 2006).

3. There is little evidence to suggest that youth placed in the juvenile justice system are routinely provided with adequate or effective mental health services.

A series of investigations by the U.S. Department of Justice (2005) into the conditions of confinement in juvenile detention and correctional facilities repeatedly found a failure on the part of the facilities to adequately address the mental health needs of youth in their care. In addition, media inquiries and reports documenting the mental health crisis within juvenile justice systems in numerous states have drawn national attention to the issue and placed additional pressure on elected officials, policy makers, and administrators to develop more effective solutions for these youth.

4. Youth with mental health disorders in the United States are increasingly seen in systems and sectors outside the traditional mental health system.

Youth with mental health needs are ending up in the juvenile justice and child welfare systems or are identified in other settings such as schools or primary health clinics (President's New Freedom Commission on Mental Health, 2003). Partnerships between the mental health system and community agencies and organizations are essential in order to reach youth who require mental health treatment but who are found in nonmental health settings (e.g., probation offices, detention centers, correctional facilities).

FOCUSING ON JUVENILE JUSTICE: A BLUEPRINT FOR CHANGE

Systems of care did not prioritize youth in the juvenile justice system, largely due to the lack of available information on how to comprehensively incorporate services for such youth into a system of care. This lack of information made it difficult for programs to establish the necessary relationships, linkages, and service strategies with the juvenile justice system to target this population of youth. This, however, changed with the development of a technical assistance document designed to provide guidance and direction to the field on improving the relationship between the juvenile justice and mental health systems to better respond to the mental health needs of youth involved with the justice system. *The Blueprint for Change: A Comprehensive Model for the Identification and Treatment of Youth in Contact with the Juvenile Justice System,* developed by the National Center for Mental Health and Juvenile Justice (Skowyra & Cocozza, 2007), offers a conceptual and practical framework for juvenile justice and mental health systems to use when developing policies and strategies designed to improve mental health services for youth involved with the juvenile justice system. It sets the highest standards for systems to work toward, summarizing what is known about the recommended ways to identify and treat mental health disorders among youth at key stages of juvenile justice processing, as well as offering recommendations, guidelines, and examples of the most productive methods for doing so. This document can easily be applied to systems of care to better integrate youth involved with juvenile justice into their programs.

Underlying Principles

The Blueprint is organized around a set of underlying principles that represent the foundation on which a system can be created that is respectful of youth and responsive to their mental health needs. They include the following:

- Youth should not have to enter the juvenile justice system solely to obtain mental health services or because of their mental illness.

- Whenever possible and matters of public safety allow, youth with mental health needs should be diverted into evidence-based treatment in a community setting.

- If diversion out of the juvenile justice system is not possible, youth should be placed in the least restrictive setting possible, with access to evidence-based treatment.

- Information collected as part of a preadjudicatory mental health screen should not be used in any way that might jeopardize the legal interests of youth as defendants.

- All mental health services provided to youth in contact with the juvenile justice system should respond to issues of gender, ethnicity, race, age, sexual orientation, socioeconomic status, and faith.

- Mental health services should address the developmental realities of youth. Children and adolescents should not be perceived or treated as little adults.

- Whenever possible, families and caregivers should be partners in the development of treatment decisions and plans made for their children.

- Multiple systems bear responsibility for these youth. A single agency may have primary responsibility at a specific time, but these youth are the community's responsibility, and thus all responses developed for these youth should be collaborative in nature, reflecting the input and involvement of the mental health, juvenile justice, and other relevant systems.

- Services and strategies aimed at improving the identification and treatment of youth with mental health needs in the juvenile justice system should be routinely evaluated to determine their effectiveness in meeting desired goals and outcomes.

Cornerstones

From the underlying principles emerged four cornerstones that form the infrastructure of the model and provide a framework for putting the underlying principles into practice. The cornerstones reflect those areas where the most critical improvements are necessary to enhance the delivery of mental health services to youth in the juvenile justice system—*collaboration, identification, diversion,* and *treatment.* The Blueprint includes a discussion of each cornerstone and detailed recommended actions that provide direction on how to address each of these four issues.

Collaboration   In order to appropriately respond and effectively provide services to youth with mental health needs, the justice and mental health systems should collaborate in all areas and at all critical intervention points within the juvenile justice continuum. Despite the large numbers of youth with mental health needs in the juvenile justice system, the current landscape of service delivery for these youth is often fragmented, inconsistent, and operating without the benefit of a clear set of guidelines specifying responsibility for the population. In the absence of such direction, a balanced solution is required, one that recognizes that an effective response must include the development of collaborative approaches involving both the mental health and juvenile justice systems. The recommended actions for addressing collaboration include the following:

1. The juvenile justice and mental health systems should recognize that many youth in the juvenile justice system are experiencing significant mental health problems and that responsibility for effectively responding to these youth lies with both of these systems.

2. The juvenile justice and mental health systems should engage in a collaborative and comprehensive planning effort to thoroughly understand the extent

of the problem at each critical stage of juvenile justice processing and to identify joint ways to respond.

3. Any collaboration between the juvenile justice and mental health systems should include family members and caregivers.

4. The juvenile justice and mental health systems should jointly identify funding mechanisms to support the implementation of key strategies at critical stages of juvenile processing to better identify and respond to the mental health needs of youth.

5. The juvenile justice and mental health systems should collaborate at every key stage of juvenile justice processing from initial contact with law enforcement to reentry.

6. Cross-training should be available for staff from the juvenile justice and mental health systems to provide opportunities for staff to learn more about each system, to understand phrases and terms common to each system, and to participate in exercises and activities designed to enhance collaboration.

Identification   The mental health needs of youth should be systematically identified at all critical stages of juvenile justice processing. The development of a sound screening and assessment capacity is critical in order to effectively identify and ultimately respond to mental heath treatment needs. Screening and assessment should be routinely performed at each youth's earliest point of contact with the justice system and should be conducted using standardized instruments. Existing standardized instruments may need to be adapted to meet the needs of specific youth populations, including minority youth and girls. For example, there is substantial evidence that youth of color—especially Black youth—are overrepresented at virtually every key processing point within the juvenile justice system (Snyder & Sickmund, 1999) in comparison with their proportions in the general population (Snyder, 2003). Many mental health screening and assessment tools currently being used with youth were originally developed with samples of youth in which the majority were non-Hispanic White (Grisso, Vincent, & Seagrave, 2005). As such, the instruments selected must consider and be appropriate for the culturally and linguistically diverse populations served. Furthermore, the results of mental health assessments should be linked to the results of risk assessments performed to help guide decisions about a youth's suitability and need for diversion to community-based services. The recommended actions for addressing identification include the following:

1. Every youth who comes in contact with the juvenile justice system should be systematically screened for mental health needs to identify conditions that require immediate response (e.g., suicide risk) and to identify those youth who require further mental health assessment or evaluation.

2. The mental health screening process should include the administration of an emergency mental health screen and a general mental health screen.

3. Access to immediate emergency mental health services should be available for all youth who, based on the results of either the emergency screen or the general screen, indicate a need for emergency services.

4. A mental health screen should be administered to any youth whose emergency mental health screen indicates a need for further assessment.

5. Instruments selected for identifying mental health needs among the juvenile justice population should be standardized, scientifically sound, have strong psychometric properties, and demonstrate reliability and validity for use with youth in the juvenile justice population.

6. Mental health screening and assessment should be performed in conjunction with risk assessments to inform referral recommendations that balance public safety concerns with each youth's need for mental health treatment.

7. All mental health screens and assessments should be administered by appropriately trained staff.

8. Policies controlling the use of screening information may be necessary to ensure that data collected as part of preadjudicatory mental health screens are not used in inappropriate ways or in any context that jeopardizes the legal interests of youth as defendants.

9. Mental health screening and assessment should be performed routinely as youth move from one point in the juvenile justice system to another (e.g., from pretrial detention to a secure correctional facility).

10. Given the high rates of co-occurring mental health and substance use disorders among this population, all screening and assessment instruments should target mental health and substance abuse needs, preferably in an integrated manner.

11. Existing screening and assessment instruments may need to be adapted for critical groups of youth, particularly youth of color and girls, pending further research.

Diversion Whenever possible, youth with identified mental health needs should be diverted into effective community-based treatment. Many youth end up in the juvenile justice system for behavior brought on by or associated with their mental health disorders. Some of these youth are charged with serious offenses, but many are in the system for relatively minor, nonviolent offenses. Given the needs of these youth and the documented inadequacies of their care within the juvenile justice system, there is a growing sentiment that whenever possible and matters of public safety allow, youth with mental health needs should be diverted into effective community treatment. Mental health experts agree that it is preferable to treat youth with mental health disorders outside of juvenile correctional settings (Koppelman, 2005). At the same time, however, both a youth's mental illness and the level of risk to community safety must be taken into account when determining whether a youth can be safely diverted into community-based treatment. It is also recognized that diversion into community-based treatment sometimes involves ongoing monitoring or supervision on the part of the juvenile justice system to ensure compliance with the terms of the referral or court order. The recommended actions for addressing diversion include the following:

1. Whenever possible, youth with mental health needs should be diverted to community treatment.

2. Procedures must be in place to identify those youth who are appropriate for diversion.

3. Effective community-based services and programs must be available to serve youth who are diverted into treatment.

4. Diversion mechanisms should be instituted at virtually every key decision-making point within the juvenile justice processing continuum.

5. Consideration should be given to the use of diversion programs as alternatives to traditional incarceration for serious offenders with mental health needs.

6. Diversion programs should be regularly evaluated to determine their ability to effectively and safely treat youth in the community.

7. More research is necessary to ensure that evidence-based interventions are culturally sensitive and meet the needs of youth of color.

8. Gender-specific services and programming should be available for girls involved with the juvenile justice system.

Treatment   Youth with mental health needs in the juvenile justice system should have access to effective treatment to meet their needs. Enormous advances have been made in this area, and evidence-based interventions are well-documented and proven effective for treating mental health disorders among youth (Hoagwood, 2005). These include psychosocial approaches such as Cognitive-Behavioral Therapy (Rhode, Clarke, Mace, Jorgensen, & Seeley, 2004), community-based approaches such as Multisystemic Therapy (Elliot et al., 1998) and Functional Family Therapy (Alexander & Sexton, 1999), and medication therapy (Jensen & Potter, 2003). However, the vast majority of mental health services that are currently available to treat youth involved with the juvenile justice system are not evidence based. More work is necessary to promote the wider use of evidence-based practices with these youth. The recommended actions for addressing treatment include the following:

1. Youth in contact with the juvenile justice system who are in need of mental health services should be afforded access to treatment.

2. Regardless of the setting, all mental health services provided to youth should be evidence based.

3. Responsibility for providing mental health treatment to youth involved with the juvenile justice system should be shared between the juvenile justice and mental health systems, with lead responsibility varying depending on the youth's point of contact with the system.

4. Qualified mental health personnel, either employed by the juvenile justice system or under contract through the mental health system, should be available to provide mental health treatment to youth in the juvenile justice system.

5. Families should be fully involved with the treatment and rehabilitation of their children.

6. Juvenile justice and mental health systems must create environments that are sensitive and responsive to the trauma-related histories of youth.

7. Gender-specific services and programming should be available for girls involved with the juvenile justice system.

CRITICAL INTERVENTION POINTS

The approaches outlined in the Blueprint were applied to the juvenile justice processing continuum to identify places within the entire continuum—from intake to reentry—where opportunities exist to make better decisions about mental health needs and treatment. This examination resulted in the identification of seven critical intervention points where the cornerstones can be addressed. These points, shown on Figure 21.1, are discussed in this section.

Initial Contact and Referral

Often, a youth's disruptive or delinquent behavior is the result of a mental health problem that has gone undetected and untreated. The problem may manifest itself in behavior that brings the youth to the attention of law enforcement. Police response at this initial contact has significant implications in determining what

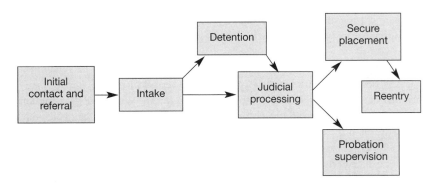

Figure 21.1. Critical intervention points in the juvenile justice processing continuum.

Box 21.1. Program examples: Initial contact and referral

The Rochester, New York, Community Mobile Crisis Team responds to calls from the police, as well as from parents and schools, regarding youth experiencing a mental health crisis in order to provide these youth with immediate access to mental health services. The team performs assessments and facilitates access to a range of intensive and coordinated mental health services that are available through Youth Emergency Services, including outpatient, home-based, and mobile mental health services. The team also conducts follow-up with the youth.

The San Francisco, California, System of Care Initiative developed a specialized training on disruptive behaviors and responses that may be linked to mental health disorders. This instruction is presented to area police officers at their training academy.

The Idaho System of Care developed a Police Pocket Guide to help officers who come in contact with youth who appear to have serious emotional disturbances.

Source: Skowyra & Cocozza (2007).

---

will happen next. Upon an encounter with a youth who appears to have a mental health problem, an opportunity exists for law enforcement to connect the youth with emergency mental health services or refer him or her for follow-up mental health screening and assessment (Box 21.1).

Intake

Intake is very often viewed as the gatekeeper to family court, thus representing an ideal opportunity to intervene early and identify the need for mental health and other types of rehabilitative services. Considering the potential influence that intake decisions can have on subsequent juvenile justice processing, it constitutes one of the most critical points within the juvenile justice continuum for applying prevention and early intervention strategies (Kelly & Mears, 1999). These strategies include the use of standardized mental health screening and assessment measures on all youth entering intake, as well as the institution of diversion mechanisms and programs so that youth in need of mental health services can be appropriately diverted into community-based treatment (Box 21.2).

Detention

Juvenile detention can be a traumatic experience for all youth, but the situation can be much worse for youth with mental health needs. Feelings of depression, anxiety, and hopelessness are heightened for all youth in detention, some of whom are experiencing their first separation from parents or caregivers, but these feelings can be even more intense for youth with mental health problems. Detention can also mean an interruption in both medication and therapeutic services

---

Box 21.2. Program example: Intake

Family Intervention Specialists (FIS) of Georgia provide intensive family intervention services to youth with mental health disorders who are at risk for out-of-home placement. At intake, specialized probation officers trained to identify mental health and substance use disorders among youth use the Massachusetts Youth Screening Instrument-2 (MAYSI-2; Grisso & Barnum, 2000) to screen all youth at intake. Youth diverted to the program undergo further evaluation and receive Brief Strategic Family Therapy as the primary intervention. Services are provided by FIS staff personnel, who work closely with probation officials throughout the period of involvement.

Source: Skowyra & Cocozza (2007).

---

for youth who receive such treatment in their community. Employing standardized mental health screening and assessment measures for all youth entering detention is critical. The institution of diversion mechanisms at detention is also recommended to identify those youth who could be safely diverted to community-based treatment. Finally, in order to ensure access to treatment, linkages between the detention center and community-based mental health providers should be established to provide treatment to youth during their detention (Box 21.3).

Judicial Processing

It is of critical importance that judges have sufficient information about a youth's mental health treatment history and current needs in order to determine how a youth's mental health disorder may have contributed to the problem behavior or

---

Box 21.3. Program example: Detention

The Bernalillo County, New Mexico, Juvenile Detention Center developed an intake process that identifies youth with mental health needs and diverts these youth to a community mental health clinic, the Children's Community Mental Health Clinic, which is located 200 yards away from the detention center. The clinic serves all youth in the county and accepts referrals from the juvenile detention center, care providers, parents, and others, thereby reducing any incentive to refer youth to detention simply to obtain mental health services. Youth brought to the detention center undergo a comprehensive intake screen to identify any mental health problems. Youth identified as in need of immediate services or further evaluation are walked to the clinic, where they receive a variety of clinical services, including individual therapy, medication management, substance abuse services, and case management. Services are provided to youth during their time in detention and then continue in their homes after they are released.

Source: Skowyra & Cocozza (2007).

offense and to make an informed dispositional decision. Ideally, information on a youth's mental health status should be collected prior to the youth's case being referred to the court for an adjudicatory hearing, and the information should be used to divert the youth to treatment earlier in the process. For many youth, however, these diversion opportunities do not exist, and the first attempt to identify any mental health concerns comes at the time when a youth has been adjudicated and intake staff personnel are developing recommendations to the court. Every effort must be made to ensure that a youth's mental status is thoroughly evaluated at this stage so that this information can be presented to the court and considered as part of the dispositional plan (Box 21.4).

Box 21.4.   Program example: Judicial processing

The Cook County, Illinois, Juvenile Court Clinic is responsible for providing a variety of services to judges and court personnel regarding clinical information in juvenile court proceedings. A multidisciplinary staff of psychologists, psychiatrists, social workers, and lawyers provide consultation regarding requests for clinical information, forensic clinical assessments, and data regarding community-based mental health resources. With a clinical coordinator present in the courtroom, the court clinic is able to provide guidance to judges and probation staff about whether an evaluation is necessary and whether a youth's needs can be met in a community-based program or setting.

Source: Skowyra & Cocozza (2007).

Secure Placement

The most restrictive sanction a juvenile court can impose entails committing a youth to a secure juvenile correctional facility. Traditional juvenile correctional facilities have not been found to be effective in running rehabilitative programs (Greenwood, Model, Rydel, & Chiesa, 1996) or at reducing recidivism (Howell, 1998). It is critical that future efforts focus on the development and implementation of evidence-based mental health treatments that can be provided to youth during their incarceration (Box 21.5).

Probation Supervision

Probation supervision is the sanction most often applied to adjudicated youth in a dispositional hearing. Often, a judge will impose a period of probation with other conditions such as participation in treatment, restitution, or community service. This represents an ideal opportunity to link a youth with treatment and simultaneously afford the leverage of the juvenile court to ensure that the youth complies with the terms of the disposition (Box 21.6).

Box 21.5.   Program example: Secure placement

Recognizing the sizable population of youth with mental health needs in their system, the Washington State Juvenile Rehabilitation Administration (JRA) created a program that incorporates recommended practice interventions for youth with mental health needs. The Integrated Treatment Model takes the evidence-based components of Functional Family Therapy, Cognitive-Behavioral Therapy, and Dialectical Behavior Therapy and uses them to provide individual treatment and skill development to youth from the point that they are admitted to the facility through their release back into the community (Juvenile Rehabilitation Administration, 2002). Staff within the facilities are extensively trained to use Cognitive-Behavioral Treatment interventions to address the multiple needs of youth and prepare them for their return home. JRA also redesigned its aftercare program, creating a new service delivery model based on Functional Family Therapy, which gears aftercare services to the entire family, not just the youth.

Source: Skowyra & Cocozza (2007).

Reentry

The goal of a placement is to successfully rehabilitate youth for their eventual return home. Critical to this is recognizing a youth's need for mental health services while in custody, providing effective treatment while a youth is in care, and ensuring that linkages are securely in place to allow for continued access to mental health care upon release. Ideally, planning for a youth's reentry into the community should begin shortly after the youth's arrival in the facility. This should include efforts to ensure the youth's enrollment in Medicaid or some type of insurance plan to pay for services once he or she is released (Box 21.7).

Box 21.6.   Program example: Probation supervision

The Integrated Co-Occurring Treatment Program in Akron, Ohio, is an intensive home-based treatment model specifically designed to treat mental health disorders and co-occurring substance use disorders among youth referred by the court as a condition of probation. Program clinicians, who work with each youth's probation officers, are available to youth and their families 24 hours per day, 7 days per week, and use individual and family therapy interventions to focus on skill development and asset building while simultaneously addressing risk reduction. Services are delivered in the home, school, and community.

Source: Skowyra & Cocozza (2007).

The Blueprint serves a dual role. It offers a plan for how mental health issues can be better addressed within the juvenile justice system as a whole, and it compartmentalizes the system into discreet points of contact, allowing commu-

---

Box 21.7. Program examples: Reentry

Project Hope, originally supported by a federal system of care grant, is an aftercare program in Rhode Island that targets youth with serious emotional disturbances who are returning to their communities from the Rhode Island Training School (RITS). All youth with a mental health diagnosis are eligible to participate. Project Hope services are obtained by youth making the transition out of the training school through the RITS clinical social worker 90–120 days prior to their discharge. Family service coordinators work closely with the clinical social worker during the time each youth is incarcerated and with each youth's probation officer when that particular youth returns to the community. Individualized service plans are modified as necessary, and a case manager is assigned to ensure implementation of the plan for a period of 9–12 months following discharge.

Manchester, New Hampshire's, System of Care initiative and Nevada's Family First and Foremost program have both adopted probation strategies that take the mental health status of youth into account when developing their probation plans. These strategies provide youth with increased opportunities to successfully comply with the terms of their probation plans.

Source: Skowyra & Cocozza (2007).

---

nities to implement the individual components of the Blueprint as a first step in system improvement. Although not a panacea, the Blueprint offers a framework that can be used by systems of care to begin the process of establishing relationships with the juvenile justice system and developing collaborative plans to better serve these youth.

JEFFERSON COUNTY COMMUNITY PARTNERSHIP: A SYSTEM OF CARE FOR YOUTH INVOLVED WITH JUVENILE JUSTICE

A system of care that has recognized youth in the juvenile justice system as a priority population is the Jefferson County, Alabama, Community Partnership Program. In 1990, Jefferson County received funding from the Alabama Department of Mental Health to provide home-based therapy and case management services to youth with serious emotional disturbances who were considered at high risk for out-of-home placement. The early success of these nontraditional services served as a catalyst for the continuing development of an interagency system of care for children, youth, and families in Jefferson County. By the mid-1990s, the county mental health authority had interagency contracts and agreements in place for direct services that allowed for the expansion of mental health service delivery into nontraditional mental health settings such as the juvenile justice and child welfare systems.

In 1997, these local collaborative efforts led to the formation of the Jefferson County Community Partnership (JCCP), and that same year, the JCCP was awarded a $5.9 million grant from SAMHSA to further develop its system of care. The grant was used to help establish four mental health diagnostic and evaluation units in Jefferson County, including two units in schools, one in the child welfare agency, and one in the family court. The Family Court Mental Health Unit was developed to identify youth coming into the court with mental health issues and to provide appropriate referral and treatment services. Its primary mission is to ensure that the least restrictive, most appropriate mental health and social services are obtained on behalf of eligible youth and their families in an effort to prevent out-of-home placement.

Continuum of Services

A full continuum of services is provided through the court unit, which serves as a port of entry. The court unit completes timely assessments of youth and their families and then develops an individualized service plan based on the results of the assessment. Eligible youth are between the ages of 5 and 21; reside in the county; have a *Diagnostic and Statistical Manual of Mental Disorders, Fourth Edition* (DSM-IV, American Psychiatric Association, 1994) diagnosis; have either a previous separation from family due to emotional or behavioral disturbance or significant functional impairments at home, school, or in the community; and are at risk of placement if services are not rendered. Referrals to the court unit typically come from probation officers or family court judges. Referrals from probation intake include delinquency cases in which charges have been filed or will be filed and cases that are diverted at intake without charges being filed.

Upon referral, a master's-level specialist performs an initial mental health and substance abuse screen to determine which youth must be referred for further evaluation. This specialist also provides mental health consultation to school personnel, probation officers, and social workers. Evaluations are conducted by either the specialist or a licensed psychologist under contract to the unit. A range of mental health services are provided directly by Court Unit staff, including psychiatric consultation; medication monitoring; emergency services; case management; outpatient therapy; and access to home-based therapy, respite care, day treatment, independent living and transitional programs, wraparound service planning, and parent and youth support groups. The youth and families involved with the court unit also benefit from agreements that the JCCP has with numerous public and private agencies to provide more traditional mental health treatment intervention services through community-based centers. In addition to the specialist, the court unit staff includes a mental health coordinator, a court liaison, a detention specialist, two full-time therapists, a part-time psychiatrist, two full-time case managers, and two parent advocates.

A key feature of the court unit is its recognition of the importance of securing family involvement in the mental health evaluation and treatment process. To help facilitate this, the court unit employs full-time parent advocates who are responsible for helping families understand, navigate, and ultimately participate in their child's mental health treatment. The parent advocates are present for the initial intake and mental health screen, and they work with families to explain the process and answer any questions they may have about the program, the system, and what they can expect to occur. The parent advocates also participate in service planning meetings with families, serve as supports to family members, and offer respite care on weekends if children and families need a break from one another.

The average length of involvement in the program is 18 months. Youth are discharged once the individualized service plan goals have been met and the terms of their probation have been completed. Many youth actually choose to remain in the program after their period of probation ends because of its accessibility and flexibility.

Consistency with the Blueprint for Change

The Jefferson County Family Court Mental Health Unit is a prime example of a system of care that exemplifies the four cornerstones of the Blueprint for Change, demonstrating that it is possible to provide comprehensive and effective services for youth involved with the juvenile justices system within a system of care.

Collaboration   The Mental Health Court Unit was conceived by a community partnership involving numerous local agencies and service providers, including the mental health authority, the juvenile court, and the county probation department. This strong interagency collaboration, led by a judge who firmly believed that youth entering family court should have access to necessary mental health care, is, in large measure, the reason the program has been so successful and has experienced such longevity. In addition to the community agencies, the program has successfully embraced families as partners and has created numerous mechanisms for families to be involved not only at the service delivery level, but also at the planning level as members of the JCCP.

Identification   One of the primary goals of the Mental Health Court Unit is to identify those youth coming into the family court who are in need of mental health services. The Mental Health Court Unit is a diagnostic and evaluation unit, and all youth referred to the unit undergo comprehensive evaluation. Although the unit also provides treatment services, mental health screening and evaluation are an essential part of the unit's intake process, serving as the basis for all subsequent treatment planning.

Diversion   The Mental Health Court Unit essentially serves as a diversion program for status offenders and delinquents who are at high risk of placement. Youth are diverted at probation intake or at court into the program for diagnostic and treatment services. The county estimates that they have diverted hundreds of youth with serious emotional disturbances from deep-end juvenile court placements.

Treatment   A unique feature of the court unit is the fact that it not only provides comprehensive evaluation services, but it also provides on-site treatment services, along with referrals for treatment in community-based mental health settings. The county has a long history of offering innovative treatments for youth, beginning with their efforts to establish a home-based treatment and case management model in the early 1990s for youth identified as at risk for out-of-home placement. Home and community-based treatment models have been found to be highly effective forms of intervention for successfully treating youth with mental health disorders in the juvenile justice system (Skowyra & Cocozza, 2007).

PRACTICAL STEPS TO INTEGRATE JUVENILE JUSTICE WITHIN SYSTEMS OF CARE

As some systems of care have demonstrated, it is possible to serve youth in the juvenile justice system within a system of care framework. The following steps can help guide this process:

1. Establish a forum for interagency discussion and collaboration.

Once there is recognition of the problem and a commitment to change, the juvenile justice and mental health systems must engage in a comprehensive and strategic planning process to address the identified problems. In order to do this, it is necessary to create or expand an existing coordinating body or task force that includes representatives from the involved systems, as well as family members and advocates. Families are critical stakeholders and should be involved in any type of collaboration involving the juvenile justice and mental health systems. Furthermore, family-run organizations can also serve as important allies in efforts to bring attention to critical issues, cultivate political will, or draw new resources to a problem.

2. Engage in a strategic planning process.

Once the interagency coordinating body or task force is in place, it is necessary to develop a strategic action plan with clear goals, objectives, and strategies for responding to the issues. A recommended first step is to designate a strong leader for the group—someone with good communication skills and a thorough understanding of the systems and the problems. Second, it is important for the group to develop a mission or policy statement that that will articulate the goal(s) for the work and guide the activities of the group. Once the mission of the group is established, it is critical to develop objectives and strategies for meeting the identified goals. Primary and secondary responsibility for follow-up on each identified objective and strategy should be clearly designated to members of the interagency coordinating body. Overall, this strategic planning process should result in the group being able to answer three primary questions: Where are we now? Where are we going? How will we get there?

3. Provide cross-training to staff from the juvenile justice and mental health systems.

Cross-training is a highly effective way to provide staff from the juvenile justice and mental health systems with the opportunity to learn more about each system, to understand phrases and terms common to each system, and to participate in exercises and activities designed to enhance intersystem collaboration. It can be particularly useful in this context because it allows staff from both systems to exchange ideas and perspectives about the treatment and supervision of youth. Cross-training can reduce barriers and create opportunities to identify common ground.

4. Implement a mental health screening and assessment mechanism.

One of the most important first steps to better respond to the mental health treatment needs among youth in the juvenile justice system is to systematically identify these needs as youth become involved with the system. A number of factors must be considered when developing a mental health screening and evaluation mechanism within a juvenile justice setting:

- The specific point of contact within the juvenile justice continuum where mental health screening will occur

- The resources available to support this effort at the identified point of contact

- The qualifications of the staff available to conduct the screenings and the evaluations

- The amount of time available for staff to perform the screening and evaluations

Instruments selected for identifying mental health needs among the juvenile justice population should be standardized, scientifically sound, have strong psychometric properties, and demonstrate reliability and validity for use with youth in the juvenile justice system.

5. Develop protocols to ensure that there are clear guidelines for follow-up on all mental health screens.

Some juvenile justice agencies or programs with established mental health screening processes have developed detailed instructions and guidelines specifying what should happen during and after the mental health screen. These protocols clarify and specify important details, leaving little room for ambiguity. They help to ensure that all staff involved with the mental health screening process clearly understand what to do in terms of administering the screen, scoring the answers, interpreting and acting on all responses, and storing and protecting the collected information (Skowyra & Cocozza, 2007).

6. Institute diversion strategies at key stages of juvenile justice system processing.

Diversion to treatment offers youth their best hope of receiving services to address their mental health needs, as well as to address the behaviors that initially brought them to the attention of the juvenile justice system. It is recognized that not all youth in contact with the juvenile justice system will need or are necessarily appropriate for diversion to community-based treatment. The population of youth for whom diversion most likely is appropriate is those youth whose mental health needs are high and whose risk to community safety, based on the results of a risk assessment, is relatively low. Procedures to identify youth appropriate for diversion to treatment must be in place. Diversion strategies can be instituted at virtually all key decision-making points within the continuum, and they can work at both the pre- and postadjudication phases of processing. It is critical that effective services be available for youth who are diverted into treatment.

7. Expand the use of evidence-based mental health practices with all youth in the juvenile justice system.

Significant advances have been made in this area, resulting in the development of interventions that are effective in treating mental health disorders among youth in the juvenile justice system. Efforts should be directed at developing the capacity to deliver these evidence-based interventions.

8. Involve families in the mental health treatment of their children.

Families can provide a strong source of support for their children, serve as advocates to make sure youth get the care they need, and work in partnership with the juvenile justice and treatment staff by providing them with information that can aid in a youth's treatment. Asking parents how they want to be involved, ensuring that they understand the adjudication process, asking them what support they may need to comply with conditions of release, and helping them obtain needed supports are all examples of ways in which the juvenile justice and mental health systems can facilitate family involvement. If families are not able to be involved with their children's treatment, it is important that steps be taken to identify caregivers or other people who could serve as advocates for the youth while they are involved with the juvenile justice system and support their involvement in treatment.

9. Create reentry programs that specifically target youth with mental health needs leaving correctional placement.

One of the key goals of juvenile correctional placements is to successfully rehabilitate youth in preparation for their eventual reintegration into society. As such, it is critical that planning for a youth's reentry to the community begin shortly after his or her arrival in placement. For youth with mental health needs, reentry planning must include the establishment of linkages with community providers to allow for continued and seamless access to quality mental health care (including medication management, if necessary) upon release. If a youth is diagnosed and treated for a mental health disorder for the first time while in the custody of the juvenile justice system, his or her family will need education about the youth's condition and support in caring for the youth upon his or her return home. In addition, reentry planning must include efforts to enroll or reactivate enrollment in Medicaid or some other type of public or private insurance program to pay for the mental health treatment services the youth will receive in the community.

10. Evaluate all new programs or policies that are created as part of a juvenile justice and mental health collaborative.

Effective mental health programs and services for youth in the juvenile justice system not only ensure that youth receive the care they need but can potentially result in cost savings by reducing future youth interaction with the justice system. To determine the effectiveness of any new program or service strategy, it is essential that an evaluation component be built into the program from the beginning. Evaluation data, both process and outcome, can help systems determine the degree to which any new initiative is successful in meeting its stated goals and objectives. Systems can use this information to jointly advocate for resources to support program continuation or expansion.

CONCLUSION

Although some systems of care have targeted the juvenile justice population, many have not, despite the existence of a persuasive body of evidence documenting large numbers of youth in the juvenile justice system with significant mental health disorders. The Blueprint for Change, the first technical assistance document of its kind, provides practical guidance and direction that can be used by systems of care to establish partnerships with the juvenile justice system that result in joint strategies to better identify and ultimately treat youth with mental health disorders. The Blueprint, combined with the system of care philosophy and approach, offers the best hope for success for a population of youth who have frequently been written off as beyond help.

REFERENCES

Alexander, J., & Sexton, T. (1999). *Functional Family Therapy: Principles of clinical intervention, assessment, and implementation.* Henderson, NV: Functional Family Therapy.

American Psychiatric Association. (1994). *Diagnostic and statistical manual of mental disorders* (4th ed.). Washington, DC: Author.

Annie E. Casey Foundation. (2003). *Reducing juvenile incarceration in Louisiana.* New Orleans: Joint Legislative Juvenile Justice Commission.

Cocozza, J. (1992). *Responding to the mental health needs of youth in the juvenile justice system.* Seattle: National Coalition for the Mentally Ill in the Criminal Justice System.

Cocozza, J. (2004, June). *Mental illness and juvenile justice: An overview of issues and trends.* Presentation at the Developing Systems of Care Training Institutes, San Francisco.

Elliot, D., Henggeler, S., Mihalic, S., Rone, L., Thomas, C., & Timmons-Mitchell, J. (1998). *Blueprints for violence prevention: Book six—Multisystemic therapy.* Boulder, CO: Center for the Study and Prevention of Violence.

Greenwood, P., Model, K., Rydel, C., & Chiesa, J. (1996). *Diverting children from a life of crime: Measuring costs and benefits.* Arlington, VA: RAND Corporation.

Grisso, T., & Barnum, R. (2000). *Massachusetts Youth Screening Instrument-2: User's manual and technical report.* Worcester: University of Massachusetts Medical School.

Grisso, T., Vincent, G., & Seagrave, D. (Eds.). (2005). *Handbook of mental health screening and assessment in juvenile justice.* New York: Guilford Press.

Hoagwood, K. (2005). *Research and policy update: Evidence-based practices for youth with mental health problems and implications for juvenile justice.* Unpublished manuscript.

Howell, J. (1998). NCCD's survey of juvenile detention and correctional facilities. *Crime and Delinquency, 44*(1), 102–109.

Jenson, J., & Potter, C. (2003). The effects of cross-system collaboration on mental health and substance use problems of detained youth. *Research on Social Work Practice, 13*(5), 588–607.

Juvenile Rehabilitation Administration. (2002, September). *Integrated Treatment Model report*. Available online at http://www.dshs.wa.gov/pdf/jra/ITM_Design_Report.pdf

Kelly, W., & Mears, D. (1999). *An evaluation of the efficiency and effectiveness of juvenile justice initial assessment and referral process in Texas*. Austin, TX: Hogg Foundation for Mental Health.

Koppelman, J. (2005). *Mental health and juvenile justice: Moving toward more effective systems of care*. Washington, DC: National Health Policy Forum.

President's New Freedom Commission on Mental Health. (2003). *Achieving the promise: Transforming mental health care in America*. Rockville, MD: Author.

Pullman, M., Kerbs, J., Koroloff, N., Veach-White, E., Gaylor, R., & Sieler, D. (2006). Juvenile offenders with mental health needs: Reducing recidivism using wraparound. *Crime and Delinquency, 52*(3), 375–397.

Rhode, P., Clarke, G., Mace, D., Jorgensen, J., & Seeley, J. (2004). An efficacy/effectiveness study of cognitive-behavioral treatment for adolescents with comorbid major depression and conduct disorder. *Journal of the American Academy of Child and Adolescent Psychiatry, 43*(6), 660–668.

Shufelt, J., & Cocozza, J. (2006). *Youth with mental health disorder in the juvenile justice system: Results from a multi-state prevalence study*. Delmar, NY: National Center for Mental Health and Juvenile Justice.

Skowyra, K., & Cocozza, J. (2007). *Blueprint for change: A comprehensive model for the identification and treatment of youth with mental health needs in contact with the juvenile justice system*. Washington, DC: U.S. Department of Justice, Office of Justice Programs, Office of Juvenile Justice and Delinquency Prevention. Available online at http://www.ncmhjj.com/Blueprint/pdfs/Blueprint.pdf

Snyder, H. (2003). *Juvenile Arrests 2001*. Washington, DC: U.S. Department of Justice, Office of Justice Programs, Office of Juvenile Justice and Delinquency Prevention.

Snyder, H., & Sickmund, M. (1999). *Juvenile offenders and victims: 1999 National Report*. Washington, DC: U.S. Department of Justice, Office of Justice Programs, Office of Juvenile Justice and Delinquency Prevention.

Stroul, B., & Friedman, R. (1986). *A system of care for emotionally disturbed children and youth*. Washington, DC: CASSP Technical Assistance Center, Georgetown University, Child Development Center.

Substance Abuse and Mental Health Services Administration. (2000, November). *System-of-care evaluation brief: Juvenile justice characteristics and outcomes of children in systems of care* (Vol. 2, Issue 2). Rockville, MD: Author. Available online at http://www.systemsofcare.samhsa.gov/newinformation/docs/2000/Nov00.pdf

Substance Abuse and Mental Health Services Administration. (2005, November/December). *SAMHSA News* (Vol. 13, No. 6). Washington, DC: Author.

Teplin, L., Abram, K., McClelland, G., Dulcan, M., & Mericle, A. (2002). Psychiatric disorders in youth in juvenile detention. *Archives of General Psychiatry, 59*, 1133–1143.

U.S. Department of Justice. (2005). *Department of justice activities under the civil rights of institutionalized persons act: Fiscal Year 2004*. Washington, DC: United States Department of Justice. Retrieved July 15, 2005, from http://www.usdoj.gov/crt/split/document/split_cripa04pdf

U.S. House of Representatives. (2004). *Incarceration of youth who are waiting for community mental health services in the United States*. Washington, DC: Committee on Government Reform.

Wasserman, G., Ko, S., & McReynolds, L. (2004). Assessing the mental health status of youth in juvenile justice settings. *Juvenile Justice Bulletin*, August, 1–7.

Wasserman, G., McReynolds, L., Lucas, C., Fisher, P., & Santos, L. (2002). The voice DISC-IV with incarcerated male youths: Prevalence of disorder. *Journal of the American Academy of Child and Adolescent Psychiatry, 41*, 314–321.

22

Services for Youth in the Child Welfare System and Their Families in Systems of Care

Jan McCarthy, Frank Rider, Caraleen M. Fawcett, and Steve Sparks

---

C hildren, youth, and families involved with the child welfare system need and deserve comprehensive, effective mental health care that builds on their individual strengths and meets their emotional and developmental needs. This chapter presents an overview of the mental health needs of children and families involved with the child welfare system and also demonstrates the link between effective mental health services and the achievement of the three major child welfare system goals—safety, permanency, and well-being. In telling Arizona's story, the chapter discusses how to work collaboratively across systems and with families to build service capacity. Voices of real families and youth, including one coauthor who has firsthand experience with the child welfare system, are offered throughout the chapter.

MENTAL HEALTH NEEDS OF CHILDREN AND FAMILIES INVOLVED WITH THE CHILD WELFARE SYSTEM

Historically, the primary focus of the child welfare system has been to protect children from abuse and neglect (i.e., safety) and to provide them with stable, permanent living situations, lifelong relationships with nurturing caregivers, and continuous relationships with family members (i.e., permanency). The system has began focusing more recently on well-being, that is ensuring that children's physical health, mental health, and educational needs are met and enhancing the capacity of parents and guardians to provide for their children's needs (McCarthy & Woolverton, 2005).

Behavioral Health Needs of Children and Families in the Child Welfare System

National statistics show that approximately 900,000 children are victims of abuse or neglect each year, and 513,000 children live in foster care (Administration for Children and Families, 2005a, 2005b). Children and youth who are placed out of their homes and who live in foster homes or group care have undergone life-shattering upheavals. At a time when they desperately need consistency and stability, they are thrown into an uncertain world of multiple placements, unpredictable contact with their siblings and families, new schools, a loss of daily routines, and the reality that they lack control over their own lives. Many feel profoundly alone and have little expectation that things will change (Children's Law Center of Los Angeles, 2007). These vulnerable and at-risk children and youth have a high prevalence of mental health needs. A review of research literature by Landsverk and colleagues (2006) suggested that between one half and three fourths of children entering foster care exhibit behavior or social competency problems that warrant mental health care. There is also evidence that this high rate of need may be anticipated for children served by child welfare who remain in their own homes (Landsverk, Burns, Stambaugh, & Reutz, 2006).

The National Survey of Child and Adolescent Well-Being (NSCAW), a longitudinal study of a nationally representative sample of youth who were subjects of reports of maltreatment investigated by child welfare agencies during 1999 and 2000, provides the first national estimates of mental health need and service use in the child welfare population. NSCAW determined that nearly half (47.9%) of the youth ages 2–14 with completed child welfare investigations ($N = 3,803$), including those living in their own homes, had clinically significant emotional or behavioral problems. The study also determined that only one fourth of these youth with mental health needs received any specialty mental health care during the previous 12 months (Burns et al., 2004).

Although these statistics apply to children of all ages in child welfare, young children bear a disproportionate share of violence and abuse in the home. Infants and toddlers experience the highest rates of child maltreatment of any age group (Groves, 2007), and, of all age groups entering foster care, the largest increase has been among young children. The effects of separation from their families and frequent placement changes can be particularly profound for very young children whose health and development may be undermined by a lack of secure and stable attachments. Problems not addressed during the earliest years of childhood can become more severe and enduring, setting the stage for additional difficulties later in life (Silver, Amster, & Haecker, 1999).

"When my 3-year-old daughter went to the foster home, she didn't know where she was or why she was there. She kept asking; no one told her. Finally, someone lied and said I was in jail. She thought they were hiding her from me and screamed at the foster mother, 'My mama is looking for me. Take me back where you picked me up, so she can find me.' She had to sleep by herself in a dark room and had nightmares. She had al-

ways slept with me. Today, she is diagnosed with ADHD and oppositional defiant disorder."
—Caraleen

Many youth age out of foster care at age 18 or 21, depending on the laws and policies of their states. Older youth in transition from the child welfare system enter adulthood with overwhelming mental health needs. The already difficult task of making the transition to independence is made more complicated— and sometimes virtually impossible—by the mental health issues these young people face (Bernstein, 2005). Of 659 foster care alumni who were 20–33 years of age at the time of one study, more than half (54.4%) had experienced clinical levels of at least one mental health problem, such as depression, social phobia, panic syndrome, post-traumatic stress disorder, or drug dependence, during the previous 12 months. Almost 20% had three or more mental health problems (Pecora et al., 2006).

"I didn't grow up a normal way or with a lot of people to support me, so I'm going to need 10 times more support now. It's a tough task. I'm not connected at all. I'm officially out there on my own, trying to survive. I need people I can talk to and rely on."
—Chris, age 21 (Bernstein, 2005)

"As I got older, I didn't want to go to therapy, I guess 'cause they were always changing my therapist and I always had a different social worker, so I wouldn't talk to people 'cause I didn't trust them."
—Erika, age 18 (Bernstein, 2005)

Among the deficits of many youth leaving foster care is the lack of abiding relationships. Having had their connections to their families of origin severed, and their subsequent connections to surrogate caretakers broken, many feel completely alone, with little expectation that things will ever be otherwise (Bernstein, 2005).

Linking Well-Being to the Achievement of Safety and Permanency

When children's physical health, mental health, and education needs are not met, and when parents do not receive the services and supports needed to care for their children or to address their own needs, it is difficult, if not impossible, to provide a stable home or to ensure safety and permanency. The Child and Family Services Review (CFSR), a comprehensive monitoring and review system designed to assist states in improving outcomes for children and families served by public child welfare systems, focuses on safety, permanency, and well-being. It acknowledges that enhancing children's healthy development and giving families the tools they need to care for their children will increase the likelihood of achieving these goals.

In a mental health analysis of the 2001–2004 CFSR process, 33 states demonstrated challenges to achieving permanency and stability for children. The complex behavioral health needs of children, along with the lack of early diagnosis, specialized providers to address needs, and well-trained and supported foster parents and social workers, led to placement disruptions, instability, and difficulty establishing and reaching permanency goals. Several states noted that children with emotional and behavioral challenges often were not considered ready for adoption, and few placement resources were available that were equipped to meet their needs. Reunification was limited by the lack of mental health and substance abuse services for parents, and reentries of children into care were attributed to the same services deficits (McCarthy, Van Buren, & Irvine, 2007). One study found that delivery of appropriate and timely mental health services may be an important element in decreasing placement instability among children removed from their homes (Hurlburt et al., 2004).

Working with Families

"At first it was hard to work on the plan. I didn't feel like I was a member of the team; most of them were strangers. It felt like they were talking over my head. So, I put my hand on the table and said, 'Please talk to me.' It was the icebreaker for me. I went to a parent support group and learned how to speak for myself. I learned how to let my emotions guide the team meeting. I found out that I could let others know that I needed help. I got a parent partner. She was my advocate. She was also an ex-addict. Her life was not always peachy creamy. I could identify with her. After the kids came home, it was not easy, but my children are doing well. I've been clean and sober for more than 8 years. I've had a job all that time. I have my kids with me, and I'm a volunteer advocate for other families. I've been there, done that, and got the T shirt. This helps when I work with other families."
—Joyce (McCarthy et al., 2005)

The best possible outcomes can be achieved in all service systems when families are engaged early in service planning. Key cross-system principles for working with families include viewing parents as experts in determining their own service needs and strengths, enhancing parents' capacity to care for their own children, listening to family voices in system-level policies and planning, working with the whole family, and supporting families as advocates and peer mentors to other families involved with child welfare.

Important considerations when working with families from the child welfare system include the following:

- Many parents who experience the stresses that lead to involvement with the child welfare system need mental health and substance abuse services and supports themselves.

- In their first contact with a family, child welfare workers engage the family around concern for the child's safety. Once parents understand the safety concerns, attention can be given to what it will take for the family to protect the child and create a safe, stable home environment that meets the child's needs.

- Children in foster care are involved with multiple families. One child might be connected with birth parents and siblings, relative caregivers, foster parents and siblings, adoptive parents, and group home staff in parenting roles, as well as social workers and court staff who have influence over their lives. The situation is even more complicated for some children who live in a succession of foster homes.

Therapists have found that what makes or breaks the treatment of children in foster care is not the work done with the children, but the alliances that they build and the services they provide to the birth parents, foster parents, and the assigned parenting figures in the social welfare and court systems (Alvarez, 2006). Everyone who works with foster children should understand the roles these individuals play in their lives, and they should ensure that they are carefully and appropriately included in decisions related to the children.

Even though many child welfare reform efforts have focused on the role of families and strengthening relationships with families, national data demonstrates that much work remains to be done. In the first round of the CFSRs, no state achieved substantial conformity with the outcome measure that states, "Parents will have enhanced capacity to meet their child's needs," which is defined as achieving the outcome for 90% of the children and families reviewed (Administration for Children and Families, 2004). In addition, "child and family involvement in case planning" was rated as an area needing improvement in 47 states.

SYSTEMIC AND PRACTICE APPROACHES

Meeting the mental health needs of children and families in the child welfare system requires both a systemic approach and specialized clinical practices. This section discusses the system of care approach and system-level findings from the CFSRs, as well as trauma-informed clinical practice approaches and evidence-based practices in child welfare.

Systems of Care

The system of care values and principles initially articulated in relation to children with serious emotional disorders are being increasingly applied in building systems of care for *all* children. By definition, a system of care is noncategorical in that it crosses agency and program boundaries. It adopts a population focus across systems, and it approaches the service and support requirements of families holistically (Pires, 2002).

Many states are using the CFSR process, especially their Program Improvement Plans (PIPs), as an opportunity to generate system change. The same practice principles that form the basis for the CFSRs are inherent in systems of care:

- Family-centered practice

- Community-based services

- Strengthening of parental capacity to protect and provide for their children

- Individualized services that respond to the unique needs of children and families

The system of care approach incorporates many improvements pursued by child welfare systems (e.g., partnering with families, building the service array, implementing financing strategies, increasing cultural competence). It is a strategy that can simultaneously address multiple items of nonconformity in states' CFSRs. As such, the system of care approach can be built into a PIP and provide a framework to help states get a complete picture of each child's situation.

Since 1992, the Substance Abuse and Mental Health Services Administration (SAMHSA) has funded more than 100 states and local communities to build systems of care to develop comprehensive community-based services and supports for children with serious emotional disorders. These grantees are guided by system of care values and principles (SAMHSA, n.d.). Sparked by the promising outcomes for families and children served by the SAMHSA program, in 2003, the Administration for Children and Families funded communities in nine states to test the effectiveness of applying system of care principles and infrastructure to the child welfare population to promote more effective collaboration among child-serving agencies and to improve CFSR outcomes (Administration for Children & Families, 2003). States have begun to recognize that the child welfare system alone cannot provide all necessary services and supports for families with children who are vulnerable to abuse and neglect and that collaboration with the mental health, substance abuse, domestic violence, education, and judicial systems, as well as the private sector, is essential.

Findings from the Child and Family Services Reviews

A recent mental health analysis of the CFSRs (McCarthy et al., 2007) uncovered the following significant challenges related to mental health services for children and families in the child welfare system and confirmed an urgent need for cross-system reform:

- A lack of accessibility to mental health assessments and services

- A lack of involvement of families in the mental health services for their own children and in system-level planning

- A lack of coordination of services across systems

- State budget deficits

- Shortages of appropriate mental health providers, especially in rural areas

- Difficulty achieving permanency and stability for children with behavioral health needs

The general findings for the 2001–2004 CFSRs determined that only one state achieved substantial conformity with the outcome "Children receive adequate services to meet their physical and mental health needs." Children's mental health was rated as an area needing improvement in 48 states (Administration for Children and Families, 2004). On a positive note, every PIP mentioned mental health issues, and 46 PIPs included goals and action steps related to mental health services, describing a number of solutions that states were pursuing to meet the mental health needs of children and families in the child welfare system.

It is important to note that only three states described how to ensure that mental health services for children and families in the child welfare system are culturally competent. This is of concern because of the disproportionate presence of children of color—especially African American and Native American children—in the child welfare system, as well as the lower use of mental health care by African American youth cited in another national study (Garland, Landsverk, & Lau, 2003).

Addressing Trauma

It is well-established that abused and neglected children suffer from short- and long-term psychological and behavioral difficulties. There is growing attention to the need to create trauma-informed child welfare systems that are responsive to the needs of vulnerable and traumatized children (Igelman, Conradi, & Ryan, 2007). The National Child Traumatic Stress Network (http://www.nctsn.org) describes services designed to reduce the impact of trauma as *trauma-informed services.* It has developed a tool to assess a child's trauma history, the severity of the child's reactions to trauma, and any related developmental concerns.

Although the most common sources of traumatic experience for children who become involved in the child welfare system are abuse, neglect, and domestic violence, many children are exposed to numerous other traumas. In addition, they are often further injured by system-induced trauma (e.g., enduring frequent placement changes, repeated and insensitive interviews, giving difficult court testimony) (Taylor, Wilson, & Igelman, 2006). The plan of creating a trauma-informed system that, at the very least, will not induce further harm to children and, at best, will support their healing involves a commitment from multiple child-serving systems, especially the child welfare and mental health systems, working in close alliance with parents.

Evidence-Based Practices

Given the traumatic life circumstances experienced by most children and youth in the child welfare system, as well as the clinical needs they exhibit, it is crucial to ensure that appropriate treatment services are provided. "The question that matters most is not whether young people get services, but whether they get better" (Bernstein, 2005). It is important to know which services and supports work for children in the child welfare system and their families.

A 2007 review of the research evidence for trauma-focused interventions for children and adolescents provides guidance about effective strategies to address emotional and behavioral problems associated with trauma (Stambaugh, Burns,

Landsverk, & Reutz, 2007). From this review, several treatment models emerged as the most supported interventions for children with histories of trauma:

- Three Cognitive-Behavioral Therapy models adapted for physical and sexual abuse for children ages 4–18 years (Trauma-Focused Cognitive Behavioral Therapy, Trauma-Focused Cognitive Behavioral Therapy for Childhood Traumatic Grief, and Abuse-Focused Cognitive Behavioral Therapy for Child Pyhsical Abuse)

- Parent–Child Interaction Therapy for children ages 4–12 years

- Child–Parent Psychotherapy for Family Violence for children up to age 5 years

- Cognitive Behavioral Intervention for Trauma in Schools for children ages 10–15 years

- Project 12-Ways/Safe Care for Child Neglect for young children

The Surgeon General's report on mental health (U.S. Department of Health and Human Services, 1999) and the California Institute for Mental Health confirm the overall effectiveness of Cognitive-Behavioral Therapy and highlight three additional evidence-based interventions that are effective for youth in foster care (Marshall, 2004):

- Multisystemic Therapy

- Treatment foster care

- Intensive case management and wraparound

Adoption and implementation of evidence-based practices is generally not cost neutral. Resources are required to develop training and quality assurance mechanisms to ensure fidelity to the model. Changes in funding structures and policies may be required, as well as investment in the organizational change management strategies that are essential for successful adoption of new practices (Wilson & Alexandra, 2005).

THE ARIZONA STORY

> "I became involved with the child welfare system after struggling with a methamphetamine addiction and becoming homeless as a result of my addiction. My 3-year-old daughter was removed to protective foster care, and I went to drug treatment. I pushed and begged and was desperate for help, even though I was scared to say so, afraid that if I cried out, I would look unstable. I was able to get into treatment really fast, unlike most people involved with child welfare. From there my journey began."
> —Caraleen

Although the 21st century opened with a worldwide sense of hope, Arizona's behavioral health, child welfare, juvenile justice, and public education systems entered the new millennium with well-documented track records of poor outcomes and sometimes disastrous failures. An almost "perfect storm" of shortcomings saw the state's public health care and behavioral health systems bound by a settlement agreement in a class action lawsuit (*JK versus Eden et al.*, 2001); child welfare system reform at the center of the new governor's platform (Arizona Office of the Governor, 2003); the juvenile corrections agency obligated in another settlement with the U.S. Department of Justice (Arizona Department of Juvenile Corrections, 2004); and the public education system ranked as the least effective in the nation from 2004 to 2006 ("Arizona Ranks as Dumbest State in the U.S.," 2006).

With virtually every discrete child-serving system in well-publicized need of reform, system builders in Arizona recognized that categorical system reform efforts were fated, at best, to limited victories, whereas noncategorical approaches to system reform had the potential to improve outcomes for the children and families who were typically involved in many of those systems at once. Enlightened in no small part by its end users—children and families—Arizona's public child-serving systems embarked on an ambitious, multidimensional effort to develop a comprehensive system of care on a statewide scale. How this work has reshaped the nexus between child welfare and behavioral health is central to Arizona's story.

Listening to and Learning from Families

"During the child welfare investigation process, I felt misrepresented, lied about, and even worse, unable to speak off the record about anything. Everything about me seemed to be misperceived and then documented."
—Caraleen

Accounts of alienation of families by child welfare and behavioral health systems are all too common. Arizona systems, like many elsewhere, tended to apply rigid, even paternalistic stances toward those they were entrusted to serve. Arizona's 2001 JK settlement agreement, the class action lawsuit that jump-started the cross-system wave of reform, was predicated on a set of 12 Principles congruent with the now well-established system of care values (Table 22.1). The first principle is the most transformative of all—*collaboration with the child and family.*

Although the JK settlement only obligated the state's public health care and behavioral health systems, it acknowledged the significant overlap of service populations among numerous systems. For example, 25% of all children enrolled in Arizona's public behavioral health system are dependent or delinquent wards of the child welfare or juvenile justice systems. This recognition was mutual, and by April 2002, through a formal memorandum of understanding, the leaders of every major child-serving system in the state had voluntarily committed the systems they managed to the same 12 Principles espoused in the JK settlement agreement.

Developing the Infrastructure   When the JK settlement agreement was initially being formulated in 2000, a Children's Executive Committee of top managers from all major child-serving systems was convened. Soon this collaborative body was developing detailed proposals to expand Arizona's array of

Table 22.1.   The 12 Arizona Principles

1. Collaboration with the child and family
2. Functional outcomes
3. Collaboration with others
4. Accessible services
5. Best practices
6. Most appropriate setting
7. Timeliness
8. Services tailored to the child and family
9. Stability
10. Respect for the child and family's unique cultural heritage
11. Independence
12. Connection to natural supports

Source: http://www.azdhs.gov/bhs/principles.pdf

Medicaid-funded supports and services, develop cross training curricula, and examine traditional points of distress where systems had historically contradicted or interfered with one another's practices. A Children's Services Collaborator position was established to galvanize these efforts.

The Children's Executive Committee then created subcommittees. One of these, the Family Subcommittee, disbanded after its very first meeting, reflecting an early strategic judgment that such a structure might actually marginalize family voices in the emerging reform. Instead, its members effectively insisted that families be invited to work on every substantive workgroup, accepting the family mantra of "Nothing about us, without us."

Birth of the Child and Family Team Concept   The Children's Executive Committee also created a Collaborative Special Teams Subcommittee that was charged with developing a common vision for an integrated, unified child and family service planning process. The subcommittee listened closely to its active family participants and eventually produced a design for a wraparound process that held promise for more effective results in serving children and families. This was the beginning of the child and family team concept in Arizona.

"When you are involved in a team that is focused on reunifying a family, everyone has to be on the same page and understand every aspect of the progress, growth, and strengths in the family. Too many times, you don't see one agency acknowledge what the other is doing with the family. This causes so much rework for a family with a long list of to-do's on their case plan. The judge had told me at my first court date, 'You have 1 year to get these things completed. Use your time wisely.' I heard his words in my sleep over and over again, but I felt like I had to wait for all those different service providers to communicate when I was already overwhelmed by the expectations and on overdrive trying to complete them."
—Caraleen

An early milestone in the development of child and family teams was the completion of a *practice improvement protocol* for the behavioral health system that served as a guide to the wraparound process (Arizona Department of Health Services, 2003). Significantly, the nine individuals who wrote the protocol represented all systems whose mandates the child and family team process would need to satisfy, and most importantly, the families it was being designed to serve. The child welfare system contributed as a coauthor its leading expert in family group decision making, which is the family engagement process that is documented in child welfare literature as a gateway to positive safety and permanency outcomes for children who are victims of abuse and neglect (see Shore, Wirth, Cahn, Yancey, & Gunderson, 2001).

Families worked on the protocol alongside expert consultants and some of the case managers who would facilitate the child and family teams. The practice improvement protocol specified that the child and family team, "Carefully consider and give substantial weight to family preferences" in formulating the service plan, acknowledging the "family's expert knowledge of their child." Foster parents and relative caregivers were given equal status as team members. Significantly, the protocol vested in the child and family team the authority to commit the resources of the involved systems to provide timely, effective, individualized services and supports. With a few medical exceptions, this includes determination of the medical necessity required to authorize Medicaid-funded behavioral health services.

As capacity for the child and family team process was building, all children involved with child welfare and juvenile justice systems—and any youth living in residential settings or at risk for such placements—were prioritized to be served by child and family teams. The protocol also required that, "When children and families are involved with multiple child-serving systems at once, then collaboration demands the team's full respect for the societal mandates of each involved system (e.g., safety, for child welfare; learning, for education)." Supported by training, the systems were soon working at both the state and local levels to flesh out detailed procedures to spell out precisely how they would offer *one family, one team, one plan.*

Family Voice in Building the Service Array   With families at the table, system leaders were gaining a new appreciation for the types of services and supports that were most helpful for their children. As with development of the child and family team process, families sat side by side with system leaders and Medicaid consultants to expand the array of covered behavioral health services. A previously limited array of traditional behavioral health services grew into a broad range of individualized direct support approaches that families needed and which could now be funded. Arizona's Division of Behavioral Health Services (ADHS) began writing service contracts to motivate and enable providers to establish personal care, living skills training, respite services, family-to-family and peer-to-peer support, therapeutic foster care (TFC) for both children and adults, supported employment, and similar flexible options.

"The turning point in my case began the day that I was invited by my assigned parent aide to attend a public forum. The people at the forum discussed creation of a community group that would consist of members of the public, along with service providers. My parent aide and I arrived at the door and looked in to see a room full of people wearing suits. Although I was somewhat intimidated by the looks of it all, still I entered the room. What came out of that meeting changed my life forever."
—Caraleen

Funding Family Organizations and Expanding Roles for Families

Intent on meeting the first JK principle, *collaboration with the child and family*, and increasingly convinced of the wisdom and expertise of families in helping to shape meaningful system improvements, Arizona's systems began to seek out and invest discretionary and special grant funds to support family and youth perspectives in a more structured, consistent way. Arizona has two family-run organizations—the Family Involvement Center in Maricopa County and MIKID (Mentally Ill Kids in Distress) statewide—that were developed to organize families' voices, to provide family-to-family support, to cultivate family leaders and system transformers, and to create new models of services and supports for formal child-serving systems. These organizations worked with the child welfare system to create family mentor and foster family mentor roles similar to the parent partner and family support partner roles that had been developed in behavioral health programs.

"A few minutes after it began, the man chairing the meeting asked if anyone else there might be willing to serve as a co-chair of this meeting. For some reason, I immediately began to stand up, but my knees began to shake, so I tried sitting down again. But my parent aide looked at me and said, 'Caraleen, if you want to stand up, then you stand.'"
—Caraleen

Multiple Roles for Families

The state's managed care organizations and service providers began to follow the lead of the state agencies and seek out, attract, utilize, pay for, support, and rely on an expanding array of key roles for families, including serving on hiring panels, verifying applicant credentials, shaping job descriptions and organizational structures, and orienting and training new hires. Arizona's behavioral health system assisted both MIKID and the Family Involvement Center to develop diversified funding as direct service providers (licensed, Medicaid-registered providers of direct support services); as system transformation agents using federal block grant and discretionary grant funding; and as training, coaching, and consultative experts contracted by regional behavioral health authorities. Arizona's child welfare and juvenile justice systems also have begun to assist with further diversifying the financial foundations of the two family-run organizations.

All Arizona child welfare workers and all behavioral health workers receive much of their initial and ongoing training from families, foster families, and increasingly from youth. Families not only complete satisfaction surveys, they also develop and facilitate those surveys, interpret them, help to staff quality improvement departments, publish findings and results in family-friendly media, and assist the system to design process improvements based on those results.

In addition, family members began to use their own strengths and experiences to help other families. Foster families began to "share parenting" with birth families. Families were beginning to imagine new futures (Madsen, 1999). Some of their former alienation from the system was evaporating, tales of success began to accumulate, and the system itself began to take notice. As Madsen (1999) noted, "In an era of cost containment and the search for more effective techniques, we may lose sight of the fact that respect is cost-effective." When systems of care harness families' enthusiasm, assets, and hopes; when they tailor supports to unique family needs; and when they stimulate families to become helpers themselves, they not only achieve better outcomes, but the budget of resources available to help is also effectively multiplied.

> "As a member of what became this community network team, I was given the one thing I had longed for . . . a listened to, credible voice. From there, I was soon traveling statewide, sharing my experiences with and concerns about the system my daughter and I had found ourselves in. People not only listened to me, but actually started to act on things. I had faithfully taken part in my substance abuse treatment, but this was the most therapeutic thing that ever happened to me. I began to feel differently about my experience. I began to feel more grateful than angry; my experience changed from a nightmare into a divine intervention. I was gradually coming to realize that the people in child welfare were not monsters. They didn't hate me. In fact, they were just like me. They had their problems, even if different ones from mine."
> —Caraleen

Youth Voice   Arizona Governor Janet Napolitano, who had made child welfare reform a cornerstone of her first term, quickly recognized the transformative nature of listening to the end users to improve public systems. She established multiple mechanisms for youth in the foster care and juvenile justice systems to offer their experiences, insights, and ideas. She also established a cross-agency Children's Cabinet in the same executive order that launched the Child Protective Services (CPS) reform and soon invited family and youth voices to influence her cabinet-level decision makers. Governor Napolitano continues to meet personally with her youth advisory board at the same frequency with which she meets with her Children's Cabinet. Youth have even become a part of the licensing review teams that the state uses to monitor its residential programs.

Bringing the Systems Together and Building Capacity

Arizona took specific progressive steps toward a common purpose across systems based on the JK settlement agreement's 12 Principles. Aligning the child welfare and behavioral health systems posed significant challenges but was approached systematically as described next.

Developing a Common Language   Key statements of values and principles were negotiated. Shared commitments to a single set of functional outcomes, to an integrated planning process for families, and to a framework that embraces the voices of youth and families at all levels of the system were agreed on and embedded in the official communications of both systems. Cross-cutting concepts were translated into the comfortable, credible language of each system to help span a cultural divide that sometimes seemed as wide as the Grand Canyon.

Frequent challenges arose. Frontline workers in both systems found themselves in lengthy work sessions, aiming to reconcile the unifying rhetoric of the JK settlement agreement with the discrepancies they continued to encounter in daily practice. The behavioral health system said the right things, child welfare workers maintained, but the words rang hollow when effective, trauma-informed healing services were not furnished in time to prevent another child's placement disruption. Child welfare workers, in the judgment of their behavioral health counterparts, were too willing to place foster children in residential treatment settings to meet their housing needs without regard to the often deleterious effects of such placements on the very children they aimed to protect.

A clinical subcommittee of the Arizona Children's Executive Committee became a sort of translation laboratory for the two systems. Arizona developed tools such as written crosswalks to help bridge the cultural divide. *Crosswalk #1—Values and Principles* reflected the congruence of the Child Welfare League of America's statement of child welfare values and principles with the 12 Arizona Principles of the JK settlement agreement. *Crosswalk #2—Child and Family Teams/Family Group Conferencing* compared the details of the various planning processes from child welfare, early childhood, developmental disabilities, and children's mental health disciplines to illustrate how the Arizona child and family team concept captured the essential components of each of these processes (Rider, 2005a, 2005b). Thus, the child and family team process became interchangeable with these other approaches as an integrated, family-engagement process to plan and deliver services and supports.

Operationalizing the Vision: Local-Level Approaches   The Memorandum of Understanding at the state executive level, which embraced the Arizona Vision and the 12 JK settlement agreement principles (including a universal set of functional outcomes for children and families), was systematically operationalized at the local level. In each region of the state, collaborative community teams developed letters of agreement addressing points of friction but primarily reinforcing and elaborating the commitment to the common purposes and beliefs that the crosswalks supported. Ultimately, the behavioral health system required successful regional contractors to negotiate detailed protocols with their child welfare, juvenile justice, and other child-serving partners, leaving little doubt about how these teams of professionals would work together in support of each family.

A strong philosophical and rhetorical foundation was embedded in policy, procedure, contracting, training, and quality measurement processes; however, its practical application demanded determined efforts to ensure that those who would operationalize the values could embrace and own the solutions. Child welfare and juvenile justice representatives joined families, adult consumers, and behavioral health professionals in evaluating managed behavioral health care organizations to ensure that their respective interests were accounted for in both contract requirements and provider commitments. Child welfare treatment experts were invited to help create the uniform, strength-based, individualized behavioral health assessment that replaced the former hodgepodge of assessment approaches previously used across the state.

Urgent Behavioral Health Response   The governor's child welfare system reform focused on partnerships with schools, health care providers, and community partners; however, its most critical partnership was with the behavioral health system. *The Arizona Republic* covered the CPS Reform process closely, and in May 2003, the newspaper ran an editorial beginning with a 5-year-old girl's grief and disorientation upon finding herself in a shelter one Friday evening after being removed from her family home to protect her from maltreatment ("Imagine you are 5 . . . And alone," 2003). Stories like hers had a profound impact, and the behavioral health system leaders invited their child welfare counterparts to take part in a series of frank conversations to figure out how to stop the pain that had touched them all. This had become personal.

Within weeks, the two systems had reviewed relevant resources (e.g., American Academy of Child and Adolescent Psychiatry & Child Welfare League of America, 2003) and conceptualized a new process by which all children would receive what became known as an *urgent behavioral health response* within 24 hours of removal to the protective custody of child welfare. A child welfare investigator must simply notify the behavioral health provider by phone—at any hour of any day—that a child is being removed to the protective custody of the state. A behavioral health clinician is then immediately dispatched to the place where the child is most comfortable to screen for immediate reactions to the maltreatment or removal situation, to provide guidance and a supportive contact for the protective caregiver, to begin the process of assessing the child's behavioral health needs, and to initiate the formation of the child and family team. Within a few days, the behavioral health clinician conducts a developmental screening for the youngest children and offers written input about visitation, placement, and services for each child that the child welfare professional can consider in formulating the initial plan for presentation to the juvenile court. This has the effect of marrying the two systems at the point of removal of the child from the home.

Child welfare and behavioral health personnel developed local protocols to best accomplish the purposes of this new process. Virtually all children in state custody qualify for Medicaid benefits, so the urgent behavioral health response is fully reimbursed as an assessment and sometimes also as a treatment activity.

Arizona's urgent behavioral health response for children entering foster care demonstrated to child welfare the good faith of the behavioral health system in wanting to understand and respond effectively to the unique needs of children and families receiving services from both systems. Furthermore, it was a strategic action in that it quickly multiplied the penetration of dependent children into the state's behavioral health system. In 2001, only 34% of dependent children had been enrolled with Arizona's regional behavioral health authorities, but by July 2006, more than 75% were enrolled. The behavioral health system was obligating itself to create significant new support and treatment capacity to meet the enduring needs and fulfill the Early and Periodic Screening, Diagnosis, and Treatment entitlements of the newly enrolled foster children. More than 12,000 children have subsequently received this urgent response service in Arizona.

Colocation   Child welfare offices were soon arranging space and communications capacity for behavioral health clinicians to colocate with them to provide immediate support as predictable behavioral health needs of children and their parents emerged. Through their colocation in child welfare intake offices, clinical professionals became exposed to the daily realities of frontline child welfare work, and more stubborn vestiges of the cultural divide between the two systems melted away. Lofty rhetoric about "our shared children" gave way to action. A common sense of urgency and shared responsibility for the well-being of the children began to blossom.

Risk-Adjusted Capitation Rates   As child and family teams began to form around these children and their families, a clearer picture emerged about their true treatment and support needs. In 2004, 9 months after the urgent response became statewide policy, the behavioral health system established a new, risk-adjusted capitation rate for dependent and delinquent children within the overall behavioral health system. In every part of the state, the capitation rate to pay for behavioral health services for these children was actuarially set at least 20 times higher than for the other 75% of children in the behavioral health system who were *not* in foster care in Arizona. The new risk-adjusted capitation rate was based on actual spending for services the children needed, and it legitimized the creation of placement stabilization teams, TFC, and other specialized supports and trauma-informed interventions for these children.

Meeting the Unique Needs of Children, Families, and Protective Caregivers: Improving and Financing Clinical Practice

> "The separation from my daughter was killing me inside. I was young, lost, and had no one to talk to about my guilt and my grief. I soon found myself faced with a daunting case plan and a ton of things to do. I did not know where to begin."
> —Caraleen

Arizona's behavioral health and child welfare systems worked together to establish a shared view of the unique behavioral health needs of children and their families in all phases of the child welfare system (from entry to exit) and of how the emerging system of care should support them. They crafted a new protocol, *Practice Improvement Protocol #15—The Unique Behavioral Health Service Needs of Children, Youth, and Families Involved with CPS*. This protocol identifies the likely treatment needs, principle-driven approaches, and recommended practices at each point along a child and family's journey in the child welfare system (Arizona Department of Health Services, 2006).

Implementing this protocol has stimulated multiple improvements in the behavioral health system and has also created accommodations for children and families served by the child welfare system:

- **Workforce development**

The state retrained its children's behavioral health workforce and undertook specific initiatives to certify clinicians in numerous evidence-based, trauma-focused skill sets and practices. ADHS supported the retraining effort with federal block grant dollars and SAMHSA discretionary grants. The ADHS curriculum on the unique behavioral health needs of children in the child welfare system was published and implemented in 2007.

- **Assessment of young children**

The behavioral health and child welfare systems joined forces with Arizona's Part C early childhood programs to incorporate comprehensive developmental screenings in a new behavioral health assessment designed collectively by the partners to be sensitive to the specific needs of infants, toddlers, and preschoolers and their caregivers.

- **Therapeutic foster care**

The state child welfare and behavioral health systems developed a joint protocol to combine federal child welfare funds (i.e., Title IV-E for room and board) with behavioral health funds (i.e., Medicaid for active treatment) to furnish high-quality TFC services for children who, only a few years ago, would have been served in inpatient, congregate residential, or even secure correctional facilities (Arizona Department of Human Services, 2007a). The number of joint TFC placements in Arizona grew from 9 in late 2003 to more than 400 by the end of 2006. In designing TFC, the two systems consulted each other and shared foster parent training curricula, including the new child welfare foster parent training that emphasizes shared parenting concepts.

> "My daughter's foster parents took the trouble to want to know me; they respected me as her mother and went out of their way to support our relationship. They knew it was best for my daughter to come home to a healthier me. In a way, she was lucky to have so many parent figures who cared enough for her to make sure we were all working toward the same thing."
> —Caraleen

- **Changes in residential treatment**

In April 2002, 100 children were in out-of-state residential treatment placements. Most of them were dependent children in state custody. Since then, the number of children in out-of-state placement has been reduced to 25. Arizona boasts one of the lowest rates of children in congregate residential placements of any state behavioral health system, attributed to the development of crisis stabilization resources, skilled behavior coaches, high-quality treatment foster care, an extensive workforce of direct support workers, and a child and family team process that blends the strengths of youth, their families, and their informal community supports with more formal clinical treatment services.

- **Adolescent substance abuse treatment services and other community-based practices**

The practice improvement protocol on the unique behavioral health needs of children involved with the child welfare system has stimulated the expansion and improvement of adolescent substance abuse treatment services, as well as trauma-informed evidence-based clinical practices and other intensive community-based practice approaches (e.g., Multisystemic Therapy, Functional Family Therapy, Brief Strategic Family Therapy, and Multidimensional Treatment Foster Care).

Increasingly, the behavioral health and child welfare systems are looking for opportunities to intervene earlier and prevent children and families from penetrating so deeply into the child welfare system. They have explored how to collaboratively expand intensive family support and preservation services to prevent children from being removed from their homes in the first place, and to expedite and reinforce their successful reunification with recovering families when removals are unavoidable.

Key Elements and Lessons Learned

1. Collaboration occurs in stages

Arizona learned that collaboration between child welfare and behavioral health includes the following important nonlinear stages: developing a shared language; becoming open to integrating the perspectives of families and other systems; creating a shared vision and purpose; guaranteeing that the public mandates of each participating system will be fully respected; identifying the recurring needs of children, their families, and protective caregivers; identifying treatment issues, themes, and effective interventions; discovering, developing, and reworking financing and human resources; tailoring individualized direct supports; developing the workforce and its clinical expertise; and leading, monitoring, measuring, and continuously improving implementation and system change.

2. Meeting resistance

System reform is not an easy process. Systems are made up of many individuals and structures that support the status quo. Arizona developed several strategies for addressing resistance:

- Use some concerted voices from inside (e.g., the Children's Services Collaborator) and outside of the organization to serve as the first seeds of change.

- Use cross-system translation and boundary expansion (*collective ownership*) techniques to introduce new information and ideas, and thus share authorship, ownership, and responsibility.

- Strategically use power and organizational pressure points to promote new behaviors.

- Embed key improvements deep into the new system culture to prevent backsliding when inevitable external changes might detract from success or impede progress.

- Frame issues in the parlance of each organization (e.g., if the organization endorses family systems theory, present the need of families who cannot remain together due to substance abuse or mental health issues and resultant family conflict) in those terms.

3.   Prioritize services for children and families involved with child welfare

In Arizona, children's services leaders invested considerable effort and time to help both the child welfare and behavioral health systems recognize that these children and families, by virtue of their experiences, have legitimate, treatable behavioral health needs. Once the behavioral health system understood this and the urgent response process created a welcoming front door to its services, the issues of financing and capacity-building had to be addressed. Because children in foster care are nearly always eligible for Medicaid, processes were designed to establish entitlement and enroll children immediately. Children in foster care and those at risk of placement in residential or juvenile justice detention settings were prioritized in the annual JK settlement plans to have child and family teams.

4.   Ensure sufficient resources

Arizona pursued several funding strategies to bring the system of care vision to reality for those involved with the child welfare system: optimizing the scope of Medicaid-covered services, obtaining a Title IV-E waiver to support expedited family reunification, securing discretionary grants, braiding funds, establishing flexible funds, and aligning contracting approaches and provider qualifications across the two systems. In addition, the child and family team process was designed to attract families' own informal resources and supports, as well as others, into the mix.

5.   Set, measure, and publicize outcomes

Arizona was able to publish data on six common cross-system outcomes by mid-2005. Consistently since then, all outcome measures have been significantly better for the children—including all foster children—involved in the first wave of child and family teams than for those not yet served by a team (Arizona Department of Health Services, 2007b). The child welfare system's 6-month reports to the Arizona Legislature confirm that significant progress is being made in virtually all areas of permanency and well-being since the implementation of these reforms.

6.   Listen to families and youth

It is essential to unleash the authentic voices of those the system is ultimately intended to serve. There are no more powerful transformation agents than youth and families who, for better or worse, will live with the results of the collective work. Systems must invite, cultivate, nurture, and cherish those voices. They will sustain the positive changes through shifts in leadership, external forces, and bureaucratic inertia.

CONCLUSION

Despite recent progress, most communities in the United States still lack well-developed systems of care. In some states, the child welfare system has essentially become the mental health system for children by providing or purchasing mental health services with child welfare funds or Medicaid funds that have been allocated to the child welfare system budget. Although this may offer a short-term solution, it saddles the child welfare system with the full responsibility for the mental health care of children who are in the system due to abuse or neglect. It also may force parents to go to the child welfare system to obtain mental health services for their children that are not available in the community. It does not build on the strengths of each child-serving system, nor does it strengthen the ability of communities to provide community-based mental health services for families and children.

A better alternative is for multiple child-serving systems to work together, along with families as partners, to create a stronger and more comprehensive community-based mental health system. The Arizona story demonstrates how one state is creating such a system.

> "I am proud to say that, after 4 years, I am still clean. My daughter and I have moved on. Now I work side by side with the same providers who once helped me, and together we are helping others who are just like I was. Sometimes I think about the different things that might have happened to me if I had not met such great people and had such life-changing events. It was the influence of compassionate hearts and the professionals working together that helped to change my attitude, and in the end I truly feel blessed."
> —Caraleen

REFERENCES

Administration for Children and Families. (2003) *Children's Bureau Demonstration Initiative: Improving child welfare outcomes through systems of care.* Available online at http://www.childwelfare.gov/systemwide/service/soc/communicate/initiative/

Administration for Children and Families. (2004). *Summary of the results of the 2001–2004 Child and Family Services Reviews: General findings from the Federal Child and Family Services Review*. Available online at http://www.acf.hhs.gov/programs/cb/cwmonitoring/results/genfindings04/genfindings04.pdf

Administration for Children and Families. (2005a). *Foster Care FY2000–FY2005 entries, exits, and numbers of children in care on the last day of each federal fiscal year*. Available online at http://www.acf.hhs.gov/programs/cb/stats_research/afcars/statistics/entryexit 2005.htm

Administration for Children and Families. (2005b). *National Child Abuse and Neglect System Report, FY 05*. Available online at http://www.acf.dhhs.gov/programs/cb/pubs/cm05/cm05.pdf

Alvarez, A. (2006). Foreword. In T.V. Heineman & D. Ehrensaft (Eds.), *Building a home within: Meeting the emotional needs of children and youth in foster care* (pp. xiii–xv). Baltimore: Paul H. Brookes Publishing Co.

American Academy of Child and Adolescent Psychiatry & Child Welfare League of America. (2003). *Policy statement on mental health and use of alcohol and other drugs, screening, and assessment of children in foster care*. Available online at http://www.aacap.org/publications/policy/collab02.htm

Arizona Department of Health Services, Division of Behavioral Health Services. (2003). *Practice improvement protocol #9: The child and family team*. Available online at http://www.azdhs.gov/bhs/guidance/cft.pdf

Arizona Department of Health Services, Division of Behavioral Health Services. (2006). *Practice improvement protocol #15: The unique behavioral health needs of children, youth and families involved with CPS*. Phoenix: Author.

Arizona Department of Health Services, Division of Behavioral Health Services. (2007a). *DBHS practice protocol: Home care training to home care client services for children*. Available online at http://www.azdhs.gov/bhs/guidance/hctc.pdf

Arizona Department of Health Services, Division of Behavioral Health Services. (2007b). *Demographic functional outcome measures: Statewide totals for T-19 clients under age 18*. Retrieved September 27, 2007, from http://www.azdhs.gov/bhs/measures/charts_0207.pdf

Arizona Department of Juvenile Corrections. (2004). *U.S. Department of Justice investigation*. Retrieved from http://www.azdjc.gov/CRIPA/CRIPAHome.htm

Arizona Office of the Governor. (2003). *Executive Order #2003-4*. Available online at http://azgovernor.gov/dms/upload/2003_4.pdf

Arizona ranks as dumbest state in the U.S. (2006, October). *Business Journal of Phoenix* Available online at http://www.bizjournals.com/phoenix/stories/2006/10/16/daily20 .html?from_rss=1

Bernstein, N. (2005). *Helping those who need it most: Meeting the mental health care needs of youth in the foster care and juvenile justice systems*. Sacramento: California Family Impact Seminar.

Burns, B., Phillips, S., Wagner, H., Barth, R., Kolko, D., Campbell, Y., et al. (2004). Mental health need and access to mental health services by youths involved with child welfare: A national survey. *Journal of the American Academy of Child and Adolescent Psychiatry, 43*(8), 960.

Children's Law Center of Los Angeles. (2007). *Making reform real: Addressing the mental health needs of children in the dependency system. Report and recommendations from the 2006 Foster Youth Mental Health Summit*. Monterey Park, CA: Author.

Garland, A., Landsverk, J., & Lau, A. (2003). Racial/ethnic disparities in mental health service use among children in foster care. *Children and Youth Services Review, 25*(5–6), 491–507.

Groves, B. (2007, Winter). Early intervention as prevention: Addressing trauma in young children. Focal point: Research, policy, and practice in children's mental health. *Research and Training Center on Family Support and Children's Mental Health*, 16–18.

Hurlburt, M., Leslie, L., Landsverk, J., Barth, R., Burns, B., Gibbons, R., et al. (2004). Contextual predictors of mental health service use among children open to child welfare services. *Archives of General Psychiatry, 61*, 1217–1224.

Igelman, R., Conradi, L., & Ryan, B. (2007, Winter). Creating a trauma-informed child welfare system. Focal point: Research, policy, and practice in children's mental health. *Research and Training Center on Family Support and Children's Mental Health*, 23.

Imagine you are 5 . . . And alone. And crying. Think you might need help? (2003, May 27). *The Arizona Republic*.

JK v. Eden et al., No. CIV 91-261 TUC JMR (D.Ariz June 26, 2001).

Kallal, J. (2006, December). Untitled presentation to the Governor's Integration Initiative Executive Committee, Phoenix, AZ.

Landsverk, J., Burns, B., Stambaugh, L., & Reutz, J. (2006). *Mental health care for children and adolescents in foster care: Review of research literature*. Seattle: Casey Family Programs.

Madsen, W. (1999). *Collaborative therapy with multistressed families*. New York: Guilford Press.

Marshall, A. (2004). *A system of care: Meeting the mental health needs of children in foster care. Best practice, next practice*. Washington, DC: National Child Welfare Resource Center for Family-Centered Practice.

McCarthy, J., Marshall, A., Collins, J., Arganza, G., Deserly, K., & Milon, J. (2005). *A family's guide to the child welfare system*. Washington, DC: Georgetown University Center for Child and Human Development, National Technical Assistance Center for Children's Mental Health.

McCarthy, J., Van Buren, E., & Irvine, M. (2007). *Child and family services review: A mental health analysis*. Washington, DC: Georgetown University Center for Child and Human Development, National Technical Assistance Center for Children's Mental Health.

McCarthy, J., & Woolverton, M. (2005). Healthcare needs of children and youth in foster care. In G.P. Mallon & P.M. Hess (Eds.), *Child welfare for the 21st century: A handbook of practices, policies, and programs* (p. 129). New York: Columbia University Press.

Pecora, P., Kessler, R., Williams, J., O'Brien, K., Downs, A., English, D., et al. (2006). *Improving family foster care: Findings from the northwest foster care alumni study*. Seattle: Casey Family Programs.

Pires, S. (2002). *Building systems of care: A primer*. Washington, DC: Georgetown University Center for Child and Human Development, National Technical Assistance Center for Children's Mental Health.

Rider, F. (2005a). *A comparison of six practice models: National Wraparound Initiative tools*. Available online at http://www.rtc.pdx.edu/nwi/tools/pdfs/Ridercomparisonofmodels wrapandothers.pdf.

Rider, F. (2005b). *Comparing behavioral health and child welfare values and principles: National Wraparound Initiative tools*. Available online at http://www.rtc.pdx.edu/nwi/tools/pdfs/RiderCW-BHValuesCrosswalk.pdf

Rubin, D., O'Reilly, A., Luan, X., & Localio, R. (2007) The impact of placement stability on behavioral well-being for children in foster care. *Pediatrics, 119*(2), 336–344.

Shore, N., Wirth, J., Cahn, K., Yancey, B., & Gunderson, K. (2001, June). *Long-term and immediate outcomes of family group conferencing in Washington State*. Available online at http://www.iirp.org/library/fgcwash.html

Silver, J.A., Amster, B.J., & Haecker, T. (Eds.). (1999). *Young children and foster care: A guide for professionals*. Baltimore: Paul H. Brookes Publishing Co.

Stambaugh, L., Burns, B., Landsverk, J., & Reutz, J. (2007, Winter). Evidence-based treatment for children in child welfare. Focal point: Research, policy, and practice in children's mental health. *Research and Training Center on Family Support and Children's Mental Health, 12–15*.

Substance Abuse and Mental Health Services Administration. (n.d.). *Comprehensive Community Mental Health Services for Children and Their Families Program* (PL 102-321). Available online at http://mentalhealth.samhsa.gov/cmhs/childrenscampaign/ccmhs.asp

Taylor, N., Wilson, C., & Igelman, R. (2006). In pursuit of a more trauma-informed child welfare system. *APSAC Advisor, 18*, 4–9.

U.S. Department of Health and Human Services. (1999). *Mental health: A report of the Surgeon General.* Rockville, MD: Author.

Wilson, C., & Alexandra, L. (2005). *Guide for child welfare administrators on evidence-based practice.* Washington, DC: American Public Human Services Association.

23

Services for Youth and Their Families in Culturally Diverse Communities

Mareasa R. Isaacs, Larke Nahme Huang, Mario Hernandez,
Holly Echo-Hawk, Ignacio David Acevedo-Polakovich, and Ken Martinez

---

Culture provides an interpretive guide for most human behavior (Bock, 1999). What is usual in one culture, such as greeting with a kiss, may be immodest or offensive in others (Singh, McKay, & Singh, 1998). This connection between culture and behavior ranges far beyond everyday issues such as the appropriateness of a given interpersonal greeting and reaches well into more serious matters such as the normalcy or aberrance of a given behavior (Bock, 1999). Stated simply, culture provides people with the background information necessary to make important decisions about what is wrong and what is right, who is normal, and who is mentally unhealthy (López & Guarnaccia, 2000).

The influence of culture on mental health is widely recognized. In the latest edition of its widely used *Diagnostic and Statistical Manual of Mental Disorders, Fourth Edition*, the American Psychiatric Association (APA; 2000) warns that mental health professionals who are not familiar with a person's cultural frame of reference are at risk for incorrectly labeling normal culturally bound variations in behavior, beliefs, or experience as mental illness. The APA's warning is consistent with the findings of the U.S. Surgeon General's supplemental report *Mental Health: Culture, Race, and Ethnicity* (U.S. Department of Health and Human Services [U.S. DHHS], 2001), which noted that one of the fundamental weaknesses of behavioral health services and research has been the failure to recognize the importance of culture in the epidemiology, conceptualization, treatment, recovery, and prevention of behavioral health disorders.

Given this context, it should not be surprising to learn that a substantial body of research examining mental health services in the United States finds significant and meaningful ethnicity-based and race-based disparities in the availability of, access to (Bui & Takeuchi, 1992; Chabra, Chavez, Harris, & Shah, 1999; Costello, Farmer, & Angold, 1997; Cunningham & Freiman, 1996;

Juszczak, Melinkovich, & Kaplan, 2003; Novins, Beals, Sack, & Manson, 2000; Novins, Duclos, Martin, Jewett, & Manson, 1999; Pumariega, Glover, Holzer, & Nguyen, 1998), quality of (Walkup, McAlpine, & Olfson, 2000; Wang, West, & Tanielian, 2000; Young, Klap, & Sherbourne, 2001), and outcomes of (Huang, 2002; U.S. DHHS, 2001) mental health care. Generally speaking, White European Americans fare better in each of these areas than do members of other racial and ethnic groups, a pattern that is particularly concerning because most mental health problems are no more prevalent or severe in these other groups than they are among White European Americans (U.S. DHHS, 2001).

These mental health service disparities are partly driven by the inability or unwillingness of publicly funded mental health systems to understand and value the need to offer services consistent with the histories, traditions, beliefs, languages, and values of diverse groups. In turn, this inability leads to other unfavorable outcomes, including misdiagnoses (Fabrega, Ulrich, & Mezzich, 1993; Kilgus, Pumariega, & Cuffe, 1995; Malgady & Constantino, 1998; U.S. DHHS, 2001; Yeh et al., 2002), increased mistrust of mental health services among members of many ethnic or racial groups, and decreased utilization of services by these same individuals (Snowden, 1998; Takeuchi, Sue, & Yeh, 1995; Theriot, Segal, & Cowsert, 2003; U.S. DHHS, 2001). Not surprisingly, the report of the President's New Freedom Commission on Mental Health (2003) cited the elimination of these disparities as one of the most important improvements needed in mental health service systems. According to the commission's report, these disparities will not be eliminated until cultural competence is recognized as an essential component of mental health care services in the United States.

This chapter provides an orientation to some of the most important issues involved in transforming mental health systems so that they are responsive to the cultural needs and social contexts of local communities. It is guided by the premise that cultural competence in mental health services occurs only when there is congruence among: 1) the direct service practices available to a community; 2) the policies, structures, and processes of the organizations supporting these direct services, and 3) a community's culture and social context (Hernandez, Nesman, Isaacs, et al., 2006). Accordingly, both direct service practices and organizational support are discussed with respect to issues involved in ensuring that both of these domains of systems of care foster congruence with a local community's culture and social context. Examples from the field are used to illustrate culturally competent approaches, and recommendations are offered for improving services to culturally diverse communities.

DIRECT SERVICE PRACTICES

This section begins with an introduction to the recent trend toward *evidence-based practices* (EBPs) in mental health services, along with some of the promises and limitations of currently available EBPs in the context of culturally diverse communities. This is followed by a description of efforts to adapt current EBPs in order to strengthen their usefulness when working with diverse clientele. The section ends with a discussion of the role that the development of *practice-based evidence* (PBE) can play in addressing some of the limitations of available EBPs in culturally diverse settings.

Evidence-Based Practices: Promises and Limitations in Diverse Communities

Early definitions of EBPs presented these primarily as interventions whose efficacy has been demonstrated through randomized clinical trials or single case studies conducted by multiple investigators in multiple sites for specific problems, populations, and settings ("Consensus Statement on Evidence-Based Programs and Cultural Competence," 2003). More advanced conceptualizations, however, make it clear that EBPs involve the incorporation of research, although not in lieu of clinical expertise and consumer values and choices. For instance, the Institute of Medicine (IOM; 2000) defined EBPs as "the integration of the best research evidence with clinical expertise and patient values" (p. 147). Similarly, the American Psychological Association (2005) stated that EBP in psychology results from the integration of the best available research with clinical expertise in the context of patient characteristics, culture, and preferences.

It is an increasingly popular belief that the dissemination of EBPs within mental health systems is equivalent to improved quality of care and will inevitably lead to improved outcomes. The very same report of the President's New Freedom Commission on Mental Health (2003) that highlights the crucial role of cultural competence in the improvement of mental health services also noted, "In a transformed mental health system, consistent use of evidence-based, state-of-the-art medications and psychotherapies will be standard practice" (p. 12). Although the wide dissemination of EBPs would appear to be a solution to the problems that members of so many U.S. ethnic and cultural groups have encountered in the mental health system, the examination of most currently available EBPs from a perspective that incorporates the broad influences of culture on behavior highlights several concerning limitations.

First, most currently available EBPs were developed without adequate inclusion of ethnic and cultural minority group members in study samples (Blase & Fixsen, 2003; Miranda et al., 2005; Sue, 1998). This means that most empirical findings regarding the efficacy or effectiveness of EBPs cannot be generalized to members of cultural or ethnic minority groups. In recognition of this concern, the National Institutes of Health (NIH; 1994) began requiring the inclusion of ethnic minority individuals in federally funded research projects; however, a review of all studies funded by National Institute of Mental Health (NIMH) in the 9 years following the enactment of this policy found that only 16% of these studies included or focused on one or more groups of minority children (Hernandez & Isaacs, 2004), a proportion that does not come close to resembling ethnic minority representation in the U.S. population. When that same review examined data for specific ethnic and cultural groups, even greater disparities emerged. For example, Latinas/os, who at that time accounted for 13% of the population, were only included in 4.6% of NIMH grants. It is important to note that, as many NIMH grants do not focus on treatment effectiveness, the actual percentage of studies targeting mental health practice for these individuals who are not White and European American is even smaller. Clearly, more mental health services research needs to focus on culturally diverse groups (Hall, 2001; Miranda et al., 2005; Miranda, Nakamura, & Bernal, 2003; Sue, 1998).

Although it is important to conduct research involving specific cultural communities, advanced approaches to culturally competent research go beyond including the members of these communities as research subjects. They also focus on more extensive partnerships that facilitate these communities' involvement in the design, implementation, and evaluation of promising and recommended practice models (Miranda et al., 2003). Two examples of EBPs that not only incorporated children and families of color in their study samples, but also began by using primarily Latina/o children and families in their development are *Brief Strategic Family Therapy* and *Family Effectiveness Training* (Szapocznik, Santisteban, Rio, Perez-Vidal, & Kurtines, 1989).

Second, there is insufficient knowledge regarding the influence of linguistic and cultural factors on the efficacy of EBPs. Even when individuals belonging to U.S. ethnic or cultural minority groups are recruited as research participants, their absolute numbers are frequently so small that linguistic and cultural factors cannot be included in the analyses (Miranda et al., 2003). It will continue to be difficult to fully understand the role of cultural factors in mental health services without drastically improved efforts to recruit adequate numbers of research participants from diverse cultural groups and without increased use of research strategies that are appropriate for small sample sizes (Miranda et al., 2003). Attention to cultural, socio-economic, ethnic lifestyle, and life span issues is also more likely when participatory research approaches are implemented (Davis, 2003).

Third, almost no attention has been paid to the influence of culture in the selection of appropriate outcomes and measures for EBPs. The first way in which this affects the relevance of EBPs in many ethnic and cultural minority communities is through a focus on outcomes that may not always be the most relevant in a given community (Hall, 2001; Rogler, 1999). For example, whereas independence is often a targeted outcome for adults and adolescents in the mental health system, functional interdependence may be a more culturally appropriate outcome of mental health interventions among many ethnic or cultural groups. The second way in which culture affects outcomes in EBP research is through its influence on measurement procedures. Although some of the outcomes that have historically been the focus of EBP research may have relevance across several ethnic or cultural groups (e.g., increased mood and energy among individuals experiencing depression, improved school performance among children with learning problems), it is important to consider that the manner in which these outcomes have been historically measured may not be appropriate across cultures.

Finally, there is a lack of theory development delineating the relationships between culture, mental health, and treatment. In addition to the influence of the many previously cited methodological shortcomings, theory development in this area is also stymied by the complexity of the relationships between culture and mental health, as well as the many important related factors that would need to be considered (e.g., acculturation, language, socio-economic status, regional effects, family variables, community variables). Moreover, given the vast diversity of ethnicities and cultures, some aspects of a theory about the relationship between culture and mental health may be universal, whereas others may be limited to certain cultures or ethnicities.

Tribal communities, in particular, have expressed serious concerns about the growing federal and state mandates that require use of EBPs. Although the stated purpose of requiring EBPs use may be grounded in the promotion of recommended practice in hopes of improving efficacy, quality of care, and outcomes, the reality is that requiring tribal community providers to use EBPs that were not designed for tribal communities is viewed by many as another form of oppression. In addition to the frequent cultural misfit between tribal community values and those reflected in EBPs, other factors exacerbate the challenge. Tribal communities are often located in isolated and remote locations, and they have few licensed and credentialed clinicians, few clinical supervisors to oversee and support EBP implementation, and few resources for training and the other expenses associated with EBPs.

Cultural Adaptation of Evidence-Based Practices

The adaptation of EBPs to specific cultural contexts is frequently proposed as one solution to the many limitations that most currently available EBPs demonstrate when applied to ethnic and cultural minority populations (e.g., Bernal, Bonilla, & Bellido, 1995; Castro & Alarcon, 2002; Constantine, 2002; Sue, 2003). Although numerous approaches to achieve this type of adaptation have been proposed, most incorporate recommendations that can be grouped into three broad strategies (Griner & Smith, 2006). The first of these is the explicit incorporation of clients' cultural values into treatment. As Griner and Smith (2006) pointed out, "Clients of color are more likely to seek out and use mental health services when their values and beliefs are congruent with the interventions provided" (pp. 532–533) (see also Coleman, Wampold, & Casali, 1995; Flaskerud & Nyamathi, 2000; Rogler, Malgady, Costantino, & Blumenthal, 1987). For example, African American clients are more likely to remain in treatment when mental health interventions are based on Afrocentric values (e.g., Banks, Hogue, Timberlake, & Liddle, 1998; Oliver, 1989).

A second adaptation strategy is to match service recipients and service providers according to their ethnic or cultural backgrounds. Matching is frequently justified on the basis that the shared cultural or ethnic heritage of the provider and recipient will facilitate understanding and foster a real time adaptation of the intervention. Although many studies do suggest that individuals who are matched in this manner are less likely to drop out of therapy and more likely to report satisfaction with services (Campbell & Alexander, 2002; Sue, 1998), the key ingredient driving these improved outcomes appears to be the service provider's ability to adapt a practice in a way that the service recipient will find palatable (Zane et al., 2005). Stated differently, it is a provider's ability to adapt a practice to a service recipient's culture, and not the provider's ethnicity or culture, that facilitates improved outcomes.

The third adaptation strategy is to employ approaches that promote cooperation with support resources that exist within clients' communities, spiritual traditions, and extended families (Armengol, 1999; Jackson-Gilfort, Liddle, Tejeda, & Dakof, 2001; Prizzia & Mokuah, 1991). For example, the intentional involvement of Latina mothers in the treatment of their children through recounting cultural folk stories led to greater reductions in presenting symptoms than traditional therapy even after 1 year of follow-up (Costantino, Malgady, & Rogler, 1986).

In practice, the careful cultural adaptation of existing EBPs involves the strategic use of many specific techniques derived from these strategies. To adapt Parent Management Training (PMT; Forgatch & Martinez, 1999; Reid, Patterson, & Snyder, 2002), a preventive EBP focused on parent training to more specifically address culturally relevant experiences of Latina/o parents and families, Martinez and Eddy (2005) first provided five Latina/o family interventionists from the community with training in unadapted PMT. Next, these interventionists joined a group of PMT and community experts focused first on evaluating the relevance of PMT's conceptual background and training techniques to the local Latina/o culture and social context and then on necessary modification of these components to increase their relevance to local Latinas/os. This team also identified new content areas that addressed culturally specific risk and protective factors (e.g., family acculturation issues) and structural barriers (e.g., discrimination). The adapted EBP was then presented to focus groups of Latina/o parents, who provided further feedback regarding necessary adaptations.

The final product consists of a group intervention involving 12 sessions. In addition to the standard content of PMT (e.g., communication, problem solving, direction giving, setting limits), the culturally adapted version includes sessions dedicated to discussing the family's Latina/o heritage, family roles, the ability to bridge cultures, and the capacity for dealing with obstacles (Martinez & Eddy, 2005). Sessions are conducted in Spanish, and they include time for a meal and social interaction, which is intended to build social support networks. Because parents in many recently immigrated Latina/o families often experience a diminished sense of influence over their families' lives as they adapt to life in the United States (Santisteban, Muir-Malcom, Mitrani, & Szapocznik, 2002), the adapted EBP focuses on increasing parental empowerment and self-efficacy. As part of this focus, the community interventionists who cofacilitate these groups are referred to as *entrenadores* (coaches), rather than by titles that would reflect *parenting expert*. Not surprisingly, given the careful attention to culturally specific factors throughout the adaptation of this EBP, subsequent research into its efficacy suggested positive results (Martinez & Eddy, 2005).

Tribal researchers have worked in concert with tribal clinicians to determine if EBPs can be culturally adapted for effective use within tribal communities. The Indian Country Child Trauma Center, part of the Oklahoma University Health Sciences Center and a member of the federal National Traumatic Stress Network, has carefully examined the manualized treatment components of a number of EBPs to determine whether each segment is meaningful within a tribal framework of values, beliefs, social protocols, purpose, and approach to healing. The center has incorporated Native American cultural conceptualizations of the world and relationships within it to culturally adapt four EBPs based on a traditional orientation to healing and well-being (BigFoot & Bonner, 2006). The Parent–Child Interaction Therapy adaptation is called Honoring Children, Making Relatives; Trauma-Focused Cognitive Behavioral Therapy is called Honoring Children, Mending the Circle; sexual behavior treatment is called Honoring Children, Respectful Ways; and a life skills development and suicide prevention and treatment program is called Honoring Children, Honoring the Future.

Reviews of the literature examining available cultural modifications to existing EBPs have generally been favorable. When Miranda and colleagues (2005) summarized published outcomes for the use of culturally adapted evidence-based treatments with ethnic minority children, they identified efficacious interventions for depression, anxiety, attention-deficit/hyperactivity disorder, and disruptive behavioral disorders. They also reviewed similar research for ethnically diverse adults and concluded that many of the established EBPs are effective for ethnic minorities, especially for African American and Latina/o populations, although much less data was available for Asian groups and Native Americans. Griner and Smith (2006) conducted a meta-analytic evaluation of 76 studies examining the effectiveness of culturally adapted interventions and found that most of these had generally strong treatment effects. In addition, interventions targeted to a specific cultural group were four times more effective than interventions provided to diverse groups of clients from a variety of cultural backgrounds, and interventions conducted in clients' native language were twice as effective as interventions conducted in English. Much of the existing literature points to a promising role for carefully conducted cultural adaptation in overcoming some of the limitations of traditional EBPs and associated disparities in behavioral health care.

Practice-Based Evidence

Although the movement toward the cultural adaptation of EBPs provides one promising direction toward cultural competence, several questions about this practice remain unanswered. For instance, how much adaptation can occur before fidelity to an EBP is jeopardized? More importantly, an over-reliance on EBPs—even those that have been successfully modified—when providing mental health services to members of ethnic or cultural minorities tends to invalidate and exclude many culturally specific interventions and traditional healing practices utilized in communities of color (Espiritu, 2003; Huang, Hepburn, & Espiritu, 2003). By definition, these practices are congruent with the cultural environment in which they are developed, and although most lack empirical support, they have often been refined through experiential and historical processes as communities continue to use those that are found to be helpful and discard those that are found to be less efficient. These experiential and historical processes yield what is referred to as *practice-based evidence* (PBE).

In the context of providing culturally competent care, it is important to note that PBE services are accepted as effective by the local community through community consensus, and they address the therapeutic and healing needs of individuals and families from a culturally specific framework. Practitioners of PBE models draw on cultural knowledge and traditions for treatment and are respectfully responsive to the local definitions of wellness and dysfunction. The practitioners can be seen as having field-driven and expert knowledge of the cultural strengths and cultural context of the community, and they consistently draw on this knowledge throughout the full range of service provision: engagement, assessment, diagnosis, intervention, and aftercare. The PBE approach includes a logic-driven selection of appropriate interventions based on a range of factors, including the cultural and historical belief systems of the community related to healing and wellness.

Despite their differing origins, PBE and EBP need not be antithetical. As demonstrated by the cultural adaptation research, EBPs that were not created with diverse populations in mind can prove useful if purposefully modified to incorporate some of this PBE. Similarly, PBE can be examined and expanded on for greater effect through careful application of scientific inquiry. In applied mental health service settings, many system of care communities have successfully combined these perspectives as a way to match service delivery to cultural help-seeking patterns, to demonstrate respect for the value of the cultural self as an integral part of wellness, and to model partnership between the medical model world view and the cultural world view (Gregory & Phillips, 1997).

For instance, the Sault Sainte Marie Band of Chippewa Indians, located in the remote upper peninsula of Michigan, offers a unique example of such fusion through a partnership between primary health care and traditional healing practices. Traditional healers partner with the tribal health services and have clinic office space for intake and healing services. The traditional healers are viewed as experts in their field, just as medical doctors are viewed as experts in their field. These healers view each other as colleagues. The practice-based practitioners (traditional healers) offer services both in the same health clinic exam rooms or in offsite locations that can better accommodate traditional practices. The end result is a partnership of services that address the medical, psychological, and traditional healing needs of the tribal consumer—all through collective attention to the value of cultural touchstones as an integral component of treatment.

ORGANIZATIONAL SUPPORT

This section introduces the concept of organizational cultural competence, which is considered essential in ensuring the accurate implementation and long-term sustainability of culturally competent direct services practices. After describing some of the most important organizational domains involved in developing culturally competent mental health services organizations, the section provides several illustrative examples of organizational cultural competence in mental health services (primarily from existing systems of care).

Domains of Organizational Cultural Competence: Infrastructure and Direct Services Support

An organization's policies, structures, and processes play a significant role in the ability to test, disseminate, and deploy culturally congruent direct service practices (both PBE and culturally adapted EBPs). Organizational cultural competence is a key factor in a variety of improved treatment outcomes, including increased access, decreased drop-out rates, decreased no-show rates for formerly underserved populations, increased client satisfaction, increased use of outpatient services, and decreased use of crisis and inpatient services (Griner & Smith, 2006; Harper et al., 2006; Hernandez, Nesman, Isaacs, Callejas, & Mowery, 2006). There are two principal domains of organizational cultural competence—*infrastructure* and *direct services support*. The infrastructure domain includes all of the broad organizational characteristics that must be adapted to support cultural competence, including the following:

- Organizational values, policies, procedures, and governance should be adapted to promote compatibility with the community and support culturally competent service practices.

- Planning and evaluation processes can contribute to cultural competence when they feature reciprocal partnerships with the community and collect data that accurately reflect the community and its cultures.

- Communication practices should be culturally competent and foster direct communication and learning within the organization and between the organization and the community.

- Human resource practices that are culturally competent include those that increase linguistic or cultural capacity and those that develop a workforce that is ethnically and culturally representative of the communities being served.

- Community outreach approaches that provide opportunities for community participation can also lead to greater cultural competence.

- Financial, technological, and other supports are also needed components of organizational cultural competence.

Direct service support, the second domain of organizational cultural competence, includes three organizational functions that are closely linked to the implementation of culturally competent direct service practices:

- *Access,* which includes all of the mechanisms that facilitate entering, navigating, and exiting needed services and supports

- *Availability,* which refers to having enough services and supports to meet the target community's needs

- *Utilization,* which refers to service use and is typically measured through factors such as the length of time in service, retention, or drop-out rates

As illustrated in Figure 23.1 (adapted from Hernandez, Nesman, Mowery, & Gamache, 2006), organizational cultural competence is achieved when there is congruence between these two domains, as well as between each of them and the culture and social context of the local population of focus. The dynamic nature of the relationships among infrastructure supports, access mechanisms, and availability of needed and appropriate services is especially important to recognize as organizations prepare to make changes to improve their cultural competence. Changes in one area may affect other areas, or the lack of change in one domain may cancel out efforts in others. Incorporating cultural competence into every aspect of the organization or system requires careful evaluation of the compatibility among an organization's policies, procedures, and values, as well as the culture and social context of the population being served.

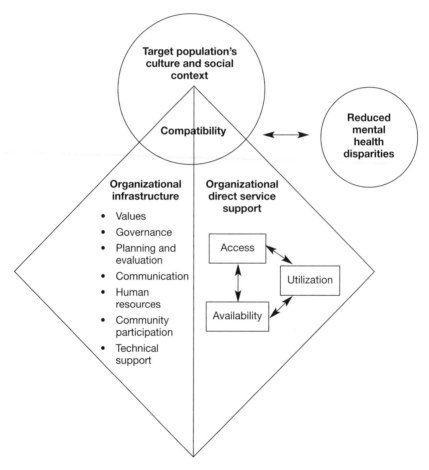

Figure 23.1. A model of organizational cultural competence in mental health services. (*Source:* Hernandez, Nesman, Mowery, & Gamache, 2006.)

Examples of Organizational Cultural Competence

Many of the principles of organizational cultural competence are evident in the daily functioning of African American Family Services (AAFS), a Minneapolis-based agency focused on the mental health needs of African Americans, particularly those afflicted with chemical dependencies. In terms of infrastructure, the first domain of organizational cultural competence, AAFS's values and principles clearly highlight its target community (local African Americans) and the need to provide services that are culturally specific. The agency has formal definitions of how cultural specificity is achieved and who comprises their target population. AAFS's planning and evaluation processes feature public meetings with their target communities, where issues affecting the local Black community and ways in which these can be addressed by AAFS are discussed. The agency's human resources practices emphasize hiring from within the community and have led to the establishment of a staff that is representative of the service population. AAFS engages in active community outreach, sponsoring and presenting informational booths at community events and fairs, developing partnerships with other local organizations, supporting staff participation on local and regional councils and committees, and engaging in close interaction with local media serving the African American population. Organizational technical support for culturally competent services is evident in many ways, including the ongoing training of existing staff. This reflects the assumption that culturally specific services result from deliberate and intentional efforts and are not necessarily achieved by focusing solely on demographic representation of the service population.

Regarding direct service support, the second domain of organizational cultural competence, AAFS encourages service access by allowing walk-in appointments, placing its offices within the community, providing expanded hours (evenings and weekends), and delivering services in a variety of settings already frequented by the community (e.g., physicians' offices, schools, other organization's service delivery sites, religious institutions traditionally important in the African American community). AAFS ensures that service availability corresponds to community needs through a process of ongoing data collection and service development. For instance, a joint needs monitoring exercise with local family courts led to an initiative that provides services around the issue of domestic violence. After identifying utilization problems among certain segments of its target population, particularly adolescents and individuals with chronic and severe mental health problems, AAFS implemented an incentive program rewarding participation with gift certificates and other appropriate inducements. These organizational characteristics support an array of services that include cultural adaptations of traditional EBPs, such as Cognitive-Behavioral Therapy and Motivational Interviewing, along with other programming more akin to PBE that arises in response to community needs and perceptions of mental health.

Another example of organizational support for culturally congruent services is found in the Tapestry system of care located in Cuyahoga County, Ohio, where

African American and Hispanic children make up the large majority of children served. Most Hispanic families are Spanish speaking. The 14 Settlement Houses founded in the late 19th century have been used as the community anchors, called Neighborhood Collaboratives, for the system of care. Tapestry's major strength in community outreach and engagement is its strategic reliance on the long-established Settlement Houses. The Neighborhood Collaboratives are based on a model of advocacy, empowerment, and self-sufficiency, and they are comfortable places where people take part in services and supports, build skills, engage in resource identification through in-house computer banks provided for families' use, and speak with parent advocates who proportionally reflect the diverse community.

Organizational cultural competence is demonstrated at the Center for Multicultural Human Services in Falls Church, Virginia. The center's vision and mission statements are operationalized in all aspects of their work. Its staff is composed of more than 80 individuals, many of whom are immigrants or refugees themselves; staff personnel speak more than 30 languages and serve more than 6,000 individuals each year in a region that contains more than 1 million immigrants. The board of directors is reflective of the populations served. Center materials are translated into most of the 30 languages. In addition to traditional clinical and school-based services, the agency's programs include services and supports for survivors of torture, trafficking, and severe trauma; immigration and human rights; legal services; transitional housing; and advanced training for culturally and linguistically diverse students in psychology, social work, and counseling. Outreach and engagement strategies include partnering with and providing space to cultural and faith-based organizations for cultural or religious celebrations such as the Vietnamese Tet Lunar New Year; funding and sponsoring cultural events, including a dance program featuring dances from many of the cultures found in their populations; founding a school for traumatized refugee Afghan children to assist them in retaining their language, culture, and history; partnering with other agencies such as Lutheran Social Services to develop a family violence prevention program for refugee populations from African countries; and partnering with local businesses such as contractors and builders to cosponsor and fund transitional housing for refugees. A key component of the Center for Multicultural Human Services is always remembering to celebrate life, culture, and language, while also dealing with the realities of trauma and illness.

The Partnership for Kids (PARK) system of care in Bridgeport, Connecticut, serves large Latina/o and African American populations, and its leadership in key management positions is reflective of the diverse community. The system of care has reached out to the Latina/o population through focus groups, and most importantly, through individual family peer-to-peer support contacts, which help to engage families and to educate them about access to services and supports. The PARK Project is school based, and families and youth are the leaders and staff who do much of the work. There are youth groups in each of the six schools involved in the system of care, facilitated by ethnically diverse youth or young adults whose roles include providing advocacy within the school setting. Family peer partners are bilingual and conduct support groups in Spanish that are held in various parts of the community, including churches. These community outreach and engagement efforts have also resulted in the successful recruitment and retention of Latina/o family and youth representation in key decision-making positions, including on the system of care's governing bodies and Cultural and Linguistic Competence Committee. The PARK Project has also integrated its cultural and linguistic competence plan with its social marketing plan to strengthen the messages and implementation of both.

The Family Voices Network system of care of Erie County, New York, has strong cultural leadership. All of the system's subcontracts mandate self and organizational cultural and linguistic competence assessments, along with required training in cultural and linguistic competence. Monetary incentives are provided to the six contracted care coordination agencies to integrate cultural and linguistic competence into individual and family service plans. All the care coordination agencies employ culturally diverse staff reflective of the populations served. In addition, the director gives recognition to individuals and agencies that meet and exceed contractual requirements through the provision of lunches and other incentives.

Rhode Island's Positive Education Partnership (PEP) system of care, which uses positive behavior interventions and supports, has formed a partnership with a local Native American tribe, which has enabled the system of care's entry into the tribal school. The entry into this cultural community was culturally respectful because staff entered as active learners. The message was "We want to learn from you." PEP supplied materials for families to create cultural art; the activity was captured by a professional photographer, who took pictures of individual families working together. During the cultural artwork, PEP integrated the development of parenting and youth skills and conflict resolution skills. This was done in a culturally congruent, strengths-based manner, using art and culture to teach useful skills in a nonthreatening way. The Native American principal of the tribal school has traveled to other tribes in the state as a PEP ambassador to assist with outreach and engagement of other tribes with PEP. In addition, PEP uses the time bank initiative led by a family organization, which is a bartering system to exchange services and supports without the traditional exchange of money. One person's time is equal to every other person's time, regardless of the service or support provided. This approach is especially culturally congruent with indigenous communities. PEP also hires culturally diverse family members as data collectors for its program evaluation.

Maine's Thrive system of care works with the significant and growing African immigrant population. The system of care staff includes African community member volunteers, including a faith-based leader, who receive stipends to help shape policies and procedures to be culturally congruent with the diverse African populations served. Thrive uses creative ways to reach out to and engage the community. For example, in the African communities from which the immigrants come, soccer is very important. The local sports field had been vandalized and was shut down. Thrive is working with the community to reopen the field to be available for cultural and sports activities. The system of care also is supporting the Muslim Women's Project. This group produced a video for Mainers to show the differences in women's roles in Africa and in the United States, with the goal of educating local residents about the struggles that African women, who often travel to the United States alone, encounter when they arrive in a very different nonagrarian, industrialized western culture. The video is intended to sensitize the locals to have a greater understanding of the cultural incongruence African women experience in this country.

The Central Massachusetts Communities of Care system has two family centers that serve as community-based hubs for entry into the system of care. Offering a welcoming environment to families and youth, these centers provide social and recreational activities, youth groups, direct services, and bilingual staff and interpreters to a large Latina/o population. They also provide care coordination services and entry into four levels of care through a simple registration process and a brief screening tool. The initial form helps families to self-identify as part of a specific ethnic or nationality group. The information is then put into a database to tailor services to the populations entering care. The family centers are staffed by family members, and the assistant director is also a family member. There are two culturally diverse youth coordinators in each family center.

RECOMMENDATIONS FOR SYSTEMS OF CARE

Two of the most important issues involved in the improvement and transformation of mental health services for children and families in the United States are the need to recognize and correct the cultural limitations of existing services and the push to disseminate and implement EBPs (President's New Freedom Commission on Mental Health, 2003). Addressing each of these issues independently of the other can create as many problems as it solves (Isaacs, Huang, Hernandez, & Echo-Hawk, 2005). A blind focus on the implementation of EBPs without acknowledgment of the limitations of the evidence supporting these, particularly in regard to their effectiveness in or generalizability to diverse ethnic groups, can render systems of care that perpetuate—and perhaps even exacerbate—existing behavioral health disparities. Similarly, a stance that unquestionably and interminably embraces all mental health practices regardless of their origin or known ability to produce favorable outcomes in any given population may also prove unlikely to render much improvement in existing mental health systems.

To achieve success, comprehensive attempts aimed at the transformation and improvement of mental health services require an intertwining of efforts to develop systems of care that utilize practices supported by research and implement efforts to effectively engage, retain, and address the needs of ethnic minority populations (Isaacs et al., 2005). As discussed, EBPs developed without reflecting the values and understanding of mental health endemic to ethnic minority populations can prove useful when carefully adapted to the cultural environment of specific target communities (Griner & Smith, 2006). Similarly, traditional mental health practices can be examined and expanded on for greater effect through the careful application of scientific inquiry (Rust & Cooper, 2007). Importantly, this comprehensive, intertwined development of systems of care is unlikely to be successful without close attention to organizational factors that support and promote culturally competent direct service practices (Hernandez, Nesman, Isaacs et al., 2006).

In any community, the development of culturally competent services must be directed by a working understanding of the manner in which mental health is perceived and pursued by members of the target population. This understanding of mental health problems from a community's perspective must incorporate the types of problems the community identifies, the community's understanding of how these problems arise, and the venues and methods for intervention recognized and obtained by the community. It should be noted that this local understanding may differ vastly from a professional understanding of the issue. For instance, professionals within mental health systems receiving many refugees from armed conflict may wish to focus on psychological trauma, which they view as arising from psychological stressors associated with war. They believe these problems are treatable by EBPs such as Cognitive Processing Therapy, in which survivors must expose themselves to stressors through detailed recounting and processing of the traumatic experience (Chard, 2005). They may additionally believe that these services are best delivered in a safe, professional setting located near many organizational supports should additional levels of treatment be needed. By comparison, many refugees from armed conflict tend to worry more about improving their functional behavior and facilitating adaptation to their new country. In these populations, psychological distancing from the memories and events related to the war experience often serves a protective and salutary psychological purpose (Wessells, 2007). When treatment is sought, it is often with traditional healers or community leaders who can perform important cultural rituals or practices interrupted or left incomplete as a result of the advent of war. Even with the best of intentions, professionals who engage in efforts to create improved systems of care without first understanding the needs and perspectives of their target populations often compromise the accessibility, engagement potential, and effectiveness of the very services they are trying to provide.

Once a working understanding of the local perceptions and practices regarding mental health is reached, an important second step is to review the available evidence examining the mental health practices (both formal and informal) already in place in the community (Rust & Cooper, 2007). As in the previously cited example regarding war and trauma, a traditional practice that is known to have a salutary effect on the mental health of certain groups can run counter to what is most frequently recommended during traditional academic training in mental health disciplines (Wessells, 2007). Considered against both the strengths and limitations of existing EBPs, an understanding of local mental health practices allows those who develop systems of care adequate leeway to incorporate traditional methods and venues for mental health promotion. In some cases, as long as existing practices are not known to have deleterious effects, their incorporation into a broader mental health services approach may be pursued and preferably accompanied by data collection efforts that examine their effectiveness. Such is the case with the example of the mental health services approaches among the Sault

Sainte Marie Band of Chippewa Indians. In other cases, existing practices may be considered during the process of culturally adapting established EBPs. This is the case in the use of Cognitive-Behavioral Therapy and Motivational Interviewing within the programs run by AAFS, where the experiences and psychological effects of discrimination and historical trauma are explored and discussed as part of adapting these interventions to the realities of the target communities.

The decision on whether to pursue the systematic development of empirical evidence around a traditional practice or adapt an existing EBP is likely to involve many factors, including the types of traditional practices available, the evidence existing that advocates for or against them, and the resources of local mental health agencies. It may be advisable to pursue the data-based refinement of existing practices that a community is already comfortable obtaining as long as these are not known to be deleterious to those who engage in them, rather than their replacement with a nonadapted EBP. This suggestion arises from the observation that a data-refined traditional practice and a culturally adapted EBP may ultimately be indistinguishable from each other, but local communities will have first been engaged before substantial efforts are implemented (Fixsen, Naoom, Blase, Friedman, & Wallace, 2005).

Finally, the successful implementation of any culturally competent approach to services will require an honest evaluation and subsequent improvement of the organizational characteristics of the mental health service institutions that are to provide these services (Harper et al., 2006; Hernandez, Nesman, Isaacs, et al., 2006). Several evaluation protocols that aid in this process are available, yet no single one appears to capture all dimensions of organizational cultural competence related to the reduction of health disparities (Harper et al., 2006). Despite the complications inherent in creating change in organizational dimensions, these changes are necessary if any implementation of culturally competent services is to achieve long-term success. Although a full discussion of practices that lead to the development of organizational cultural competence in mental health systems of care is beyond the scope of this chapter, there are excellent resources available that expand on the concepts introduced here and ground them in actual practice. These include seminal documents on cultural competence within systems of care by Cross, Bazron, Dennis, and Isaacs (1989) and Isaacs and Benjamin (1991), along with a volume edited by Hernandez and Isaacs (1998) on promoting cultural competence within children's mental health services. More recent works include Harper and colleagues' (2006) enlightening review of organizational infrastructure practices associated with cultural competence, and Hernandez, Nesman, Isaacs, and colleagues' (2006) monograph on culturally competent organizational practices related to direct service support.

CONCLUSION

In the contemporary United States, members of ethnic minority groups have faced a disproportionate mental health burden, arising in great measure from mental health systems that do not recognize the limitations of existing mental health practices and do not actively engage in efforts to overcome such limitations (President's New Freedom Commission on Mental Health, 2003; U.S. DHHS, 2001). This chapter has outlined the foundational information required for the development of systems of care that provide the best possible care to all children and families, regardless of ethnic, religious, national, cultural, linguistic, or socio-economic background. The mental health profession has developed an adequate understanding of factors driving inequitable care and perpetuating behavioral health disparities. Implementation of the strategies presented in this chapter will help to ensure that, in view of increasing ethnic diversity in the United States, the mental health needs of growing segments of the national population will no longer go misunderstood and unmet.

REFERENCES

American Psychiatric Association. (2000). *Diagnostic and statistical manual of mental disorders* (4th ed.). Washington, DC: Author.

American Psychological Association. (2005). *The APA policy statement on evidence-based practice*. Retrieved March 30, 2006, from http:// www.apa.org/practice/ebp.html

Armengol, C.G. (1999). A multimodal support group with Hispanic traumatic brain injury survivors. *Journal of Head Trauma Rehabilitation, 14,* 233–246.

Banks, R., Hogue, A., Timberlake, T., & Liddle, H. (1998). An Afrocentric approach to group social skills training with inner-city African American adolescents. *Journal of Negro Education, 65,* 414–423.

Bernal, G., Bonilla, J., & Bellido, C. (1995). Ecological validity and cultural sensitivity for outcome research: Issues for the cultural adaptation and development of psychosocial treatment with Hispanics. *Journal of Abnormal Child Psychology, 23,* 67–82.

BigFoot, D.S., & Bonner, B.L. (2006). *Honoring Children, Mending the Circle*. Norman, OK: University of Oklahoma Health Sciences Center, Indian Country Child Trauma Center.

Blase, K.A., & Fixen, D.L. (2003). *Evidence-based programs and cultural competence*. Retrieved December 6, 2004, from http://nirn.fmhi.usf.edu/resources/index.cfm

Bock, P.K. (1999). *Rethinking psychological anthropology: Continuity and change in the study of human action* (2nd ed.). Prospect Heights, IL: Waveland Press.

Bui, K., & Takeuchi, D.T. (1992). Ethnic minority adolescents and the use of community mental health care services. *American Journal of Community Psychology, 20,* 403–417.

Campbell, C.I., & Alexander, J.A. (2002). Culturally competent treatment practices and ancillary service use in outpatient substance abuse treatment. *Journal of Substance Abuse Treatment, 22,* 109–119.

Castro, F.G., & Alarcon, E.H. (2002). Integrating cultural variables into drug abuse prevention and treatment with racial/ethnic minorities. *Journal of Drug Issues, 32,* 783–810.

Chabra, A., Chavez, G.F., Harris, E.S., & Shah, R. (1999). Hospitalization for mental illness in adolescents and the use of community mental health care system. *Journal of Adolescent Health, 24,* 349–356.

Chard, K. (2005). An evaluation of cognitive processing therapy for the treatment of post-traumatic stress disorder related to childhood sexual abuse. *Journal of Consulting and Clinical Psychology, 73,* 965–971.

Coleman, H.L.K., Wampold, B.E., & Casali, S.L. (1995). Ethnic minorities' rating of ethnically similar and European American counselors: A meta-analysis. *Journal of Counseling Psychology, 42,* 55–64.

Consensus Statement on Evidence-Based Practice and Cultural Competence. (2003). Conclusions from March 2003 meeting sponsored by the National Implementation Research Network of the Louis de la Parte Florida Mental Health Institute at the University of South Florida and the Annie E Casey Foundation, Tampa, FL.

Constantine, M.G. (2002). Predictors of satisfaction with counseling: Racial and ethnic minority clients' attitudes toward counseling and ratings of their counselors' general and multicultural counseling competence. *Journal of Counseling Psychology, 49*, 255–261.

Costantino, G., Malgady, R.G., & Rogler, L H. (1986). Cuento therapy: A culturally sensitive modality for Puerto Rican children. *Journal of Consulting and Clinical Psychology, 54*, 639–645.

Costello, E.J., Farmer, E.M.Z., & Angold, A. (1997). Psychiatric disorders among American Indian and white youth in Appalachia: The great mountains study. *American Journal of Public Health, 87*, 827–832.

Cross, T.L., Bazron, B.J., Dennis, K.W., & Isaacs, M.R. (1989). *Towards a culturally competent system of care (Vol. I): A monograph on effective services for minority children who are severely emotionally disturbed.* Washington, DC: Georgetown University Child Development Center, CASSP Technical Assistance Center.

Cunningham, P.J., & Freiman, M.P. (1996). Determinants of ambulatory mental health service use for school-age children and adolescents. *Mental Health Services Research, 31*, 409–427.

Davis, K. (2003). The disparity hypothesis: An overview of current research findings on mental health of people of color in the United States. In American College of Mental Health Administrators (Eds.), *Reducing disparity: Achieving equity in behavioral health services. Proceedings of the 2003 Santa Fe Summit.* Santa Fe, NM: American College of Mental Health Administrators.

Espiritu, R. (2003). *What about promotoras, shamans, and kru khmers? The need to expand the evidence base for diverse communities.* Washington, DC: National Technical Assistance Center for Children's Mental Health, Georgetown University Child Development Center.

Fabrega, H., Ulrich, R., & Mezzich, J.E. (1993). Do Caucasian and Black adolescents differ at psychiatric intake? *Journal of the Academy of Child and Adolescent Psychiatry, 32*, 407–413.

Fixsen, D.L., Naoom, S.F., Blase, K.A., Friedman, R.M., & Wallace, F. (2005). *Implementation research: A synthesis of the literature* (FMHI Publication #231). Tampa: University of South Florida, Louis de la Parte Florida Mental Health Institute, National Implementation Research Network.

Flaskerud, J.H., & Nyamathi, A.M. (2000). Attaining gender and ethnic diversity in health intervention research: Cultural responsiveness versus resource provision. *Advances in Nursing Science, 22*, 1–15.

Forgatch, M.S., & Martinez, C.R., Jr. (1999). Parent management training: A program linking basic research and practical application. *Journal of the Norwegian Psychological Society, 36*, 923–937.

Gregory, S.D., & Phillips, F.B. (1997). Of mind, body, and spirit: Therapeutic foster care—an innovative approach to healing from an NTU perspective. *Child Welfare, 76*, 127.

Griner, D.G., & Smith, T.S. (2006). Culturally-adapted mental health interventions: A meta-analytic review. *Psychotherapy: Theory, Research, Practice, and Training, 43*, 531–538.

Hall, G.C.N. (2001). Psychotherapy research with ethnic minorities: Empirical, ethical, and conceptual issues. *Journal of Consulting and Clinical Psychology, 62*, 502–510.

Harper, M., Hernandez, M., Nesman, T., Mowery, D., Worthington, J., & Isaacs, M. (2006). *Organizational cultural competence: A review of assessment.* Tampa: University of South Florida, Louis de la Parte Florida Mental Health Institute, Research and Training Center for Children's Mental Health.

Hernandez, M., & Isaacs, M.R. (Vol. Eds.). (1998). *Systems of care for children's mental health series: Promoting cultural competence in children's mental health services.* Baltimore: Paul H. Brookes Publishing Co.

Hernandez, M., & Isaacs, M. (2004). *Promises and challenges of evidence-based practices: A review and analysis of the NIMH CRISP database, 1995–2003.* Draft paper prepared for the National Alliance of Multi-ethnic Behavioral Health Associations, Washington, DC.

Hernandez, M., Nesman, T., Isaacs, M., Callejas, L.M., & Mowery, D. (Eds.). (2006). *Examining the research base supporting culturally-competent children's mental health services.* Tampa: University of South Florida, Louis de la Parte Florida Mental Health Institute, Research and Training Center for Children's Mental Health.

Hernandez, M., Nesman, T., Mowery, D., & Gamache, P. (2006). Introduction and overview. In M. Hernandez et al. (Eds.), *Examining the research base supporting culturally-competent children's mental health services* (pp. 1–17). Tampa: University of South Florida, Louis de la Parte Florida Mental Health Institute, Research and Training Center for Children's Mental Health.

Huang, L. (2002). Reflecting on cultural competence: A need for renewed urgency. *Focal Point, 16,* 4–7.

Huang, L.N., Hepburn, K., & Espiritu, R. (2003). *To be or not to be evidence based: Data matters* (Vol. 6). Washington, DC: National Technical Assistance Center for Children's Mental Health, Georgetown University Child Development Center.

Institute of Medicine. (2000). *Crossing the quality chasm: A new health system for the 21st century.* Washington, DC: National Academies Press.

Isaacs, M.R., & Benjamin, M. (1991). *Towards a culturally competent system of care (Vol. II): Programs which utilize culturally competent principles.* Washington, DC: Georgetown University Child Development Center, CASSP Technical Assistance Center.

Isaacs, M.R., Huang, L.N., Hernandez, M., & Echo-Hawk, H. (2005). *The road to evidence: The intersection of evidence-based practices and cultural competence in children's mental health.* Baltimore: National Alliance of Multi-Ethnic Behavioral Health Associations.

Jackson-Gilfort, A., Liddle, H.A., Tejeda, M.J., & Dakof, G.A. (2001). Facilitating engagement of African American male adolescents in family therapy: A cultural theme process study. *Journal of Black Psychology, 27,* 321–340.

Juszczak, L., Melinkovich, P., & Kaplan, D. (2003). Use of health and mental health services by adolescents across multiple delivery sites. *Journal of Adolescent Health, 32,* 108–118.

Kilgus, M.D., Pumariega, A.J., & Cuffe, S.P. (1995). Influence of race on diagnosis in adolescent psychiatric inpatients. *Journal of the American Academy of Child and Adolescent Psychiatry, 34,* 67–72.

López, S.R., & Guarnaccia, P.J. (2000). Cultural psychopathology: Uncovering the social world of mental illness. *Annual Review of Psychology, 51,* 571–598.

Martinez, C.R., Jr., & Eddy, J.M. (2005). Effects of culturally adapted parent management training on Latina/o youth behavioral health outcomes. *Journal of Consulting and Clinical Psychology, 73,* 841–851.

Malgady, R.G., & Constantino, G. (1998). Symptom severity in bilingual Hispanics as a function of clinician ethnicity and language of interview. *Psychological Assessment, 10,* 120–127.

Miranda, J., Bernal, G., Lau, A., Kohn, L., Hwang, W., & LaFromboise, T. (2005). State of the science on psychosocial interventions for ethnic minorities. *Annual Review of Clinical Psychology, 1,* 113–142.

Miranda, J., Nakamura, R., & Bernal, G. (2003). Including ethnic minorities in mental health intervention research: A practical approach to a long-standing problem. *Culture, Medicine, and Psychiatry, 27,* 463.

National Institutes of Health. (1994). *NIH guidelines on the inclusion of women and minorities as subjects in clinical research.* Retrieved March 30, 2006, from http://grants.nih.gov/grants/policy/emprograms/overview/women-and-mi.html

Novins D.K., Beals J., Sack W.H., & Manson S.M. (2000). Unmet needs for substance abuse and mental health services among Northern Plains American Indian adolescents. *Psychiatric Services, 51*, 1045–1047.

Novins, D.K., Duclos, C.W., Martin, C., Jewett, C., & Manson, S.M. (1999). Utilization of alcohol, drug, and mental health treatment services among American Indian adolescent detainees. *Journal of the American Academy of Child and Adolescent Psychiatry, 38*, 1102–1108.

Oliver, W. (1989). Black males and social problems: Prevention through Afrocentric socialization. *Journal of Black Studies, 20*, 15–39.

President's New Freedom Commission on Mental Health. (2003). *Achieving the promise: Transforming mental health care in America, final report* (Pub. No. SMA-03-3832). Rockville, MD: U.S. Department of Health and Human Services.

Prizzia, R., & Mokuah, N. (1991). Mental health services for Native Hawaiians: The need for culturally relevant services. *Journal of Health and Human Resources Administration, 14*, 44–61.

Pumariega, A.J., Glover, S., Holzer, C.E., & Nguyen, N. (1998). Utilization of mental health services in a tri-ethnic sample of adolescents. *Community Mental Health Journal, 34*, 145–156.

Reid, J.B., Patterson, G.R., & Snyder, J. (2002). *Antisocial behavior in children and adolescents: A developmental analysis and model for intervention.* Washington, DC: American Psychological Association.

Rogler, L.H. (1999). Methodological sources of cultural insensitivity in mental health research. *American Psychologist, 54*, 424–433.

Rogler, L.H., Malgady, R.G., Costantino, G., & Blumenthal, R. (1987). What do culturally sensitive mental health services mean? The case of Hispanics. *American Psychologist, 42*, 565–570.

Rust, G.R., & Cooper, L.A. (2007). How can practice-based research contribute to the elimination of health disparities? *Journal of the American Board of Family Medicine, 20*, 105–114.

Santisteban, D.A., Muir-Malcolm, J.A., Mitrani, V.B., & Szapocznik, J. (2002). Integrating the study of ethnic culture and family psychology intervention science. In H.A. Liddle, D.A. Santisteban, R.F. Levant, & J.H. Bray (Eds.), *Family psychology: Science-based interventions.* Washington, DC: American Psychological Association.

Singh, N.N., McKay, J.D., & Singh, A.N. (1998). Culture and mental health: Nonverbal communication. *Journal of Child and Family Studies, 7*, 403–409.

Snowden, L. (1998). Managed care and ethnic minority populations. *Administration and Policy in Mental Health, 25*, 581–592.

Sue, S. (1998). In search of cultural competence in psychotherapy and counseling. *American Psychologist, 53*, 440–448.

Sue, S. (2003). In defense of cultural competency in psychotherapy and treatment. *American Psychologist, 58*, 964–970.

Szapocznik, J., Perez-Vidal, A., Hervis, O.E., Brickman, A.L., & Kurtines, W.M. (1989). Innovations in family therapy: Strategies for overcoming resistance to treatment. In R.A. Wells & V.J. Giannetti (Eds.), *Handbook of brief psychotherapies.* New York: Plenum Publishing.

Szapocznik, J., Santisteban, D., Rio, A.T., Perez-Vidal, A. & Kurtines, W.M. (1989). Family effectiveness training: An intervention to prevent problem behavior in Hispanic adolescents. *Hispanic Journal of Behavioral Sciences, 11*, 4–27.

Takeuchi, D.T., Sue, S., & Yeh, M. (1995). Return rates and outcomes from ethnicity-specific mental health programs in Los Angeles. *American Journal of Public Health, 85*, 638–643.

Theriot, M.T., Segal, S.P., & Cowsert, M.J., Jr. (2003). African Americans and comprehensive service use. *Community Mental Health Journal, 39*, 225–237.

U.S. Department of Health and Human Services. (2001). *Mental health: Culture, race, and ethnicity.* Rockville, MD: Author.

Walkup, J.T., McAlpine, D.D., & Olfson, M. (2000). Patients with schizophrenia at risk for excessive antipsychotic dosing. *Journal of Clinical Psychiatry, 61,* 344–348.

Wang, P.S., West, J.C., & Tanielian, T. (2000). Recent patterns and predictors of antipsychotic medication regimens used to treat schizophrenia and other psychotic disorders. *Schizophrenia Bulletin, 26,* 451–457.

Wessells, M. (2007). *Child soldiers: From violence to protection.* Cambridge, MA: Harvard University Press.

Yeh, M., McCabe, K., Hurlburt, M., Hough, R., Hazen, A., Culver, S., et al. (2002). Referral sources, diagnoses, and service types of youth in public outpatient mental health care: A focus on ethnic minorities. *Journal of Behavioral Health Services and Research, 29,* 45–60.

Young, A.S., Klap, R., & Sherbourne, C.D. (2001). The quality of care for depressive and anxiety disorders in the United States. *Archives of General Psychiatry, 58,* 55–61.

Zane, N, Sue, S., Chang, J., et al. (2005). Beyond ethnic match: Effects of client-therapist cognitive match in problem perception, coping orientation, and therapy goals on treatment outcomes. *Journal of Community Psychology, 33,* 569–585.

V

Future Directions for Systems of Care

24

Workforce Implications

Issues and Strategies for Workforce Development

Joan M. Dodge and Larke Nahme Huang

The workforce stands at the heart of transforming mental health delivery systems for children and their families. Without careful attention to ensuring the presence of high-quality workers who are prepared and trained in the skills and competencies needed to work in today's environment, the task of transformation becomes difficult, if not impossible. Workforce development is a necessary and critical strategy for transformation.

For many years, state and local agencies, community organizations, and professional associations across the United States have faced major challenges in educating, training, and retaining a quality mental health workforce. Workforce development concerns are evident within nearly every discipline and among many of the stakeholder groups that address mental health disorders in adults, children, youth, and their families. Workforce development is finally being recognized as a major *lever of change* in transforming the service delivery systems for those needing mental health services. Levers of change, or *leverage points,* are those places in a complex system where a small shift in one thing can produce cascading changes throughout the system (Meadows, 1999). Workforce strategies, including effective recruitment, retention, and training practices, must be seen as levers of change in transforming systems of care (President's New Freedom Commission on Mental Health, 2003).

Nationwide, many innovative efforts are addressing workforce challenges occurring at community, state, and national levels. These comprise multipronged efforts by stakeholders to address the mental health workforce crisis. This chapter outlines unique issues and challenges for the health and human service delivery workforce in the children's mental health field. It also describes workforce development goals and some of the creative responses implemented by individuals, organizations, and agencies to ensure that a quality workforce is in place for children and youth and their families. In addition, the chapter outlines four key transformation strategies that are significant levers of change to advance workforce development.

WORKFORCE CHALLENGES IN CHILDREN'S MENTAL HEALTH

For the field of children's mental health, significant and complex challenges for the workforce are created by a number of factors, including demographic and epidemiological trends; significant changes in service systems; and increased expectations for partnerships with families, cultural and linguistic competence, cross-system collaboration, evidence-based interventions, and accountability in service delivery.

Demographic trends in children's mental health bring new challenges to workforce development, including a growing and increasingly diverse population of youth. By the year 2030, there will be 83.2 million individuals under the age of 18 in the United States, a 16% increase over the 2000 census figures (U.S. Department of Health and Human Services [U.S. DHHS], 2002). In 2000, four diverse groups—African American, Latino, Asian American, and American Indian—amounted to 39% of all American children (U.S. Bureau of the Census, 2000). By 2015, growth rates among these groups are expected to far surpass those of non-Hispanic White youth, whose population will actual decrease by 3% (Snyder & Sickmund, 1999). Twelve percent of the current U.S. population was born outside the country, raising the potential for linguistic isolation from existing helping systems (U.S. Bureau of the Census, 2000).

Epidemiological trends present another challenge for workforce development, with research suggesting an increasing prevalence of mental health disorders among children and youth and increasing rates of multiple diagnoses and complex problems. In the United States, 1 child in 5 has a diagnosable mental health disorder (Friedman, Katz-Leavey, Manderscheid, & Sondheimer, 1998), and 1 child in 10 has a serious emotional disturbance that causes substantial impairment in functioning at home, at school, or in the community (National Advisory Mental Health Council, 2001). Increasing numbers of very young children are being referred to treatment agencies for help with social-emotional disturbances (Pottick & Warner, 2002). At least one third of the children being served by the U.S. mental health system are diagnosed with two or more psychiatric disorders (Warner & Pottick, 2004). Increasing numbers of youth are identified with co-occurring mental health and substance abuse disorders (Pottick, 2002), and increasing numbers of children are identified with co-occurring developmental disabilities and mental health disorders (Emerson, 2003). In addition, youth involved with other child-serving systems often have mental health problems. Fifty to seventy-five percent of youth involved with the juvenile justice system are estimated to have mental health needs (Cocozza & Skowyra, 2002). Studies estimate that approximately 48% of youth in the child welfare system have significant emotional or behavioral problems (Burns et. al., 2004). In spite of the high prevalence of mental health disorders, only 20% of the children with mental health needs receive services or supports, and for many of these children, the services are inadequate (U.S. DHHS, 2001a).

Not only are the characteristics of the child and youth population changing, but the service delivery environment is changing as well. Since the 1980s, there have been dramatic changes in how services and supports are provided for children and youth with complex needs and their families—changes that are attributable, in part, to the system of care concept and philosophy. Workers are expected to enter the children's mental health field with new and different competencies and to apply their knowledge and skills in rapidly changing environments. There often are substantial gaps in the core competencies of providers in the children's mental health workforce, as well as a mismatch between their educational preparation and the actual requirements for service delivery. In fact, significant concerns have been expressed that preservice academic education bears little relation to the demands of actual work with children and families in the community (Meyers, Kaufman, & Goldman, 1999). Few professionals receive adequate training in the values, skills, and attitudes consistent with systems of care that call for partnerships with families, cultural competence in service delivery, comprehensive cross-agency interventions, individualized care, and home and community-based service approaches (England, 1997; Hansen, 2002; Morris & Hanley, 2001; Pires, 1996). Many training programs continue placing emphasis on clinical impairment and symptom reduction, as opposed to focusing on the strengths of children and their families and improving their functional status. In addition, there is a lag time between development of evidence-supported interventions and their implementation in the field.

Another change in the children's mental health field that poses challenges for workforce development is reflected in the new roles for families in all aspects of service delivery. Clinical professionals are no longer always viewed as the sole experts but rather as individuals with expertise who must work in partnership with the families whose children are in treatment. Families are seen as bringing expertise and in-depth experience, not only about their own children's suffering and the concomitant stresses on the family, but also about policies and practices that can truly meet families' needs. When families are equal decision makers, they may request support services such as respite care or in-home aides that are quite different from the outpatient therapy or day treatment that mental health clinicians typically are trained to provide (Duchnowski, Kutash, & Friedman, 2002).

Increasing the cultural and linguistic competence of the workforce is another challenge for the future. The Surgeon General's Report, *Mental Health: Culture, Race, and Ethnicity,* emphasized the role of culture in providing services to diverse ethnic and racial populations, as well as the severe shortage of providers in the core mental health professions trained to work with these populations (U.S. DHHS, 2001b). As the population shifts and more youth of color are in need of mental health services, training programs must better address their needs by developing and disseminating training on culturally and linguistically effective practices in mental health care delivery. Although an increasing body of knowledge (U.S. DHHS, 2001b) and new tools for training exist (Cross, Bazron, Dennis, & Isaacs, 1989; Trader-Leigh, 2002), the political and academic will has been slow to mobilize.

Challenges with collaboration and systems thinking must also be addressed to prepare the workforce of tomorrow. The application of systems thinking to understand the multiple components of a child's life requires a team approach to services and is a fundamental change from traditional categorical training (Meyers et al., 1999). Most professional education and training programs have curricula dictated by professional associations that tend to be siloed and discipline specific. In reality, community-based care is built on interagency collaboration and service integration, requiring individuals from different disciplines and systems to value one another and work together to develop coordinated services and individualized care for children and their families. Rarely are professionals or paraprofessionals taught how to meaningfully collaborate with each other.

Accountability and using what works are new expectations in the changing service delivery environment. Providers are increasingly expected to incorporate evidence-based practices into their work with children and families; however, there are significant gaps between the development of evidence-based interventions, the adaptation of these interventions to diverse populations and real-world settings, the education and training of providers in these practices, and their implementation in the field. In addition, there are new expectations of the children's mental health workforce to demonstrate positive outcomes in their work with children and families. Linking various performance measures to the work of individual practitioners and organizations is an essential component of an accountability structure for the children's mental health workforce.

A number of policy reports have highlighted these workforce challenges. The Surgeon General's report on mental health (U.S. DHHS, 1999) described the crisis in the children's mental health workforce, both in terms of critical shortages of providers and the need for training in the new models of care emerging through system reforms and research on treatment effectiveness. The Institute of Medicine (2001) noted the importance of preparing the workforce required for a revamped health care system. The President's New Freedom Commission on Mental Health (2003) provided a blueprint for transforming the delivery of mental health services based on changes in values; skills; attitudes; the incorporation of demonstrably effective treatments; and shifting services from traditional inpatient, outpatient, and residential treatment to home and community-based services and supports. To achieve this transformation, the commission recognized the urgent need to address workforce issues.

WORKFORCE DEVELOPMENT ACTION PLAN

In response to workforce challenges, the Substance Abuse and Mental Health Services Administration (SAMHSA) commissioned the Annapolis Coalition (a nonprofit organization) to develop a plan on workforce development that encompassed the breadth of the field, was national in scope, and could serve as a resource to states and communities to plan strategies for implementation. *An Action Plan on Behavioral Health Workforce Development* (Hoge et al., 2007) was shaped by a comprehensive planning process involving multiple stakeholder groups and was designed to stimulate, inform, and guide individuals, agencies, organizations, and sectors of the mental health field as they develop their own detailed workforce action agendas. The final action plan has a set of seven action goals, each with specific objectives and action steps. Each of these goals is discussed in this chapter, and relevant issues for children and their families are high-lighted. In addition, examples of emerging, innovative strategies to address the goal are described.

> *Goal 1*: Significantly expand the role of individuals in recovery and their families, when appropriate, to participate in and ultimately direct or accept responsibility for their own care. Provide care and supports to others and educate the workforce.

Implications for Children's Mental Health Workforce

Family-directed care is a radical change from traditional practice and represents a bold step in transforming mental health service delivery, making it more responsive to the needs of families and children with emotional, behavioral, and substance use disorders. Whereas previously, families had been blamed for their children's disorders, families should now be viewed as partners in interventions, as well as in program planning and policy development. Families are an untapped resource, poised to expand the capacity of the workforce in children's mental health care. To achieve this goal, the workforce requires training to work in a manner consistent with the guidelines for family-driven, youth-guided systems developed by the Child, Adolescent, and Family Branch at the Center for Mental Health Services in partnership with the Federation of Families for Children's Mental Health.

Examples of Workforce Development Strategies

The Maryland Coalition of Families for Children's Mental Health, the Maryland state chapter of the Federation for Families for Children's Mental Health, provides training to family members to fulfill four different roles:

1. Family advocates

2. Family navigators

3. Family support partners in wraparound services

4. Family members as cotrainers

The coalition has identified nine core competencies for family workers:

1. Theoretical knowledge

2. System of care expertise

3. Family support skills

4. Knowledge of laws and policy

5. Cultural competence

6. Communication skills

7. Organization skills

8. Advocacy skills

9. Values

Training includes a Family Leadership Institute, which offers 6 months of intensive training and uses a standardized curriculum to train family navigators and family support partners. Ongoing supervision following these training programs is also provided (J. Walker, personal communication, March 22, 2007).

Tennessee's Voices for Children (TVC), a statewide Federation of Families chapter, has developed a number of strategies in which family members, including youth, have partnered with state universities at both the undergraduate and graduate levels to educate individuals who will be working with children with mental health needs and their families. Youth members of TVC's Youth Council have given presentations to undergraduate students at several universities, as well as to the American Psychiatric Association. Family members have also given presentations to graduate students in psychology and accompanied physicians on grand rounds at the local psychiatric hospital to provide a family perspective (C. Bryson, personal communication, April 2, 2007).

In North Carolina, SUCCESS for Children and Families, a local family organization, has been involved with the University of North Carolina at Greensboro (UNCG) in an interdisciplinary system of care course that is cross-listed in the departments of nursing, psychology, counseling, human development, and social work. This semester-long, interdisciplinary training, which is financially supported by UNCG's Center for Youth, Family, and Community Partnerships, uses family members as coteachers with university faculty, providing graduate and undergraduate students with an understanding of family-driven and youth-guided issues in a system of care. In addition, family members with SUCCESS and North Carolina Families United, the statewide family organization, offer two other training programs codesigned and cotaught by family members with agency personnel through contracts with the state of North Carolina and UNCG—a 2-day training program for individuals from multiple child-serving agencies on child and family teams from a family perspective and a training program to inform families on how to select mental health and substance abuse service providers within their managed care system (L. Jones, personal communication, April 9, 2007).

Goal 2: Expand the role and capacity of communities to effectively identify their needs and promote behavioral health and wellness.

Implications for Children's Mental Health

Children and adolescents with mental health needs are rarely identified and served exclusively in the mental health specialty system. Rather, they are identified and treated in schools, primary care facilities, child care facilities, recreational settings, child welfare and juvenile justice agencies, and other systems that are not specifically designed to meet the mental health needs of children. In each of these settings or systems, there are increased efforts to screen, identify, and intervene early in an effort to prevent the onset or the exacerbation of mental health problems. For the children's mental health field, a public health approach that includes the concepts of prevention, early intervention, and treatment is applicable to this goal of expanding the capacity of communities to promote behavioral health and identify needs throughout the developmental stages of childhood. This approach requires the engagement of a broader workforce than just specialty mental health practitioners. This broader workforce includes many professionals and paraprofessionals in various settings in the community that are often closest to the children and their families and who may be the only individuals that address mental health and co-occurring problems at their earliest stages, both by age and severity. Enlisting de facto providers in other child-serving settings and systems (e.g., education, child care, recreation, child welfare, primary care, juvenile justice) requires a set of core competencies for these workers to practice promotion of social-emotional well-being and effective early intervention. Training based on these core competencies is needed for community providers to fulfill this role for children and youth at all stages of the developmental spectrum (infants and young children through adolescents and young adults).

Communities must also understand the role of stigma related to mental illness, not only for those who are suffering from a mental health disorder but also for those who may practice in the field. Public education and antistigma campaigns should be piloted and implemented in states and communities, as well as educational campaigns with positive messages identifying incentives and rewards for working in the children's mental health field to attract students. In addition, communities must help their business partners to understand the implications of mental health disorders as economic issues that affect employee productivity and to ensure that relevant needs are addressed in benefit packages. For example, Employee Assistance Program professionals need training to identify and intervene early in child and family mental health issues that affect workers' performance.

Examples of Workforce Development Strategies

Two major child-serving systems that provide community-based training for the de facto workforce on social-emotional well-being, prevention, and early intervention of mental health problems are the early care system for young children up to age 5 years and the public education system for older children. An example of efforts in the early childhood arena is being led by the Center on the Social and Emotional Foundations for Early Learning (CSEFEL), which has developed training modules based on evidence-based practices to address the social-emotional needs of young children. CSEFEL works with states to develop a cadre of experienced trainers who will use this evidence-based curriculum to build and sustain these skills among the early care and education workforce in communities. In addition, each state will identify model sites to implement the CSEFEL model (R. Kaufmann, personal communication, June 30, 2007).

For older children, a number of states are training school personnel in Positive Behavioral Interventions and Supports (PBIS). The Illinois PBIS Network (2005), a component of the Illinois Statewide Technical Assistance Center, describes PBIS as a "proactive systems approach for creating and maintaining safe and effective learning environments in schools, and ensuring that all students have the social/emotional skills needed to ensure their success at school and beyond." PBIS provides strategies that focus on schoolwide interventions for all students, secondary interventions for high-risk students and individual (i.e., tertiary) strategies for students with complex needs. The Illinois PBIS Network builds the skills and capacity of PBIS district and school-based leadership teams throughout the state by providing training, coaching, and technical assistance. The focus is on assisting schools to develop structures for teaching expected behaviors and social skills; creating student behavioral and academic support systems; and applying data-based decision making to discipline, academics, and social-emotional learning at the school, district, regional, and state levels. The Illinois PBIS Network promotes family and community involvement at all levels of implementation. The network has designed a comprehensive statewide PBIS training program that includes specific training for new teams, coaches, targeted interventions, school-based wraparound, data management, and functional assessment of behavior. It also has a training and technical assistance series that focuses on each particular level of intervention (universal, secondary, and tertiary) and includes all of the informational topics that are critical to understanding and implementing that level (L. Eber, personal communication, August 12, 2007).

In addition to training other child-serving systems, a number of states are creating structures and programs that are developing the capacity of the workforce—both professional and paraprofessional—throughout their regions and communities. In Indiana, the state-funded Technical Assistance Center for Systems of Care and Evidence-Based Practices for Children and Families assists communities in building local systems of care for children with or at risk for mental health disorders which involve both mental health and partner child-serving systems. The center's approach includes individualized ongoing community coaching, community and regional workshops, an annual statewide training conference, a newsletter, and a listserv (J. McIntyre, personal communication, March 5, 2007).

The Mental Hygiene Administration of the Maryland Department of Health and Mental Hygiene, is developing a certificate program at the University of Maryland to train community mental health professionals at the master's level and above in early childhood mental health. A second certificate program is being created through the Maryland Association of Resources for Families and Youth in partnership with the University of Maryland to train mental health paraprofessionals in community-based service delivery (A. Zachik, personal communication, May 2, 2007).

Goal 3: Implement systematic recruitment and retention strategies at the federal, state, and local levels.

Implications for Children's Mental Health

Although the specialty mental health professions are expected to grow over the next decade (McRee et al., 2003), shortages still exist for serving certain target populations, including children and youth with serious emotional disturbances. In addition, many clinicians work in private clinic or office-based settings rather than in more natural settings, do not work in public sector programs, and do not have the competencies needed to work within systems of care. Significant shortages of child psychiatrists, psychologists, and social workers have been reported in many states, especially in rural areas (Manderscheid & Berry, 2006). In addition, the field needs to increase the number of bicultural and bilingual providers and also ensure that all providers receive the training needed to provide culturally and linguistically competent services to diverse populations regardless of the provider's racial, ethnic, cultural, or linguistic background (Hoge et al., 2007) Thus, focused attention on recruitment, retention, and training strategies is essential to ensure high-quality service delivery.

Examples of Workforce Development Strategies

One recruitment recommendation that emerged through the work of the Annapolis Coalition was to address the critical shortage of child and adolescent psychiatrists by expanding the Triple Board Program for medical students interested in pediatrics and child and adolescent psychiatry. Doubling the number of slots in this program will increase the workforce with physicians trained in pediatrics, general psychiatry, and child and adolescent psychiatry by some 20 new specialists per year, which could represent a significant increase over 10 years.

Beginning in 1996, the Maryland Department of Health and Mental Hygiene, Mental Hygiene Administration has funded the Maxie Collier Scholars program at Coppin State University, a historically Black university in Baltimore City. The program's purpose is to recruit and mentor students of color into careers in children's mental health. Students in psychiatry, psychology, social work, and nursing are selected and are mentored by a graduate school professor in their field of interest through undergraduate school and into their graduate studies. During the summer, internships in the children's mental health field are offered. The Maxie Collier Scholars receive an enriched academic background, monetary stipends each academic semester, graduate school preparation, internship experiences, opportunities to attend mental health conferences and workshops, and access to a network of career placement resources. Students must commit to pursuing a career in Maryland's mental health system and have a stated interest in the mental health needs of the African American population (A. Zachik, personal communication, May 2, 2007).

The state of Alaska, which has been designated a mental health professional shortage area and has a projected 47.3% increase in the need for behavioral health professionals, recruits and meets workforce needs in rural areas by hiring, training, supervising, and funding rural human service workers in villages. This unique program is a partnership among the University of Alaska at Fairbanks; the Alaska Department of Health and Human Services, Division of Behavioral Health; and the Native Health Corporations, with the goal of developing a counselor in every village. The training provides academic and career ladders for students who live in communities throughout the state, many of which are isolated and remote, to work in the behavioral health field. Funding support and supervision are provided to students who may begin at an associate or certificate level and then continue their education into the bachelor's and master's levels.

> *Goal 4:* Increase the relevance, effectiveness, and accessibility of training and education.

Implications for Children's Mental Health

The mental health workforce serving children and their families should be educated and trained to work in a manner consistent with nationally agreed-on core competencies that prepare them to: 1) respect and partner with youth and families; 2) provide individualize care; 3) work across agencies and systems; 4) provide culturally and linguistically competent services; 5) conduct strengths-based assessments that are linked to individualized service planning and service provision; 6) partner with natural supports; 7) collaborate across professions and disciplines; 8) use developmentally appropriate evidence-based and recommended practices across the spectrum from promotion and prevention to early intervention and treatment; and 9) work in a collaborative and consultative role to nonspecialty mental health providers, agencies, and systems. These areas comprise the basic attitudes and skills needed to function effectively within systems of care.

There are often deep-seated philosophical and conceptual differences in mental health care with respect to schools of practice, philosophies, and perspectives about services among the various child-serving disciplines and communities of practice. To reach consensus on core competencies across these groups is a challenging task. The "guild" mentality is deeply ingrained in the mental health field and promotes a sense of "professional preciousness" (Sarason, 1973) that can get in the way of identifying core competencies that are relevant across disciplines. Professional associations are usually involved in the licensing and accreditation process for their respective disciplines and are important targets for change strategies around education and training. A place to start would be to work with professional associations toward achieving consensus on core competencies consistent with the previously cited elements; developing a training curriculum related to core competencies that can be implemented nationwide; implementing effective transfer strategies to ensure that these competencies are disseminated, understood, and put into practice through preservice and in-service training programs across all disciplines; and evaluating the core competencies training curriculum and transfer strategies. Having a foundational set of core knowledge, skills, and attitudes needed for the children's mental health workforce would ensure: 1) basic standards for quality among all practitioners, 2) a shared language and set of skills across disciplines and service systems, 3) a framework for accountability and continuous improvement for providers, and 4) guidance for consumers and families in establishing their expectations of care.

Examples of Workforce Development Strategies

The Michigan Association for Infant Mental Health developed specialty competencies for individuals working with infants, toddlers, and their families. Based on four levels of skill and knowledge, these specialty competencies have become the basis for professional endorsement and serve as qualifications for hiring. A graduate certificate program in Infant Mental Health at the Merrill Palmer Institute of Wayne State University is reflective of these competencies and interdisciplinary in nature. Graduates come from their own specific disciplines but are trained to work within the infant and early childhood mental health field, with their training linked to this established set of specialty competencies (Meyers, 2007).

Another example of education and training linked to established competencies is given at Southern New Hampshire University, which offers a unique, competency-based graduate program in Community Mental Health. This training is specifically designed to prepare individuals for work in community-based mental health settings for children and adults and is targeted at diverse groups of potential students, including: 1) current staff working in the mental health and substance abuse fields who desire certificate- or master's-level education; 2) staff working in related services (e.g., child welfare, juvenile justice, schools, corrections, family support services, vocational rehabilitation, specialized housing services); 3) mental health consumers in recovery and family members who are interested in becoming mental health service providers; and 4) members of the general public who might be interested in a career in the mental health field.

All courses offered through the Southern New Hampshire University Program in Community Mental Health are based on a comprehensive set of core competencies identified as most critical for working with adults with psychiatric disabilities, children and adolescents with severe emotional disturbances and their families, and individuals with co-occurring psychiatric and substance abuse disorders. These competencies were developed in collaboration with Vermont's mental health system and modified using the experience of other groups nationally. All courses in the program include not only professional perspectives, but also the perspectives of service users and family members. The program is designed for adult learners on campus in Manchester, New Hampshire and off campus at distance learning sites in Milwaukee, Madison, Green Bay, and Wausau, Wisconsin; Burlington, Vermont; and Anchorage, Alaska. In addition to the coursework, two 300-hour internships are required. The program works with state licensing boards to meet their educational requirements for licensing.

Competency-based distance learning and the use of web-based technologies to increase accessibility to training have exciting possibilities for the future. One training program that uses a distance learning approach based on identified competencies within a system of care approach is the Graduate Certificate in Children's Mental Health with an Emphasis on Systems of Care offered by the Department of Child and Family Studies at the Louis de la Parte Florida Mental Health Institute at the University of South Florida. Initiated in 2006, the certificate program is a collaboration with partners in other universities through the Systems of Care Professional Training Consortium that provides a values-infused and empirically based education to individuals who work in agencies and systems that serve children and youth with mental health needs and their families. The program is delivered through a variety of distance learning methodologies for graduate students seeking specialized training in children's mental health, as well as other professionals needing new skills and knowledge to be future leaders in the children's mental health arena (C. MacKinnon-Lewis, personal communication, April 3, 2007).

Another innovative example of training using a distance learning approach is the one designed by TVC for potential respite care providers. This web-based, 7-week curriculum is a collaboration with Middle Tennessee State University that provides training to individuals who are interested in becoming respite providers. The program has a training coordinator who screens for basic requirements and then provides frequent ongoing support to the students. Students are given a Certificate of Continuing Education from Middle Tennessee State University (C. Bryson, personal communication, April 2, 2007).

Goal 5: Actively foster leadership development among all segments of the workforce.

Implications for Children's Mental Health

The importance of effective leadership in developing a vision for change, initiating change, and sustaining change is essential to transforming the children's mental health system. Many government, family, and advocacy leaders describe their roles as "putting out fires" rather than as leading a movement of transformation (E.B. Kagen, personal communication, May 16, 2007). In both small community-based programs and large agencies or organizations that are working for transformed care for children and their families, leadership plays a critical role in identifying the vision and values for services and supports, training and supervising personnel, reflecting on the interaction between individuals and organizations, instilling an attitude of appreciative inquiry and growth, and cultivating individual and organizational resiliency. Thus, leadership development is critical to a transformation agenda, requiring skilled, effective leaders at state and local levels.

Examples of Workforce Development Strategies

The National Technical Assistance Center for Children's Mental Health at the Georgetown University Center for Child and Human Development developed the *Leadership in Systems of Care Training Program*, a curriculum that offers a variety of learning opportunities for leaders at multiple levels to enhance their skills, provide fresh perspectives, and gain new knowledge to lead change and transformation efforts. This leadership training curriculum, which has also been adapted for family leaders, provides leaders throughout the children's mental health field with an opportunity to take a step back from their day-to-day responsibilities and deepen their knowledge of the nature of leadership, examine their roles as leaders in system transformation, and provide strategies to support their continued growth and development as leaders. This leadership training curriculum is designed for families and professionals at the national, state, territorial, tribal, local, and neighborhood levels of systems of care who are committed to expanding their own leadership capacity. Topics include distinguishing leadership from management, developing strategies for shared leadership between formal and informal leaders, and highlighting the role of shared vision and values in a time of intensive change. Participants also have the opportunity to apply these concepts during the training to a current leadership challenge they are facing in the field (Kagen & Hepburn, 2006).

Goal 6: Enhance the infrastructure available to support and coordinate workforce development efforts.

Implications for Children's Mental Health

Without an infrastructure to address workforce issues, it is unlikely that federal, state, or local governments can effectively transform the systems that are in place to serve children and their families with mental health issues. Structures, strategic plans, training, and fiscal mechanisms that ensure that new workers are well-educated as they enter the workplace, coupled with mechanisms to provide them with in-service training and opportunities for growth as they continue in their employment, are essential for quality care. Infrastructure components include— but are not limited to—workforce development plans and structures, data collection, strategies for recruitment and retention, collaborations between child-serving agencies and public higher education (state universities, community colleges), funding mechanisms and incentives, and public awareness of opportunities for employment in children's mental health.

Creating the infrastructure for workforce development is not without significant challenges. Challenges include: 1) building consensus for a shared set of competencies that are value-based, cross-discipline, and cross-system, which challenges the entrenched "guild" mentality of professional disciplines; 2) differing beliefs about the value of family and youth involvement and family and youth partnerships in directing care; 3) the opposition of state regulatory authorities to providing feedback on the monitoring and regulation of providers of mental health care; 4) resistance among university and academic departments to providing input regarding curriculum development and core competencies; and 5) difficulty identifying financing mechanisms to support a workforce development infrastructure.

Examples of Workforce Development Strategies

In spite of the obstacles, a number of states and communities have increased their infrastructures for workforce development. In 2005, the National Technical Assistance Center for Children's Mental Health at Georgetown University, in collaboration with the Subcommittee on Leadership and Workforce of the Children, Youth, and Families Division of the National Association of State Mental Health Program Directors completed an environmental scan to assess states' status on workforce infrastructure. Questions related to the overall importance of workforce development as perceived by the state directors of children's mental health and the development of core competencies, state workforce plans, statewide training structures and programs, recruitment and retention strategies, and relationships with institutions of higher education. At the time of this scan, most respondents felt that workforce development was important in the implementation of quality services (65%) but felt that resources were often inadequate. Some states (e.g., New Mexico, Michigan, Vermont) have worked on the creation of competencies for individuals working with the infant and early childhood population, whereas other states (e.g., Pennsylvania, Connecticut, Maryland) have identified cross-disciplinary and cross-agency core competencies for professionals and paraprofessionals serving children with mental health needs and their families. Some states have developed a statewide workforce development plan or are in the process of developing one. In addition, a number of states have supported a statewide training structure that is specifically charged with increasing the capacity of the workforce for children with mental health needs and their families. Examples of these structures include the Pennsylvania CASSP Institute, the Technical Assistance Center for Systems of Care and Evidence-based Practices for Children and Families in Indiana, and the Innovations Institute in Maryland. Some of these structures have resulted in stronger linkages between the state public mental health authority and public institutions of higher education.

> *Goal 7:* Implement a national research and evaluation agenda on behavioral health workforce development.

Implications for Children's Mental Health

Another recommendation calls for regular and systematic data collection on the children's behavioral workforce, citing this as essential to creating a quality workforce. Tracking information about providers can be an important role for professional associations, as well as for payers. Data about the need for services and service utilization also are needed to inform workforce development plans and strategies.

Examples of Workforce Development Strategies

There has been increased recognition of the need for data on human resources in the mental health disciplines, including psychiatrists, psychologists, social workers, and psychiatric nurses. A basic data set was published in *Mental Health, United States 1998* (Manderscheid & Sonnenschein, 1998), with updated information in the most recent edition, *Mental Health, United States 2004* (Manderscheid & Berry, 2006) that also includes counselors, marriage and family therapists, psychosocial rehabilitation counselors, school psychologists, pastoral counselors, and applied and clinical sociologists. A chapter entitled *Mental Health Practitioners and Trainees* provides important information on mental health practitioners, using data elements that are comparable across the various specialty disciplines and collected through the professional associations for each discipline. Although each specialty is not broken down to reflect professionals who work primarily with children and adolescents, this data set provides a comprehensive snapshot of the current status of human resources in the major mental health disciplines, identifies overlapping trends across the disciplines, and calls for policy makers to work together to improve the quality of information in this important area (Manderscheid & Berry, 2006).

The American Academy of Child and Adolescent Psychiatry (AACAP) has recognized the need for data and has made an effort to generate information on the child and adolescent psychiatry workforce. In 1999, AACAP formed a task force to examine the status of the workforce of child and adolescent psychiatrists and to establish the recruitment of medical students and residents into child and adolescent psychiatry as a primary priority. AACAP then formulated a 10-year recruitment initiative with a strategic plan focusing on four areas—data, education, access, and advocacy.

AACAP collected data from medical schools and child and adolescent psychiatry training programs on faculty resources and students' exposure to the field. Data were collected from first-year psychiatry residents on their decisions to enter the field of child and adolescent psychiatry, and additional data were gathered on current child and adolescent psychiatrists regarding patient demographics and consultation. In addition, AACAP collected informal information indicating that a supply of board-certified pediatricians who have exited the field for various reasons may be interested in child and adolescent psychiatry. After reviewing this information, AACAP developed and submitted a proposal to the Accreditation Council on Graduate Medical Education (ACGME) and the American Board of Psychiatry and Neurology to receive approval for a 3-year integrated training track in adult and child and adolescent psychiatry for individuals who are eligible for the pediatric boards or board-certified pediatricians. Additional data are being collected on pediatricians with an interest in retraining in child and adolescent psychiatry.

In 2007, AACAP's Steering Committee on Workforce Issues held a 5-year evaluation of its progress in all four areas of the strategic plan. The largest success reported was a 12% increase in the number of residents entering the field of child and adolescent psychiatry from 2002–2007 (ACGME, 1999–2006); however, a 2006 study documented continuing shortages of child and adolescent psychiatrists nationwide (Thomas & Holzer, 2006). The AACAP Committee agreed to continue its focus on data, recruitment, advocacy, access, and education until 2012 with attention to understanding how medical students and residents make career decisions and to studies on practicing child and adolescent psychiatrists (K. Kroeger Ptakowski, personal communication, May 8, 2007).

IMPLICATIONS FOR THE FUTURE AND NEXT STEPS

Many challenges and strategies related to the workforce crisis in children's mental health have been discussed, but several strategies have the potential to be major levers of change that could make a significant difference if applied strategically (Institute of Medicine, 2006). The following areas represent four major transformative strategies that could significantly improve the future workforce for children's mental health care.

Developing Value-Based Core Competencies to Align with the System of Care Approach

Much has been accomplished in the children's mental health field since the 1980s with the articulation of the values and conceptual framework for a comprehensive, community-based system of services and supports. The challenge for today and the future, however, is operationalizing these values and ensuring that the workforce has the requisite values, knowledge, skills, and attitudes that are essential to deliver high-quality services within the system of care framework.

The children's mental health field must identify core competencies (attitudes, skills, and knowledge) for all disciplines and levels of workers—professional and paraprofessional—that focus on system of care values and principles. Furthermore, specialty competencies in specific disciplines must be expanded so that these competencies are aligned with the system of care philosophy. These core competencies need to be articulated around the values of: 1) respecting the strengths of the child and family and partnering with them; 2) individualizing care; 3) demonstrating collaborative work across agencies and systems; 4) implementing culturally and linguistically competent services; 5) drawing on and partnering with natural supports in the community; 6) partnering across professions and disciplines; 7) understanding and using developmentally appropriate evidence-based and recommended practices in mental health promotion, prevention, early intervention, and treatment; and 8) working in consultative roles with nonspecialty mental health providers and agencies such as personnel in primary health care, education, child care, child welfare, and juvenile justice settings.

Developing an agreed-upon set of value-based core competencies for various roles within the workforce would serve multiple purposes by: 1) ensuring a level of care and quality among all practitioners; 2) ensuring a shared language and set of knowledge and skills across disciplines and service systems; 3) facilitating accountability and continuous professional and provider improvement; and 4) helping consumers and families in their expectations of care. These core competencies could then be linked to education (preservice and graduate) and training (in-service) opportunities, as well as serve as the basis for licensure and certification of practitioners and the accreditation of education and training programs. At the same time, payers of services could be convinced of the need for these identified core competencies to ensure good outcomes and accountability by linking the competencies with performance measures and client outcomes.

Expanding the Pool of Providers

The workforce of the future for children's mental health services must include an expanded pool of providers. First, the workforce must include not only providers who are professionals in mental health disciplines, but also the many professionals and paraprofessionals across the multiple child-serving systems that affect the lives of children with mental health needs. In addition, providers must represent diverse cultural and ethnic groups, and they must also demonstrate the necessary knowledge and skills to work with diverse populations of children and families.

Furthermore, the pool of providers must include family members. One of the most transformative elements for providers is the expanded roles of families and family organizations in all aspects of service delivery. Family members provide a great deal of care for their own children, often seeing themselves as the "silent army" waiting to partner with professional providers (Huang, Macbeth, Dodge, & Jacobstein, 2004). In addition, many family members have taken on more formal roles in systems of care, including organizing advocacy efforts, serving on policy and advisory bodies at state and local levels, planning and evaluating services, and serving as trainers at both preservice and in-service levels. Some family organizations are serving the children in their communities by becoming providers of direct services and supports, as well as by providing training and peer support to other family members.

As the field has moved in the direction of family-directed care, there has been a significant shift in power between the child and family needing services and the professional or paraprofessional service providers. Training programs must focus on how to work with families as partners, demonstrate genuine respect for families and diverse lifestyles, and harness family strengths and capacities. To be effective, individuals working with children and families must learn to subordinate their own egos and status; listen, reflect, and synthesize information; acknowledge different areas of expertise; and create and sustain effective service planning teams.

Expanding the role of families by promoting their involvement in all aspects of the system, including being educated and trained to provide services and supports as part of the workforce itself, ensures that stronger decision-making partnerships will develop between family members and their providers. This role expansion for families is especially important in diverse communities, including rural communities, where the need to train and develop a local workforce is critical.

Planning Strategically and Developing an Infrastructure Focused on the Workforce

Policy makers, planners, and other key stakeholders within state mental health and other child-serving systems, universities, family organizations, and community organizations must specifically and strategically address workforce issues within their own communities and states. Strategic and systemic thinking by a committed group of partners could lead to the design of comprehensive work-force plans created to address the multiple and complex components of workforce development. Ideally, strategic plans for workforce development should involve multiple child-serving systems, have a multidisciplinary focus, consider a variety of providers such as family partners, establish collaborative relationships between public systems and institutions of higher education, and address complex financ-ing issues. Critical attention in planning should focus on ensuring a diverse work-force and on creating education and training opportunities to increase culturally and linguistically relevant attitudes, knowledge, and skills. Important to the im-plementation of workforce plans is the creation of structures within states or com-munities that provide leadership in building workforce capacity.

Whether these structures are training centers, institutes, steering committees, or advisory bodies, they can organize the various functions involved in workforce development and may provide actual competency-based training and education for professionals, paraprofessionals, and family members. Structures that provide train-ing to multiple audiences on evidence-based or promising practices, cultural and linguistic competence, family and youth partnerships, and leadership skills have the potential to serve as major levers of change for their service delivery systems.

Developing New Models for Education and Training Using Technology

The future of systems of care requires new models for educating and training the workforce. It is crucial to better utilize current technology for training across dis-ciplines and distances, and also to create new ways to use emerging technology to better serve children and families. Although many states, communities, universi-ties, and organizations are already moving ahead with the use of audio and video conferencing for large groups, one-on-one web casting, and web-based trainings, there is still much to learn about the use of these technologies to ensure a well-educated workforce. In addition, increased use of information technology is es-sential for additional functions in the children's mental health system, including organizing data and health records; assisting in service provision (e.g., telehealth); monitoring outcomes and the performance of providers; and increasing access to training for professionals, paraprofessionals, and family members through dis-tance learning methodologies.

CONCLUSION

If the children's mental health field is to make a major transformative shift, the many complex questions that are inherent in ensuring a quality, well-educated workforce must be seriously addressed. Agencies, organizations, and individuals at multiple levels must begin to implement the seven action goals set forth in the action plan and develop their own unique strategies relevant to each goal. In addi-tion, beginning conversations on how to implement the four transformative strategies (competencies, expanded providers, infrastructure development, and new models for education and training) is an important starting point for developing a workforce that will be better equipped to meet the mental health needs of children and families in the future.

REFERENCES

Accreditation Council on Graduate Medical Education (ACGME). (1999–2006). *ACGME Resident Census.* Chicago: Author.

Burns, B.J., Philips, S.D., Wagner, H.R., Barth, R.P., Kolko, D.J., Campbell, Y., et al. (2004). Mental health need and access to mental health services for youth involved with child welfare: A national survey. *Journal of American Academy of Child and Adolescent Psychiatry, 43*(8), 960–970.

Cocozza, J., & Skowyra, K., (2002) Youth with mental health disorders: Issues and emerging responses. *Office of Juvenile Justice and Delinquency Prevention Journal, 7*(1), 3–12.

Cross, T., Bazron, B., Dennis, K., & Isaacs, M. (1989). *Towards a culturally competent system of care* (Vol. I). Washington, DC: Georgetown University Child Development Center, CASSP Technical Assistance Center.

Duchnowski, A., Kutash, K., & Friedman, R. (2002). Community-based interventions in a system of care and outcomes framework. In B. Burns & K. Hoagwood (Eds.), *Community treatment for youth: Evidence-based interventions for severe emotional and behavioral disorders* (pp. 16–37). New York: Oxford University Press

Emerson, E. (2003). Prevalence of psychiatric disorders in children and adolescents with and without intellectual disability. *Journal of Intellectual Disability Research, 47*(1), 51–58.

England, M. (1997). Training the existing workforce. *Administration and Policy in Mental Health, 25,* 23–26.

Friedman, R., Katz-Leavey, J., Manderscheid, R., & Sondheimer, D. (1998). Prevalence of serious emotional disturbance: An update. In R. Manderscheid & M. Henderson (Eds.), *Mental health, United States 1998* (pp. 110–112). Rockville, MD: Substance Abuse and Mental Health Services Administration.

Hansen, M. (2002). *The need for competencies in children's public mental health services: A CASSP discussion paper of the Pennsylvania CASSP Training and Technical Assistance Institute.* Hoboken, NJ: John Wiley & Sons.

Hoge, M.A., Morris, J.A., Daniels, A.S., Stuart, G.W., Huey, L.Y., & Adams, N. (2007). *An action plan on behavioral health workforce development.* Cincinnati, OH: Annapolis Coalition on the Behavioral Health Workforce.

Huang, L., Macbeth, G., Dodge J., & Jacobstein, D. (2004). Transforming the workforce in children's mental health. *Administration and Policy in Mental Health, 32*(2), 161–187.

Illinois PBIS Network. (2005). *What is PBIS?* Retrieved August 8, 2007, from http://www.pbisillinois.org.

Institute of Medicine. (2001). *Crossing the quality chasm: A new health system for the 21st century.* Washington, DC: National Academies Press.

Institute of Medicine. (2006). *Improving the quality of health care for mental and substance-use conditions: Quality chasm series.* Washington, DC: National Academies Press.

Kagen, E.B., & Hepburn, K.S. (Eds.). (2006). *Leadership in systems of care: A training curriculum.* Washington DC: Georgetown University Center for Child and Human Development, National Technical Assistance Center for Children's Mental Health.

Manderscheid, R.W., & Berry, J.T. (Eds.). (2006). *Mental health, United States 2004.* Rockville, MD: Substance Abuse and Mental Health Services Administration.

Manderscheid, R.W., & Sonnenschein, M.A. (Eds.). (1998). *Mental health, United States 1998.* Washington, DC: U.S. Government Printing Office.

McRee, T., Dower, C., Briggance, B., Vance, J., Keane, D., & O'Neil (2003). *The mental health workforce: Who's meeting California's needs? A report of the California workforce ini-*

tiative. San Francisco: University of California, San Francisco, Center for the Health Professions, California Workforce Initiative.

Meadows, D. (1999). *Leverage points: Places to intervene in a system*. Hartland, VT: Sustainability Institute.

Meyers, J. (2007). Developing the workforce for an infant and early childhood mental health system of care. In B.A. Stroul & R.M. Friedman (Series Eds.) & D.F. Perry, R.K. Kaufmann, & J. Knitzer (Vol. Eds.), *Systems of care for children's mental health series: Social and emotional health in early childhood: Building bridges between services and systems* (pp. 97–119). Baltimore: Paul H. Brookes Publishing Co.

Meyers, J., Kaufman, M., & Goldman, S. (1999). Promising practices: Training strategies for serving children with serious emotional disturbance and their families in a system of care. *Systems of Care: Promising Practices in Children's Mental Health* (1998 Series, Vol. V). Washington, DC: American Institutes for Research, Center for Effective Collaboration and Practice.

Morris, J., & Hanley, J. (2001). Human resource development: A critical gap in child mental health reform. *Administration and Policy in Mental Health, 28*, 219–227.

National Advisory Mental Health Council Workgroup on Child and Adolescent Mental Health Intervention Development and Deployment. (2001). *Blueprint for change: Research on child and adolescent mental health*. Rockville, MD: National Institute of Mental Health.

Pires, S. (1996). Human resource development. In B.A. Stroul & R.M. Friedman (Series Eds.) & B.A. Stroul (Vol. Ed.), *Systems of care for children's mental health series: Children's mental health: Creating systems of care in a changing society* (pp. 281–297). Baltimore: Paul H. Brookes Publishing Co.

Pottick, K. (2002). *Children's use of mental health services doubles, new research—policy partnership reports. Update: Latest Findings in Children's Mental Health*. Policy report submitted to the Annie E. Casey Foundation, New Brunswick, NJ.

Pottick, K., & Warner, L. (2002). *More than 115,000 disadvantaged preschoolers receive mental health services. Update: Latest Findings in Children's Mental Health*. Policy report submitted to the Annie E. Casey Foundation, New Brunswick, NJ.

President's New Freedom Commission on Mental Health. (2003). *Achieving the promise: Transforming mental health care in America. Final report* (DHHS Pub. No SMA-03-3832). Rockville, MD: Author.

Sarason, S. (1973). *The creation of settings and future societies*. San Francisco: Jossey-Bass.

Snyder, H., & Sickmund, M. (1999). *Juvenile offenders and victims: 1999 national report*. Washington, DC: Office of Juvenile Justice and Delinquency Prevention.

Thomas, C., & Holzer, T. (2006). The continuing shortage of child and adolescent psychiatrists. *Journal of the American Academy of Child and Adolescent Psychiatry, 45*(9), 1023–1031.

Trader-Leigh, K. (2002). *Building cultural competence: A took kit for workforce development*. Washington, DC: Joint Center for Political and Economic Studies.

Warner, L.A., & Pottick, K.J. (2004). More than 380,000 children diagnosed with multiple mental health problems. *Latest Findings in Children's Mental Health*. Report submitted to the Annie E. Casey Foundation.

U.S. Bureau of the Census. (2000). *Census data reports and profiles*. Retrieved July 2005, from http://www.census.gov/main/www/cen2000.html

U.S. Department of Health and Human Services. (1999). *Mental health: A report of the Surgeon General*. Rockville, MD: Author.

U.S. Department of Health and Human Services. (2001a). *Report of the Surgeon General's conference on children's mental health: A national action agenda*. Washington, DC: Author.

U.S. Department of Health and Human Services. (2001b). *Mental health: Culture, race, and ethnicity—A supplement to mental health: A report of the Surgeon General*. Rockville, MD: Author.

U.S. Department of Health and Human Services. (2002). *Trends in the well-being of America's children and youth*. Rockville, MD: Author.

25

Policy Implications

New Directions in Child and Adolescent Mental Health

Sybil K. Goldman, Beth A. Stroul,
Larke Nahme Huang, and Chris Koyanagi

This chapter focuses on future policy directions in child and adolescent mental health. The policy framework presented goes beyond an emphasis on children with serious emotional disturbances to a broader vision of a public health approach that aims to prevent mental health problems and create conditions that promote positive social-emotional health and well-being for all children. Achieving this vision will require a transformation of policies and the current service delivery system and will involve addressing both prevention and treatment. There has been significant progress made in understanding how to build comprehensive, community-based systems of care to improve services and outcomes for children and youth with serious emotional disturbances. The challenge is to incorporate the values, principles, and lessons learned from systems of care into an overarching public health framework that promotes health, prevents disability, and treats those in need of services based on the best available science of what is effective.

ROLE OF PUBLIC POLICY IN SERVICE DELIVERY

Achieving this transformation of the nation's mental health system will require major shifts in public policy. There are numerous definitions of the term *public policy* in the literature. One definition describes it as authoritative decisions made in the legislative, executive, or judicial branches of government that are intended to direct or influence the actions, behaviors, or decisions of others (Longest, 1998). A more general definition is a system of laws, regulatory measures, courses of action, and funding priorities concerning a given topic promulgated by government entities at national, state, and local levels or by tribal authorities. Policy strategies such as legislation, executive orders, judicial decisions, regulations, contracts, memoranda of understanding, and funding mechanisms are levers of change that determine to whom and by what means services are delivered and fi-

----

nanced (Georgetown University National Technical Assistance Center for Children's Mental Health, 1999).

The public policy context for a service delivery system typically is based on prevailing principles and values that, in turn, affect the management and structure of programs, which then affect program operations and, ultimately, program impact (Friedman, 2001a; Usher, Gibbs, & Wildfire, 1995). Policies decide eligibility criteria, create organizational structures, establish financing and reimbursement arrangements, dictate the types of interventions, set standards, and determine outcomes to be monitored and accountability procedures (Friedman, 2001a). Many of the public policies that have affected children's mental health since the 1980s have been based on system of care values and principles. Recent policy documents have confirmed the system of care philosophy and approach, but they also have highlighted areas that need improvement and represent new directions, most notably a stronger focus on mental health promotion, prevention, and early intervention (President's New Freedom Commission on Mental Health, 2003; U.S. Department of Health and Human Services [U.S. DHHS], 1999b; U.S. Public Health Service, 2000).

NEW DIRECTIONS IN CHILD AND ADOLESCENT MENTAL HEALTH POLICY

Recent Policy Recommendations

Since the late 1990s, several high-level bodies have articulated and reaffirmed needed reforms in mental health policy and service delivery. In 1999, the first-ever Surgeon General's Report on Mental Health represented a major landmark, documenting the state of scientific advances in mental health and setting forth a policy vision for the future. *Mental Health: A Report of the Surgeon General* (U.S. DHHS, 1999b) called for a public health approach to mental health, underscored the need for a developmental perspective for understanding and treating mental health disorders in children, highlighted the importance of addressing risk and protective factors to prevent mental health disorders and promote healthy development, and synthesized the evidence base for services across the life span. In 2000, as a follow-up to this report, the U.S. Surgeon General convened a conference on children's mental health that resulted in a national action agenda, which established children's mental health as a national priority and delineated action steps to organize and coordinate services in the child's cultural and community context (U.S. Public Health Service, 2000).

In 1999, the U.S. Supreme Court's groundbreaking Olmstead decision signified another policy milestone supporting the goal of providing care for children with mental health needs in their homes and communities. The Supreme Court specified that the institutionalization of individuals with disabilities who, given appropriate supports, could live in the community is a form of discrimination. The intent of the Olmstead decision is consistent with the system of care philosophy—avoiding out-of-home placements to the greatest extent possible and returning children to their home communities in a timely way with appropriate services and supports in place (Lezak & Macbeth, 2002). The need for such legal action underscores the large number of individuals with disabilities who still do not receive home and community-based services despite a federal focus on building systems of care (Angold, Erkanli, Egger, & Costello, 2002; Leaf et al., 1996).

The Substance Abuse and Mental Health Services Administration's (SAMHSA) *Report to Congress on the Prevention and Treatment of Co-Occurring Substance Abuse Disorders and Mental Disorders* confirmed what many researchers and practitioners in the fields of both mental health and substance abuse had been finding for some time—high rates of co-occurring mental health and substance use problems in both youth and adults (U.S. DHHS, 2002). Studies increasingly report that most youth referred for substance abuse treatment have at least one co-occurring mental health problem, and in a mental health clinical population, substance abuse disorders range from 50% to 80% (Kessler et al., 2005; Myers, Brown, & Mott, 2004; Turner et al., 2004; Wilens et al., 1994). The SAMHSA report suggested that there is a window of opportunity to implement prevention strategies for children and adolescents to prevent or mitigate substance use and mental health disorders and also highlighted the need for policy reforms to address this reality.

In 2002, the second Presidential Commission on Mental Health was created—24 years after the first such commission—with a specific mandate to study the existing mental health service delivery system and make recommendations for improvements that will enable adults with serious mental illness and children with serious emotional disorders to live, work, learn, and fully function in their homes, schools, and communities. In 2003, the President's New Freedom Commission on Mental Health issued its report entitled *Achieving the Promise: Transforming Mental Health Care in America.* The report presented 6 goals and 19 recommendations that, in aggregate, would begin to change how mental health care is organized, financed, and delivered in order to achieve the goal of recovery, resilience, and a life in the community where both adults and children can thrive:

- *Goal 1*—Americans understand that mental health is essential to health.

- *Goal 2*—Mental health care is consumer and family driven.

- *Goal 3*—Disparities in mental health services are eliminated.

- *Goal 4*—Early mental health screening, assessment, and referral to services are common practice.

- *Goal 5*—Excellent mental health care is delivered and research is accelerated.

- *Goal 6*—Technology is used to obtain mental health care and information.

A children's subcommittee of this commission was established to study the challenges and make recommendations for achieving these goals for children. Although the mandate of the commission focused on interventions for children with serious disorders, the subcommittee expanded the focus to include preventive and early interventions for children at risk for mental health disorders, as well as the promotion of mental health for all children.

In 2006, a study by the Institute of Medicine on Improving the Quality of Health Care for Mental and Substance-use Disorders identified six priority areas for reform of the American mental health care system for both adults and children. These priorities specified the need for: 1) patient-centered mental health care, 2) the application of evidence and quality improvement tools to mental health care, 3) coordination and integration of mental health care with general health care and other sectors, 4) the use and development of technology in mental health care, 5) the development of the mental health workforce to support necessary changes, and 6) the development of funding mechanisms and market incentives to leverage change.

These recent reports, coupled with two decades of experience implementing systems of care, provide a vision and a blueprint for policy directions to improve the lives of children who are at risk or who suffer from mental health problems in the United States. The reports emphasize a number of common themes including the importance of care being driven by families and consumers, including youth; the elimination of racial, ethnic, and geographic disparities in care; the emphasis on home and community-based services and supports; the interconnectedness between health, mental health, and substance abuse; support for a public health approach to mental health; and policies and services informed by the advances in research and science, including prevention research.

Policy Framework for a
Public Health Approach to Mental Health

The policy vision and framework that emerges from these influential reports is a mental health system rooted in a public health model that promotes positive mental health and the overall social, emotional, and cognitive well-being of all children across the developmental life span. Children's mental health *is* a public health concern. Prevalence studies show that approximately 1 in 5 U.S. children (20%) has a diagnosable mental health disorder, and 1 in 10 youth has a disorder severe enough to cause substantial impairment in functioning at home, at school, or in the community (Shaffer et al., 1996). Suicide is the third leading cause of death among youth ages 15–24 (Anderson & Smith, 2003).

Research indicates that multiple risk and protective factors contribute to the mental well-being of children or can result in a range of mental illnesses. According to the Surgeon General's Report, the field of prevention has developed to the point that the reduction of risk, the prevention of onset, and early intervention are realistic possibilities (U.S. DHHS, 1999b). Thus, it is both logical and humane to intervene early in children's lives before problems are established and become intractable. The science of early childhood development, compellingly presented in the Institute of Medicine's *From Neurons to Neighborhoods* (Shonkoff & Phillips, 2000), makes a strong case for the effectiveness of early interventions in the first years of life.

The public health approach is characterized by a concern for the health of a population in its entirety, and it focuses not only on traditional areas of diagnosis, treatment, and etiology, but also on epidemiologic surveillance of the health of the population at large, health promotion, disease prevention, and access to and evaluation of services (Davis, 2002; Last & Wallace, 1992; U.S. DHHS, 1999b).

Core elements of a public health approach include (Elliott, Hamburg, & Williams, 1998):

- Community-based methods for identifying the sources of the problem and taking a population-based perspective

- Epidemiological data and analyses for identifying patterns of risk and protective factors

- Ongoing surveillance and tracking of the problem and the identified risk and protective factors to establish trends in prevalence and incidence

- The designing of community-based interventions based on systematic analysis of the problem to reduce or eliminate risk factors and enhance protective factors

- The evaluation and monitoring of interventions to establish and improve effectiveness

- Public education to share information about the problem and effective or ineffective interventions

These strategies, more commonly applied to physical health concerns, need to incorporate a mental health focus, which includes building an understanding and awareness of the risk and protective factors for mental illness and mental health; mobilizing national, state, and community resources to gather data; effectively tracking and intervening to prevent mental illness; undertaking a public awareness campaign dedicated to mental health promotion and early intervention; and providing treatment, rehabilitation, and recovery-oriented services for individuals already diagnosed with mental health disorders.

In its pioneering publication on prevention of mental health disorders, the Institute of Medicine presented a model that spans a full spectrum of mental health interventions for mental health disorders compatible with a public health approach. Shown in Figure 25.1, the spectrum includes universal prevention interventions targeted at an entire population group; selective preventive interventions targeted to individuals or a subgroup whose risk of developing mental or behavioral disorders is significantly higher than average; indicated preventive interventions directed at individuals who are already showing signs or symptoms that foreshadow a mental or behavioral disorder; treatment for those in need of care and intervention; and maintenance care for those with longer-term disabilities.

Building the policy framework for a public health approach requires addressing multiple fronts, often simultaneously. New alliances must be forged between such sectors as public health, maternal and child health, mental health, substance use, early childhood, and education. Bridges must be built between prevention and treatment systems. Financing and intervention strategies must be aligned. Research on the effectiveness of both prevention and treatment interventions must be accelerated, especially studies focused on interventions for diverse communities and populations.

At the same time that policies are shifting to implement a public health approach to mental health, it is also essential that policies continue to support and build on the reforms and progress in children's mental health service delivery since

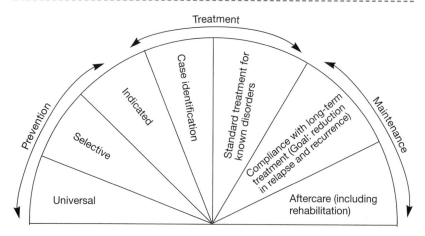

Figure 25.1. Institute of Medicine's Mental Health Intervention Spectrum for Mental Disorders. (From Mrazek, P.J., & Haggerty, R.J. [Eds.]. [1994]. *Reducing risks for mental disorders: Frontiers for preventive intervention research* [p. 23]. Washington, DC: National Academies Press; reprinted by permission.)

the 1980s, especially for those children and adolescents with serious and complex emotional disorders and their families. Significant work has been accomplished in children's mental health through systems of care to implement the values and principles of a high-quality and effective service delivery system (Stroul, 2002). Both national and community evaluations have shown that positive outcomes for children with severe disorders and their families have been achieved through the implementation of systems of care (Center for Mental Health Services, 2001). The fundamental values, principles, and key components of a system of care are relevant and essential to a public health approach and the continuum of promotion, prevention, and treatment. Within a public health construct, systems of care also provide a model for organizing and delivering a comprehensive array of interventions and supports for that population of children with mental health disorders requiring treatment. However, there continue to be significant gaps in the implementation of systems of care and the reforms needed to improve service delivery strategies and outcomes. The following section outlines important policy priorities and highlights potential strategies to address these critical areas (Huang et al., 2005).

POLICY PRIORITIES

The policy priorities delineated next provide a standard of care and implementation strategies to ensure high-quality and accessible mental health systems for children and their families in communities across the nation.

Family- and Youth-Centered Care and Partnerships

Policy priority: Policies should be designed to support families, substitute families, and other primary caregivers and to ensure that they are respected partners in all aspects of the system.

The family is the most important and lifelong resource in a child's life and is responsible for the child from both a legal and moral perspective. Families should be integrally involved in the planning, delivery, and evaluation of services and supports for their own child and family and should be provided with meaningful choices of services and providers. When the natural family is not involved, efforts are needed to reach out to engage and support the surrogate or substitute family or other caregivers (Stroul & Friedman, 1996). Beyond their integral role in service planning and delivery for their own child and family, new roles are emerging for families that involve them as partners in policy making; system planning, management, and implementation; research, evaluation, and quality improvement; and training and teaching in universities and other professional development settings (McCammon, Spencer, & Friesen, 2001; Sabin & Daniels, 1999).

With the emphasis placed on consumer-driven care, new roles are also emerging for youth to be engaged in treatment decisions and in leadership roles to plan and shape services and systems of care. Youth with emotional and mental health disorders have organized nationally to create Youth M.O.V.E. (Motivating Others Through Voices of Experience). For adults with mental illness, there is an increasing body of research showing the effectiveness of peer-to-peer services for recovery (Yanos, Primavera, & Knight, 2001). These findings have relevance for young people as well.

Given the challenges faced by families of children with emotional disorders in conjunction with the research documenting the positive impact of their involvement, policies are needed to foster family participation as partners in service delivery as well as at the system level; provide information and a constellation of formal and informal family support services (e.g., education and training, peer support, home aides, respite care); eliminate the need to relinquish custody to receive necessary care; and enhance the capacity of family organizations to provide information, support, and advocacy. These policies should be supported by expanding funding to family organizations and by providing coverage for family support services in public and private insurance.

Culturally and Linguistically Competent Care

Policy priority: Services and supports should be equitable and responsive to the cultural and linguistic characteristics of the populations served.

The United States is a nation of diverse races, ethnicities, and cultures. The problems of unmet need and inappropriate care are particularly severe for children from racially and ethnically diverse backgrounds. As former Surgeon General David M. Satcher noted, "It is essential that our nation continues on the road toward eliminating racial and ethnic disparities in the accessibility, availability, and quality of mental health services" (U.S. DHHS, 2001, vii). Within the children's mental health field, a major effort has been made to promote the development of culturally competent services and systems (Cross, Bazron, Dennis, & Isaacs,

1989; Hernandez & Isaacs, 1998). Some progress has been made, but more work must be done to achieve equity in access, quality, and outcomes for people of color (U.S. DHHS, 2001). Children of color tend to receive mental health services in more restrictive and coercive settings, such as juvenile justice and child welfare systems, than through schools or mental health settings (Alegria, 2000). African American youth receive less treatment in schools and more in restrictive residential treatment centers (Firestone, 1990). African American and Latino children have the highest rates of unmet need (Ringel & Sturm, 2001), and, although they are identified and referred at the same rates as the general population from primary care, they are less likely to receive specialty mental health services or medications (Kelleher, 2000). American Indian/Alaska Native adolescents and young adult males have the highest suicide rate of all groups (Centers for Disease Control and Prevention, 2007). Latino and Asian adolescent girls have among the highest rates of depression and experience more barriers to care (Commonwealth Fund, 1998). Many families, particularly those who have immigrated to this country, speak limited English, creating an extra barrier to effective care and a need for linguistic competence in mental health and related systems.

Given the number of different racial and ethnic groups in the United States, as well as the heterogeneity within each group, there is no simple solution to addressing the many service delivery challenges. It is essential, however, that policies and strategic plans to address these disparities be developed and implemented and that they be based on the voices, views, and recommendations of representatives of diverse racial and ethnic groups. Thus, federal, state, and local agencies should work with diverse ethnic and racial leadership, organizations, families, and consumers to develop policies and strategies to remove structural, linguistic, cultural, and financial barriers and improve access to quality care. These efforts should address key needs including consistent racial and ethnic data collection, evaluation of disparities reduction programs, minimum standards for culturally and linguistically competent behavioral health services, locally determined benchmarks and indicators for culturally competent care, reimbursement policies for culturally based interventions and alternative care, and greater diversity within the workforce that reflects the populations being served.

Individualized, Customized Care

Policy priority: Services should be individualized and guided by a comprehensive single plan of care for each child and family that incorporates a focus on strengths, as well as on problems and needs, to guide the types and combination of services and supports that will be provided.

Research on children with emotional disorders has clearly demonstrated that they are a diverse group in terms of diagnostic characteristics, strengths and needs, level of functioning, family strengths and issues, co-occurring conditions, values and beliefs, and involvement with service systems (Angold, Costello, & Erkanli, 1999; Friedman, Kutash, & Duchnowski, 1996; McGonaughy & Skiba, 1993;

Silver et al., 1992). In response to this variability, a strong focus on the development of individualized and culturally competent service plans has developed in
the children's mental health field (Behar, 1986; Goldman, 1999; Lourie, Katz-
Leavy, & Stroul, 1996; VanDenBerg, 1999). Such an approach, often referred to as
the *wraparound process* (VanDenBerg, 1999), seeks to build a comprehensive treatment plan based on the special strengths, needs, and goals of each child and family,
utilizing both formal services and resources in the child and family's natural support system. Research has documented individualized care as promising (Bruns,
Hoagwood, & Mrazek, 1999), and the application of this model in practice has
grown rapidly around the country. The Institute of Medicine's Committee on
Quality of Health Care in America called on private and public purchasers, health
care organizations, clinicians, and patients to work together to customize care
based on patients' needs and values, stating, "The system of care should be designed to meet the most common types of needs but have the capability to respond
to individual patient choices and preferences" (Institute of Medicine, 2006, p. 78).

As purchasers and providers of services, states and communities should ensure that each child with a complex emotional disorder has an individualized,
single plan of care that addresses the child and his or her family's needs across life
domains and also incorporates services and supports from all needed agencies and
systems. These plan types should be developed by multidisciplinary child and
family teams, and the family and youth should assume a key partnership role with
providers in the development, implementation, and monitoring of the plan
(Bruns, Suter, Burchard, Force, & Leverentz-Brady, 2004).

Comprehensive Home and Community-Based Services and Supports

Policy priority: A broad array of home and community-based services and
supports should be available and responsive to the biological, neurologi-
cal, psychological, and social aspects of children's mental health problems and supportive of the multiple areas of functioning in a child's life.

Children belong in their homes and in their communities, and thus every effort
should be made to keep them there. A broad array of services and supports should
be accessible to children and families. These services should be provided in the
least restrictive, clinically appropriate setting, and they should emphasize natural
settings where children spend the most time (e.g., with their families, in schools,
in primary health care settings, in child care, in other child-serving settings and
systems). If placement in an out-of-home setting is the only viable option, concerted efforts must be made to return children to their homes and to community
settings as soon as is appropriate.

Since the 1980s, there has been a substantial growth in services other than
traditional office-based outpatient therapy and residential or inpatient care. These
services include intensive home-based services, day treatment, mentoring, respite
care, wraparound, therapeutic foster care, and others. Based on an analysis of

mental health service use and expenditures, since the 1990s, there has been a documented shift toward outpatient care (Sturm et al., 2001); however, significant service gaps in the continuum of care for children and their families remain. In many communities, overreliance on out-of-home and out-of-community treatment options and overemphasis on traditional psychotherapeutic interventions still exist. Despite widespread interest in home, school, and community-based services and supports, the capacity to provide many of these services is lacking, and investments in service capacity development have been insufficient to ensure access to a broad array of services and supports in communities (Stroul, Pires, & Armstrong, 2001). Service gaps are also perpetuated by the outdated mental health benefits provided by many insurance carriers, which include little coverage for the home and community-based services that could replace costly out-of-home treatment.

Federal and state governments should provide incentives and work in partnership with families and the private sector to encourage the investment of resources to build a full range of home and community-based services and supports. State plans for comprehensive coordinated care for children should be developed. Financial and other resources should be provided to support the start-up or retooling costs for such services. In addition, a model benefit design that includes a comprehensive array of treatments, services, and supports that also promotes the use of evidence-based interventions should be developed and widely disseminated. Reimbursement policies and other program funding mechanisms also need to be redesigned to serve as an incentive to utilize an array of home and community-based service alternatives.

Cross-System Coordination and Financing

Policy priority: Coordination should occur to rationalize and better align service delivery and financing across the multiple systems that share responsibility for children with mental health challenges and their families.

The mental health system is a maze that defies easy description. Responsibility is spread over a complex patchwork of programs operated by federal, state, and local governments and the private sector that provide and pay for treatment, services, and supports. To further complicate matters, each entity has different mandates, missions, service settings, financing streams, eligibility rules, and requirements. This fragmentation is compounded exponentially for children because of the range of additional child-serving systems responsible for children with emotional and behavioral disorders. Child welfare, public health, mental health, substance abuse, early childhood, developmental disabilities, juvenile justice systems, and particularly the schools are involved in the delivery and funding of mental health and other services to children; however, they are often sharply divided by differing policies, procedures, and philosophies (Knitzer & Yelton, 1990; Wishmann, Kates, & Kaufmann, 2001). Education, child welfare, and juvenile justice systems provide and pay for significant amounts of mental health services, often more than the specialty mental health system, although they are not specifically designed to be mental health delivery systems (U.S. Public Health Service, 2000).

The confusion and cost shifting resulting from the involvement of so many agencies often creates insurmountable systemic barriers to effective and comprehensive service delivery. Recent data have confirmed that youth in the juvenile justice and child welfare systems have high rates of mental health disorders, often with co-occurring substance abuse disorders, but they receive few mental health services (Claussen, Landsverk, Ganger, Chadwick, & Litrownik, 1998; Cocozza & Skowyra, 2000; Friedman & Simmons, in press; Garland et al., 2001; Lyons, Baerger, Quigley, & Griffen, 2001; Teplin, 2002). Federal, state, and community policies need to support cross-system collaboration in order to provide a comprehensive array of services that includes those that will meet mental health and substance abuse needs in whatever system the child or youth enters.

Further complication at the policy, system, and practice level exists because some children and families are covered through employer-based commercial insurance programs, which in the absence of parity with physical health coverage, typically cover brief, short-term services and a narrow, fairly traditional range of outpatient and inpatient care. Families with private insurance who exhaust their coverage or who need services not available through their private carriers must turn to the public systems for services. In some states, families must go through the painful process of relinquishing custody of their children to become eligible for intensive mental health services in public systems (Giliberti & Schulzinger, 2000).

Public payers play an essential role for youth with serious emotional disorders. These children are overrepresented in families who have low incomes, public insurance, or no insurance at all. Almost one third of these children (31%) are covered by Medicaid or the State Child Health Insurance Program (S-CHIP), another 11% receive other publicly funded services, and 14% are uninsured (Mark & Buck, 2006). Nearly half (44%) of all youth with serious mental health disorders have private insurance, which, as noted, tends to be extremely limited and generally requires high out-of-pocket copayments for mental health services (Mark & Buck, 2006).

The focus on a multisector, multilevel approach to system transformation has been identified as essential if significant change is to take place in mental health services (Ferlie & Shortell, 2001; Ringeisen, Henderson, & Hoagwood, 2003); however, coordinating the delivery and financing of services to support a vision of a comprehensive community-based system of care is a formidable task. As a first step, each state government should plan and implement a comprehensive cross-agency plan for prevention, early intervention, and treatment for children's mental health that clarifies responsibility among the child-serving systems. Implementing collaborative efforts to deliver community-based services and supports, revising rules that impede service delivery, and aligning the financing to support prevention and treatment should be integral aspects of this endeavor. A critical component of such planning should be revising funding policies related to children's mental health to support a full array of home and community-based services and supports.

Effective efforts have been deployed by various states and local communities to draw on multiple funding streams and create innovative financing strategies for systems of care (Bruns, Burchard & Yoe, 1995; Kamradt, 2000; VanDenBerg & Grealish, 1996). Hayes (2002) described financing strategies through which states and communities could make better use of resources and improve child and family outcomes by shifting funds from higher cost placements (e.g., out-of-state residential care) to lower cost programs and services (e.g., intensive in-home services). The system could then reinvest the funds that were saved in new or alternative supports and services that are equally, if not more, effective; maximize federal and state revenues by utilizing programs that provide funding contingent on state, local, or private match (e.g., Medicaid); create more flexibility by pooling funds from several agencies into a single unified funding stream; or create new dedicated revenue streams (e.g., establish a children's trust fund from a state's share of the national tobacco settlement, raise dedicated taxes, such as mil levies). In the current climate of limited resources and major shortfalls in state budgets, maximizing the benefits from available funds requires flexibility at the federal and state level, combining resources in innovative ways, and reshaping spending practices for dollars that are already in the system (Koyanagi, Boudreaux, & Lind, 2003).

Despite the success of a few innovators to merge the funding from the diverse streams for children's mental health, a more rational policy would be to close the gaps in the current streams and align the program objectives to focus on meeting the needs of each individual child and family. For example, legislation requiring private insurers and S-CHIP to cover mental health services to the same extent as they cover medical or surgical benefits would greatly ease access for children with mild or moderate mental health disorders and prevent their families from having to seek publicly funded services. Medicaid could be revised to create a service category for intensive home and community-based mental health services that requires states to cover appropriate evidence-based practices (e.g., Multisystemic Therapy, family education, therapeutic foster care, intensive in-home services, skills building, behavioral therapy) for those with emotional disorders. In addition, Medicaid rules could allow families of very young children to be treated as a family unit regardless of the eligibility status of the caregivers and also use more appropriate diagnostic tools for infants and toddlers. Within all public programs, the disincentives for access to community services should be removed, and barriers that discourage the use of residential services such as screening and diversion as appropriate should be put in place. Importantly, public mental health systems could place greater attention on children's mental health, and both legislative and executive branches could provide significantly increased resources to meet children's needs.

Prevention, Early Identification, and Early Intervention

Policy priority: Services and supports should emphasize prevention, early identification, and intervention for children of all ages to maximize positive outcomes. Early childhood mental health programs must be implemented to prevent the negative developmental trajectories documented in research.

The Surgeon General's report on mental health set the stage for the incorporation of prevention, early identification, and early intervention services into a spectrum of mental health interventions (U.S. DHHS, 1999b). Yet there are significant barriers that have hampered efforts to translate what is known about prevention and early intervention into action, including: 1) the lack of a clear infrastructure for the delivery of preventive and early intervention services that, by their nature, cut across agencies, disciplines, service delivery systems, and outcome domains; 2) few training opportunities for families, teachers, health practitioners, and mental health clinicians to learn how to reliably screen and assess children, how to connect them and their families with services, and how to deliver effective services; 3) resources for prevention and early intervention services that are limited, fragmented, categorical, and a low priority in overstretched systems; 4) a lack of public advocacy by families for prevention and early intervention services; and 5) inadequate testing of the relevance of specific interventions for different cultural and socioeconomic groups (Mrazek, 2002).

An important starting point to increase the focus on prevention, early identification, and early intervention would be the establishment of an infrastructure at the federal and state levels and in every community to plan, coordinate, and support the development and implementation of these services. In the mental health system, planning and resources have largely been devoted to youth with the most serious and complex disorders, with little attention or funding devoted to the early identification and prompt intervention for mental health problems in multiple settings or to the promotion of positive mental health and the prevention of mental health disorders. Many children and families must wait until their problems have reached serious or crisis proportions before they can receive help. Prevention and early identification and intervention (i.e., intervening early in the course of a mental health problem) offer the best opportunity to maximize the likelihood of positive outcomes, and policies should be directed at wide-scale implementation of prevention and early intervention efforts. Policies for prevention, promotion, and early intervention need to reflect the fact that children rarely come in contact with mental health providers before they have a problem. Schools, pediatric offices, and other childhood programs are the best locations for these types of services.

Of particular concern is strengthening early childhood interventions. Despite research that shows a disturbingly high prevalence of emotional and behavioral disorders among young children (Lavigne et al., 1996), this population has been neglected. Emerging neuroscience reveals the impact of environmental factors on brain development and early psychosocial behavior, and it makes the convincing argument that early detection, assessment, and treatment can prevent the escalation of mental health problems (Shonkoff & Phillips, 2000). There are increasing data on the effectiveness of mental health services and supports for young children that focus on the parent (Olds et al., 1998), the child (Cowen et al., 1996), or the parent–child interaction (Eyberg et al., 2001). Group-based (Greenberg, Domitrovich, & Bumbarger, 2001) and multicomponent interventions (Ramey & Ramey, 1998) also have empirical support, and mental health consultation to early childhood programs has shown promising results (Donahue, 2002).

Thus, a national effort focusing on the mental health needs of young children and their families should be implemented, including educating parents and providers about the importance of the first years of a child's life for developing a foundation for healthy social and emotional development; creating greater awareness about mental health problems in young children; implementing a comprehensive approach to early screening, assessment, and intervention in natural early childhood settings; educating and training professionals in effective intervention and treatment approaches for young children and their families; and eliminating disincentives and barriers, particularly in diagnostic and financing systems, to serving this population.

Integration of Behavioral Health and Primary Care

Policy priority: A focus on behavioral health care should be incorporated into primary health care systems to identify the need for behavioral health interventions, to connect children and their families with appropriate behavioral health services and supports, and to better coordinate health and behavioral health services.

Integrating behavioral health into primary health care represents a critical component of an overall strategy to move toward a public health approach. The World Health Organization (WHO) reported that as the ultimate stewards of health systems, governments must take responsibility for ensuring the integration of mental health treatment into the health system (WHO, 2001). Primary care is the opportune point of entry to identify risks and to initiate services to children and youth who have or are at risk for having behavioral health problems (Huang, Freed, & Espiritu, 2006; Kaye, 2006; Rosman, Perry, & Hepburn, 2005). Understanding the role of primary care in providing quality screening, identification, and intervention is essential for improving services and outcomes for children and youth. One of the key recommendations of the President's New Freedom Commission on Mental Health (2003) is that screening for mental health disorders be incorporated in primary health care across the life span and that individuals in need be connected to treatment and supports.

The American Academy of Pediatrics (AAP) has played a leadership role in articulating the importance of pediatricians in the healthy development of children and in defining the concept of a *medical home*, through which the medical care of infants, children, and adolescents should be accessible, continuous, comprehensive, family centered, coordinated, compassionate, and culturally effective (AAP, 2002). Delivered or directed by well-trained physicians, such comprehensive care is broadly defined as preventive, acute, and chronic care services that include screenings, developmental assessments, counseling, and appropriate referrals. The U.S. Department of Health and Human Services' Healthy People 2010 goals and objectives call for all children with special health care needs (*including mental health*) to receive regular ongoing comprehensive care within a medical home (U.S. DHHS, 1999a). Numerous barriers, however, hinder full implementation of this concept, including inadequate financing, a lack of infrastructure, a lack of practitioner skills within both primary care and mental health, and communication and confidentiality issues (Stroul, 2007). Recommendations for better linking primary care and mental health services include creating state-level steering committees to enhance the provision of behavioral health services within primary care settings; establishing guidelines and memoranda of understanding; passing parity laws that reimburse behavioral health similarly to health care and reimbursement systems that pay pediatricians for mental health care; providing financial incentives to primary care providers to undertake more thorough screening and follow-up related to behavioral health; developing financing strategies that support braiding funding streams and collaborative, integrated models of care (e.g., colocation of services, behavioral health consultation to primary care providers, referral arrangements); implementing Medicaid reforms to improve behavioral health screening under the Early and Periodic Screening, Diagnosis and Treatment (EPSDT) Program; financing compensation for care coordination between medical homes and systems of care; improving training and certification and licensing requirements involving preservice and continuing education for physicians in behavioral health and for mental health professionals working in primary care settings; and developing cross-system communication, information-sharing, and data collection and sharing strategies (Stroul, 2007).

Mental Health Services in Schools

Policy priority: The mental health needs of youth in the education system should be more fully recognized and addressed, and effective approaches for providing mental health services and supports to youth in schools should be developed, evaluated, and disseminated, including strategies for prevention, early identification, early intervention, and treatment.

Every day during the school year, more than 52 million children attend 114,000 schools in the United States (Jamieson, Curry, & Martinez, 2001). The mission of schools is to educate *all* students, and to ensure academic achievement, schools have identified the need to attend to the health and emotional well-being of their students. Recognizing that children receive more services through schools than any other public system, strengthening mental health services in schools offers a strategic opportunity to provide effective services to many children (Hoagwood & Erwin, 1997).

Nationally, children with emotional and behavioral disorders in special education have the highest drop-out rates (50.6%) and the next to lowest rate of graduating with a standard diploma (41.9%) of any group of children with disabilities in schools (U.S. Department of Education, 2001). The Individuals with Disabilities Education Act (IDEA) Amendments of 1997 (PL 105-17) have been an important vehicle for addressing the needs of children with emotional disorders. Revisions and appropriate technical assistance should be undertaken to assist states and communities to implement IDEA more effectively to ensure that all children with emotional and behavioral disorders receive the assessments, services, and supports that will enable them to be successful in school.

There is increasing evidence that school mental health programs improve educational outcomes by decreasing absences, reducing discipline referrals, and improving test scores (Jennings, Pearson, & Harris, 2000). In addition, school-based wraparound approaches have been proven effective in significantly reducing restrictive out-of-school and out-of-home placements (Eber, Osuch, & Redditt, 1996). Positive Behavior Support has become one of the most frequently used and promising interventions within schools, focusing part of its work on the entire school, part on children at risk, and part on children with significant problems that have already been identified (Horner & Carr, 1997; Sugai et al., 2000). Thus, a continuum of mental health services should be provided in schools, including prevention, early identification, early intervention, and treatment. Furthermore, mental health services should be provided through school health centers, and funding for school-based mental health services should be included in Medicaid and other federally funded health, mental health, and education programs.

Practices Based on Evidence, Clinical Judgment, and Family Preference

Policy priority: Children and families should be informed of and given access to evidence-based practices, and when the scientific basis is incomplete, services should be guided by experience, clinical judgment, and family preference.

Many states and communities continue to offer traditional services as opposed to community-based care. They also have difficulty adopting evidence-based services and supports, and fail to incorporate knowledge from biopsychosocial research into services and policy. There is an accumulating evidence base in children's mental health supporting home and community-based services approaches, but there is a lag in the dissemination of evidence-based practices and their incorporation into clinical practice. Furthermore, despite the progress that has been made, many interventions have not as yet been tested on the highly diverse population of children with multiple needs, problems, and co-occurring conditions who are typically served within public systems (Friedman, 2001b; Friedman & Hernandez, 2002; Shirk, 2001).

An important step toward improving the effectiveness of services and supports is the development, dissemination, and implementation of interventions supported by scientific evidence. The availability of such interventions provides families with the ability to make informed choices about the services they would like to receive, provides practitioners with the opportunity to learn new and improved approaches, and most important, has the potential to significantly improve outcomes. The challenge is promoting not just the dissemination of these interventions in an effective manner, but also their implementation with fidelity, thus moving science to services.

At the same time, it is important to recognize that children and their families are highly heterogeneous with a diverse set of strengths and needs. Families and youth should be able to choose the interventions that will work for them. Evidence-based interventions are not available for all problems and needs, and even when available, they do not work uniformly with all families. Jensen (2001) emphasized that it is essential not to lose sight of the importance of using best clinical consensus and experience in working collaboratively with families to make decisions about services where an evidence base has yet to be developed. It also is important that there be support for innovative efforts to develop new interventions at the same time as evidence-based practices are being disseminated, to identify promising practices that are emerging in communities around the country that may be candidates for evaluation, and to broaden the concept of evidence-based interventions to include evidence-based *processes* that may cut across a number of clinical interventions, such as relationship building or skill building or the individualized, wraparound approach to service delivery (Chorpita, 2003; Friedman, 2003; Weisz, Sandler, Durlak, & Anton, 2005).

Trauma-Informed Services

Policy priority: Policies should promote the recognition of the role trauma plays in child and adolescent mental health problems, and effective interventions should be provided to prevent and treat trauma.

An increasing body of research confirms a strong correlation between trauma and mental health disorders. The Adverse Childhood Experiences study, a collaboration between the Centers for Disease Control and Prevention and the Kaiser Health Plan's Department of Preventive Medicine, is designed to examine the childhood origins of many of the nation's leading health and social problems. Findings suggest that stressful or traumatic childhood experiences such as abuse, neglect, witnessing domestic violence, or growing up with substance abuse or mental illness, parental discord, or crime in the home are common pathways to social, emotional, and cognitive impairments and lead to increased risk or unhealthy behaviors and disability (Anda, 2006). Advances in neuroscience are showing that serious adverse factors in childhood can disrupt neurodevelopment and have lasting effects on brain structure and function. The problems that arise from adverse childhood experiences call for an integrated approach toward addressing these significant risk factors.

The National Child Traumatic Stress Network (NCTSN), funded by SAMHSA, supports research and provides information and technical assistance on the impact of trauma on children, as well as effective interventions to prevent and treat trauma. An NCTSN survey found that the vast majority of children served by the network (78%) have been exposed to multiple or prolonged trauma (Spinazzola et al., 2003). Findings further revealed that initial exposure typically occurs early, with an average age of onset of 5 years old. As a result, a Task Force on Complex Trauma of the NCTSN recommended that policy makers: 1) advocate for recognition of complex trauma as a public health problem affecting millions of children in the United States annually; 2) engage in policy efforts aimed at closing the gap between the needs of children and families affected by complex trauma and available resources; 3) increase awareness of the fact that effective interventions for children exposed to complex trauma can be implemented and that these interventions need to be integrated across the systems in which children who are affected are located; 4) influence the creation and design of federal, state, and foundation service, training, and research grants to increase understanding of interventions and access to resources; 5) support funding for evidenced-based prevention and intervention programs integrated across federal, state, and local agencies; and 6) advocate for strategies to improve clinical diagnosis, treatment guidelines, and third-party reimbursement for services provided to children with complex trauma (Cook, Blaustein, Spinazzola, & van der Kolk, 2003).

Workforce Development

Policy priority: Policies are needed to support the creation of an adequate workforce for child and adolescent mental health services, addressing the number of professionals and frontline workers, along with the values and competencies, needed to achieve a transformed approach to improving children's mental health.

To address the need for a workforce well prepared to implement systems of care, preservice and in-service training must be shifted to the new philosophy based on the inclusion of families and youth as partners in service delivery. This is a shift away from an almost exclusive focus on office and clinic-based practice to a greater emphasis on individualized home and community-based service approaches and the role of collaboration across disciplines and agencies in service planning and delivery. Training must include strengths-based approaches, individualized care, culturally and linguistically competent care, and the clinical advances embedded in evidence-based and promising practices (Friedman, 1993; Morris & Hanley, 2001).

For mental health staff working with children and families, a transformed service delivery system would offer expanded roles and approaches to care. To fulfill these roles, the workforce needs training that goes beyond the clinical treatment of disorders. Staff must also develop an ability to harness the strengths of the child, partner with families and youth in treatment planning and decision making, and consult and collaborate with providers in other child-serving systems. Personnel must be prepared to work in nonmental health settings, such as schools, early childhood, primary care, juvenile justice, and child welfare. Training in evidence-based practices is increasingly important, as consumers, families, and payers are committed to getting services that work based on science or the recommended clinical consensus. With significant disparities in access, quality, and outcomes of services for diverse ethnic and racial populations, the workforce must be diverse, and staff must become better trained to work with children and families from many different cultures and backgrounds. Training must enhance cultural competence, and the field must create specific incentives and strategies to recruit and train culturally and linguistically diverse practitioners to work in systems of care.

In a transformed system for children's mental health, research roles will expand with the movement toward evidence-based practices and the need to build the science base for promising field-initiated approaches. Thus, workforce development policies also should be directed at increasing the pool of qualified researchers in children's mental health.

Accountability, Performance Measurement, and Quality Improvement

Policy priority: There should be a clear focal point for responsibility and accountability for children's mental health care. Services and systems of care should be guided by standards for access, quality of care, and performance measures of service delivery and outcomes to reduce inappropriate and ineffective care and produce data for continuous improvement of services and supports.

Children's mental health services and systems have suffered from a lack of reliable, practical, policy-relevant data and accountability mechanisms to guide decision making and quality improvement at both the system and service delivery levels. A major impediment to accountability in the multiple systems and agencies that serve children and families—and a starting point for accountability systems—has been a general failure to develop theories of change that clearly define the population of concern, goals, intended outcomes, and strategies for achieving the intended outcomes (Hernandez & Hodges, 2001). In addition, data systems at state and local levels are frequently inadequate to support decision making and are poorly integrated across child-serving systems. Medicaid data on children's mental health services are particularly weak. Ongoing data collection is essential to inform administrators and other stakeholders in the system about how well the system is meeting its goals and to aid in decision making and resource allocation.

At the service delivery level, consistent with the President's New Freedom Commission on Mental Health (2003), agreement is emerging on emphasizing functional outcomes for children with mental health problems—they should be at home, living productively in their community, in school, and out of trouble and demonstrate improved and stable mental health (Hernandez & Hodges, 2001; Osher, 1998; Rugs & Kutash, 1994). Communities, however, have not developed clear theories of change with specific outcomes and indicators to assess progress, and this has impeded efforts to make services and systems more accountable. Although child- and family-level outcome data are an important part of accountability and continuous quality improvement, it must be recognized that unless data are also collected on who the system is serving and how they are being served, it is difficult to interpret such outcome data.

The development of strong internal accountability and continuous quality improvement procedures requires good information systems within the guidelines of the Health Insurance Portability and Accountability Act (HIPAA) of 1996 (PL 104-191), clearly conceptualized theories of change, reliable measures, feedback systems that incorporate the data to review progress and determine if changes are needed, and collaboration from numerous stakeholders in defining goals and selecting relevant measurement strategies. The children's mental health field could benefit greatly from a federal–state partnership that provides leadership, information, and technical assistance on how to best implement procedures to improve accountability and quality in mental health service delivery to children and their families.

CONCLUSION

Research and widespread consensus of leaders in the field of children's mental health have converged in recent years to support a policy agenda that embraces prevention, early intervention, and treatment for children and youth with or at risk for mental health, substance use, and other developmental problems. To achieve this goal, national, state, and local policy makers will need to build the political will to invest in a public health approach to ensure the health and well-being of this nation's children for the future. A public education campaign on why this approach makes sense from both a human and fiscal perspective, and what it will take to implement it, will be essential to building this political will. Collaboration, commitment, and financing strategies across the multiple systems that need to be engaged in this effort will also be critical. To bring about this transformation of the country's prevention and service system will require policy makers and other stakeholders to utilize the diverse array of policy vehicles available; to apply the knowledge gained from research, evaluation, and implementation of prevention, early intervention, and system of care initiatives; and to implement strategic solutions to the multiple policy priorities outlined in this chapter.

REFERENCES

Alegria, M. (2000). Health service disparities: Access, quality, and diversity. In *Report of the Surgeon General's conference on children's mental health: A national action agenda.* Washington, DC: U.S. Public Health Service.

American Academy of Pediatrics. (2002). Policy statement: The medical home—medical home initiatives for children with special needs project advisory committee. *Pediatrics, 110,* 184–186.

Anda, R. (2006). *The health and social impact of growing up with alcohol abuse and related adverse childhood experiences: The human and economic costs of the status quo.* Handout developed for the Board of Scientific Advisors to the National Association for Children of Alcoholics, Rockville, MD.

Anderson, R.N., & Smith, B.L. (2003). Deaths: Leading causes for 2001. *National Vital Statistics Report, 52,* 1–86.

Angold, A., Costello, E.J., & Erkanli, A. (1999). Comorbidity. *Journal of Child Psychology and Psychiatry, 40*(1), 57–87.

Angold, A., Erkanli, A., Egger, H.L., & Costello, E.J. (2002). Stimulant treatment for children: A community perspective. *Journal of the American Academy of Child and Adolescent Psychiatry, 39*, 975–984.

Behar, L. (1986). Changing patterns of state responsibility: A case study of North Carolina. *Journal of Clinical Child Psychology, 14*(3), 188–195.

Bruns, E., Burchard, J., & Yoe, J. (1995). Evaluating the Vermont system of care: Outcomes associated with community-based wraparound services. *Journal of Child and Family Studies, 4*, 321–339.

Bruns, E.J., Hoagwood, K., & Mrazek, P.J. (1999). Effective treatment for mental disorders in children and adolescents. *Clinical Child and Family Psychology Review, 2*, 199–254.

Bruns, E.J., Suter, J.C., Burchard, J.D., Force, M., & Leverentz-Brady, K. (2004). Assessing fidelity to community-based treatment for youth: The wraparound fidelity index. *Journal of Emotional and Behavioral Disorders, 12*, 69–79.

Center for Mental Health Services. (2001). *Annual Report to Congress on the Evaluation of the Comprehensive Community Mental Health Services for Children and Their Families Program, 2001*. Atlanta: ORC Macro.

Centers for Disease Control and Prevention, National Center for Injury Prevention and Control. (2007). *Web-base injury statistics query and reporting system (WISQARS)*. Data retrieved January 3, 2007, from http://www.cdc.gov/ncipc/wisqars.

Chorpita, B. (2003, August). *Connecting the evidence base to practice: What it takes to get there*. Paper presented at the meeting on Evidence-Based Practice in Children's Mental Health, National Association of State Mental Health Program Directors, Fort Lauderdale, FL.

Claussen, J.M., Landsverk, J., Ganger, W., Chadwick, D., & Litrownik, A. (1998). Mental health problems of children in foster care. *Journal of Child and Family Studies, 7*, 283–296.

Cocozza, J., & Skowyra, K. (2000). Youth with mental health disorders: Issues and emerging responses. *Juvenile Justice, 7*(1), 3–13.

Commonwealth Fund. (1998). *The Commonwealth Fund survey of the health of adolescent girls*. New York: Author.

Cook, A., Blaustein, M., Spinazzola, J., & van der Kolk, B. (Eds.) (2003). *Complex trauma in children and adolescents*. Los Angeles and Durham, NC: National Child Traumatic Stress Network.

Cowen, E., Hightower, A., Pedro-Carroll, J., Work, W., Wyman, P., & Haffey, W. (1996). *School-based prevention for children at risk: The primary mental health project*. Washington, DC: American Psychological Association.

Cross, T., Bazron, B., Dennis, K., & Isaacs, M.R. (1989). *Towards a culturally competent system of care*. Washington, DC: Georgetown University Child Development Center.

Davis, N.J. (2002). The promotion of mental health and the prevention of mental and behavioral disorders: Surely the time is right. *International Journal of Emergency Behavioral Health, 4*, 3–29.

Donahue, P. (2002). Promoting social and emotional development in young children: The role of mental health consultants in early childhood settings. In *Kauffman Early Education Exchange* (Vol. 1, pp. 64–79). Kansas City, MO: Ewing Marion Kauffman Foundation.

Eber, L., Osuch, R., & Redditt, C. (1996). School-based applications of the wraparound process: Early results on service provision and student outcomes. *Journal of Child and Family Studies, 5*, 83–99.

Elliott, D.S., Hamburg, B.A., & Williams, K.R. (1998). *Violence in American schools: A new perspective*. Cambridge, UK: Cambridge University Press.

Eyberg, S., Funderbunk, B., Hembree-Kigin, T., McNeil, C., Querido, J., & Hood, K. (2001). Parent–child interaction therapy: One- and two-year maintenance of treatment effects in the family. *Child and Family Behavior Therapy, 23*(4), 1–20.

Ferlie, E., & Shortell, S.M. (2001). Improving the quality of health care in the United Kingdom and the United States: A framework for change. *The Millbank Quarterly, 79*(2), 281–316.

Firestone, B. (1990). Information packet on use of mental health services by children and adolescents. Rockville, MD: Center for Mental Health Services Survey and Analysis Branch.

Friedman, R.M. (1993). Preparation of students to work with children and families: Is it meeting the need? *Administration and Policy in Mental Health, 20,* 297–310.

Friedman, R.M. (2001a). *A conceptual framework for developing and implementing effective policy in children's mental health.* Tampa: University of South Florida, Research and Training Center for Children's Mental Health.

Friedman, R.M. (2001b). The practice of psychology with children, adolescents, and their families: A look to the future. In J.N. Hughes, A.M. LaGreca, & J.C. Conoley (Eds.), *Handbook of psychological services for children and adolescents* (pp. 3–22). New York: Oxford University Press.

Friedman, R.M. (2003, August). *Direction for the future: Developing data-based and value-based systems of care that incorporate effective practice.* Paper presented at the meeting on Evidence-Based Practice in Children's Mental Health, National Association of State Mental Health Program Directors, Fort Lauderdale, FL.

Friedman, R.M., & Hernandez, M. (2002). The national evaluation of the Comprehensive Community Mental Health Services for Children and Their Families Program: A commentary. *Children's Services: Social Policy, Research, and Practice, 5*(1), 67–74.

Friedman, R.M., Kutash, K., & Duchnowski, A.J. (1996). The population of concern: Defining the issues. In B.A. Stroul & R.M. Friedman (Series Eds.) & B.A. Stroul (Vol. Ed.), *Systems of care for children's mental health series: Children's mental health: Creating systems of care in a changing society* (pp. 69–80). Baltimore: Paul H. Brookes Publishing Co.

Friedman, R., & Simmons, D. (in press). Prevalence of social, emotional, and mental disorders in the juvenile justice population. In J. Cocozza & K. Skowyra (Eds.), *The mental health needs of juvenile offenders: A comprehensive review.* Washington, DC: Office of Juvenile Justice and Delinquency Prevention.

Garland, A.F., Hough, R.L., McCabe, K.M., Yeh, M., Wood, P., & Arons, G. (2001). Prevalence of psychiatric disorders in youth across five sectors of care. *Journal of the American Academy of Child and Adolescent Psychiatry, 40,* 409–418.

Georgetown University National Technical Assistance Center for Children's Mental Health. (1999). *Types of policy strategies to modify service systems for children and their families.* Annapolis, MD: Author.

Giliberti, M., & Schulzinger, R. (2000). *Relinquishing custody: The tragic result of failure to meet children's mental health needs.* Washington, DC: Bazelon Center for Mental Health Law.

Goldman, S.K. (1999). The conceptual framework for wraparound. In B.J. Burns & S.K. Goldman (Eds.), *Systems of care: Promising practices in wraparound for children with serious emotional disturbance and their families* (pp. 9–16). Rockville, MD: Substance Abuse and Mental Health Services Administration.

Greenberg, M., Domitrovich, C., & Bumbarger, B. (2001). The prevention of mental disorders in school-aged children: Current state of the field. *Prevention and Treatment, 4*(5) [electronic journal]. Retrieved January 12, 2005, from http://journals.apa.org/prevention/volume4/pre0040001a.html

Hayes, C. (2002). *Thinking broadly: Financing strategies for comprehensive child and family initiatives.* Washington, DC: The Finance Project.

Health Insurance Portability and Accountability Act (HIPAA) of 1996, PL 104-191, 42 U.S.C. §§ 201 *et seq.*

Hernandez, M., & Hodges, S. (Vol. Eds.). (2001). *Systems of care in children's mental health series: Developing outcome strategies in children's mental health.* Baltimore: Paul H. Brookes Publishing Co.

Hernandez, M., & Isaacs, M. (Vol. Eds.). (1998). *Systems of care in children's mental health series: Promoting cultural competence in children's mental health services.* Baltimore: Paul H. Brookes Publishing Co.

Hoagwood, K., & Erwin, H. (1997). Effectiveness of school-based mental health services for children: A 10-year research review. *Journal of Child and Family Studies, 6(4),* 435–451.

Horner, R.H., & Carr, E.G. (1997). Behavioral support for students with severe disabilities: Functional assessment and comprehensive intervention. *Journal of Special Education, 31,* 84–104.

Huang, L.N., Freed, R., & Espiritu, R.C. (2006). Co-occurring disorders of adolescents in primary care: Closing the gaps. *Adolescent Medicine, 17,* 453–467.

Huang, L.N., Stroul, B., Friedman, R., Mrazek, P., et al. (2005). Transforming mental health care for children and their families. *American Psychologist, 60,* 615–627.

Individuals with Disabilities Education Act Amendments (IDEA) of 1997, PL 105-17, 20 U.S.C. §§ 1400 *et seq.*

Institute of Medicine. (2001). *Crossing the quality chasm: A new health system for the 21st century.* Washington, DC: National Academies Press.

Institute of Medicine. (2006). *Improving the quality of health care for mental and substance-use disorders.* Washington, DC: National Academies Press.

Jamieson, A., Curry, A., & Martinez, G. (2001). *School enrollment in the United States: Social and economic characteristics for students. October, 1999* (Report No. P20533). Washington, DC: Bureau of the Census.

Jennings, J., Pearson, G., & Harris, M. (2000). Implementing and maintaining school-based mental health services in a large, urban school district. *Journal of School Health, 70,* 201–205.

Jensen, P. (2001, November). *Indicators and early identification in children's mental health: Identifying acceptable indicators.* Paper presented at the 17th Annual Rosalyn Carter Symposium on Mental Health Policy, Carter Center, Atlanta, GA.

Kamradt, B.J. (2000). Wraparound Milwaukee: Aiding youth with mental health needs. *Juvenile Justice Journal, 7(1),* 19–26.

Kaye, N. (2006). *Improving the delivery of health care that supports young children's healthy mental development: Early accomplishments and lessons learned from a five-state consortium.* Portland, ME: National Academy for State Health Policy.

Kelleher, K. (2000). Primary care and identification of mental health needs. *Report of the Surgeon General's Conference on Children's Mental Health: A national action agenda.* Washington, DC: U.S. Public Health Service.

Kessler, R., Berglund, P., Demler, O., et al. (2005). Lifetime prevalence and age-of-onset distributions of DSM-IV disorders in the National Comorbidity Survey Replication. *Archives General Psychiatry, 62,* 593–602.

Knitzer, J., & Yelton, S. (1990). Collaboration between child welfare and mental health. *Public Welfare, 2,* 24–34.

Koyanagi, C., Boudreaux, R., & Lind, E. (2003). *Mix and match: Using federal programs to support interagency systems of care for children with mental health care needs.* Washington, DC: Bazelon Center for Mental Health Law.

Last, J.M., & Wallace, R.B. (Eds.). (1992). *Maxcy-Rosenau-Last Public Health and Preventive Medicine* (13th ed.). Norwalk, CT: Appleton and Lange.

Lavigne, J.V., Gibbons, R.D., Christoffel, K.K., Arend, R., Rosenbaum, D., et al. (1996). Prevalence rates and correlates of psychiatric disorders among preschool children. *Journal of the American Academy of Child and Adolescent Psychiatry, 35,* 205–214.

Leaf, P.J., Alegria, M., Cohen, P., Goodman, S., et al. (1996). Mental health service use in the community and schools: Results from the four-community MECA study. *Journal of the American Academy of Child and Adolescent Psychiatry, 35(7),* 889–897.

Lezak, A., & Macbeth, G. (Eds.). (2002). *Overcoming barriers to serving our children in the community.* Rockville, MD: U.S. Department of Health and Human Services.

Longest, B.B., Jr. (1998). *Health policy making in the United States.* Chicago: Health Administration Press.

Lourie, I.S., Katz-Leavy, J., & Stroul, B.A. (1996). Individualized services in a system of care. In B.A. Stroul & R.M. Friedman (Vol. Eds.) & B.A. Stroul (Series Ed.), *Systems of care for children's mental health series: Children's mental health: Creating systems of care in a changing society* (pp. 429–452). Baltimore: Paul H. Brookes Publishing Co.

Lyons, J., Baerger, D., Quigley, J., & Griffin, E. (2001). Mental health service needs of juvenile offenders: A comparison of detention, incarceration, and treatment settings. *Children's Services: Social Policy, Research, and Practice, 4*(2), 69–85.

Mark, T.L., & Buck, J.A. (2006). Characteristics of U.S. youths with serious emotional disturbance: Data from the national health interview survey. *Psychiatric Services, 57*(11), 1573–1578.

McCammon, S., Spencer, S., & Friesen, B. (2001). Promoting family empowerment through multiple roles. *Journal of Family Social Work, 5*(3), 1–24.

McGonaughy, S., & Skiba, R. (1993). Comorbidity of externalizing and internalizing problems. *School Psychology Review, 22,* 421–436.

Morris, J.A, & Hanley, J.H. (2001). Human resource development: A critical gap in child mental health reform. *Administration and Policy in Mental Health, 28*(3), 219–227.

Mrazek, P.J. (2002). *Enhancing the well-being of America's children through the strengthening of natural and community supports: Opportunities for prevention and early mental health intervention.* Paper prepared for the Subcommittee on Children and Families, President's New Freedom Commission on Mental Health, Washington, DC.

Mrazek, P.J., & Haggerty, R.J. (Eds.). (1994). *Reducing risks for mental disorders: Frontiers for preventive intervention research.* Washington, DC: National Academies Press.

Myers, M., Brown, S., & Mott, M. (1995). Preadolescent conduct disorder behaviors predict relapse and progression of addiction for adolescent alcohol and drug abusers. *Alcohol Clinical Experimental Research, 19,* 1528–1536.

Olds, D., Henderson, C., Cole, R., Eckenrode, J., Kitzman, H., Luckey, D., et al. (1998). Long-term effects of nurse home visitation on children's criminal and antisocial behavior. Fifteen-year follow-up of a randomized controlled trial. *Journal of the American Medical Association, 280*(14), 1238–1244.

Olmstead v. L.C., 527 U.S. 581 (1999).

Osher, T.W. (1998). Outcomes and accountability from a family perspective. *Journal of Behavioral Health Services and Research, 25*(2), 230–232.

President's New Freedom Commission on Mental Health. (2003). *Achieving the promise: Transforming mental health care in America. Final report.* Rockville, MD: U.S. Department of Health and Human Services.

Ramey, C., & Ramey, S. (1998). Prevention of intellectual disabilities: Early interventions to improve cognitive development. *Preventive Medicine, 27*(2), 224–232.

Ringeisen, H., Henderson, K., & Hoagwood, K. (2003). Context matters: Schools and the "research to practice gap" in children's mental health. *School Psychology Review, 32*(2), 153–168.

Ringel, J., & Sturm, R. (2001). National estimates of mental health utilization and expenditure for children in 1998. *Journal of Behavioral Health Services and Research, 28*(3), 319–332.

Rosman, E.A., Perry, D.F., & Hepburn, K.S. (2005). *The best beginning: Partnerships between primary health care and mental health and substance abuse services for young children and their families.* Washington, DC: Georgetown University National Technical Assistance Center for Children's Mental Health.

Rugs, D., & Kutash, K. (1994). Evaluating children's mental health service systems: An analysis of critical behaviors and events. *Journal of Child and Family Studies, 3*(3), 249–262.

Sabin, J., & Daniels, N. (1999). Public-sector managed behavioral health care: III. Meaningful consumer and family participation. *Psychiatric Services, 50*(7), 883–885.

Shaffer, D., Fisher, P., Dulcan, M., et al. (1996). The NIMH Diagnostic Interview Schedule for Children Version 2.3 (DISC-2.3): Description, acceptability, prevalence rates, and performance in the MECA study. *Journal of the American Academy of Child and Adolescent Psychiatry, 35*, 865–877.

Shirk, S.R. (2001). The road to effective child psychological services: Treatment processes and outcome research. In J.H. Hughes, A.M. LaGreca, & J.C. Conoley (Eds.), *Handbook of psychological services for children and adolescents* (pp. 43–59). New York: Oxford University Press.

Shonkoff, J., & Phillips, D. (2000). *From neurons to neighborhoods: The science of early childhood development.* Washington, DC: National Academies Press.

Silver, S.E., Duchnowski, A.J., Kutash, K., Friedman, R.M., Eisen, M., Prange, M.E., et al. (1992). A comparison of children with serious emotional disturbance served in residential and school settings. *Journal of Child and Family Studies, 1*(1), 43–59.

Spinazzola, J., Ford, J., van der Kolk, B., et al. (2003). *Complex trauma in the National Child Traumatic Stress Network.* Paper presented at the 19th Annual Meeting of the International Society for Traumatic Stress Studies, Chicago.

Stroul, B.A. (2002). *Issue brief—Systems of care: A framework for system reform in children's mental health.* Washington, DC: Georgetown University Child Development Center, National Technical Assistance for Children's Mental Health.

Stroul, B.A. (2007). *Integrating mental health services into primary care settings—Summary of special forum held at the 2006 Georgetown University Training Institutes.* Washington, DC: Georgetown University Center for Child and Human Development, National Technical Assistance for Children's Mental Health.

Stroul, B.A., & Friedman, R.M. (1996). The system of care concept and philosophy. In B.A. Stroul & R.M. Friedman (Series Eds.) & B.A. Stroul (Vol. Ed.), *Systems of care for children's mental health series: Children's mental health: Creating systems of care in a changing society* (pp. 3–22). Baltimore: Paul H. Brookes Publishing Co.

Stroul, B.A., Pires, S.A., & Armstrong, M.I. (2001). *Health care reform tracking project: Tracking state managed care reforms as they affect children and adolescents with behavioral health disorders and their families.* Tampa: University of South Florida, Research and Training Center for Children's Mental Health.

Sturm, R., Ringel, J., Bao, C., Stein, B., Kapur, K., Zhang, W., et al. (2001). National estimates of mental health utilization and expenditures for children in 1998. In National Advisory Mental Health Council Workgroup on Child and Adolescent Mental Health Intervention Development and Deployment, *Blueprint for change: Research on child and adolescent mental health* (p. 93). Rockville, MD: National Institute of Mental Health.

Sugai, G., Horner, R.H., Dunlap, G., Hieneman, M., Lewis, T.J., Nelson, C.M., et al. (2000). Applying positive behavior support and functional behavior assessment in schools. *Journal of Positive Behavior Interventions, 2*, 131–143.

Teplin, L.A. (2002). *Psychiatric disorders in youth in juvenile detention.* Paper presented at the 15th Annual Research Conference, a System of Care for Children's Mental Health: Expanding the Research Base, University of South Florida, Tampa.

Turner, W., Muck, R., et al. (2004). Co-occurring disorders in the adolescent mental health and substance abuse treatment systems. *Journal of Psychiatric Drugs, 36*, 451–461.

U.S. Department of Education. (2001). *Twenty-third annual report to Congress on the implementation of the Individuals with Disabilities Education Act: Results.* Washington, DC: Author.

U.S. Department of Health and Human Services. (1999a). *Healthy people 2010.* Washington, DC: U.S. Public Health Service.

U.S. Department of Health and Human Services. (1999b). *Mental health: A report of the Surgeon General.* Rockville, MD: U.S. Public Health Service.

U.S. Department of Health and Human Services. (2001). *Mental health: Culture, race, and ethnicity. A supplement to mental health: A report of the Surgeon General.* Rockville, MD: U.S. Public Health Service.

U.S. Department of Health and Human Services. (2002). *Report to Congress on the preven-tion and treatment of co-occurring substance abuse disorders and mental disorders*, Rockville, MD: Substance Abuse and Mental Health Services Administration.

U.S. Public Health Service. (2000). *Report of the Surgeon General's conference on children's mental health: A national action agenda*. Washington, DC: Author.

Usher, C.L., Gibbs, D.A., & Wildfire, J.B. (1995). A framework for planning, implement-ing, and evaluating child welfare reforms. *Child Welfare, 74*, 859–876.

VanDenBerg, J. (1999). History of the wraparound process. In B.J. Burns & S.K. Gold-man (Eds.), *Promising practices in wraparound for children with serious emotional distur-bance and their families* (pp. 1–6). Washington, DC: Center for Effective Collaboration and Practice, American Institutes for Research.

VanDenBerg, J., & Grealish, M. (1996). Individualized services and supports through the wraparound process: Philosophy and procedures. *Journal of Child and Family Studies, 5*, 7–21.

Weisz, J., Sandler, I., Durlak, J., & Anton, B. (2005). Promoting and processing youth mental health through evidence-based prevention and treatment. *American Psychologist, 60*(6), 628–648.

Wilens, T., Biederman, J., Spencer, T., et al. (1994). Comorbidity of attention-deficit dis-order and psychoactive substance use disorders. *Hospital Community Psychiatry, 45*, 421–435.

Wishmann, A., Kates, K., & Kaufmann, R. (2001). *Funding early childhood mental health services and supports*. Rockville, MD: Substance Abuse and Mental Health Services Ad-ministration.

World Health Organization. (2001). *The world health report 2001: Mental health: New understanding, new hope*. Geneva: Author.

Yanos, P.T., Primavera, L.H., & Knight, E.L. (2001). Consumer-run service participation, recovery of social functioning, and the mediating role of psychological factors. *Psychi-atric Services, 52*(4), 493–500.

26

Research and Evaluation Implications

Using Research and Evaluation to Strengthen Systems of Care

ROBERT M. FRIEDMAN AND NATHANIEL ISRAEL

San Aggra County is a semi-rural American county. It is a large county land-wise, and has one mid-sized city (population 75,000), where much of the population resides. The remaining residents live in sparsely populated frontier areas, interspersed with small towns. The county is slowly losing its population, and hence its tax base, to Metroplex, a large city (population 750,000) approximately 90 miles away. Although many multigenerational families have been leaving the county, the Latino population in San Aggra has grown substantially since the 1990s. Proportionately, there are fewer young families in San Aggra than there were 10 years ago, but this trend is largely being offset as younger Latino families continue to settle there.

In San Aggra, service providers in the mental health and child welfare sectors depend heavily on Medicaid dollars to fund services. The state recently introduced privatized managed care into the public children's service system, so private companies now contract out many of the mental health and child welfare services formerly provided by the public system.

Relationships among providers are collegial, but there is the sense that certain sectors and agencies are privileged over others. More dollars have been allocated for spending on juvenile justice, while the child welfare system's budget has been cut. In addition, school administrators, although concerned about a few children's behavior problems in class, have stopped providing in-school mental health services in order to focus their resources on improving students' standardized test scores. The recent introduction of privatized managed mental health care has reduced the number of therapy sessions that children in the public mental health sector are able to receive. With all of these changes, there is a general sense that resources are tight and that professionals have to work around the formal system in order to get adequate resources for families with children with mental health concerns.

There are several interagency councils that meet on a regular basis in San Aggra County to discuss children's issues. The meetings typically are congenial and collegial, but they have not resulted in the development of any comprehensive plans or the creation of any new programs. There was an effort to create an interagency staffing process for children who are involved with multiple service sectors and represent an especially serious challenge. This has more or less faded away as attendance grew erratic.

There is a local chapter of a nationally based parent advocacy organization that provides valuable educational and support services for families. Representatives of this organization participate in interagency council meetings, and they have become more outspoken over time. This has generated a very favorable response from several members of the councils, but the response has been less favorable from others, particularly providers.

When the director of the children's public mental health system found that there was an opportunity to apply to the Center for Mental Health Services for a grant to establish a system of care for children with serious mental health challenges and their families, she quickly realized that it could bring critical service dollars into the community. With the help of an outside consultant, she cowrote the grant, gathering input from friends and colleagues in other systems, primarily the child welfare system. When the community received the grant a year later, there was an undercurrent of both surprise and relief; service dollars had been found, and the system would be shored up! Stakeholders set about convening a board to decide how to fund their services while keeping to the requirements of the grant.

The preceding vignette provides one brief example of a children's mental health service delivery system and the community context in which it operates. Such systems are based in diverse communities, serve different populations, have unique goals and resources, are based on varying values and conceptual frameworks, and are composed of many different parts—some resulting from careful planning and others resulting from the self-organization of independent agents. Furthermore, these parts each have multiple connections, and virtually every component, as well as the overall context, is dynamic, changing in both predictable and unpredictable ways.

The very complexity of these systems creates great challenges for those who wish to systematically study them. Examiners must go beyond traditional research and evaluation methods and approaches. This chapter examines the complexity of systems of care and offers suggestions for conducting research and evaluation.

As Patton pointed out in a 1980 discussion of different research models, "The debate and competition between paradigms is being replaced by a new paradigm—a paradigm of choices. The paradigm of choices recognizes that different methods are appropriate for different situations" (pp. 19–20). This chapter is based on the premise that the situation of concern is how to study complex systems, such as systems of care, and how to gather data that can be used to improve them.

GOALS AND QUESTIONS

As part of the context, it is important to offer an overall goal for the systems of care that are being studied. The overall goal, consistent with the recommendation of the Transformation Work Group of the Child, Adolescent, and Family Branch of the Center for Mental Health Services (2005), is to provide access to effective care for all children with mental health challenges and their families in accordance with system of care values and principles. The particular challenge at the system level is to provide the needed resources, infrastructure, and policies to achieve this goal, and to align them with recommended practice to ensure that access to effective care is achieved, which results in positive outcomes for children and families.

Given this overall goal and the role of the system level, it is suggested that there are three main questions for research and evaluation to address:

1. How well are systems of care achieving their desired goals? Furthermore, are there particular areas that have been successful and others in need of improvement? For example, are systems of care providing effective services for those families who actually receive services, but not providing access to care for the overall population? Are they providing access to effective care for one group of children and families but not for others?

2. How might we improve performance, both within systems of care in individual communities and nationally? How can systems of care do a better job at achieving their goals?

3. How effective are systems of care overall?

The third question has occupied considerable attention in the field (Bickman et al., 1995; Bickman, Noser, & Summerfelt, 1999; Brannan, Baughman, Reed, & Katz-Leavy, 2002; Holden, Friedman, & Santiago, 2001; Rosenblatt, 1998; Stroul, 1993). It is not the purpose of this chapter to review the research findings on this question. In fact, the point has been made that, for several reasons, the children's mental health system of care field needs to move beyond this question to focus more on the first two questions (Friedman, 2007). There will always be service delivery systems. Services cannot exist in the absence of a system that provides policies, resources, and regulatory mechanisms. This is true not only for children's mental health but also for all educational and human services.

Furthermore, there appears to be widespread agreement at the federal and state levels that system of care values and principles should be the foundation for service delivery systems. This has been reflected in the report of the President's New Freedom Commission on Mental Health (2003), in special reports done by states (Friedman, 2002), and in most states' legislative and executive branch policies (Evans & Armstrong, 2003). The disappointment and frustration in children's mental health has to do with the challenge of implementing effective systems, not with the values that serve as their foundation.

Given the inevitability that services will be embedded in a system, as well as the widespread agreement on system of care values and principles, the key questions become how well are we doing in a particular community, group of communities, or state and how can we do better. The issue of the overall effectiveness of a general concept called *systems of care* is of less relevance than the issue of doing the best job possible of serving children and families in various communities.

The mental health care system is very much like other fields, such as education or business. Although educators may be interested in a general way in how well the educational system is doing nationally and may learn some valuable lessons from looking elsewhere, their primary concern is how they can do a better job at educating the children in their community. In business, the question is not how well is the economy doing overall, or how well competitors' businesses are doing, but "How can this business be as successful as possible?"

It should be noted that there are many separate components within systems of care. Some of these are at the practice level, some are at the organizational level, and some are at the system level. Research and evaluation can make important contributions to understanding how these components are functioning. This, however, is not the primary focus of this chapter. This chapter does not review research and evaluation methods for studying particular clinical interventions, nor does it examine research findings on particular practice-, organizational-, or system-level interventions. Rather, the focus is on the entire system of care.

Langhout (2003) distinguished between what she calls *particularistic* or *specific* research versus more *holistic* or *pattern-focused* research. Particularistic research, according to this formulation, involves more microlevel studies of well-described independent variables. Holistic, or pattern-focused, research is more macro in its approach, and particularly looks at the connections between different components, the context in which the study takes place, and the pattern of relationships that emerge. The latter type of research is examined here, not because the other research is not valuable, but because of the relevance of more pattern-focused research to the topic at hand—how to study and improve complex systems.

One type of research with particular relevance to the second question is called *action research*. It has its origins in the 1940s with a social psychologist named Kurt Lewin. The title comes from linking the action to solve the problem with the research. The research is highly contextualized within the particular organization or system that has the problem, and the process of study is cyclical, involving a "nonlinear pattern of planning, acting, observing, and reflecting on the changes in the social situations" (Noffke & Stevenson, 1995, p. 2). Although the term *action research* is not used frequently in the children's mental health field, efforts at data-based decision making in which the problem is studied in the organizational or system context in which it takes place, and in which data are used for purposes of improvement, bear great similarity to Lewin's action research.

The national evaluation of the system of care grant program of the Center for Mental Health Services has placed an increased focus on continuous quality improvement procedures. A protocol for gathering such data has been collected in a participatory manner, and data collection is currently underway. Early indications are that, in some communities, these data, which can be used to make comparisons across time and with other communities, are proving to be very useful.

It should be noted as well that there is an increasing trend in human services to systematically and routinely gather various types of information on system performance (Barwick & Ferguson, 2007; Green, 2001; Hodges, Woodbridge, & Huang, 2001). These data are then used as part of what is sometimes called an *internal evaluation* or *performance measurement* process, also intended for the purpose of ongoing system improvement. There are many different terms being used to describe similar processes, but the key point is the importance of gathering practical information on a regular basis to help strengthen the functioning of the overall system, organization, or program.

FOUNDATION FOR RESEARCH AND EVALUATION IN SYSTEMS OF CARE

In addition to clarity about goals, it is suggested that a three-part foundation for research and evaluation in systems of care comprising values and principles, conceptual framework for systems, and theory of change should be established to maximize the impact.

Values and Principles

The values and principles that serve as a foundation for systems of care, originating with the monograph that first laid out a general blueprint for such systems (Stroul & Friedman, 1986), have been described throughout this book. The important point is that they should serve as a foundation not only for system development but also for research and evaluation. For example, if the values and principles emphasize a family-driven system, families should be involved in developing the research or evaluation agenda and methods, as well as helping to interpret the results. The field of participatory action research has been particularly clear about emphasizing this aspect of systems of care (McTaggart, 1991; Turnbull, Friesen, & Ramirez, 1998; Whyte, 1991). Similarly, cultural competence is critical to service and system development, and thus it is also critical to research and evaluation. If the principle of tailoring services to build on the strengths and meet the needs of each individual is basic to systems of care, should it not be incorporated into research and evaluation?

This is not to suggest that researchers and evaluators do not possess specialized technical knowledge. Clearly they do, and this knowledge must be capitalized on. It can, however, be done in a participatory, collaborative way that is consistent with system of care values and principles, or it can be done in an expert-driven, top-down way that is inconsistent with system of care values and principles.

A particular challenge is presented for evaluations of multisite programs. Although system of care values and principles emphasize the importance of community-driven evaluations, the funding source for a multisite evaluation, for understandable reasons, often seeks to have data on cross-site performance of an intervention. Community-level input may be sought and obtained at the stage of developing the evaluation, and this is very helpful in the process. Typically, however, the data collection requirements for the evaluation emerge through a hierarchical process. The impact of this deviation of evaluation methods from system of care values clearly needs to be studied. The risks are that it may result in the use of measures or data collection procedures that are inappropriate for particular communities (Granger, 1998), that there will be community resistance to participating in the process, or that the evaluation will inadvertently work against conveying a message of community ownership. The evaluation may not be neutral in this regard. Its very existence in a manner that is inconsistent with system of care values and principles may adversely affect the success of the intervention because it works against communities that perceive themselves to be in the driver's seat for the initiative. Although not always the case, multisite national evaluations may result in communities failing to gather data of great local relevance because they are too busy focusing on data for a multisite evaluation.

It is noteworthy in this regard to point out that in a study of successful comprehensive community initiatives conducted for the Department of Health and Human Services, it was found that, in many instances, the initiative started at a grass roots level in response to a local need, and that local leaders specifically refused external funding in the early stages so that they could clearly continue following their own agenda and methods (Gray, Duran, & Segal, 1997).

Conceptual Framework

In traditional research and evaluation designed to study interventions, the intervention essentially serves as the independent variable, and it is hypothesized that if it is effective, it will result in a change in one or more outcome measures or dependent variables. In traditional research, it is important that the characteristics of the independent variable be clearly and thoroughly specified, that they be measured in objective terms, and that they be static. Under such conditions, it then becomes possible for the intervention to be replicated.

Such is a model—often used in research on interventions at the child and family level—where dosages of medications may be spelled out clearly and perhaps medication algorithms as well, or where detailed and thorough treatment manuals are used to ensure that interventions are applied with fidelity. Through such careful specification of the independent variable, it is hoped that generalizable knowledge (i.e., knowledge not dependent on context) will be developed.

Although the merits of this argument can be debated for interventions at the child and family level, there clearly are problems with this approach for studying interventions at the community system level. As pointed out with the vignette, such interventions are multifaceted, evolving, difficult to measure, and dynamic. In fact, the very concept of a system implies that the whole is greater than the sum of its parts, and the interconnections are often as important as the components. As described in Chapter 3, both systems' dynamic modeling and complexity theory emphasize the fact that a characteristic of such systems is that the relationships between actions and outcomes are often nonlinear and hard to predict.

In her article entitled "Dancing with Systems," Meadows (1999) pointed out that, "Self-organizing, nonlinear, feedback systems are inherently unpredictable. They are not controllable. They are understandable only in the most general way. The goal of foreseeing the future exactly and preparing for it perfectly is unrealizable" (p. 1). Similarly, in discussing the dynamic nature of interventions, Patton (1994) indicated that program designers:

> Never expect to arrive at a steady state of programming because they're constantly tinkering as participants, conditions, learnings, and context change. They don't aspire to arrive at a model subject to summative evaluation and generalization. Rather, they aspire to continuous progress, ongoing adaptation, and rapid responsiveness . . . they assume a world of multiple causes, diversity of outcomes, inconsistency of interventions, interactive effects at every level—and they find such a world exciting and desirable. (1994, p. 313)

Based on contributions from the fields of organizational development, systems dynamic modeling, and complexity theory, there are some concepts that, when taken together, offer an alternative model to that of a static, measurable independent variable related in linear ways to a dependent variable. This alternative model emphasizes that:

- Systems are iterative, evolving, changing, dynamic, and always emerging.

- Systems typically involve feedback loops—some by design and some not—and may include adjustments based on the feedback.

- An understanding of systems requires an understanding of not only the individual components, but also of the relationships, connections, and integrative mechanisms among agents.

- Systems are affected by contextual issues that frequently change.

- Causal relationships are often nonlinear and complex.

- Within complex systems, a key to understanding is studying recurring patterns and identifying implicit and explicit rules.

- Values, principles, goals, and culture are often the key to what happens.

- There is no one objective system. The rules, policies, connections, values, and culture may look different to various agents. Thus, the system exists in the eye of the beholder.

Such a conceptual framework for a system that varies so dramatically from a traditional research framework has important implications for how research and evaluation is conducted. In a traditional model, periodic changes in the way in which the system operates may present a major challenge to clearly measuring and specifying the intervention. From a perspective of complexity theory and complex adaptive systems, such changes may not only be inevitable, but they may represent positive adaptations. Rather than being a challenge that may compromise the experimental design, they may be the essence of system or organizational development and may contribute to its success. Efforts to maintain the independent variable as a static phenomenon may create a major obstacle to success.

Theories of Change

The concept of a theory of change is one of the integrative mechanisms within a system (Hernandez & Hodges, 2003a, 2003b; Weiss, 1995). It specifies the population of concern, the desired outcomes, and the methods for trying to successfully achieve the outcomes for the population of concern. It is intended to be created in a participatory way including many stakeholders, consistent with system of care values and principles.

A theory of change provides an important starting point for research and evaluation efforts. Often, researchers and evaluators either participate in the development of the theory or ask questions that are designed to help clarify it. This serves as an important mechanism for focusing the attention of the researcher and evaluator. If the theory of change says that a key process within a system is the development of individualized, strength-based, culturally competent treatment plans that are regularly reviewed and modified, then this may become a major focus of the evaluation efforts. If a theory of change indicates that strong collaboration between different service sectors is essential to success, then presumably an evaluation would study the development, maintenance, and periodic change in the relationships between the potential partners.

If the theory of change says that important activities consistent with complex adaptive systems are to promote connections between key agents, to support efforts by these agents to self-organize, and to prepare to take advantage of unanticipated opportunities that may arise, then these activities become important aspects of the data collection. If change and adaptation brought about through a periodic reflective process based on performance data is part of the theory of change, then this becomes a focus for the research and evaluation.

The essential point is that the process of developing a theory of change helps stakeholders clarify the goals they are trying to achieve and what they think it may take to achieve that. It also helps researchers focus their efforts. If the goal of the data collection is to improve the system, as in utilization-focused evaluation (Patton, 1997), rather than to reach general conclusions about whether systems of care work overall, then the observations and findings of the evaluation team can be regularly funneled to the system stakeholders for the purpose of strengthening the system.

Theories of change that are developed in communities as they initiate a system change effort help clarify goals and strategies. It is essential, however, that such theories not become static documents that fail to account for changes that take place (Granger, 1998). Part of the challenge for systems of care is to deal with transitions—both expected and unexpected—within a community system. These can be due to changes in personnel, budget, particular service sectors, and policies at the state or federal level, as well as media attention, desired or otherwise. Although these changes may not affect the goals of the initiative, they may very well affect the strategies developed to reach those goals.

It is also important that theories of change reflect the multiple levels involved in a system of care and show the relationships among them. The idea that changes at one level of a system (e.g., the system level) will directly affect another level (e.g., the practice level) needs to be examined closely within a system of care. If it is anticipated that a change at the policy level will affect the practice level, thereby resulting in better child and family outcomes, then the chain of logic behind this reasoning must be explained. Although policies designed to improve collaboration among different service sectors may have a number of benefits, within a theory of change process, community stakeholders may be challenged to explain why they believe that policy-level change will result in changes at the practice level or with child and family outcomes. Indeed, the growing field of implementation suggests that policy-level change is not sufficient to create behavioral change among frontline practitioners who are charged with implementing the policy. Rather, consistent and ongoing coaching, modeling, and feedback are required to create enduring system and behavioral change at the practice level (Fixsen, Naoom, Blase, Friedman, & Wallace, 2005).

The type of evaluation that is proposed for systems of care is designed to provide important data on a regular, ongoing basis in order to understand how well a local system of care is doing in relation to its desired outcomes and its theory of change. The purpose is to facilitate data-based decision making for purposes of system improvement in real time as the system develops. This contrasts with more summative evaluations in which the purpose is to assess the overall effectiveness of an intervention in achieving its goals after a period of time has elapsed. Summative evaluations to determine whether something works can be helpful, and these are certainly needed in some instances, but they typically fail to provide timely process information about the usefulness of different system adaptations that are implemented in response to changes in local conditions or data indicating inadequate performance in particular areas (for a related argument, see Lipsey, 1993). Because summative evaluations do not provide practical, timely, actionable information, they often end up as reports that get placed on bookcases and are never used (Patton, 1997).

IMPLICATIONS AND EXAMPLES

The first implication of this approach is that there should be clarity about the purpose of a research or evaluation effort. As suggested, the development of generalizable knowledge is an important purpose for research, but the main purpose of research and evaluation within communities seeking to develop as effective a system as possible is to gather information that will be of help in the system's development and ongoing improvement. As important as the development of generalizable knowledge may be, the purpose of a public human services system is to provide effective services for the identified local population of concern, and thus all evaluation efforts should be aligned with that purpose.

The evaluation efforts in turn should be consistent with system of care values and principles, the conceptual framework for the system development effort, and the theory of change. Selected research and evaluation methods should be consistent with these entities and also feasible and of practical use. This section describes some methods that can be used in carrying out this type of research and evaluation. It should be noted that there are other references that describe approaches that can be used for conducting children's mental health services research that are more geared toward establishing generalizable knowledge (e.g., Reich & Bickman, 2005).

Assessing the Fidelity of Practice with System of Care Values and Principles

Hernandez, Vergon, and Mayo (Chapter 13) discussed the development of an instrument to assess direct practice in systems of care. The System of Care Practice Review (SOCPR) is based on the view that the best indicator of whether a community is operationalizing system of care values and principles comes from the feedback provided by those individuals who are served by the system. By examining how youth and families are served, one can get an overall sense of how well the system is functioning.

This approach illustrates several of the concepts that have been presented. First, the SOCPR was specifically designed to measure adherence or fidelity to system of care values and principles. With input from many stakeholders, questions were developed that address the degree to which system of care values and principles (e.g., community-based care, cultural competence) were actually implemented in direct services.

Second, although the unit of analysis is an individual family, the procedure captures the viewpoints of multiple participants within each family. Data are gathered through semi-structured, open-ended interviews with 4–5 individuals per family, including a youth (depending on the developmental stage), parent, and care manager, as well as through a review of case records. The selection of multiple informants and the use of open-ended interviews ensure that several voices are heard on the degree to which direct practice is adhering to system of care values and principles. This has proven very useful, as it is not unusual to find that parents and care managers have different perspectives on the degree to which family strengths were incorporated in a treatment plan or the degree to which families were afforded choice of services or providers.

Third, the SOCPR incorporates both qualitative and quantitative information. The interviews, with their open-ended responses, provide a rich set of qualitative data from multiple perspectives. Trained interviewers then use this information to give overall quantitative ratings of the degree of practitioner fidelity to system of care values and principles.

Fourth, if incorporated as a regular part of a system of care's performance measurement and internal evaluation process, this approach provides practical information regarding the extent to which practice aligns with values on a regular, timely basis. The information may show, for example, that even though collaboration among some service sectors is strong, it may need to be strengthened among others. Alternately, it may show that treatment plans are not adequately incorporating individuals who represent a particular family's natural support system. This information can be used to make specific adaptations to bring system practice in line with system of care values.

Another part of direct practice that has attracted considerable research attention, as well as attention within local theories of change, is the treatment planning process. Research on treatment planning processes has indicated that services that actually take place within communities are inconsistent with either the system of care's own values and principles or recommended practice (Walker, Koroloff, & Schutte, 2003). An instrument, the Wraparound Observation Form, has been developed to assess the treatment planning process through direct observation (Epstein et al., 1998; Epstein et al., 2003). The form has also been modified by others (Davis, Dollard, & Vergon, 2005). Several communities in Arizona, Florida, and North Carolina (Cook, Kilmer, DeRusso, Vishnevsky, & Meyers, 2007; Davis & Dollard, 2004) have invested considerable resources in the study of how this process was being carried out in their jurisdictions. This is another example of identifying an important component of an effective system through a theory of change and analysis of system values, thereby leading to close examination of the methods through research with the goal of developing and maintaining a high-quality treatment planning process. These efforts are consistent with the overall focus on determining the extent to which interventions are applied with fidelity at the practice level.

Tracking Performance of Relevant Outcomes

Information about system performance from measures such as the SOCPR and the Wraparound Observation Form can also be viewed longitudinally. The field of system dynamics suggests that a starting point can be the identification of a small set—perhaps only one—of system relevant outcomes of concern to all major system stakeholders. In the case of systems of care, the use of out-of-home care is an example of an outcome of interest to multiple stakeholder groups. The identification of such a system-level outcome of interest is critical in that it introduces a common metric by which performance across changing programs and policies and systems can be measured. Tracking this indicator over time allows one to see a snapshot of system development over time.

This snapshot can be augmented by a description of critical system events (e.g., changes in policy) listed on the timeline. Thus, on one axis, viewers can see critical system events and adaptations, and on the other axis, they can see the tracking of system performance over time in meeting a commonly desired outcome. The resulting graphic provides a story of system development that draws on the strengths of narrative traditions and the use of quantitative outcome indicators. This method was used to document performance in the Hawaii system of care, as well as events related to their current level of performance (Daleiden, Chorpita, Donkervoert, Arensdorf, & Brogan, 2006). In this way, overall system performance is contextualized and easily communicated to multiple audiences.

This longitudinal tracking of performance in which quantitative data is combined with narrative and contextual information has been used to measure system performance in other contexts. In response to class action lawsuits (e.g., the R.C. lawsuit in Alabama, the Felix lawsuit in Hawaii), systems have developed performance monitoring systems designed to demonstrate to families and to the courts that they are shifting system performance in accordance with statutes and the requirements of settlement agreements (Bazelon Center for Mental Health Law, 1998; Chorpita & Donkervoet, 2005). The focus of the R.C. lawsuit was on improving services and outcomes for children in the foster care system with mental health challenges. *Performance testing*, a procedure developed by Groves (1994) that is similar to the SOCPR, was used on a regular basis to see how the system was functioning at the individual child and family level, as well as how system functioning changed over time. To gather the perspectives of system- and organizational-level stakeholders on system functioning, interviews were conducted with key community informants on a frequent basis. This was presented along with aggregate, quantitative data on such dimensions as the number of children in care, their length of time in care, and their placement types. This combined information had practical value, was useful from an accountability standpoint, and was also helpful in determining when the conditions of the class action lawsuit had been adequately met.

Model Building

Another approach that is consistent with the conceptual framework of systems dynamic modeling and complexity theory is model building. One can take the outcome of interest as a starting point for building a model of how individuals flow through a system and how the diverse activities within the system create system performance.

One quantitative model of system performance is called a Systems Dynamics Model (SDM) (Sterman, 2001). To build an SDM, one starts by defining a system outcome of interest. Relevant stakeholders then describe all the potential decision points or actions that contribute to this particular outcome. For instance, out-of-home care admissions may result from a number of actions. These could include the lack of less intensive levels of care available in specific settings that lead to increasingly serious behavior problems; funding incentives to use out-of-home care; the lack of stakeholder awareness of the availability of other treatment resources; or fear of the consequences of leaving a potentially dangerous child in the community.

Generating such a model, and finding data to populate each proposed contributor to system performance, requires the presence of a diverse group of stakeholders that represent decision makers at each decision point. Synthesizing the input of this group of stakeholders and building a System Dynamics Model are tasks that often allow stakeholders to think about system performance in new ways. Decisions that occur for stakeholders at one level of the system are often poorly understood by stakeholders at another level. Similarly, the process by which decision makers choose to take action is also often poorly understood. Because of this, the gathering and sharing of data about the types of decisions encountered by stakeholders and the rules governing such decisions is often very useful for decision makers at every level of the system. These kinds of models are being used in other public health efforts, such as diabetes prevention and care, and hold great promise for understanding the effects of decision making at multiple levels on system performance for systems of care (Homer & Hirsch, 2006; Jones et al., 2006).

Examining Decision-Making Rules

Models such as Systems Dynamics Models can provide opportunities for the examination and understanding of processes within systems of care, as well as for taking appropriate follow-up action. If, as the model is populated, there are particular points where the flow of children and families through the system is surprising or problematic, follow-up interviews with relevant individuals in the system can be held to try to gain an enhanced understanding of what is transpiring and corrective strategies can be implemented as needed. This interviewing may reveal implicit decision rules that are governing behavior in the system that would otherwise be unknown. It may be that even though a particular service has been set up specifically to help keep families together and avoid an out-of-home placement, it is not being used for those children and families most in need of this type of intervention. Potential referring staff may be operating under an implicit rule of protecting themselves by making referrals of children at risk of committing violent acts for out-of-home care outside of the local community, rather than taking the risk of maintaining a child within his or her community. It may be that referral patterns and flow through the system are being affected by an implicit rule of protecting the reputation of the agency, even if a child and another agency may suffer and despite explicit proclamations of the desire and intention to be collaborative. The combination of modeling with ethnographic interviewing (Agar, 2004) can be particularly helpful in understanding the implicit rules in a system so that they can be addressed and altered while monitoring the effect of such alterations on overall system performance.

As systems of care develop, the decision rules adopted by individuals at each level of the system are intended to more closely align with the philosophy that frames all systems of care. Thus, over time, the probability should decrease that decisions at the administrative, supervisory, or frontline staff levels will encourage the use of services or providers not in synch with system of care values. Given the multitude of policies, organizations, and individuals involved in systems of care, it is anticipated that there will be frequent changes. Focusing on decision-making rules and processes that should be present across all programs, levels of administration, and collaborating agencies and organizations can maximize adherence to the system of care approach. Thus, generating data and creating models that link decision rules and outcomes allows evaluators to track system development and to communicate about system performance in useful ways.

Using Intensive Case Studies

An additional approach to internal evaluation is through the use of intensive case studies. Case studies are in-depth descriptions of individual cases based on information gathered from multiple sources using multiple methods in naturalistic settings (Murray, 1992; Thompson, 2000; Yin, 2003). Such case studies incorporate the following features:

- Information from multiple perspectives

- Longitudinal information about system change over time

- Contextual information, including information about changes in leadership, policy, and practices over time or in community conditions

- Quantitative and qualitative data

- Information about outcomes and processes at all levels of the system

- Information about adherence to both system of care values and principles and the theory of change

- Information that examines the connections between system parts, the implicit and explicit rules of the system, and the flow of individuals through the system

Such case studies provide comprehensive and rich information that can be used both to validate the successes of a system and to identify areas in need of improvement. They typically involve outside consultants with expertise in ethnographic research and system evaluation. These case studies can focus on an entire system of care or just on particular parts of a system (e.g., how successfully it is providing rapid access to care for those in need). Again, the intent is to gather data that can be used to provide information about system processes and performance—data that can be used to improve the overall level of the system's effectiveness.

CONCLUSION

This chapter has provided a conceptual framework for research and evaluation within systems of care, offering examples of methods and approaches that are consistent with this framework. The essential emphasis as systems of care continue to develop is on research and evaluation efforts that examine both system processes and outcomes for the purpose of continuous improvement. Doing so will provide local communities with evaluation data that are both timely and relevant and that support the efforts of systems of care to adapt and progress in ways that best meet the needs of children and adolescents with mental health challenges and their families.

REFERENCES

Agar, M. (2004). We have met the other and we're all nonlinear: Ethnography as a nonlinear dynamic system. *Complexity, 10,* 16–24.

Barwick, M., & Ferguson, B. (2007). Continuous quality improvement and data-based decision-making in children's mental health: A system of care perspective. In C.C. Newman, C.J. Liberton, K. Kutash, & R.M. Friedman (Eds.), *A system of care for children's mental health: Expanding the research base, 19th annual proceedings* (pp. 377–381). Tampa: University of South Florida, Louis de la Parte Florida Mental Health Institute.

Bazelon Center for Mental Health Law. (1998). *Making child welfare work: How the R.C. lawsuit forged new partnerships to protect children and sustain families.* Washington, DC: Author.

Bickman, L., Guthrie, P.R., Foster, E.M., Lambert, E.W., Summerfelt, W.T., Breda, C.S., et al. (1995). *Evaluating managed mental health services: The Fort Bragg Experiment.* New York: Plenum Press.

Bickman, L., Noser, K., & Summerfelt, W.T. (1999). Long-term effects of a system of care on children and adolescents. *The Journal of Behavioral Health Services & Research, 26*(2), 185–202.

Brannan, A.M., Baughman, L.N., Reed, E.R., & Katz-Leavy, J. (2002). System of care assessment: Cross-site comparison of findings. *Children's Services: Social Policy, Research, and Practice, 5,* 37–56.

Chorpita, B.F., & Donkervoert, C. (2005). Implementation of the Felix Consent Decree in Hawaii. In R.G. Steele & M.C. Roberts (Eds.), *Handbook of mental health services for children, adolescents, and families* (pp. 317–332). New York: Springer.

Cook, J.R., Kilmer, R.P., DeRusso, A., Vishnevsky, T., & Meyers, D. (2007). Assessment of child and family team functioning using the participant rating form. In C.C. Newman, C.J. Liberton, K. Kutash, & R.M. Friedman (Eds.), *A system of care for children's mental health: Expanding the research base, 19th annual proceedings* (pp. 317–322). Tampa: University of South Florida, Louis de la Parte Florida Mental Health Institute.

Daleiden, E.L., Chorpita, B.F., Donkervoert, C., Arensdorf, A.M., & Brogan, M. (2006). Getting better at getting them better. *Journal of the American Academy of Child and Adolescent Psychiatry, 45,* 749–756.

Davis, C.S., & Dollard, N. (2004). *Team process and adherence to wraparound principles in a children's community mental health care system of care.* Unpublished manuscript, University of South Florida, Louis de la Parte Florida Mental Health Institute.

Davis, C.S., Dollard, N., & Vergon, K. (2005). Negotiating practice: The use of communication to construct family centered care in a community mental health system of care. In C.C. Newman, C.J. Liberton, K. Kutash, & R.M. Friedman (Eds.), *A system of care for children's mental health: Expanding the research base, 17th annual proceedings* (pp. 169–172). Tampa: University of South Florida, Louis de la Parte Florida Mental Health Institute.

Epstein, M.H., Jayanthi, M., McKelvery, J., Frankenberry, E., Hardy, R., Dennis, K., et al. (1998). Reliability of the wraparound observation form: An instrument to measure the wraparound process. *Journal of Child and Family Studies, 7,* 161–170.

Epstein, M.H., Nordness, P.D., Kutash, K., Duschnowski, A., Schrepf, S., Benner, G., et al. (2003). Assessing the wraparound process during family planning meetings. *Journal of Behavioral Health Services and Research, 30,* 352–362.

Evans, M.E., & Armstrong, M.I. (2003). *Understanding collaboration in systems of care.* Presentation at the 16th Annual Research Conference—A system of care for children's mental health: Expanding the research base, University of South Florida, Louis de la Parte Florida Mental Health Institute, Tampa.

Fixsen, D.L., Naoom, S.F., Blase, K.A., Friedman, R.M., & Wallace, F. (2005). *Implementation research: A synthesis of the literature.* Tampa: University of South Florida, Louis de la Parte Florida Mental Health Institute.

Friedman, R.M. (2002). *Child and adolescent mental health: Recommendations for improvement by state mental health commissions:* Tampa: University of South Florida, Louis de la Parte Florida Mental Health Institute.

Friedman, R.M. (2007). *Conceptualization and measurement of systems of care.* Presentation at the 20th Annual Research Conference—A system of care for children's mental health: Expanding the research base, University of South Florida, Louis de la Parte Florida Mental Health Institute, Tampa.

Granger, R.C. (1998). Establishing causality in evaluations of comprehensive community initiatives. In K. Fulbright-Anderson, A.C. Kubisch, & J.P. Connell (Eds.), *New approaches to evaluating community initiatives: Vol. 2. Theory, measurement and analysis* (pp. 221–246). Washington, DC: The Aspen Institute.

Gray, B., Duran, A., & Segal, A. (1997) *Revisiting the critical elements of comprehensive community initiatives.* Unpublished manuscript.

Green, R.S. (2001). Improving service quality by linking processes to outcomes. In B.A. Stroul & R.M. Friedman (Series Eds.) & M. Hernandez & S. Hodges (Vol. Eds.), *Systems of care for children's mental health series: Developing outcome strategies in children's mental health* (pp. 221–238). Baltimore: Paul H. Brookes Publishing Co.

Groves, I. (1994). *Performance and outcome review.* Tampa: University of South Florida, Louis de la Parte Florida Mental Health Institute.

Hernandez, M., & Hodges, S. (2003a). Building upon the theory of change for systems of care. *Journal of Emotional and Behavioral Disorders, 11*(1), 19–26.

Hernandez, M., & Hodges, S. (2003b). *Crafting logic models for systems of care: Ideas into action.* Tampa: University of South Florida, Louis de la Parte Florida Mental Health Institute.

Hodges, S., Woodbridge, M., & Huang, L.N. (2001). Creating useful information in data-rich environments. In B.A. Stroul & R.M. Friedman (Series Eds.) & M. Hernandez & S. Hodges (Vol. Eds.), *Systems of care for children's mental health series: Developing outcome strategies in children's mental health* (pp. 239–255). Baltimore: Paul H. Brookes Publishing Co.

Holden, E.W., Friedman, R., & Santiago, R. (2001). Overview of the national evaluation of the Comprehensive Community Mental Health Services for Children and Their Families Program. *Children's Services: Social Policy, Research, and Practice, 5*(1), 57–66.

Homer, J.B., & Hirsch, G.B. (2006). System dynamics modeling for public health: Background and opportunities. *American Journal of Public Health, 96*(3), 452–458.

Jones, A.P., Horner, J.B., Murphy, D.L., Essien, M.D., Milstein, B., & Seville, D.A. (2006). Understanding diabetes population dynamics through simulation modeling and experimentation. *American Journal of Public Health, 96,* 488–494.

Langhout, R.D. (2003). Reconceptualizing quantitative and qualitative methods: A case study dealing with place as an exemplar. *American Journal of Community Psychology, 32,* 229–244.

Lipsey, M.W. (1993). Theory as method: Small theories of treatments. In L.B. Sechrest & A.G. Scott (Eds.), *Understanding causes and generalizing about them: No. 57. New directions for program evaluation* (pp. 5–38). San Francisco: Jossey-Bass.

McTaggart, R. (1991). Principles for participatory action research. *Adult Education Quarterly, 41,* 168–187.

Meadows, D. (1999). *Dancing with systems.* Available online at the Sustainability Institute web site, http:www.sustainabilityinstitute.org/pubs/Dancing.html

Murray, A. (1992). Early intervention program evaluation: Numbers or narratives? *Infants and Young Children, 4*(4), 77–88.

Noffke, S.E., & Stevenson, R.B. (1995). *Educational action research: Becoming practically critical.* New York: Teachers College Press.

Patton, M.Q. (1980). *Qualitative evaluation methods.* Thousand Oaks, CA: Sage Publications.

Patton, M.Q. (1994). Developmental evaluation. *Evaluation Practice, 15,* 311–319.

Patton, M.Q. (1997). *Utilization-focused evaluation: The new century text* (3rd ed.). Thousand Oaks, CA: Sage Publications.

President's New Freedom Commission on Mental Health. (2003). *Achieving the promise: Transforming mental health care in America, final report* (Pub. No. SMA-03-3832). Rockville, MD: U.S. Department of Health and Human Services.

Reich, S., & Bickman, L. (2005). Research designs for children's mental health services research. In M.E. Epstein, K. Kutash, & A. Duchnowski (Eds.), *Outcomes for children and youth with emotional and behavior disorders and their families: Programs and evaluation best practices* (pp. 71–100). Austin, TX: PRO-ED.

Rosenblatt, A. (1998). Assessing the child and family outcomes of systems of care for youth with serious emotional disturbance. In M.H. Epstein, K. Kutash, & A. Duchnowski (Eds.), *Outcomes for children and youth with behavioral and emotional disorders and their families: Programs and evaluation best practices* (pp. 329–362). Austin, TX: PRO-ED.

Sterman, J.D. (2001). Systems dynamics modeling: Tools for learning in a complex world. *California Management Review, 43*(4), 8–25.

Stroul, B. (1993). *Systems of care for children and adolescents with severe emotional disturbances: What are the results?* Washington, DC: Georgetown University Child Development Center.

Stroul, B., & Friedman, R.M. (1986). *A system of care for children and youth with severe emotional disturbances.* Washington, DC: Georgetown University Child Development Center, CASSP Technical Assistance Center.

Thompson, J.R. (2000). Reinvention as reform: Assessing the national performance review. *Public Administration Review, 60*(6), 508–521.

Transformation Work Group (2005). *Transformation work group report.* Unpublished manuscript, Council for Collaboration and Coordination of the Child, Adolescent, and Family Branch, Center for Mental Health Services, Substance Abuse and Mental Health Services Administration, Rockville, MD.

Turnbull, A.P., Friesen, B.J., & Ramirez, C. (1998). Participatory action research as a model for conducting family research. *JASH, 23*(3), 178–188.

Walker, J.S., Koroloff, N., & Schutte, K. (2003). *Implementing high-quality collaborative individualized support planning: Necessary conditions:* Portland, OR: Portland State University, Research and Training Center on Family Support and Children's Mental Health.

Weiss, C.H. (1995). Nothing as practical as good theory: Exploring theory-based evaluation for comprehensive community initiatives for children and families. In J.P. Connell, A.C. Kubisch, L.B. Schorr, & C.H. Weiss (Eds.), *New approaches to evaluating community initiatives: Concepts, methods, and contexts* (pp. 65–92). Washington, DC: Aspen Institute.

Whyte, W.F. (Ed.). (1991). *Participatory action research.* Thousand Oaks, CA: Sage Publications.

Yin, R.K. (2003). *Case study research: Design and methods* (3rd ed.). Thousand Oaks, CA: Sage Publications.

Index

Page references to boxes, figures, and tables are indicated by *b*, *f*, and *t*, respectively.